AF674237

Oral Drug Delivery Technology

Second Edition

Oral Drug Delivery Technology

Second Edition

Aukununu Jithan

Ph.D. (USA)

Mother Teresa College of Pharmacy,
Hyderabad, India.

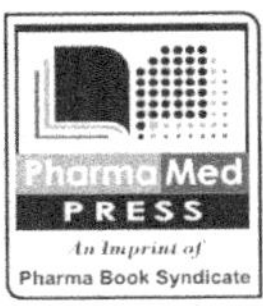

PharmaMed Press

An imprint of Pharma Book Syndicate

A unit of BSP Books Pvt. Ltd.

4-4-309/316, Giriraj Lane,
Sultan Bazar, Hyderabad - 500 095.

Published by

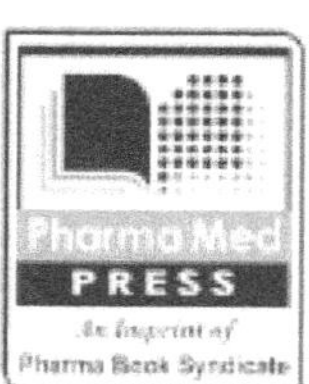

PharmaMed Press

An imprint of Pharma Book Syndicate

A unit of BSP Books Pvt. Ltd.

4-4-309/316, Giriraj Lane, Sultan Bazar, Hyderabad - 500 095.

Phone: 040-23445605, 23445688; Fax: 91+40-23445611

ISBN: 978-93-85433-24-5 (HB)

Dedicated to

My
Beloved Parents

Shri. Aukunuru Jagan Mohan Rao and
Smt. Indira

Preface to Second Edition

Since the release of the first edition of this book, several things changed. Generic market in India, especially oral formulations has doubled. We are now supplying generic drugs to several countries of the world. Rules of their acceptance into respective markets have rigidified. Exploratory pharmaceutics in India is still receiving lukewarm attention. However, this is slowly changing in big pharmaceutical companies in India. Now companies are trying to introduce new drugs into global markets. Strong preformulation teams, intelligent formulators, proficient regulatory managers, superior production managers are now needed more than before. This edition has been modified to cater the needs of pharmaceutical professionals in the above mentioned areas in a better way. Although central theme of this edition remained the same as that of the first edition, the following changes have been executed:

1. The structure of the book is revamped to give a more elegant look and comprehensive overview. Several chapters have been revised and expanded to provide greater insight.
2. The entire chapter on oral formulations has been given a totally new look. Description of all types of oral formulations has been included in this one chapter.
3. A chapter on process validation has been added.
4. Chapters on safety and toxicity of new drug substances and Pharmaceutical statistics have been deleted to bring more attention to pharmaceutics and industrial pharmacy.

Again, this book is intended for B.Pharm, M.Pharm and Ph.D. students as well as for industrial personal. It could be used as a reference book as well as text book.

In addition, I also wish to acknowledge several people. I wish to thank my wife, Gaddam Lakshmi and my baby Anjani for co-operating during the preparation of this edition. I wish to thank Anil Shah Ji for publishing my books and Naresh Daver for executing the preparation of this second edition. Special thanks to Dr. Ravi Pillai, my boss at Ranbaxy Ltd., who allowed me to write this book while I was working for him.

- Author

Preface to First Edition

In the recent years oral drug delivery has been making rapid progress that new concepts are introduced into the subject very routinely. This could be mainly attributed to the accelerated drug discovery process. Oral drug delivery in terms of research has also been improving at the same pace. However, this subject is not being adopted quickly into B.Pharma and M.Pharma curricula. Students are still reading the older concepts. What a scientist is doing in the industry is not being taught at B.Pharma and M. Pharma levels. This state of affairs is cutting the root of pharmacy education and is likely to undermine the standard pharmacy graduates, as the focus has been Industrial Pharmacy at this time in India. What is required today is a textbook of reasonable size, including the essentials of drug discovery, formulation development, oral drug delivery and regulatory affairs, in the current perspective. This book is an attempt in that line.

I have made an humble attempt to present the subject in a lucid manner and have taken all humanly possible care to avoid mistakes.

I thank my colleagues, friends and family for their help and encouragement. I am especially thankful to Prof. Dr. D.R. Krishna, Dean, University college of Pharmaceutical Sciences, Kakatiya University, for his foreword to the Book.

- Author

Contents

CHAPTER 1

NEW DRUG SUBSTANCES

- **Introduction**
- **New Drug Substance: Definition**
- **Lead Identification and Optimization**
- **Procurement of New Drug Substance**
- **Molecular Optimization**
- **Conclusions**

Introduction

Most drugs currently marketed are selected after several years of investigations and trials. Generally, in the selection of pharmaceutical solids, the combined efforts of chemists, biologists, molecular biologists, pharmacologists, toxicologists, statisticians, physicians, pharmacists, pharmaceutical scientists, and engineers are needed. Now-a-days team effort and well-defined strategies right from the beginning of project initiation to the drug reaching the market are executed. This consumes several years of hard work and enormous amount of capital. Occasionally, lot of the efforts is wasted because of improper planning and wrong methodologies. Thus, drug discovery is a challenging process.

Drug development can be simply classified into synthetic compounds, molecular modifications, semi-synthetic compounds and natural products. Although plant based therapy has been in practice in eastern countries like India and China for several centuries, isolation of active ingredient from these well known plants is novel. There is evidence that this kind of *natural product therapy* in western countries also existed. As a whole, this field is not progressing much because a high rate of failures is reported with some of the active compounds tested. *Synthetic compounds* have been in medical practice for only 70 years. At the end of Second World War, with a lot of casualties reported in the war and also because of several diseases like plague afflicting western countries and with several accidental discoveries, synthetic chemicals were introduced into medicine. Quickly these compounds proved to be very successful as therapeutic agents. The other area is the modification of the synthetic compounds. Some of the recent introductions into the synthetic chemistry with the advent of high-throughput screening are highly potent molecules. However, these molecules suffer from several disadvantages including very low solubility, poor permeability, toxicity etc. *Chemical modifications* such as salt formation, prodrugs etc. were found to be helpful in reducing the disadvantages. Finally, *semi-synthetic compounds:* This class of compounds includes antibiotics like semi-synthetic penicillins and anti-cancer molecules like flavopiridol. These are synthetic modifications in a fermented or a plant derived compound. Drugs obtained as microbial end products have been in the market for several years. The most famous of these molecules is penicillin and its derivatives. Currently several penicillins are in the market for the treatment of various cancers, fungal diseases, bacterial diseases and viral diseases. Plant-derived products are currently a fashion in the pharmaceutical research. These products existed in ancient India for thousands of years. Till allopathy was introduced, pharmacists in the Indian subcontinent used these products to treat the people. As mentioned before, Ayurveda is very sophisticated and only very efficient practitioner or pharmacist was able to use its therapy rightly. Current knowledge about Ayurveda is mostly drawn from relatively later writings, primarily the Charaka Samhita (approximately

1500 BC), the Ashtang Hridayam (approximately 500 AD), and the Sushrua Samhita (300-400 AD). Active leads are generally extracted from well known plant drugs.

New Drug Substances

Any chemical substance with new therapeutic value could be called a "New Drug Substance". As mentioned previously it could be a synthetic compound, natural product or a semi-synthetic compound. According to the FDA, *any drug that is recognized among experts, qualified by scientific training and experience, as being safe and effective under the conditions recommended for its use is termed a "new drug"*. Several definitions of new drug substances could be found in the literature.

Lead Identification and Optimization

Lead identification and optimization is an important aspect of new drug substance development. A "lead compound" is the basic structure that elicits some pharmacological action against the target disease. In earlier times, leads were identified by random synthesis of a series of molecules, their pharmacological activity determined and the structure-activity relationship (SAR) established for this series of molecules. The lead would be modified as per the pharmacological results. The goal is to enhance the potency and to obtain better therapeutic agents of this series of compounds. However, this used to be a tedious process in drug discovery. With advanced technologies such as high-throughput synthesis and screening techniques, innovations were introduced into the lead identification and optimization. The molecular targets for a disease generally are proteins, may be enzymes, receptors or structural proteins. Since proteins are important targets for a disease either in drug discovery or diagnosis, pharmaceutical companies are currently investing hugely on protein targeted drug design and discovery. The target proteins are isolated to pure state and the crystal structure determined. Lead is then identified by predictions based on *in-silico* techniques and optimized. These molecules could be synthesized and screened.

The bottom line in the current drug discovery process is the rapid and accurate lead optimization. This requires tremendous expertize in medicinal chemistry, synthetic chemistry, formulation technology, bioscreening and pharmacology. Currently, experts use proprietary and third party tools and QSAR (Quantitative Structure Activity Relationship) modeling for relating the key calculated molecular descriptors (physicochemical, topological, structural, ADME-related (ADME stands for Absorption, distribution, metabolism and elimination) and others) with specific biological activity in assessing lead optimization techniques. Because of the enormous database currently available, a single small unit at one location will not be able to handle such a decision. Several third party tools such as commercial outsourcing facilities could clearly decipher their know-how of *in silico* lead optimization techniques. The resulting outcome is an efficient drug discovery process.

The design of molecules in the current *in silico* techniques is based on knowledge of biochemistry, the understanding of interaction of ligands with proteins, affinity generating structure elements (AE) substructures involved in interaction with target proteins, chemistry-perception and the characterization of molecules. The basic precept in such a design is different characterizations of molecules leads to different molecular representation spaces and the same set of molecules could have vastly different distributions in its various representation spaces. When the target knowledge is zero, diverse libraries are generated using *in silico* techniques. If pharmacophore is known focused libraries are developed. In this case pharmacophore based libraries are generated. A structure-based design is used if protein X-ray crystallographic study has given a known target structure. Random drug-like libraries involve expanding the corporate compound collection by suitable acquisitions, and enumerating virtual libraries and choosing diverse sets using, for example, Genetic Algorithms (GA). Pharmacophore based libraries can also be developed by traditional medicinal chemistry skills.

The other important area in lead discovery and optimization is proteomics. Proteomics is the study of proteins and its application in several scientific areas including drug discovery and development. Proteins are important targets of drug discovery. In several disease states, the protein expression is altered. This is one of the reasons for the evolution of proteomic techniques. The identification, characterization and quantification of all proteins involved in a particular pathway, organelle, cell, tissue, organ or organism that can be studied in concert to provide accurate and comprehensive data about that system. When scientists can accurately and dependably identify and understand the activity of these protein systems, the underlying characteristics of disease and wellness will be clearly deciphered. The same principle holds true for protein alteration expressions in disease state models. Thus, proteomics has the potential to revolutionize the development of innovative clinical diagnostics and pharmaceutical therapeutics. For example, a specific configuration of proteins in liver tissue could define a particular tumor, or a successful regression of that tumor, in response to therapy and thus amenably, this is the underlying top principle in the role of recent therapy discovery.

The techniques in proteomics fathom from the identification of thousands of proteins in a particular model system, to the detailed analysis of the 3D structure, possible modifications/isoforms, and function of a single protein. All these factors are very contributing to the drug discovery in all its stages. The stages include target identification, target validation, drug design, lead optimization, and pre-clinical and clinical development. Currently high throughput proteomics is aiding this process of drug development. High-throughput proteomics are able to identify potentially hundreds to thousands of protein expression changes in model systems following perturbation by drug treatment or disease. This lends itself particularly well to target identification in drug discovery process. However, this data analysis and validation of potential protein targets is a time-consuming and labor-intensive process. Identification of proteins is only beginning to assume importance in rapid drug discovery process. Identification of appropriate protein in a disease state as well as a suitable molecule with thorough binding or targeting properties to the protein of interest is not only time consuming but also may be very costly. In these situations, the best alternative is to use the existing database of proteins and drug molecules of interest and proceed with drug discovery process. Several biochemical methods are currently in place in the identification of the proteins that are altered during disease state. The most common method used in biochemistry labs is two-dimensional gel electrophoresis. It is very effective at identifying protein expression changes in a system. Currently high throughput techniques are used in proteomic technologies. In a recent technique, each protein is terminally tagged and digested, and then only the terminal peptides are isolated and sequenced, allowing for rapid identification of an entire proteome. This technique is termed as protein sequence tags (PST).

Apart from the lead optimization using binding of ligands to the proteins of interest, parallel synthesis techniques is a part in the lead optimization process. A range of innovative methods using computer software is currently used in speeding up solution phase synthesis that further accelerates lead optimization. Synthesis of batches of 100 compounds at one time using stem-reflux or stem-cool stirrer hotplates or MTP blocks is reported. Purification is a processing step in the synthesis. Current high throughput purification methods include simple "lollipop" technique, membrane technology to separate aqueous and organic phases, the use of resin based scavenging agents, parallel centrifugation, parallel solvent blow-down and parallel cartridge based chromatography. As per one report, because of the introduction of these techniques there has been a 10-fold increase in assay productivity since 1995. The other methods use biocatalytic and chemoenzymatic techniques. The technique worth mentioning to describe is solid phase synthesis and its modifications.

Thus, in tandem with in silico techniques, synthesis of compounds is also initiated. New techniques are leading to the rapid synthesis of compounds. Solid-phase organic synthesis (SPOS) is an important tool in the field of synthetic chemistry. The basics of this synthetic process for the generation of new chemicals were adopted from solid-phase peptide synthesis. In this method, the substrates are attached to a solid support (polystyrene, polyethylene glycol, cellulose, controlled pore glass, etc.). The reaction is achieved in this state and subsequently the reactants and the products are detached from the support by using specific techniques. The purification of this mixture of products is achieved using several separation and analytical techniques and a library of chemicals is generated. Most commonly used and one of the earliest supports is polystyrene cross-linked with divinylbenzene (PS-DVB). Because of its hydrophobicity and steric hindrances, PS-DVB does not provide environment that is solution like. Thus, currently several new supports are being investigated. The new supports are aimed at achieving enhanced product isolation, compound purity and would also support solution-phase synthesis resulting in faster reaction rates through rapid diffusion and reaction mobility. Cross-linking of SPOS with polyethylene glycol (PEG) was the major addition to the art of solid-phase polymer synthesis. The spacer PEG determined the properties of the solid-phase support. This increased the hydrophilicity and conferred flowing solvent-like properties along with mechanical and physico-chemical properties more ideal compared to that of SPOS. Several factors like bead size, nature of the polymer, the lipophilicity, its porosity all affect the effectiveness of the synthesis. Basically, with optimum properties, a resin behaves like a micro-reactor. The reactions are rapid and selective in this micro-reactor.

Now-a-days pharmaceutics scientists play a major role in lead optimization. Once leads are procured after synthesis, pharmacological activity is quickly determined. This is generally accomplished in pharmacology labs. Usually this information is obtained with NCEs (new chemical entities) solubilized in DMSO (dimethylsulfoxide) or other similar easy formulations either in cell culture or small animal models. Without pharmacological or toxicological evaluation, the complete activity or safety of a lead, as per the regulatory agencies demands is not established. Thus, its pharmacological activity is first investigated. Further, it reaches pharmaceutical technology group for toxicological and pharmacological evaluation. As a first step, the preformulators prepare a dosage form to be used for preclinical toxicological studies. A lowest and highest possible dose will be incorporated into the formulation and administered into the animal. The maximum toxicological dose will be identified. Subsequently, this formulation will be tested for its activity in animal models. Dose-dependency of the activity is the first priority. Based on the pharmacology and toxicology results, few compounds will be selected from the library of leads. These compounds will be further developed. Scientists from exploratory pharmaceutics then take up the challenging issue of the formulation development.

Once a compound is obtained in pure form, the solid-state characterization becomes important. At the end of synthesis and purification, solid drug substances display a wide and unpredictable solid-state properties. Any change in these forms is not a big issue after synthesis. The project could be dropped at a later date. However, the appearance of these crystals during processing and upon storage of the final product would be an important issue. As per New Drug Application (NDA) guidelines, a new drug application should contain information on solid-state properties of a drug particularly, when bioavailability is an issue. Appropriate analytical procedures should be used to detect various solid-state forms such as polymorphs, hydrates, desolvated solvates and amorphous forms, as part of regulatory requirements.

Procurement of New Drug Substances

Modern drugs are either synthesized, extracted or semi-synthetic. However, a systematic drug development is valid yet for only synthetic compounds. These compounds could be synthesized using the very routine laboratory techniques or with the help of modern high throughput techniques. Once the lead for a disease is identified and it is optimized its synthesis in large quantities is initiated. High throughput synthetic techniques are recently introduced into the field of synthetic chemistry. The identification of new leads and the optimization of the synthetic techniques saw a new growth in this area. Lately, several new procedures developed have resulted in enhanced productivity of pharmaceutical industry. The recent innovations in synthetic chemistry such as solid/liquid phase synthetic techniques have reduced reaction times and often result in improved yields compared to solution state synthesis. These polymer-based synthetic techniques are able to generate large library of diverse chemicals in a rapid and parallel manner. In addition, the current screening techniques are very sophisticated and often times very efficient thereby making the drug discovery process very productive.

Molecular Optimization

Once the pharmacology and toxicology are determined, final formulation development, clinical trial and market potential formulation development are subsequently pursued. However, the molecules that are lately being synthesized are very poorly water-soluble. As such, the formulation development is a big issue with these molecules. Thus, it is currently a routine practice in big pharmaceutical companies to develop the formulations for these types of molecules and then proceed to the next step of toxicological evaluations. This may be time consuming. However, the studies may become leads to quick formulation development for such poorly insoluble molecules that may enter the lab later. In any case either of the methods depending on the convenience could be preceded.

Prior to the development of formulations, the first criterion is the physical characterization and optimization of the molecule. This helps in the formulation development process. A physical pharmacist develops a formulation. The short-term stability of this molecule is determined. This ensures that the formulation would be stable during the course of preclinical toxicological evaluations. If the molecule is not stable, a different formulation is attempted till a stable short-term formulation is developed. The other problem that may be encountered is the low bioavailability of the molecule being tested with the formulation developed. In these circumstances, desired concentration of the drug in the plasma is not obtained to elicit its biological activity. Definitely when biological activity is not elicited, toxicological manifestations are also not observed. In any of these situations, the best solution is the development of a parenteral intravenous formulation. This helps in determining direct toxic dose of a drug in the model of interest. Generally this formulation is a solution. A suitable solvent in which the drug dissolves should be identified. The other possibility is the development of a suitable formulation to enhance the bioavailability of the drug. Thus, if there is any problem with the drug substance, although demonstrating good pharmacological property, the formulations used in the early toxicology or mechanistic pharmacology investigations a intravenous dosage form is preferred. In this case the drug has to be soluble in water or any other suitable solvent. On the other hand, if any of the techniques and methods do not assist in the investigations, the best alternative is to modify the drug to change its physico-chemical properties or select an optimum physical form with suitable properties. These modifications could result in salts, prodrugs, suitable physical forms (solvates, polymorphs, hydrates) or even new analogs may emerge from the modification efforts. Thus, the investigations into the molecular modifications of a drug entity to make it optimum to demonstrate pharmacological and therapeutic activity would be of interest and innovation for drug development scientists. These modifications to the original molecule can be called as molecular optimization.

Although the above modifications are the likely possibilities, the very commonly tested derivatizations are salts and prodrugs. Salt formation results in the removal of an acidic or basic group from a molecule and thereby enhances the dissolution of this counter ion in water and thus likely enhances the bioavailability. For instance, ephedrine hydrochloride is formed by the addition of a proton to form an ionized drug molecule that is then neutralized with a counter ion (Ephedrine hydrochloride is prepared by addition of a proton to the basic secondary nitrogen atom on ephedrine resulting in a protonated drug molecule that is neutralized with a chloride ion). In general, organic salts are more water-soluble than the corresponding un-ionized molecules, and hence, offer a simple means of increasing dissolution rates and possible improvement in the bioavailability. Ample literature is available with regard to the prodrugs. Along with salt formation, prodrug synthesis is also one of the techniques to alter the physico-chemical properties of a drug substance to enhance the formulation and biopharmaceutic developments. Uptil today, most prodrugs are esters or amides designed to increase lipophilicity. One of the first investigated prodrugs is a morphine analog. These prodrugs are synthesized to enhance the brain permeation of morphine and other CNS (central nervous system) agents. The main characteristics of prodrugs include the rate of hydrolysis, formulation stability, bioavailability and tissue permeation. These are discussed in detail elsewhere in this textbook. Each of the techniques for molecular optimization; selection of suitable physical form, selection of suitable solid form, suitable salt form and development of prodrugs is discussed below.

Selection of a suitable solid form

Solid state of the drug is also an important aspect of molecular optimization. Once it is established that a molecule is a promising candidate for future investigations, its synthesis procedure in large quantities will be developed. This step is called bulk drug synthesis. In most instances, bulk synthesis of a chemical entity is developed in parallel with preformulatory investigations. Generally, a drug candidate is not thoroughly characterized during this stage. However, if synthesis steps are achieved by the end of all preformulation studies and the bulk synthesis yields a different tougher solid substance (a polymorph, a hydrate, a clathrate etc.) and if the bioavailability of this substance is different from the already investigated physical form of the drug, it is likely that all the preclinical toxicological studies have to be repeated with the new physical drug substance or a new bulk synthetic process for this molecule has to be developed. Thus, synthesis procedure for a suitable solid form is important. There are several other reasons why a suitable solid form has to be selected. The selection of a suitable solid form of the drug substance is a vital step in pharmaceutical development. Given that a drug substance can exist in multiple solid forms, including polymorphs, hydrates, solvates, salts, co-crystals, and amorphous, and that each of them have different properties that can affect bioavailability, solubility, dissolution rate, stability and manufacturability, the appropriate evaluation and comparison of the properties of the solid forms in a rigorous and effective manner requires extensive expertise, knowledge and a good methodology Thus, solid form of the new chemical entity has to be thoroughly investigated.

Because of the various reasons mentioned above, it is definitely very important to know the various types of solid forms a drug could exist in. This would be of future help in sorting out any problem that might have arised during the storage conditions of the formulations. The first step in this investigation is to obtain various physical forms by the recrystallization of the drug from various solvents. These solvents include water, methanol, ethanol, propanol, isopropanol, acetone, acetonitrile, ethylacetate, hexane and mixtures, if appropriate. Cooling hot saturated solutions or partly evaporating clear saturated solutions could also obtain new crystal forms. Crystal habit and the internal structure of a drug could affect bulk and physicochemical properties, which range from flowability to chemical stability. Two terms are described in defining a crystal. One *habit* and the other, *crystal structure*. Both of them are separate. The description of the outer appearance of a crystal is the habit and the molecular arrangement within the solid is termed the internal structure. The crystal habits could be platy, equant (massive); needle (acicular); bladed; tabular and prismatic. A single internal structure can have several different habits, depending on the environment for growing crystals. A change in the internal structure alters the crystal habit. However, chemical changes such as salt formation would lead to a change in the internal structure and the external habit. It has to be noted that various crystal structures, habit as well as internal structure, exist for a single molecule. In addition, the physical, physico-chemical, physiological and the pharmacological properties of these individual polymorphs are different. Thus, a drug substance's visual appearance and its microscopic view are to be thoroughly investigated to avoid any future problems associated with the clinical substance to reduce the expenditure invested by a pharmaceutical company on a single chemical entity. The internal structure could classify a drug into either a crystalline or an amorphous solid. Crystals are characterized by repetitious spacing of constituent atoms or molecules in three-dimensional array, whereas amorphous forms have atoms or molecules randomly placed in a liquid. Amorphous forms are typically prepared by techniques like rapid precipitation, lyophilization, or rapid cooling of liquid melts. Solubilities of amorphous solids are higher than crystalline forms because of the higher thermodynamic energy of amorphous forms than corresponding crystalline forms. The major problem associated with the existence of different physical forms for a single drug is the transition of one physical form to the other upon storage or during processing. Generally, amorphous solids revert to more stable crystalline forms during formulation development or storage.

Crystal form of drug substances influences the physical, chemical and mechanical properties of drugs. Therefore, solid-state properties of drugs and the excipients are to be done to obtain consistent product performance. As mentioned before, the first aspect investigated is the physical nature of a new chemical entity. This ensures the commonness of the New Chemical Identity

(NCI) used for various purposes. This includes synthesis and formulation development. Immediately after it is received, a pharmaceutical scientist looks the NCI under a microscope. This will give an indication of the physical form of the drug. The drug substances as looked under a polarized microscope are either isotropic or anisotropic. Isotropic substances have single refractive index. Amorphous drugs like supercooled glasses and noncrystalline solid organic compounds, or substances with cubic crystal lattices, such as sodium chloride, are isotropic material. Under cross-polarized filters, these isotropic substances do not transmit light, and they appear black. Substances with more than one refractive index are anisotropic and appear bright with brilliant colors (birefringence) against the black polarized background. The differences in the refractive indices and the crystal thicknesses result in the different colors of a crystal. Anisotropic substances have either two (uniaxial) or three principle refractive indices (biaxial). Most drug substances are biaxial, corresponding to either orthorhombic, monoclinic or triclinic crystal system. Only a well-trained crystallographer can identify the crystal nature of a biaxial system or a drug substance. One refractive index should be enough to describe a crystal structure. However, proper orientation and exposure of crystals under a microscope along with its crystallographic axes is required to define a crystal properly. Orientation also affects the crystal identification under the microscope. This requires good training. However, regular scientists could investigate the routine microscopic investigations such as crystal habit and observe transitions induced by heat or solvents. With the presence of organic solvents or water in a crystal, there is always a question to a pharmaceutical scientist to define the characteristic feature of a drug substance. The presence of water or organic solvent either resulting during synthetic steps or during formulation development or storage affects the function of the pharmaceutical formulation effects the properties of new drug substances. When solvent molecules exist in a crystal lattice and form molecular adducts, the substance is called a solvate. If the solvent is water, the molecular adducts are called as hydrates. Hydrates are very common with most of the pharmaceutical formulations because of the omnipresence of water in all the pharmaceutical formulations. Desolvated solvate is a crystal from which the solvate is removed intentionally or unintentionally and the crystal retains its solvate structure. However, this is not always the case. Some times crystals are more rigid than the other forms of drugs.

A drug's bioavailability, formulation development, solubility changes and stability depend on the physical structure of the drug. As such, polymorphism could be defined as the ability of a compound to crystallize as more than one distinct crystalline species with different internal lattices. As mentioned before, this sometimes makes things complicated for new drug development. The well-known example is the existence of chloramphenicol palmitate as three different crystalline forms and one amorphous form. It was found that three formulations demonstrated different bioavailabilities suggesting this to be a key phenomenon in chloramphenicol development. The other example is the anticonvulsant drug carbamazepine. This drug exists in solid state as three polymorphic anhydrous forms and as a dihydrate. It is practically insoluble in water and is marketed as a tablet. Wet granulation is the technique that is used in the development of granules for such a drug to be used for tablet compression. Examples of other drugs that are known to exist as polymorphs are mebendezole, theophylline, dihydroepiandrosterone, and tenoxicam. Several properties such as melting point, density, hardness, crystal shape, optical properties and vapor pressure are influenced by the physical states of a drug. Some of these properties can be used in investigating polymorphic nature of a drug. Because of all these variations, a suitable solid state of a drug should be identified very early on. Techniques such as microscopy, fusion methods, differential scanning calorimetry, infrared spectroscopy, x-ray diffraction, scanning electron microscopy, thermogravimetric analysis and dissolution/solubility studies are used in the assay of the physical forms of drugs. A specific technique should be fine to investigate the physical nature. However, it is always advisable to use several alternative techniques to perfectly confirm the physical nature of drugs so as to reduce the cost of formulation development and as such, drug development process. Some of these techniques were in place for over several years. Inspiteof the availability of a lot of information on these techniques, new techniques are always investigated to improvise the formulation development process with new chemical entities. Differential scanning calorimetry (DSC) is the best technique for detecting solvates. This is because of the heat change involved in the desolvation, esp. for hydrates. However, DSC alone does not indicate the existence of solvates. The analytical data obtained from nuclear magnetic resonance spectroscopy (NMR) and thermogravimetric analysis (TGA) indicates the existence of solvates. DSC then becomes good technique for analyzing solvates and determining the percentage of the solvates present. General protocols can be followed when deciding an optimum physical form for the drug substance. As indicated previously different physical forms are investigated very early on, they are characterized and also known to the pharmaceutical scientist. A decision tree for polymorphic forms and hydrates (solvates can be developed). These decision trees are generally based on physical form consistency, the dissolution, critical relative humidity values, and transition points. Consistency of the API solid state under the influence of environment destabilizing factors such as exposure time, ultraviolet light, pH, moisture, temperature, and pharmaceutical processing operations like milling, compression and compaction should be investigated so as to select optimum physical form. There are a set of rules for selection of suitable solid form. These are described below.

The first choice of API for a solid drug formulation is the anhydrate of active substance (free acid, free base or neutral compound). Anhydrates together with salts form the majority of all drug formulations. If the anhydrate for some reason is not suitable (e.g. it is little soluble, unstable, has complicated polymorphism etc.), then possible hydrates are monitored. The hydrate is most frequent a solvate containing water molecules in its crystal structure. Water molecules can be incorporated in the structure in a stoichiometric manner (stoichiometric hydrates) or non-stoichiometrically (non-stoichiometric hydrates), For the formulation stable stoichiometric hydrates in a lower stage of hydration are chosen in which water molecules are bound to molecules of the active substance by H-bonds. The dehydration of a stoichiometric hydrate often results in the collapse of the crystal structure and the origin of an amorphous phase. Non-stoichiometric hydrates are not suitable for the formulation because the water content in them changes with the partial pressure of water vapour in the ambience and with temperature a thus they difficult to define. In non-stoichiometric hydrates, water is not bound very firmly, it rather fills present cavities in the structure without forming Hbridges.The dehydration of non-stoichiometric hydrates does not result in the origin of an amorphous phase but a crystalline anhydrate originates. Other solvates (with the exception of ethanol solvates) are not used for the formulation but can be used as important precursors. For instance polymorhs which are otherwise difficult to attain can be obtained by their desolvation. Stability is another important issue when a hydrate is selected as the final molecular form. The stability of the system anhydrate/hydrate depends on the ambient relative humidity. Many active substances form hydrates, often in a various degree of hydration and stability. If the hydrate is the more stable in the system anhydrate/hydrate then the hydrate has all available reliable proton donors and acceptors better satiated compared to anhydrate (Etters rule). For instance ergot alkaloid tergurid exists as an anhydrate, a twothird hydrate and a monohydrate, and the stable phase is the monohydrate Formulations from hydrates are not very frequent and represent only several per cent of the total number of APIs (e.g. chloral hydrate, levofloxacin hemihydrate, terpin hydrate and others). The reason is their thermal instability and possibility of the potential dehydration during drying. Of excipients, much used is the lactose monohydrate.

Selection of a suitable polymorphic form also is some times very important. Compounds can exist in different crystalline forms. Among pharmaceutical molecules, the most frequent case is dimorphism (existence of two different polymorphs). A well-known example is the patent litigation between pharmaceutical companies Glaxo and Novopharm over two polymorphs of ranitidine hydrochloride, which decreases the production of stomach acid, or the problems of the company Abbot Laboratories concerning two polymorphs of ritonavir – an inhibitor of HIV-protease. Since polymorphs differ by their crystal structures, they differ by their properties, of which solubility and dissolution rate are the most important. A typical ratio of solubility of two polymorphs is less than two, but there are exceptions, e.g. polymorphs of premafloxacin I/III or polymorphs of chloramphenicol A/B have this ratio larger than 10. Thus it can happen that a less soluble polymorph does not even reach the minimum medicinal concentration in blood.

Amorphous compound are also some times preferred over crystalline compounds because of the advantages they offer for this drug. Amorphous forms are thermodynamically metastable which results from the disordering of their inner structure on molecular level. Compared to ordered crystalline phases, amorphates have better molecular mobility which results in a better dissolution profile and thus a better oral bioavailability. On the other hand this is compensated by lower chemical and physical stability (shorter expiration) and by greater demands on production and storing (e.g. protecting atmosphere). Current formulations from amorphous phases include asthma medicine, e.g. zafirlukast (Accolate, Astra-Zeneca), quinapril hydrochloride (Accupro, Accupril, Pfizer), anti-fungal drug itraconazole (Sporanox, Janssen-Cilag) or nonsteroidal anti-inflammatory drug indomethacin (Indocin, Merck). In solid drug formulations, amorphates are stabilized by suitable excipients (e.g. PVP, trehalose, sorbitol,etc.). Another type of molecular optimization leads to the formation of cocrystals. Cocrystals are at present the most dynamically developing group of solid pharmaceutical substances. The definition of the term "pharmaceutical cocrystal" is still under discussion, but essentially it is a multi-component compound that is formed between a molecular or ionic API and a cocrystal former that is a solid under ambient conditions.

Selection of Suitable Salt Form

Salt selection is the important step in the development process initiated very early on. Before even toxicology studies are initiated. This is because if in toxicology studies it is determined that the salt form that was used was not appropriate; the entire studies should be repeated. Toxicology studies are generally time consuming and expensive. But what is the need to prepare salts. The unionized (free) form of weak acids and bases may not be ideal molecular forms for development. Very early on salts can be synthesized and tested. Analog selection was based on the in vitro activity, however, today a blend of developmental issues such as salt formation are surfacing. Thus, salt screening is performed very early on. Salt selection affects several physical properties of the API. Salts have different physical properties than their free forms. Selection explores whether a particular salt might have properties that are more appropriate than the parent. Improving oral absorption by increasing the dissolution is one main reason for prepare salts. It is important that a suitable physical form of a particular salt form has to be selected. More details about the salt formation are described in another chapter of this book. However, the minute details of molecular optimization with this technique will be discussed here. Very early on permeability, solubility (Cs) and pKa, the intrinsic properties of the molecules are determined. The major dependent variables, absorption and consistency of the API, can be manipulated, optimized and balanced in salt selection. For a given acid or base form of a drug different salts will be synthesized and then a suitable salt form for further development will be selected. This is called salt selection. A general protocol for the salt selection (optimization) has been recently proposed. It is called as a three-tier system (2) and is described as below:

Tier 1: Hygroscopicity

Tier 2: Thermal analysis and x-ray diffraction

Tier 3: Accelerated solid-state stability

Tier 1 eliminates any form with excess moisture sorption desorption characteristics. Only good candidates progress to the next step. In the second tier, changes in the crystal structure are examined under extremes of moistures condition using any of the techniques previously described for the physical forms which include thermal analysis or x-ray diffraction. This is to detect desolvation or aqueous phase transformation problems. Aqueous solubility is also determined at this stage to address dissolution problems. The best candidates for formulation and manufacturing are considered here and the only good candidates proceed to tier-3. In this tier, accelerated thermal and photostability testing is carried. This is a time consuming process. Drug-excipient compatibility with commonly used excipients is also performed at this stage. If tier 3 eliminates all the salts synthesized, newer salts can be considered. The entire salt screening process can be reevaluated. Although these are the general rules that have been proposed, deviations are also possible and optimization of molecule for salt development should be carefully performed. For example, the HCl salt of ranitidine due to its hygroscopicity would not have been selected in this three tier approach, however, it is the most successful salt in the market. This emphasizes a need for prioritizing the salt selection process so that a wide range of development issues should be considered and addressed as early as possible. If a hydrochloric acid has much better absorption properties than the free base but is hygroscopic, it is better to deal with this problem. Otherwise, bioavailability may be compromised when more stress is given to the consistency of the physical form. The free base/acid forms are generally not preferred in this three tier approach unless all alternatives have failed despite its potentially favourable dissolution in gastric fluids and its sensitivity to particle size reduction with a reactive sink.

Prodrugs

Prodrugs are one way to optimize the molecular properties of new drug substances. Basically, they come under structural modification for molecular optimization. There are several reasons for the development of prodrugs. A separate chapter is devoted for prodrugs in this book and is thus not discussed here in detail. A brief overview for pharmaceutics student will be presented here. Often NCEs have adequate biological activity but do not have the required physical properties to become a drug. For orally administered drugs, the compounds need to dissolve and then permeate across the gastrointestinal tract. For intravenous drugs, the compound must have adequate solubility in the vehicle as well as in the blood for the reasons of safety. Prodrugs are one of the methods to solve safety issues and property design problems and should be considered very early on in the drug discovery stages. Poor membrane permeability, poor solubility, and poor dissolution are the problems that can be addressed using prodrug approach. Prodrug design has also been used to reduce the toxicity. Lets discuss absorption.

The three factors that inhibit the passage of a drug molecule through biological membranes are:

(a) Charge,
(b) water of hydration and
(c) molecular size.

To enhance the permeability, now scientists are exploring prodrugs to exploit membrane transporters. There are several membrare transporters on the membranes which can be utilized to enhance the permeability of molecule. For instances, nucleoside prodrugs can be synthesized for a given drug to aid its transport across the membrane using nucleoside transporters. Similarly, peptide transporters can be utilized. Recently, some of the structural requirements of the plasma membrane peptide transporter, PEPT1 has been elucidated. Thus, prodrugs which utilize this transporter can be synthesized with improved absorption. The antiviral agent valcyclovir is a prodrug of acyclovir. It has been observed that the H-bonding of guanidine molecule of valcyclovir may enhance its PEPT1 absorption. Reducing ionization using prodrug strategy can also increase the absorption of the drug. For instance, most factor Xa inhibitors used for preventing the activation of thrombin and blood clots have utilized a highly charged group either guanidine or amidine group. These groups however have reduced oral bioavailability because of the charge. One strategy to over come this bioavailability is to have prodrugs with reduced charge. Once they reach systemic circulation, they convert back to the original drugs. Water of hydration can be reduced with prodrugs to enhance the oral bioavailability. Impact of strong H-bonds between NCE polar groups and water provides barrier for absorption. By converting the original drug to a lipophilic prodrug, the water barrier can be removed and thereby enhancing the oral absorption. As the molecular size increases, the permeability decreases. A prodrug with reduced molecular size can be synthesized to enhance its permeability.

Using prodrugs for solubility enhancement can take atleast two different pathways:

(a) increasing water solubility,
(b) decreasing crystal packing.

Fosphenytoin is an injectable prodrug of phenytoin. It is freely soluble and rapidly cleaved back to phenytoin upon injection. The aqueous solubility of the parent drug is 20-25 mcg/ml while that of the prodrug is 88000 mcg/ml. Such enhancement in solubility can also decrease the pain at site of the injection. Parecoxib sodium is a prodrug of valdecoxib with enhanced solubility. The increase in the solubility is because of the disruption of H-bonding and crystal packing as well as increasing pKa. Prodrugs can increase the dissolution of the parent drug. Fosamprevanir is a prodrug of amprevanir with enhanced dissolution and then bioavailability. Amprevanir is formulated with large amounts of excipients for optimum dissolution and bioavailability. This made 8 capsules to be administered twice or thrice a day with 1200 mg dosing.

Conclusions

New drug research is currently in a good swing. New methods are being innovated and placed. The trend for the past 100 years in pharmaceutical therapy is synthetic molecules. Their clinical testing, pharmaceutical testing and the synthesis procedure were all slower and thus the process consumed several years before the drug entered the market. On the other hand, currently these processes have become high throughput i.e., high-speed processes. The older techniques were very robust and history has proved that they are effective. However, the new high-throughput screening techniques are still in the development and transitional state. Before the total introduction of these techniques into drug research, it would take several years for continuous and robust development of methods in this area. Some of these techniques are currently fruitful and some are promising for further considerations. However, the goal of this chapter is to introduce facts about the discovery of new chemical entities. In addition several other areas are being introduced into new drug discovery process. These include microbial and plant products.

Questions for Practice and Exercise

1. What constitutes the body of team involved in the selection of pharmaceutical solids? Briefly, elucidate the role of each specialist in such a selection process.
2. Explain about a new drug substance.
3. Explain the different solid-state characterization techniques used in new drug substance discovery.
4. What are the different types of solid states of drugs?
5. How do you perform the molecular optimization of an API?
6. How is salt screening used in the molecular optimization of an API?
7. How is a suitable solid form for a drug substance selected?
8. Explain structural modification as a tool for molecular optimization of an API.

References

1. Gu CH, Grant DJ. Estimating the relative stability of polymorphs and hydrates from heats of solution and solubility data. J Pharm Sci. 2001 Sep;90(9):1277-87.
2. Morris KR et al. Int J Pharm. 1994:105:209.
3. Bahumil Kratochvil. Solid forms of pharmaceutical molecules. www.imc.cas.cz/nmr/projeckt/ws/springer. Date:15/7/2012.

Bibliography

1. The Practice of Medicinal Chemistry, Second Edition, Edited by Camille Georges Wermuth, Elsevier Publications, 2003.
2. Foye`s Principles of Medicinal Chemistry, Fifth Edition, David A. Williams and Thomas L. Lemke, Lippincott Williams & Wilkins, 2002.
3. The Theory and Practice of Industrial Pharmacy, Third Edition, Edited by Leon Lachman, Herbert A. Lieberman, and Joseph L. Kanig, Lea & Febiger Publications, 1986.

4. Physical Pharmacy: Physical Chemical Principles in the Pharmaceutical Sciences, Third Edition, Alfred Martin, James Swarbrick and Arthur Cammarata, Lea & Febiger Publications, 1983.

5. Pharmaceutical Dosage Forms and Drug Delivery Systems, Seventh Edition, Howard C. Ansel, Loyd V. Allen, Jr., and Nicholas G. Popovich, Lippincott Williams & Wilkins, 1999.

6. Molecular Modelling: Principles and Applications, Second Edition, Authored by Andrew Leach, Pearson Education Ltd., 1999.

7. Protein-Ligand Interactions: From Molecular Recognition to Drug Design (Methods and Principles in Medicinal Chemistry), First Edition, Edited by Hans-Joachim Böhm and Gisbert Schneider, Wiley VCH, 2003.

8. Combinatorial Library Design and Evaluation: Principles, Software Tools, and Applications in Drug Discovery, First Edition, Edited by Arup K. Ghose and Vellarkad N. Viswanadhan, Marcel Dekker Inc., 2001.

9. High-throughput synthesis: Principles and Practices, First Edition, Edited by Irving Sucholeiki, Marcel Dekker Inc., 2001.

10. Remington: The Science and Practice of Pharmacy. 21st Edition. Philadelphia, PA. Lippincott Williams & Wilkins. 2005.

11. Bahumil Kratochvil. Solid forms of Pharmaceutical molecules. www.imc.cas.cz/nmr/projectkt/ws/springer. Date 15-7-2012.

CHAPTER 2

BIOTECHNOLOGY PRODUCTS

- **Introduction**
- **Classification**
    - Hormones
    - Vaccines
    - Monoclonal Antibodies
    - Blood Factor Therapeutics
    - Interferons
    - Interleukins
    - Antisense Oligonucleotides, DNA and RNA
- **Formulation Strategies**
    - Conventional Oral Dosage Forms
    - Pegylation
    - Microparticles and Nanoparticles
    - Liposomes
- **Computer Aided Design**
- **Preclinical and Clinical Trial Products**
- **FDA Regulations**
- **Conclusions**

Introduction

Biotechnology products are the drugs or other medically useful compounds that are productions or modifications of products that use living organisms (e.g., microorganisms, fungus, plant tissue culture). As per one report more than 350 biotech drug products and vaccines are currently in clinical trials. These products are targeting various cancers, Alzheimer's disease, cardiovascular disease, diabetes, multiple sclerosis (MS), AIDS and arthritis. Although in its infancy with disease management, several diagnostic kits are made of biotechnology end products. Currently, there are more than 4,000 biotech companies. These are either located in Japan or in USA. Most of these are medium scale companies and are with limited size and finances. Collaborations of these medium scale companies with multi-national companies have also resulted in the accelerated development of these products and the companies. At one stage, several biotechnology companies produced several products with very optimistic and promising viewpoint. However, with the elimination of many of the products from clinical stages, the viewpoint of pharmaceutical industries is currently in a different angle. The reason for their elimination may be either very high hopes initially laid, high cost requirement, lack of suitable delivery system, not reading the market views carefully, or overconfidence of the scientists involved in these projects. However, the research resulted in the generation of several new sciences and methodologies along with a very few products in the market currently. However, a brief overview is presented in this chapter.

In terms of contributions by different countries, Japanese biotechnology companies have played a key role in innovations in this area by themselves and also by collaborations for over several decades. The US and European markets also invested hugely on biotechnology products. The US biotech industry spent US $15.6 billion on research and development in 2001, which greatly exceeds the amount spent by foreign biotech industries. The number of biotech companies in the US has steadily been growing over the past several years. There were 1231 companies with 79,000 employees in 1992 and by 2001 there were 1457 companies with 191,000 employees. There are currently about 1800 biotech companies in Europe, as per one report. However, after several innovations, enormous capital and lot of people working in this area, there needs a lot of progress. This industry could be considered still in infancy. Currently, other countries like India and China are seeing enormous progress. The objective of this book chapter is to elucidate the basic concepts of important biotechnology products along with some of the basics about their delivery.

Classification

Biotechnology products could be classified in several ways. In this book, they are classified as Hormones, Vaccines, Interferons, Interleukins, Monoclonal Antibodies, Blood Factor Therapeutics and Genes and Related Material. Most of the products are proteins, peptides, steroids and DNA and RNA like structures. Structural details and the synthesis methods are not discussed in this chapter.

Hormones

Hormones have a very significant role in human system. Hormonal regulation is a function of central nervous system. Any deficiency results in diseases characterized by a lack of that particular hormone. Several natural hormones and their synthetic modifications are currently in the market for various purposes.

The central nervous system regulates body functions in two fundamentally different ways,

1. Direct innervation of organs by the sympathetic and parasympathetic nervous system. Responses are essentially instantaneous - within fractions of a second and
2. Indirect control by products of the endocrine system.

Endocrine control is not instantaneous, instead requires seconds or longer to produce a physiological response. This control is performed by hypothalamus, pituitary gland, endocrine organs (thyroid, adrenals, gonads, and pancreas) and organs like kidneys, heart and arteries. Hypothalamus produces stimulatory and inhibitory releasing factors that act upon the anterior pituitary gland. In addition, hormones like oxytocin and vasopressin are produced in hypothalamus. Pituitary gland produces peptide hormones that target various endocrine and non-endocrine targets. Hormones were one of the first therapeutic agents of human origin to be investigated for clinical applications. Several benefits were found with hormonal therapy. The main use of the hormonal therapies is during their deficiencies. Hormones of central nervous system include growth hormone, thyrotropin, corticotropin, follicle stimulating hormone, luteinizing hormone, prolactin, vasopressin, oxytocin, melanocyte stimulating hormone, corticotropin-like intermediate lobe peptide, ACH 18-39 AA, enkephalins and endorphins. These are the main hormonal products. Proopiomelanocorticotropin (POMC) peptide/hormone gives rise to ACTH, β-lipotropin (b-LPH), α- and β-MSH, enkephalins, and endorphins in different cells. POMC is regulated by dopamine and serotonin in the intermediate pituitary and by CRH in the anterior pituitary gland. Some of the hormones are currently marketed and are in clinical trials for various diseases. A few of these are described here.

Human growth hormone

Human growth hormone is essential for growth. The deficiency of this hormone results in reduced growth in children. Genentech, Inc. (USA) markets the hormone as Protropin. Somatrem (Protropin) is a biosynthetic, single polypeptide chain of 192 amino acids, produced by a recombinant DNA procedure in *E.coli*. This drug consists of one more amino acid (methionine) than the natural occurring human growth hormone. This hormone stimulates linear growth by affecting the cartilaginous growth areas of long bones. It also stimulates growth by increasing the number and size of skeletal muscle cells, influencing the size of organs, and increasing red cell mass through erythropoietin stimulation. It is administered intramuscularly or subcutaneously. Currently, research efforts have been directed to developing non-invasive hGH delivery systems to overcome the pain of injection, lipoatrophy at the site of injection, and to increase patient compliance, thereby improving the quality of life for the patient. Different controlled, repeated and sustained delivery systems like microparticles and nanoparticles are currently being investigated to deliver Human Growth Hormone. The other route is lung delivery. The lungs represent a relatively unexploited route of delivery for large therapeutic molecules that would otherwise be delivered parenterally. The lungs also represent an attractive route for drug delivery mainly due to the high surface area for absorption, thin alveolar epithelium, and extensive vascularization. However, the research in this area is in very initial stages. Another issue is that hGH is susceptible to various degradation processes including aggregation, deamidation, oxidation, reduction, and hydrolysis. These routes and delivery systems could avoid these problems with the current growth hormone therapy researches.

Corticotropin

Corticotropin has been used in the treatment of various conditions. Several companies currently supply it as a therapeutic agent. Some of the uses include diagnostic testing of adrenocortical function, treatment of nonsuppurative thyroiditis, hypercalcemia associated with cancer, acute exacerbations of multiple sclerosis, tuberculous meningitis when accompanied by antituberculous chemotherapy, trichinosis with neurologic or myocardial involvement, and treatment of glucocorticoid responsive rheumatic, collagenous, dermatologic, allergic, ophthalmic, respiratory, hematologic, neoplastic and gastrointestinal tract diseases. The recent discovery in this area is for its use in the treatment of infantile spasms. Recent information about corticotropin (ACTH) in the treatment of infantile spasms and evaluation gave answers to some of the questions and addressed several issues including

1. the efficacy of doses of ACTH in comparison with other drugs, especially with vigabatrin, and the efficacy in patients with tuberous sclerosis;

2. tolerability; and
3. long-term outcome. In two studies conducted, high doses were not more effective than low doses but were more effective in another study. Definitely corticotropin has a therapeutic role in this very rare disease.

Estrogens

Estrogens like other steroid hormones, are potent actors in the cardiovascular system. Since half the population have high levels of estrogen most of their lives it is plain that estrogen has a variety of beneficial physiologic functions. Clinical studies, however, have demonstrated that a specific formulation of a combination of potent estrogens and metabolites is not a magic bullet, but induces both positive and negative impacts on different organ systems. More research into the mechanistic actions of estrogens in specific pathways in individual cell types is necessary to determine appropriate therapeutic interventions to replace the loss of positive effects of estrogens while minimizing the negative effects in postmenopausal women. New information has emerged showing that estrogen has both beneficial and detrimental effects. Further mechanistic studies and use of well defined forms of estrogens and selective estrogen receptor modulators will continue to provide novel mechanistic information that will likely lead to the development of new avenues for therapeutic interventions.

Growth factors

Growth factors are proteins that bind to receptors on the cell surface, with the primary result of activating cellular proliferation and differentiation. Many growth factors are quite versatile, stimulating cellular division in numerous different cell types while others are specific to a particular cell-type. The currently marketed growth factor is recombinant human platelet-derived growth factor for topical adjunctive therapy for diabetic ulcers. Endogenous platelet-derived growth factor increases the proliferation of cells that repair wound and form granulation tissue. This factor promotes the chemotactic recruitment and proliferation of cells involved in wound repair and increasing the formation of granulation tissues.

Thyrotropin

Thyrotropin is used diagnostically to determine subclinical hypothyroidism or low thyroid reserve, to differentiate between primary and secondary hypothyroidism, and to differentiate between primary hypothyroidism and euthyroidism in patients whose thyroid function has been suppressed by the administration of thyroid replacement therapy. Thyrotropin is also used to aid in detection of remnants and metastases of thyroid carcinoma, and to demonstrate the presence of dormant thyroid tissue in patients with a toxic adenoma that has suppressed surrounding normal thyroid tissue.

Gut hormones

Gut hormones are useful in the treatment of obesity and associated problems. Obesity is the main cause of premature death in the UK. Worldwide its prevalence is accelerating. It has been hypothesized that a gut nutriment sensor signals to appetite centres in the brain to stop food intake at the end of filling. Gut hormones have been identified as an important mechanism for this. Ghrelin stimulates, and glucagon like peptide-1, oxyntomodulin, peptide YY (PYY), cholecystokinin and pancreatic polypeptide inhibits appetite. At physiological postprandial concentrations they can alter food intake markedly in humans and rodents. In addition, in obese humans fasting levels of PYY are suppressed and postprandial release is reduced. Administration of gut hormones might provide a novel and physiological approach in anti-obesity therapy and also may be helpful in ulcers. Most likely the ulcers that are caused in juveniles some time evanesce when they grow up. The reason may be the alteration and normalization of the hormonal levels with the increase in the age.

Vaccines

Vaccines are the very common and one of the first pharmaceutical products to be used in the human beings. Basically these products increase the immunity of the body against a particular disease or a pathogen and hence reduce the mortality against the respective disease or the pathogen. Very occasionally boosters are administered into the body to continuously produce immunity. Currently, pharmaceutical companies are not that much keen on the generation of vaccines because of the likely losses encountered by pharmaceutical companies owing to the reduction of the incidence of the disease states in the human beings with vaccine administration. However, in some disease occasions, for the benefit of society and patient bill reductions, vaccines are inevitable. Also, in these conditions prevention is better than cure. Examples of such conditions are polio, tuberculosis, diphtheria, AIDS and all kinds of cancers. In the earlier days and even today most commonly these products are produced by injecting the pathogen or a disease state in a harmless manner and thus resulting in the generation of resistance to the body. Occasionally, a vaccine product may be an antigen in the case of a pathogen or a peptide in the case of a cancer or other such disease. These may be derived from an animal or a microorganism. However, with these products, the techniques routinely in practice are costly and tedious. On the other hand, genetic engineering is used very often to produce these products in the present scenario. A revolution in the biotechnological development of vaccines would be needed as scheduled at very rapid rate to increase the marketing of the entire group. A couple of examples to illustrate biotechnology vaccines will be discussed here.

Cancer is a very severe disease afflicting human kind at this time. Chemotherapy is very commonly used in the treatment of cancer. However, currently **cancer vaccines** are slowly gaining prominence. Comprehension and regulatory investigations on immune systems in recent times resulted in rapid strides in research in this area and further in the development of cancer vaccines. The current cancer therapies have their deleterious effects on the normal tissues as the major toxic side effect. On the other hand, cancer vaccines could avoid these side effects and may result in the very effective therapies. A pathogen as in the example of bacterial or viral infections has antigens generally on the surface, which are recognized by the human immune system. According to the opportunity, these pathogens cause diseases. In some the disease effects may be elicited and in other the disease may not be seen. This phenomenon has intrigued scientists over several years leading to the basic investigations in immunology. As mentioned before a pathogen is recognized by the immune system as an antigen. Once these antigens are recognized, different cells of immune system produce antibodies against the respective pathogen. A vaccine consists of immunity raised against a specific pathogen by a clinical person by administering a product generated or marketed by a pharmaceutical person. The principle of generation of vaccines is similar with cancer vaccines with little difference. The basic understanding of this difference would help in better acknowledging the science behind the development of cancer vaccines. The major difference between microbial pathogens and tumors as potential vaccine targets is that cancer cells are derived from the host, and most of their macromolecules are normal self-antigens present on normal cells. To take advantage of the immune system's specificity, one must find antigens that clearly mark the cancer cells as different from host cells, limiting the number of antigens available. The game in the development of the cancer vaccines is the recognition of these membrane proteins from a bush of proteins that are specific to cancer cells and further utilize these proteins in the development of vaccines.

Generally, tumor antigenic proteins are expressed on the surface of the tumor cells. In disease states antibodies are developed for these cell surface antigens and are used in the natural immunity. Additionally, many potential tumor antigens are not expressed on the surface of tumor cells and thus are inaccessible to antibodies. The immune system has evolved a solution to this problem: the MHC antigens (HLA molecules in humans) that act as an internal surveillance system to detect foreign or abnormal proteins made inside the cell. A sampling of all proteins synthesized in the cell is cleaved by proteasomes into short fragments (peptides) that are transported into the endoplasmic reticulum. There, the peptides are loaded onto newly synthesized class I MHC molecules, such as HLA-A, -B, and -C. The peptide-MHC complexes are transported to the cell surface for recognition by the T cell receptors (TCRs) of $CD8^+$ T lymphocytes, such as CTLs (natve cytotoxic T lymphocytes). Thus, CTLs recognize short peptides, 8–10 amino acid residues in length, arising from the proteasomal degradation of intracellular proteins and able to bind to class I HLA molecules. For this reason, CTLs are not limited to tumor antigens expressed intact on the cell surface but can detect any abnormal protein synthesized in the cell, greatly expanding the range of tumor antigens detectable by the immune system. Furthermore, CTLs play an important role in the rejection of transplanted organs and tissues, analogous to tumors as foreign or abnormal human cells invading the host. Thus, although monoclonal antibodies have clearly shown therapeutic efficacy in certain cancers (e.g., trastuzumab, rituximab, alemtuzumab), most cancer vaccine strategies have focused on induction of CTLs that lyse tumor cells. Recent understanding of the mechanisms of activation and regulation of $CD8^+$ T cells has given new life to tumor immunology. Notwithstanding the critical role of $CD8^+$ T cells, induction of tumor-specific $CD4^+$ T cells is also important not only to help $CD8^+$ responses, but also to mediate antitumor effector functions through induction of eosinophils and macrophages to produce superoxide and nitric oxide.

For naive $CD8^+$ T lymphocytes to be activated initially, or "primed," they generally require presentation of antigens by professional APCs, such as DCs. DCs express high levels of costimulatory molecules, such as CD80 and CD86, which can make the difference between turning off the CTL precursor and activating it. DCs also secrete critical cytokines such as IL-12 and IL-15 that contribute to CTL activation and memory. In addition, a number of regulatory mechanisms that dampen the immune response are exploited by tumors to escape immunosurveillance. These mechanisms include the inhibitory receptor CTLA-4 on the T cells themselves and negative regulatory cells such as the $CD25^+CD4^+$ regulatory T cell and also certain types of $CD4^+$ natural killer T (NKT) cells that inhibit tumor immunosurveillance. Major hurdles in developing cancer vaccines include: identification of antigens that focus on the exquisite specificity of the immune system on cancer cells without harming normal cells; development of methods to induce an immune response sufficient to eradicate the tumor, in the face of self-tolerance to many tumor antigens; and overcoming mechanisms by which tumors evade the host immune response. An extensive listing of the known tumor-associated antigens is available, and more are being discovered. Tumor antigens can be categorized into four groups:

(a) antigens unique to an individual patient's tumor;

(b) antigens common to a histologically similar group of tumors;

(c) tissue-differentiation antigens; and

(d) ubiquitous antigens expressed by normal and malignant cells. These categories and the two major strategies used to identify tumor antigens are described in several review articles and major textbooks published in this area. The following two figures adopted from Berzofsky et al., 2004 very well describe the modes of developments of cancer vaccines.

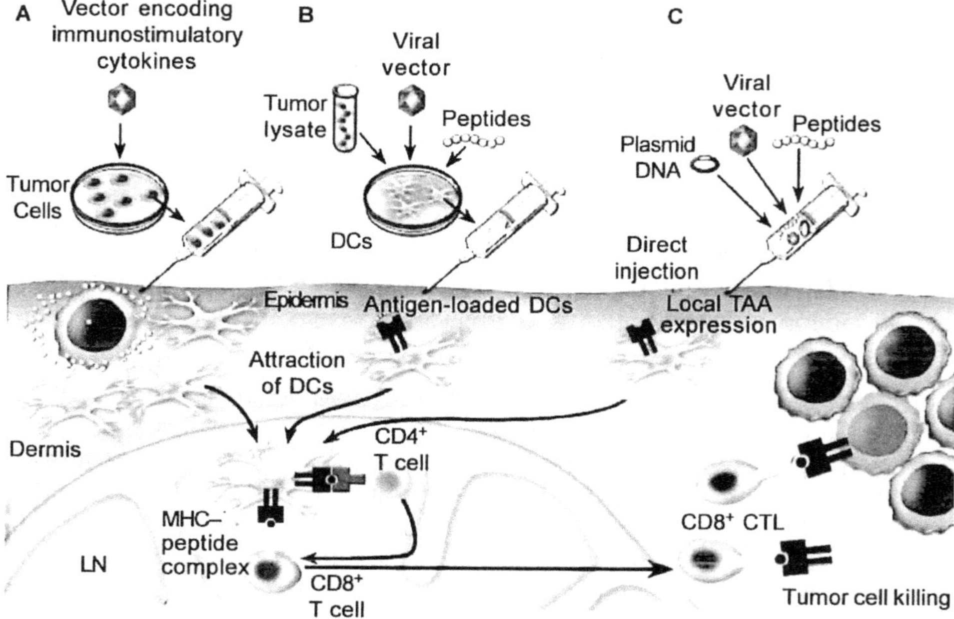

Figure 2.1

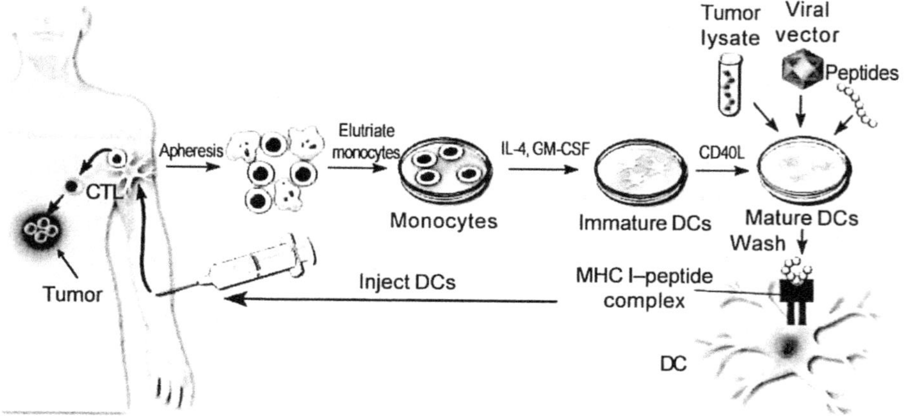

Figure 2.2

Research on the development of cancer vaccines was in vogue among cancer researchers for quite some time. In laboratory animals like rat, the results demonstrated promise and the vaccines have successfully stimulated the immune system. However, research was not always fruitful in human beings. However, recent results demonstrated more promising results. Several reasons could be mentioned for the unfruitful results. Some reasons include:

- There was a tremendous variation in the immunity and more often patients had very low immunity and the immune system was not able to react to the vaccines
- Often the chemistry of tumor patients is not the same as that of healthy patient and in these situations there is compromise in the tumours of the cancer patients and thus reduced stimulation to the vaccine
- Not all the tumor cells are the same and often some cells are more resistant than other cells and thus proper dosage optimization is not yet achieved. Thus, more resistant cells are not affected by the vaccine.

The other observation is that not enough doses were used in the clinical trials with these vaccines to demonstrate an outward response. However, the future picture shows to be rosy.

The currently marketed and the other ideal example for a recombinant vaccine is the **vaccine for Hepatitis B**. Hepatitis B virus (HBV) (previously known as the serum hepatitis virus) infection is a major cause of acute and chronic hepatitis, cirrhosis, and primary hepatocellular carcinoma worldwide as known to several scientists over several years since very ancient times. Now hepatitis has a recombinant vaccine. It is estimated that more than 200 million persons are chronically infected with HBV worldwide, and up to 80% of new liver cancer cases each year are attributable to HBV infection. The best treatment currently available is to give immuno-suppressants by prophylaxis. Because of the huge mortality a vaccine was developed. This vaccine was commercially available in the USA since 1982. In 1986, a recombinant vaccine was licensed and a different recombinant vaccine was licensed in 1989.

A basic tenet of vaccinology is that the prophylactic vaccine induces immunity. Thus, an immune state must be possible. In the case of HBV, the immune state is indicated by the presence of antibodies against HBsAg (the hepatitis B surface antigen), also known as the anti-HBsAg IgG. This neutralizing antibody is also known as the correlate of immunity. Thus, any effective vaccine for HBV must the production of anti-HBsAg IgG in the host. Vaccines against HBV were first made from the serum of people who had been HBV infected and subsequently cleared the infection. Because these individuals naturally produced anti-HBsAg IgG and then cleared the infection, they were immune to re-infection with HBV. The serum from these individuals was taken and purified antibody was passively administered to others in order to induce immunity. Although this strategy works in a theoretical manner, there are complications including supply shortage and host rejection of the foreign antibody.

In the early 1980's, researchers discovered a new way to produce this antibody utilizing recombinant DNA technology. In an infected individual, HBsAg is present in two forms: as a protein on the surface of the 42nm virion (also called the Dane particle) and as a secreted 22nm particle that is a hollow sphere of surface antigen. Using the yeast *Saccharomyces cerevisiae*, researchers created a vector that contained the coding sequences for this surface antigen of HBV, HBsAg. The key to this success was that the yeast assembled this 22nm protein in the same way that excess surface antigen assembles and is secreted in humans. Therefore, the artificial surface antigen resembled the naturally occurring particle. One reason finding an alternate vector for expression of these surface antigen genes was so important in creating an effective vaccine was that this 22nm particle could be administered safely to humans. Because the 22nm particle contains the surface structure of HBV but does not contain the DNA of the actual virus, humans exposed to this product could produce their own anti-HBsAg IgG without any risk of being infected by HBV itself. Because the host was now producing his own antibody rather than passively receiving it from another individual, immunity was more likely to be long-lived and more effective. With the advent of recombinant DNA technology and the creation of the yeast vector, it was possible to create the first safe, effective recombinant vaccine for human use.

Monoclonal Antibodies

Most of the vaccines and other biotechnology agents are proteins or peptides. Vaccines are generally antibodies. Monoclonal antibodies are some times vaccines. However, not all monoclonal antibodies are vaccines. These could be used as therapeutic and diagnostic agents. Antibodies have two very important characteristics. First, they are extremely specific; that is each antibody is produced from same cell type and attacks one particular antigen. These are called monoclonal antibodies. The important applications of monoclonal antibodies are in the treatment of human diseases like cancer, viral infections and autoimmune disorders. The market and research for these therapeutic agents is tremendously increasing with several products already in the market. Some examples in the market include muromonab-CD3-Orthoclone (OKT3), satumomab pendetide – oncoscint CR/OV kit, rituximab (rituxan), transtuzumab (herceptin), palivizumab (synagis), daclizumab (zenapax), basiliximab (simulect) and inflixinad (remicade). Currently, altogether, they have very less market. However, keeping in view the rise of disease states, the potential may definitely increase. The second antibodies, once activated by diseases, continue to confer resistance against that disease; classic examples are the antibodies to the childhood diseases chickenpox, rabies and measles. The fundamentals of vaccinology involve the second class of antibodies. These are not monoclonal and generally a group of antibodies clubbed together. As a memory stored in the human immune system, they are generated to a specific opportunistic microorganism or a cancer cell and not to a specific protein. Thus, the entire design of the individual cells becomes important. Rather than fighting with a specific protein, this results in the generation of several proteins because of the recognition of several protein targets on the cells. These are called polyclonal antibodies.

It is the first trait of antibodies, their specificity, which makes these antibodies very valuable. These antibodies are useful not only therapeutically; they are also helpful in the diagnosis of a wide variety of illnesses. These monoclonal antibodies can detect the presence of drugs, viral and bacterial products, and other unusual or abnormal substances in the blood. Realizing the importance and potential of the monoclonal antibodies in the utility, much time was spent on this class of therapeutic agents. As a whole, these could be defined as homogenous sets of immunoglobulins with well-defined specificity and biochemical characteristics. These products were introduced into clinical practice in the early 1980's, and since then their use has rapidly expanded. Most of the side effects observed with first-generation murine antibodies have been successfully overcome with the advent of humanized (chimeric or CDR-grafted) and more recently fully human antibodies.

Monoclonal antibody technology is helpful in therapy because of several other advantages, which could be clearly described using the following advantages for immunotherapy to cancer,

1. Immune reaction directed destruction of cancer cells,
2. Interference with the growth and differentiation of malignant cells,
3. Antigen epitope directed transport of anti-cancer agents to malignant cells,
4. Anti-idiotype vaccines;
5. Development of engineered (humanized) mouse monoclonals for anti-cancer therapy and
6. A variety of different agents (e.g. toxins, radionuclides, chemotherapeutic drugs) have been conjugated to mouse and human monoclonal antibodies for selective delivery to cancer cells. A few of the products currently in the market are henceforth discussed.

OKT3

OKT3 is a drug sometimes used for "acute" organ rejection - meaning rejection that occurs suddenly and threatens to destroy a new organ very quickly. It may also be used to prevent rejection during the first 10 to 14 days after surgery in patients who have serious side effects with other immunosuppressive drugs. OKT3 is made of a specially engineered monoclonal antibody that can target certain cells and stop their attack. It is an antibody to the T3 antigen of human T cells - those cells that directly attack a new organ. OKT3 prevents or reverses graft rejection by blocking the T cells and stopping their work. It has been available for general use since 1986. Reversal of rejection occurs in about 95 percent of patients given the drug. The major problem has been with side effects.

Colon cancer is the second most common cause of cancer mortality. Ovarian cancer is the most common gynecologic malignancy cause of death in women. A labeled monoclonal antibody attaches to a tumor-associated antigen and allows these tumor masses to be imaged or treated, depending on the radionuclide used. **Indium-111 satumomab** pendetide was the first labeled monoclonal antibody to be approved by the Food and Drug Administration (FDA) for tumor imaging. It is reactive with most colorectal and ovarian cancers, as well as other cancers.

Rituximab

Rituximab is an intravenous drug that is used to treat B-cell non-Hodgkin's lymphoma. Tumor cells (like most normal cells) have receptors on their surfaces. Molecules on the outside of the cell can attach to these receptors. When they do, they can cause changes to occur within the cells. One receptor, present in more than 90% of B-cell non-Hodgkin's lymphomas, is called CD20. Molecules that attach to CD20 can affect the growth and development of the tumor cells and, sometimes, the production of new tumor cells. Rituximab is a man-made antibody that was developed using cloning and recombinant DNA technology from human and murine (mice or rat) genes. Rituximab is thought to attach to the CD20 receptor and cause the tumor cells to disintegrate (lyse). In some non-Hodgkin's lymphomas, it also prevents the production of more tumor cells. The FDA approved Rituximab in 1997.

Herceptin

Herceptin (Trastuzumab) is a recombinant DNA-derived humanized monoclonal antibody that selectively binds with high affinity in a cell-based assay (K_d = 5 nM) to the extracellular domain of the human epidermal growth factor receptor 2 protein, HER2. The antibody is an IgG_1 kappa that contains human framework regions with the complementarity-determining regions of a murine antibody (4D5) that binds to HER2. The humanized antibody against HER2 is produced by a mammalian cell (Chinese Hamster Ovary [CHO]) suspension culture in a nutrient medium containing the antibiotic gentamicin. Herceptin is the first humanized antibody approved for the treatment of HER2 positive metastatic breast cancer. Herceptin is designed to target and block the function of HER2 protein overexpression. Research has shown that women with HER2 positive metastatic breast cancer have a more aggressive disease, greater likelihood of recurrence, poorer prognosis and approximately half the life expectancy of women with HER2 negative breast cancer.

Daclizumab

Daclizumab is an immunosuppressant drug used to prevent the body from rejecting a transplanted organ. It is typically used to lower the body's natural immunity in patients who receive kidney transplants. Daclizumab works by preventing the white blood cells from getting rid of the transplanted kidney. The effect of daclizumab on the white blood cells may also reduce the body's ability to fight infections. Daclizumab (Zenapax®) (molecular wt = 144kd.) is a humanized monoclonal antibody (IgG1) produced by recombinant DNA technology. It gained FDA approval in Dec 1997. It is known by several other names including HAT (Humanized Anti-Tac), SMART anti-Tac, anti-CD25, and humanized anti-IL2-receptor. It was developed and patented by Protein Design Laboratories (Mountain View, CA) and it is marketed by Hoffman LaRoche (Nutley, NJ).

Infliximab

Infliximab is a recently approved drug (known by brand as Remicade) that treats Crohn's disease patients with moderate to severe cases. However, the U.S. Food and Drug Administration allow its use as only a last resort. The patient must receive standard treatment with mesalamine, corticosteroids, and immune-suppressive agents first. If these drugs are not effective, then infliximab can be used. The purpose of the drug infliximab is to prevent inflammation with anti-tumor necrosis factor substances. This particular drug blocks the activity of an inflammatory chemical in the tissue called tumor necrosis factor (TNF). Excessive TNF seems to lead to increased inflammation and damage in the tissues in disorders like Crohn's disease and rheumatoid arthritis. Because infliximab blocks TNF, it is known as “anti-TNF”.

Blood Factor Therapeutics

As the advances in the area of recombinant DNA technology and transgenic protein production along with the development of cheaper economical and efficient protein purification techniques, protein drugs were made cost-effective and commercially viable. However, not much success in this area has been in the oversight. One of the earlier protein products developed with the help of recombinant technologies is Blood Products or also called as blood factor therapeutics. The recombinant blood products that are currently on the market include Factor VII (NovoSeven; Novo Nordisk), Factor VIII (Helixate; Aventis Behring), Factor IX (BeneFix; Genetics Institute) and Protein C (Ceprotin; Baxter).

Cascade of role of various blood factors is depicted in the Figure 3. A lack or deficiency of any of these factors could result in pathological situation that would lead to no clotting and eventually death. In addition, a recent report from the American Thrombotic Association underscores the severity of such blood-clotting disorders, ranking them as the major causes of death over AIDS and cancer. About 80% of hemophiliacs use recombinant proteins with only 20% using plasma concentrates.

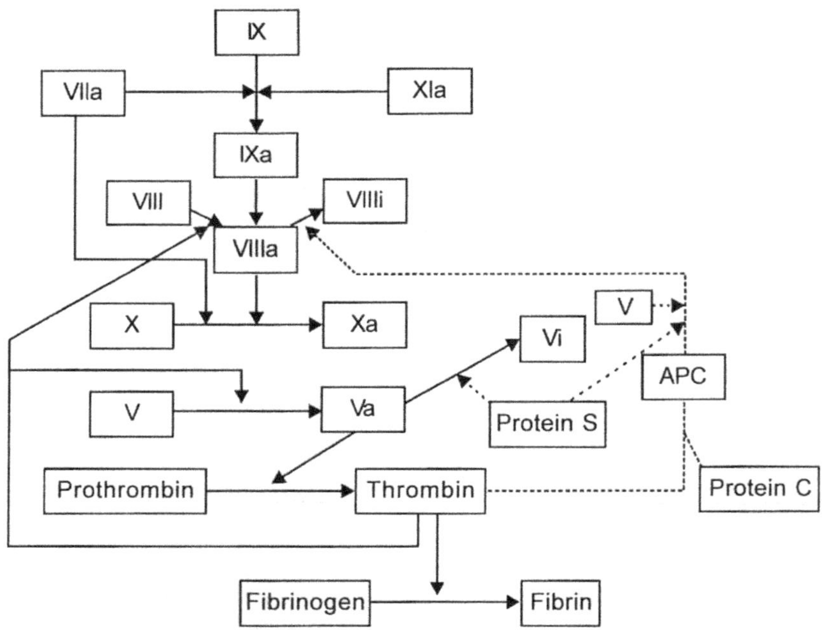

Figure 2.3

Interferons

In 1957, two British scientists, Alick Isaacs and Jean Lindenmann, found that infected chick embryo cell released a naturally produced glycoprotein that allowed noninfected cells to resist viral infection. These two scientists termed this protein as interferon, because it was initially looked like "to interfere with the transmission of infection." These molecules do not fight the virus straight but aids in the increase in the immunity to the host. It was initially thought that these molecules are panacea for cancer. However, this proved to be false. As a class, interferons are a part of the large immune regulatory network within the body that includes lymphokines, monokines, growth factors, and peptide hormones. Interferons are classified into two types – type I interferons (alpha and beta), which share the same molecular receptor, and type II (gamma or immune), which has a different receptor. The recent discovery of several other molecules has confidently cut short the initial prominence given to these molecules. However, two of these molecules are currently in the market. These are Interferon beta-1b marketed as Betaseron and Interferon beta-1a marketed as Avonex. Interferons are currently very popular because of the variegated therapeutic roles.

Apart from the current marketed interferons, several pegylated interferons are currently actively investigated to treat various other diseases. Pegylated interferon therapy for the treatment of chronic hepatitis-C virus provides significant increases in sustained virological response rates compared with standard interferons. This is in the very early stages of research and market. Two pegylated interferons are now available and are used in conjunction with ribavirin, an antiviral nucleoside used in the treatment of viral diseases, to maximize response rates in infected patients. The two-pegylated interferons, peginterferonalpha-2a and peginterferonalpha-2b, differ substantially in terms of their chemical and structural characteristics, pharmacokinetic and pharmacodynamic properties, and dosing and administration. A full understanding of the differences between the two drugs is important to maximize the clinical benefits. Controlled studies designed to characterize the effects of the two drugs on viral kinetics and sustained virological response rates are emerging and may help to shed additional light on the use of these compounds in patients with chronic hepatitis C. In addition, these interferons are used in the treatment of several other diseases. Interferon-inducible, double-stranded RNA-dependent protein kinase PKR is well known as an early cellular responder to viral infection. Activation of PKR has been associated with a number of downstream cell stress and cell death events, including a generalized shutdown of protein translation, activation of caspase-8, participation in JNK and p38 MAPK pathways, activation of NF-kappaB, etc. Recently, the activation of PKR has also been described in several neurodegenerative diseases, including Huntington disease, Alzheimer disease (AD), and amyotrophic lateral sclerosis. Although the relationship between PKR and these diseases is still unclear, the overlaps between known functions of PKR and biochemical events that occur in these neuropathologies are discussed here. The interferons (IFN) are proteins that have antiviral, antiproliferative and immuno-modulating effects, and in the central nervous system these effects are mediated through the opiate receptors and the dopaminergic system. There is evidence that AD may be related to certain prion diseases and certain viruses, and that the IFN system has become deteriorated in this condition. Thus, recent studies have focused in the use of interferons in the treatment of Alzheimer's disease.

Interleukins

Cytokines have been in the focus of scientific interest for more than a decade now. Vast literature is available. Some cytokine therapies are already used as part of clinical practice, ranging from early exploratory trials to well-established therapies that have already received approval. Interleukin-10 first identified as cytokine synthesis inhibiting factor (CSIF) produced by macrophages as the major source is a crucial important agent for immunoregulation and led to its use in first clinical trials. The powerful immunomodulatory properties of IL-10 and the promising results from IL-10 delivery on the course of several inflammatory diseases in experimental models induced the interest on clinical application of IL-10. Human recombined IL-10 has been tested in healthy volunteers, patients with Crohn's disease, rheumatoid arthritis, psoriasis, hepatitis C injection, HIV infection, and for the inhibition of therapy associated with cytokine releases in organ transplantation and Jarisch-Herxheimer reaction. In phase I clinical trials, safety, tolerance, pharmacokinetics, pharmacodynamics, immunological, and hematological effects of single and multiple doses of IL-10 administration resulted in well toleration without serious side effects at lower doses to higher doses, with mild to moderate shivers and flu-like symptoms with higher doses upon intensive treatment.

IL-10 is a pluripotent cytokine with potent effects on numerous cell populations in particular circulating and resident immune cells as well as epithelial cells. Thus, it becomes an important broad effector molecule in immunoregulation/host defense. Initially, it was found that it mainly mediates suppressive functions. However, more recent data suggested that it has stimulatory properties in certain cell populations also. Thus, IL-10 could be considered more as immunoregulator rather than immunosuppressive. Apart from these IL-10 was found to be useful in the treatment of several life-threatening immunological diseases as mentioned before, viz., rheumatic arthritis, Crohns diseases, transplant patients, chronic hepatitis-C, human immunodeficiency virus and probably AIDS, respectively.

Antisense Oligonucleotides, DNA and RNA

Innovations in molecular biology, biotechnology and related fields resulted in genetic therapy. This could include therapy using DNA, RNA and antisense oligonucleotides. Therapy with DNA and RNA could be called gene therapy and therapy with antisense oligonucleotides could be called antisense therapy. **Antisense technology** is based on a simple and rational principle of Watson-Crick complementary base pairing of a short oligonucleotide with the targeted mRNA to downregulate the disease-causing gene product. The initial clinical results were quite encouraging and thus lead to the progress of this class of pharmaceuticals. One product **Vitravene** is already in the market. This product is an antisense oligonucleotide useful in the treatment of diabetic retinopathy and related diseases. Currently antisense oligonucleotide therapy targeting bcl-2, BCR-ABL, C-raf-1, Ha-ras, c-myc, PKC, PKA, p53 and MDM2, mostly useful in the treatment of cancers is actively being pursued. Most of these are cancer-causing genes. While the first-generation phosphorothioate antisense oligonucleotides are in clinical trials, a number of factors, including sequence motifs that could lead to unwanted mechanisms of action and side effects, have been identified. As a result, a number of chemical modifications to obtain second generation of antisense oligonucleotides with reduced side effects are currently in preclinical and clinical set up.

Gene carrying chromosomes are the basic physical and functional units of heredity. Genes are specific sequences of bases that encode instructions to produce proteins. Although genes get a lot of attention, the main end products: proteins are important. These are the main functionalities of a cell. Similarly, the other gene related products are RNAs. These are the products before the protein between DNA and the proteins. When genes are altered, the encoded proteins are unable to carry out their normal functions resulting in genetic disorders. Several approaches could be used to correct the end results including protein therapies, peptide therapies, antibiotics, antisense therapy etc. However, all the methods are transient and some times results in severe side effects. In these situations, it was realized a decade or two decades ago, that gene therapy/correction would be one approach. The other approach is the injection of RNA into the cells. However, with a lot of research, several techniques have been introduced. Thus, gene therapy is a technique for correcting defective genes responsible for disease development. The therapy could also be called **DNA therapy**. The approaches in gene therapy include

1. A normal gene may be inserted into a nonspecific location within the genome to replace a nonfunctional gene.
2. An abnormal gene could be swapped for a normal gene through homologous recombination.
3. The abnormal gene could be repaired through selective reverse mutation, which returns the gene to its normal function, and
4. The regulation (the degree to which a gene is turned on or off) of a particular gene could be altered. Research on these lines is still being progressed. The other aspect in this area is RNA therapy. RNA interference or gene silencing may be a new way to treat Huntington's disease. Short Double-stranded RNA (short, interfering RNAs or siRNAs) is used in the

degradation of RNA of a particular sequence inside a cell. If a siRNA is designed to match the RNA copied from a faulty gene, then the abnormal protein product of that gene will not be produced. Similarly, new gene therapy approach repairs errors in messenger RNA derived from defective genes. Technique has potential to treat the blood disorder thalassaemia, cystic fibrosis, and some cancers. The last techniques consist of **RNA therapy**.

Formulation Strategies

Oral delivery of biotechnology drugs still is a problem to chase. Most of the biotechnology products cited in this chapter are administered by parenteral route. On the other hand drug delivery systems are aiding their oral delivery. Delivery systems for biotechnology products are helpful in solving formulation, pharmacokinetic, toxicity and inefficacy problems. Formulation is a major problem associated with biotechnology products. This is because of the physical and chemical instability in the formulation approaches currently undertaken. In addition, immunogenecity is a major issue. After administration by either oral or intravenous route, the antibodies formed against a therapeutic protein can result in serious clinical effects, such as loss of efficacy and neutralization of the endogenous protein with essential biological functions. This is particularly true with recombinant human proteins. The extent of the presence of degradation products in a protein formulation could also influence immunogenecity. The extent to which the presence of degradation products in protein and biotechnology formulations influences their immunogenicity is also a very important factor. Oral route of delivery can be attempted for biotechnology drugs. Tablets and capsules are the most common formulation strategies for oral administration. However, the main problem after oral administration is the degradation and lack of poor absorption across the intestines. Thus, research on their delivery has been initiated.

Conventional Dosage Forms

Conventional dosage forms consist of tablets and capsules. Due to the high structural fragility, hydrophilicty and molecular weight, proteins, DNA, vaccines, hormones and monoclonal antibodies after oral administration undergo unsatisfactory absorption through the mucosa. In addition, oral administration results in rapid elimination from the circulation. This seriously compromises therapeutic applicability and performance. In addition, during the transit through the intestinal tract, these molecules are inactivated by the high acidity of the stomach, the nutrients and secreted enzymes. If all the dosage forms are clubbed together, 40% of medications are tablet dosage forms. Because of the convenience of manufacture, ease of controlling the release, long lasting nature, patient compliance, tablets are the very suitable oral dosage forms. However, in case if the manufacture is not possible with a particular protein due to any physical instability during the manufacture of a tablet, a capsule dosage form would be the preferred dosage form. This dosage form would avoid degradation due to the manufacture processess such as compaction and compression. Apart from these advantages, capsule dosage forms offer several other advantages. As a whole, both these oral formulations are helpful for the oral delivery of the biotechnology products along with offering several other advantages.

Depending on the drug carrier matrix and the auxiliary agents used, peptide or protein liberation could be adjusted to delay or prolonged release. Some of the polymers used as drug carrier matrices for tablets form a gel after contact of liquids of the mucosal membranes, thereby acting as bioadhesive and sustained action dosage forms. Most of the biotechnology products currently administered, are applied after parenteral routes of administration. This route is associated with inconvenience because of pain, fear and risks. Currently, the research from injectable to non-invasive and from injectable to oral conversions is in high demand. As mentioned before, tablets and capsules are the very common approaches for oral delivery of these biotechnology products. Pharmaceutical technologies to overcome barriers after oral administration include the use of 1) enzyme inhibitors, 2) permeation elevators, and 3) multifunctional polymers. The excipients thus attempted should give cohesiveness to the tablet formulation, should give powderability to the drug polymer conjugates, flowability to fill in capsules and tablet machines etc. Multifunctional polymers not only give permeation increase, compactability, swelling behaviour, but also mucoadhesive properties. As such this area is very novel, couple of simple examples will be illustrated henceforth.

Insulin

Insulin is a protein hormone used in the treatment of diabetes. It is a stable protein after intravenous administration. However, it is profoundly degraded in the intestinal fluids. Calceti et al., 2004 investigated an oral formulation for insulin. As a first step, insulin-monomethoxypoly (ethylene glycol) derivatives were obtained by the preparation of mono- and di-terbutyl carbonate insulin derivatives, reaction of available protein amino groups with activated 750Da PEG and, finally, amino group de-protection. This procedure allowed for obtaining high yield of insulin-1PEG and insulin-2PEG. After subcutaneous administration, these two types of insulin maintained native biological activity. Using *in vitro* studies, it was demonstrated that PEGylation increased insulin's stability towards proteases. Insulin-1PEG was formulated into mucoadhesive tablets constituted by the thiolated polymer poly (acrylic acid)-cysteine. The therapeutic agent was released slowly from these tablets within 5 hours. *In vivo*, by oral administration to diabetic mice, the glucose levels were found to decrease by about 40% since the third hour from administration and the biological activity was maintained up to 30 hours. According to these results, the combination of PEGylated insulin with a thiolated polymer used as drug carrier matrix might be a promising strategy for oral insulin administration. In a different study, Bernkop-Schnurch et al., (2004) investigated various new polymers for insulin oral delivery. In recent years, thiolated polymers have become alternatives in the arena of non-invasive peptide delivery. These polymers are generated by the immobilisation of thiol-bearing ligands to mucoadhesive polymeric excipients. By formation of disulfide bonds with mucus glycoproteins, the mucoadhesive properties of these polymers are improved up to 130-fold. Due to formation of inter- and intramolecular disulfide bonds within the thiomer itself, dosage forms such as tablets or microparticles display strong cohesive properties resulting in comparatively higher stability, prolonged disintegration times and a more controlled release of the embedded peptide drug. The permeation of peptide drugs through mucosa was also improved by the use of thiolated polymers. Additionally some thiomers exhibit improved inhibitory properties towards peptidases. Tablets including thiomer and pegylated insulin, for instance, resulted in a pharmacological efficacy of 7% after oral application to diabetic mice. This is a very promising result and further studies could lead to tablet and capsule dosage forms for biotechnology drugs.

Snoeck V (2003) investigated the efficacy and feasibility of an oral **enterotoxigenic vaccine** to prevent enterotoxigenic Escherichia Coli (ETEC). This vaccination is used to prevent enterotoxigenic Escherichia coli (ETEC) induced postweaning diarrhoea, which mostly occurs in the piglets. At the moment of weaning, the piglets need active mucosal immunity. This group investigated the feasibility of oral vaccination of suckling piglets against F4+ETEC infection with F4 fimbriae. The investigation also included enteric-coated pills for the vaccine. Oral vaccination with enteric-coated pellets of F4 fimbriae was compared to vaccination with F4 fimbriae in solution. The pellet form was more effective than the solution form. The use of an enteric-coat was more effective likely because of the protection from inactivation by milk factors and degradation by enzymes and bile compared to a solution form.

Pegylation

Pegylation is generally used to facilitate i.v. administration of proteins. As this is an important technology in biotechnology, it is worth mentioning here. Mobile nontoxic PEG chains are conjugated to biotherapeutics to improve their therapeutic and formulation benefits. After pegylation, generally, the hydrodynamic volume is increased, thereby increasing the plasma retention time, solubility, and shields the antigenic determinants on the drug from detection by the immune system. One major challenge is the chemical conjugation and the other major challenge is ideal conjugation to improve the properties and not shield the active aminoacids and the structures in a natural or a biotechnological protein. Pegylation technology at this time uses linker-less conjugation methods to reduce the toxicity or immunogenicity.

PEG conjugates are usually prepared by techniques that employ random derivatization of lysine residues. The overall utility of these methods is limited, due to the heterogeneity and decreased bioactivity of the products. Therefore, the development of a method for site-specific pegylation of proteins is required. Most commonly the thiol-selective pegylation at a cysteine residue by site-directed mutagenesis is used to obtain maleimide-based or haloacetic-based PEG derivatives. Although this type of coupling is superior to other modification methods with respect to both the specificity and the rate of the reaction, there are several limitations to this method which include

1. The unmodified or modified form of a genetically-engineered mutant may have a different structure and function, as compared to the native protein,
2. A cysteine mutant may form disulfide isomers with intact cysteine residues, which would decrease the yield of the properly folded form and
3. *N*-maleimide derivatives, although considered to be sulfhydryl group-specific, may react at a much slower rate with amino and imidazoyl groups in the range of pH 7 to 8. Several other methods are available to form PEG conjugates. An example of pegylation of a protein commercially available with therapeutic benefits is pegylated interferon.

Type I interferons (IFNs)

Type I interferons (IFNs) are proteins that initiate antiviral and antiproliferative responses. Interferons are clinically important, and several subtypes of IFNα2 have been approved as drugs for the treatment of hepatitis B and C, as well as for cancers such as chronic myelogenous leukemia and hairy cell leukemia. IFNα2 are administered intramuscularly, subcutaneously, or intravenously, resulting in different pharmacokinetic profiles. In any mode, the administered cytokine is rapidly inactivated by body fluids and tissues and cleared from the blood plasma several hours following administration. The major routes of IFNα2 elimination from the circulatory system are proteolysis, receptor-mediated endocytosis, and kidney filtration. Prolonging the maintenance dose of IFNα2 in circulation is a desirable clinical outcome. A nonreversible, 12 kDa PEG- IFNα2 was approved as a therapeutic conjugate in 2001. It was administered once a week to hepatitis-C patients. This modified version facilitated a sustained antiviral response rate of 24%, as opposed to a 12% response rate obtained by the native cytokine. Although, the covalent attachment of PEG chains to proteins prolongs their lifetime *in vivo,* this process results in a dramatic reduction or even loss of biological and pharmacological activities. For example, 40 kDa PEG- IFNα2 has only 7% of the activity of the native cytokine, calling for higher doses to be administered. Furthermore, PEG-IFN does not readily penetrate all the tissues; while 12 kDa PEG- IFNα2b is widely distributed, 40 kDa PEG- IFNα2a is restricted to the blood and the interstitial fluid. This major drawback was recently overcome by designing a PEG- IFNα2 conjugate capable of generating native IFNα2 at a slow rate under physiological conditions. Thus, a variety of conjugates of interferons for various purposes could be synthesized and used. Likewise conjugates for various biotechnology drugs could be procured.

Nanoparticles and Micro particles

Controlled drug delivery technology represents one of the frontier areas of pharmaceutical formulation science. These delivery systems offer numerous advantages compared to conventional dosage forms, which include improved efficacy, reduced toxicity, and improved patient compliance and convenience. Of the different dosage forms reported, nanoparticles and microparticles attained much importance, due to a tendency to accumulate in inflamed areas of the body. Nano and microparticles for their attractive properties occupy unique position in drug delivery technology. Different polymers are currently used in the formulation and manufacture of nanoparticles and microparticles. Most of the times these are biodegradable. Nanoparticles are the particles of the size range in nanometers and microparticles are the particles in micrometers. Literature evidence suggests that these nanoparticles are taken up by phagocytosis and endocytosis and by different mechanisms after oral administration. Thus, the systemic delivery of nanoparticles is possible after oral administration. On the other hand, microparticles are mainly used for sustained release of drugs and biotechnology products. These microparticle ranges from 1μ to 100μ. Some times they are also produced in sizes larger than 100 μ that may be called just as particulates. The degradation times are larger for biodegrable microparticles than nanoparticles and thus are used for sustained release. However, reports also indicate that they could be used for vaccine delivery after oral administration. These microparticles act as adjuvants for vaccines. The payer's patches in the intestines are found to generate immunological responses and some times stimulate immunological cascade in the systemic circulation. Currently, ample literature is available with regard to micro- and nano-particles. Several products are already in the market. An example of a nanoparticle formulation development of a commercially available protein is the nanoparticle formulation for human calcitonin.

Salmon Calcitonin Nanoparticles

Salmon calcitonin nanoparticles were recently developed to protect this drug from gastrointestinal degradation. Salmon calcitonin, a polypeptide hormone consisting of 32 amino acids, plays a crucial role in both bone remodeling and calcium homeostasis. Currently, sCT is administered by injection or intranasally for the treatment of osteoporosis. Because sCT needs to be given on a daily basis over a long period of time, oral administration is a much more desirable route of administration for the convenience of patients. Apart from susceptibility to intestinal degradation, the inherent low permeability of proteins and peptides through the GI membrane results in an extremely low absorption percentage via the oral route. Therefore, the focus of the study was to develop an effective oral salmon calcitonin nanoparticle formulation.

Many previous studies have shown that nano- and microparticles are easily taken up by a group of localized endothelial cells in the small intestine, especially by the tissue called Peyer's patch. One of the major mechanisms for facile absorption of microparticles in the oral route is endocytosis process by M cells in the Peyer's patch. An M cell is a specialized cell for taking up nutrients and foreign materials through the endocytic mechanism. The endocytic mechanism is influenced by several factors, such as size and surface charge of microparticles, type of ligand attached to microparticles, and types of materials comprising microparticles. Although the exact endocytic mechanism and pathway are still unclear, biodegradable poly (lactic-*co*-glycolic acid) (PLGA) micro- and nanoparticles are being popularly exploited to increase the bioavailability of poorly absorbed macromolecular drugs, including proteins, peptides, and vaccines. However, it has been very difficult to prepare PLGA nano- and microparticles encapsulating a sufficient amount of hydrophilic protein and peptide drugs for oral delivery. Protein and peptide drugs are generally encapsulated in the PLGA nano- and microparticles by a double-emulsion solvent evaporation method. This formulation method often produced relatively large PLGA microspheres in a micrometer-scale range, which were unsuitable for the purpose of an endocytic cellular delivery. Generally, for these purposes, nanoparticle formulation is ideal.

Liposomes

Liposomes are of considerable commercial interest in drug and vaccine delivery. Liposomes are very well known and their structures and properties have been very thoroughly researched. These are made out of phospholipids. Essentially they are uni- or multi-lamellar lipid/water structures with diameters in the micron range. They can be formulated to incorporate a wide range of materials as a payload either in the water or in the lipid compartments. Using a variety of techniques, different liposomes could be formulated and classified. Conveniently liposomes could be classified into multilamellar, large unilamellar and small unilamellar vesicles. These are classified according to the methods of preparation. Multilamellar vesicles consist of phospolipid bilayers as in an onion, while unilamellar vesicles consist of one layer of phospholipid bilayer. The drug could be incorporated into hydrophilic core or hydrophobic phospholipid bilayer. Liposomes have been very actively investigated for over 40 years. However, keeping in view, several disadvantages such as the leak of the drug and reduced half-life in the systemic circulation compared to microparticles or nanoparticles, they went out of the center stage. With enormous literature backup, currently they are gaining prominence and in addition because of the generation of several new genetic engineering products such as DNA and synthesis of new cationic polymers, they are again gaining lime-light. Some liposome products are already in the market. A recent investigation of a successful story of liposomal DNA will be described henceforth.

Oral (intragastric) liposome-mediated DNA immunization

Oral (intragastric) liposome-mediated DNA immunization was recently investigated by Perrie et al., 2002 with successful results. Plasmid DNA pRc/CMV HBS encoding the S (small) region of hepatitis B surface antigen (HBsAg) was incorporated by the dehydration–rehydration method into Lipodine™ liposomes composed of 16 µmoles phosphatidylcholine (PC) or distearoyl phosphatidylcholine (DSPC), 8 µmoles of (dioleoyl phosphatedylethanolamine (DOPE) or cholesterol and 4 µmoles of the cationic lipid 1,2-dioleoyl-3-(trimethylammonium propane (DOTAP) (molar ratios 1 : 0.5 : 0.25). Incorporation efficiency was high (89–93% of the amount of DNA used) in all four formulations tested and incorporated DNA was shown to be resistant to displacement in the presence of the competing anionic sodium dodecyl sulphate molecules. This is consistent with the notion that most of the DNA is incorporated within the multilamellar vesicles structure rather than being vesicle surface-complexed. Stability studies performed in simulated intestinal media also demonstrated that dehydration–rehydration vesicles (DRV) incorporating DNA (DRV(DNA)) were able to retain significantly more of their DNA content compared to DNA complexed with preformed small unilamellar vesicles (SUV–DNA) of the same composition. Moreover, after 4h incubation in the media, DNA loss for DSPC DRV(DNA) was only minimal, suggesting this to be the most stable formulation. Oral (intragastric) liposome-mediated DNA immunisation studies employing a variety of DRV(DNA) formulations as well as naked DNA revealed that secreted IgA responses against the encoded HBsAg were (as early as three weeks after the first dose) substantially higher after dosing with 100µg liposome-entrapped DNA compared to naked DNA. Throughout the fourteen week investigation, IgA responses in mice were consistently higher with the DSPC

DRV(DNA) liposomes compared to naked DNA and correlated well with their improved DNA retention when exposed to model intestinal fluids. To investigate gene expression after oral (intragastric) administration, mice were given 100μg of naked or DSPC DRV liposome-entrapped plasmid DNA expressing the enhanced green fluorescent protein (pCMV.EGFP). Expression of the gene, in terms of fluorescence intensity in the draining mesenteric lymph nodes, was much greater in mice dosed with liposomal DNA than in animals dosed with the naked DNA. These results suggest that DSPC DRV liposomes containing DNA (Lipodine™) may be a useful system for the oral delivery of DNA vaccines.

Computer Aided Design

Bioinformatics, chemi-informatics and computer aided drug design are very routinely used techniques in drug design. These techniques are also applied for the design of biotechnology drugs. Assigning coding genes in genome is one of the major challenges in genomics. Several groups all over the world are currently involved in this research aspect. The key in all the biotechnology drugs is the gene. Thus, computer aided design basically consists of the design of gene, locating the probable gene in a nucleotide, design of corresponding RNAs and design of corresponding antisense oligonucleotides. Several techniques such as fourier transformations are currently used in the design of the software for this kind of design. In the design of peptide and protein drugs, different sets of software, methods and tools are available. A simple example of the design of vaccines will be described henceforth. Identification of peptides that elicit a T cell response plays a vital role in vaccine design. It is well established that MHC peptide binding is prerequisite for T-cell recognition (TCR) but not all MHC peptides binding site do not recognize the T cells. Groups are currently working to develop new methods for prediction of T-cell epitopes in antigen sequences. Recently, a server for predicting MHC binding sites has been developed. The prediction method used in this server is based on matrix optimization techniques (MOT). Two major databases

(i) MHCBN which consists MHC binders/non-binders and T cell epitopes;

(ii) BCIPEP consists B cell epitopes have been developed based on the prediction of T cell epitopes and MHC binders in antigen sequences. The aims of these projects are to identify the potential vaccine candidates for subunit vaccine design. Similary, a variety of softwares and computer programs are currently being investigated all over the world using a variety of techniques.

Preclinical and Clinical Trial Products

Preclinical stages of biotechnology products itself is very challenging. Most of the products are generated using cell culture and tissue culture studies. Immunogenecity generated out of these products thus at the very early extraction and synthesis stage is very important. Identification of a therapeutic protein itself is very crucial. Identification of the protein from a variety of proteins would sometimes pose severe problems. Several techniques like western blotting, Northern blotting, gel electrophoresis, column separation techniques are currently used in the purification process. This is some times very tedious and laborious. If a protein or any other biotechnology products have physical and formulation stability, then it is fine and the preclinical studies are very perfect. However, if the stability of the products were compromised in the formulation development stages, it would definitely impact the preclinical studies. The challenges lie in the stable formulation development and then investigate these preclinical formulations.

Currently several of the biotechnology products are in preclinical and clinical trial investigations. Although, vaccines for several diseases are in the market for some time including genetically engineered vaccines, for cancer therapy, success was not yet noticed. One case study of a clinical trial of a ***cancer vaccine*** that better illustrates an ideal kind of biotechnology vaccine will be presented henceforth here. This example is regarding a lymphoma cancer vaccine. B-cell lymphoma affects an estimated 41,000 Americans each year according to a survey in 1990s. This is a cancer of the lymph glands generated by misbehaved B cells (white blood cells). These are the very early producers of body's disease-fighting antibodies. According to one survey perhaps in 25,000 of patients, the cancer is a low-grade lymphoma (slow-growing tumors with a high rate of recurrence). The first results of the study were published in October 1999 issue of Nature medicine. In a very small group of patients a clear anti-tumor effect was observed after vaccination over the course of five years, according to the researchers at the Nationals Cancer Institute. National Cancer Institute (NCI) then launched a large-scale randomized, Phase III clinical trial with a custom-made vaccine from patient's own tumors.

The vaccine was created by fusing the tumor cells of the individual patients to antibody-producing mouse cells that act as mini-factories, churning out large quantities of tumor proteins into the tissue culture media. The protein of interest is collected from the tissue culture fluid – in this case a receptor molecule on the outer coating of the immune systems B cells. The receptor molecule is "exquisitely specific for this type of tumor because it is an immunoglobulin," And since it is unique to a given B cell, any tumor derived from that malignant B cell will have this [receptor molecule] marker. The vaccine mixture also included a highly immunogenic carrier protein and an "adjuvant" or immune system booster. In this study, patients received an initial injection, followed by booster shots for four months. 18 of 20 patients who were vaccinated against this common blood-cell tumor remained in complete remission on an average of four years after vaccine therapy without any evidence of microscopic disease. The patients who were selected in this study had minimal disease or were in a chemotherapy-induced first remission before the vaccine was administered. Currently, large-scale clinical trial study in a large group of patients is in progress.

FDA Regulations

Structural features are one of the major problems associated with immunogenecity. The mechanisms by which protein therapeutics or infact any genetic product can induce antibodies as well as the models used to study immunogenicity and the basic concepts of immunogenecity are very important. For a protein product, the chemical structure (including amino acid sequence, glycosylation, and pegylation) can influence the incidence and level of antibody formation. Moreover, it is shown that physical degradation (especially aggregation) of the proteins as well as chemical decomposition (e.g., oxidation) may enhance the immune response. This is the main issue a new drug application has to be taken in consideration during FDA applications with regard to genetic engineering products. The other issue is the safety and toxicity, which are mostly in similar lines as described in the chapter on safety of new chemical entities.

Conclusions

As such, the biotechnology products because of the concepts and challenges attracted pharmaceutical scientist for over several decades. Several drawbacks in the beginning stages were challenges. However, the recent innovations are helping in eliminating these challenges and would be crucial for further development of biotechnology products, not in a contorted way but straight, honest and precise manner. The presence of ample literature currently further helps in this regard.

Questions for Practice and Exercise

1. Write a brief note on the following:
    1. Human Growth Hormone
    2. Corticotropin
    3. Estrogens
    4. Growth Factors
    5. Thyrotropin
    6. Gut Hormones

2. Write a brief note on the following:
   (a) Cancer Vaccines
   (b) vaccine for Hepatitis B
   (c) OKT3
   (d) Rituximab
   (e) Herceptin
   (f) Daclizumab
   (g) Infliximab
3. Write a brief note on the following:
   (a) Blood factor therapeutics
   (b) Interferons
   (c) Interleukins
   (d) Antisense Oligonucleotides
4. Write a brief note on the following:
   (a) Formulation Strategies
   (b) Conventional Dosage Forms
   (c) Pegylation
   (d) Nanoparticles and Microparticles
   (e) Liposomes
5. Write a brief note on the Engineering and Technology Associated with the production and isolation of cancer vaccines.
6. What is fermentation process? What are its uses?
7. Illustrate with suitable examples how a fermentation process could be used for pharmaceutical production.
8. Using a suitable drug example illustrate a fermentation (biotechnology) process including the production, selection and optimization.
9. Write a detailed technical note on a fermentation process.
10. Write a brief note on the following:
    (a) Production of Monoclonal Antibodies
    (b) Production of Cancer Vaccines
    (c) Production of Antisense Oligonucleotides
    (d) Production of DNA and RNA
    (e) Production of Tumor Antigens

References

1. Berzofsky JA, Terabe M, Oh S, Belyakov IM, Ahlers JD, Janik JE, Morris JC. Progress on new vaccine strategies for the immunotherapy and prevention of cancer.J Clin Invest. 2004 Jun;113(11):1515-25. Review.
2. Snoeck V, Huyghebaert N, Cox E, Vermeire A, Vancaeneghem S, Remon JP, Goddeeris BM. Enteric-coated pellets of F4 fimbriae for oral vaccination of suckling piglets against enterotoxigenic Escherichia coli infections.Vet Immunol Immunopathol. 2003 Dec 15;96(3-4):219-27.
3. Perrie Y, Obrenovic M, McCarthy D, Gregoriadis G. Liposome (Lipodine)-mediated DNA vaccination by the oral route. J Liposome Res. 2002 Feb-May;12(1-2):185-97.
4. Calceti P, Salmaso S, Walker G, Bernkop-Schnurch A. Development and in vivo evaluation of an oral insulin-PEG delivery system. Eur J Pharm Sci. 2004 Jul;22(4):315-23.

Bibliography

1. Immunogenetics and Artificial Antigens, Revised Edition, Authored by R. Petrov, R. Khaitov, and R. Ataullakhanov, Nauka Publishers, 1987.
2. Pharmaceutical Biotechnology, First Edition, Authored by AK Saluja, HN Kakrani, and SS Purohit, Agrobios (India) Publications, 2003.
3. Production Technology of Recombinant Therapeutic Proteins, First Edition, Authored by Chiranjib Chakraborthy, Biotech Books, 2004.
4. Applied Antisense Technology, First Edition, Edited by CS Stein and AM Kreig, Wiley-Liss Publications, 1998.
5. Pharmaceutical Dosage Forms and Drug Delivery Systems, Seventh Edition, Authored by H.C. Ansel, L.V. Allen, and N.G. Popovich, Lippincott Williams & Wilkins, 1999.
6. Quality Control, Seventh Edition, Authored by DH Besterfield, Prentice Hall, 2003.
7. The Theory and Practice of Industrial Pharmacy, Third Edition, Edited by Leon Lachman, Herbert A. Lieberman, and Joseph L. Kanig, Lea & Febiger Publications, 1986.
8. Pharmaceutical Biotechnology, Second Edition, Edited by DJA Crommelin et al., CRC Press, 2002.

CHAPTER 3

EVALUATION OF EARLY DEVELOPMENT CANDIDATES: PHYSICAL PROPERTIES

- **Introduction**
- **Physical properties**
    - Specific surface area
    - Hygroscopicity
    - Bulk density and flow properties
    - Crystallization
- **Physico-chemical properties**
    - pKa
    - Solubility analysis
    - Partition coefficient
    - Dissolution rate
    - Solid state stability
    - Solution stability
- **Regulatory considerations**
- **Conclusions**

Introduction

The pace of introduction of new chemical moieties into the market has tremendously increased over the past two decades. In recent times, because of the advent of high throughput methods in drug synthesis and screening, it is likely that several new molecules will be introduced into the market in near future. It thus becomes imperative to devise effective means of reducing the cost of the entire process of bringing a molecule into the market. In the early stages of any project it is important to adequately characterize both the drug substance and the excipients. This reduces the risk of undesirable findings during clinical and manufacturing stages. Any alteration in the drug substance would require fresh investigations including bioequivalence studies. This is the key issue a pharmaceutical scientist has to keep in mind always when dealing with new chemical entities **(New Drug Substances)** and the corresponding products. Alternatively, although there is lot of information available for generic drugs, new polymorphs are always investigated to improve the properties. In these two issues the study of physical properties of drug substances becomes essential. In this respect, innovations are always in place whatever the drug candidate is: whether old, new, plant product, microbial product or an animal product.

Once a compound is identified to be most likely new chemical entity for further investigation based on the preliminary pharmacological screening of the compound, it is categorized as an exploratory compound. A simple solution form, a suspension form, an IV solution, a tablet form or a capsule form for this exploratory chemical based on the convenience is developed and used for further investigations. Physical and physico-chemical studies will be performed. If this exploratory compound is a tougher molecule, then a systematic investigation is accomplished. Otherwise, a simple tentative formulation is developed for preliminary investigations. Judicious selection and investigation depends on the experience of the scientist who is screening. The training received by the personnel incharge is also very important. If things go wrong at this stage with a very potent new chemical entity, then lot of income goes waste. In the past, a simple tentative formulation was developed and used for early toxicological and pharmacological screening. Further, the preformulation, formulation and clinical investigations are systematically investigated till the final stages of drug reaching the market. Currently, because of the introduction of several high-throughput screening techniques, the physico-chemical properties are obtained in hand in hand with the high throughput synthesis of new chemical entities. These high throughput synthesis techniques are developed after several years of constant investigations of the scientists in this area.

To develop a solution, a suspension, a syrup or an emulsion, the information of physico-chemical properties such as solubility, pK_a and partition coefficient, would be required. To develop a tablet, a capsule or any other solid dosage form solid-state properties the information such as specific surface area, flowability, particle size, bulk density, etc. would be required. Thus, the study of these properties is essential to develop a decent formulation for a novel chemical entity, right from the beginning to the end of drug development. The following reasons for the evaluation of the physical properties of early developmental candidates could be furnished:

1. Reducing the time and cost of introducing a molecule into the market.
2. Selection of an appropriate form of the drug substance, such as salt form, prodrugs etc.
3. Selection of application type (e.g. oral, dermal or injectable).
4. Selection of the form of delivery (e.g. quick acting or slow release).
5. Increasing the ease of product development.
6. Reducing undesirable findings during clinical phases.
7. Release of the best drug into the market.

This chapter deals with the solution and solid-state properties of a new chemical entity in detail to be used for product development. Thorough examination of these properties at the initial stages pays in a long run for a promising therapeutic agent.

Physical Properties

Specific surface area, hygroscopicity, bulk density, flow properties, crystallization are the physical properties to be investigated for new drug substances.

Specific Surface Area

Surface area properties of a drug particle affect the dissolution and chemical reactivity of a drug substance. These properties include size, shape and surface morphology of a drug substance. The smaller the particles, the better are the bulk flow and formulation homogeneity. The simplest way to measure the particle size is to use a microscope. However, it is tedious to measure the average particle size with such techniques. The best way is to use photomicrographs and hemacytometer slides. Particles with a large specific area are good adsorbents for the adsorption of gases and of solutes from solution. The other factor that is also important is the particle shape. Generally, a sphere has minimum surface area per unit volume. The more asymmetric a particle is, the greater the surface area per unit volume. For a collection of particles that are not spherical, which is the case with drug powders, the diameter that is related to the surface area or volume through a correction factor is to be considered. Since these surface properties affect the homogeneity, content uniformity and dissolution properties of a tablet form, which ultimately affects the bioavailability, these properties have to be thoroughly evaluated during toxicological stages before clinical trials are preceded so that perfect correlation is obtained between the bioavailability data with a formulation when the studies are transferred from toxicology studies to clinical studies. Accordingly, sophisticated methods are currently used. These include adsorption methods and air permeability methods. Quantasorb, manufactured by the Quantachrome Corporation USA, is one instrument used to obtain surface area measurements. A mixture of helium and nitrogen is passed through the sample; helium is inert and is not adsorbed on the powder surface while nitrogen is adsorbed on the powders. A thermal conductivity instrument attached to the instrument measures the conductivity associated with the adsorption, which in turn indicates the size of the particles. In air permeability technique, the resistance to the flow of a fluid, such as air through a plug of compacted powder is used to determine the surface area of the powder. The greater the surface area of the powder the greater is the resistance offered to the flow of the air. An example of such an instrument is "The fisher subsieve sizer"

Hygroscopicity

The amount of water adsorbed on the surface of drug particle influences the solid-state stability as well as the flow properties and compactibility of a drug substance. Thus, this property of the drug substance becomes crucial for investigations. Some chemicals such as sodium chloride are deliquescent and totally absorb moisture to completely dissolve. But it is a different situation with drug substances. Most drugs are partially hygroscopic. Provided the opportunity, the first property to be determined for a new drug characterization is to measure its hygroscopicity. Alternatively, these properties could be studied later, after preformulation is accomplished. The stability of a solid drug depends on the hygroscopicity of a particular solid state of a drug, which in turn depends on the type of the crystal or physical form of the drug that in turn depends on the synthetic techniques or the recrystallization method for that particular drug. The hygroscopicity of a substance is determined by exposing the compound to different humidity conditions for specific time intervals and then assaying for water content using Karl-Fischer reagent etc. The other instrumental method that could be used to measure the hygroscopicity is the gas chromatography. Dynamic water sorption (DWS) that requires very little amount of compound for handling is also used in the hygroscopicity measurements at above +25°C.

Hygroscopicity most of the times affects the compactibility of new drug substances. Promise holds when hygroscopicity of an NCE would be very less or totally void. Compactability as a property is affected by compressibility, adhesive/cohesive interactions and mechanical properties of the components. For instance, paracetamol, an analgesic compound is a poorly compactable drug. Its monoclinic crystal form and its poor plastic deformation explain the poor compaction behavior of paracetamol. Water content also influences the compactibility, suggesting that hygroscopicity is one of the key issues in the development of tablet dosage forms. The mechanism of water absorption in most of the cases is either hydrate formation or site-specific adsorption. The greater the compactibility, the better are the tablet properties. Many attempts were tried to increase the compactibility of a tablet substance. In this regard the reduction of hygroscopicity of a drug substance is very crucial. This can be achieved by obtaining drug crystals by using altered synthetic or recrystallization techniques. Thus, generally anhydrous forms of APIs are preferred.

Bulk Density and Flow Properties

Bulk density is an essential pharmaceutical property to be thoroughly investigated for a new chemical entity. This is because of its importance in capsule filling and tablet compression. Apparent high bulk density will not allow a capsule to be filled in the specific volume and in addition during tablet compression, the tablets would not be compressed either because of the rebound effect or because of the bulk volume occupied by the tablet powder in the die. Bulk density along with flow properties of a drug substance occupies major investigation problems, which have to be sorted out as early as possible in the formulation development. These problems can be very evident in tablet and capsule formulation with drugs having high apparent bulk densities. Experimentally, the true density is determined by suspending drug particles in solvents of various densities and in which the compound is insoluble. In these measurements, wetting and pore penetration are enhanced by the addition of a small quantity of surfactant to the solvent mixtures. After vigorous shaking, the samples are centrifuged briefly and then left to stand undisturbed until floatation or settling has reached equilibrium. The sample that remains suspended corresponds to the true density of the material. One way of avoiding this density problem for a new chemical entity is to use wet granulation and then punch the tablets or fill the granules in a capsule. However, this is not always helpful. There are some very tough drugs that are not amenable to compression because of their bulk density properties. In addition, currently, direct compression of new chemical entities is in full practice. This saves time and the cost invested in the solid dosage manufacture. If a drug has very high bulk density, it may not be used in a direct compression process. The drug has to be modified so as to obtain bulk drug with good compressibility properties. The other aspect in this regard is the utility of these properties in modern solid dosage form technology.

In modern solid dosage form technology (capsules and tablets), the current practice is to prepare dosage forms with reduced excipient content. Technology that reduces the size of the dosage form, improves the compressibility of the solid drug, its flowability and enhances the aesthetics as desirable. This was not the case with older drugs that needed huge amounts of excipients. Wet granulation process was routinely used to manufacture drug excipient granules, which were subsequently punched to form ideal drug tablets that are marketed even in the developed countries and are approved by United States Pharmacopoiea (USP), British Pharmacopoiea (BP) and Japanese Pharmacopoiea (JP). In this regard, flow properties of drugs become very important. One factor on which flow properties depend is hygroscopicity. The best example in this regard is the development of aspirin crystals by Wang et al., 2003 with very low excipient content. Aspirin, a traditional antipyretic analgesic has been used in clinical treatment for over 100 years. Because of the innovation of aspirin's potential utilities it is still very hot in the market accordingly. However, because of its poor stability, compressibility and flowability aspirin formulation is still a problem. Wang et al., using Wurster fluidized bed developed aspirin granules with good flow properties. The resulting granules possessed excellent flowability, suitable size, good compressibility, and high drug content that will help to decrease the amount of excipients required to miniaturize solid dosage forms.

Crystallization

Crystallization is a common phenomenon in pharmaceutical processing right from the manufacturing of Active Pharmaceutical Ingredient (API) (new drug substance) to the storage of the final formulation approved. In this context, systematic investigations of crystallization phenomenon would be of a definite interest to a pharmaceutical scientist. Crystallization process can be termed as a metastable thermodynamic state. This occurs because any substance or events tend to stabilize to reach the lowest possible thermodynamic state. This state of any substance is termed as a metastable state. This metastable state is either intentionally or unintentionally created either by supersaturation, in the crystallization of desired solid-state modifications, and in the control of solid-phase conversions during isolation, manufacturing, storage, and dissolution. Examples of metastable states include solid solutions, freeze-concentrated solutions, solutions of weak acids or bases exposed to a pH change, solutions prepared by dissolving a solid-state modification with a higher solubility (higher free energy), and residual solutions during filtration, granulation, and drying. Cystallization mechanism and kinetics determine the extent of this phenomenon. Thus, such an investigation is worth pursuing. The factors that can apparently affect crystallization include molecular or ionic transport, viscosity, supersaturation, solubility, solid-liquid interfacial tension, and temperature.

Nucleation kinetics is experimentally determined from measurements of nucleation rates, induction times and metastability zone widths (the supersaturation or under-cooling necessary for spontaneous nucleation) as a function of initial supersaturation. Currently, molecular simulations from the data obtained from the solution and crystal structure of drug substances is used in establishing the crystal structure of a new chemical entity. Molecular association processes in supersaturated systems is obtained by laser Raman spectroscopy and laser light scattering is used in the identification of prenucleation clusters and growth units under well-defined experimental conditions. Raman and fluorescence spectroscopic techniques are capable of providing information about the solution structure or the species present in solutions.

Physico-chemical Properties

Several physico-chemical properties of new leads have to be investigated very early on. These could include pK_a, solubility analysis, partition coefficient, dissolution rate, solid-state stability, and solution state stability.

pK_a

pK_a determinations of a new chemical entity are important because this controls solubility and consequently the oral absorption of a molecule in a given solution, formulation or body fluid. In the pH ranges from 1 to 10, the solubility and consequently oral absorption could be altered by orders of magnitude with changing pH. pK_a is the pH at which 50% of a substance is ionized. Buffer, temperature, ionic strength, and cosolvents affect the pK_a values. Incorporation of cosolvents in pK_a measurement instrument methods is important because of the likely poor solubility and possible precipitation of these compounds in aqueous media. This is especially true with the currently synthesized poorly soluble new chemical entities. Potentiometric and spectrophotometric methods are the popular methods used in the determinations of pK_a\`s of new chemical entities. Currently, GlpK_a instrument is in the market for the determination of pK_a's of new chemical entities. This instrument measures the potentiometric pK_a of a compound. The advantage offered by the current GlpK_a instrument is that, the assays are fully automated; temperature and ionic strengths are monitored during the runs and four-line cosolvent options available. The following solvents could be used in GlpK_a measurements with 0.15 M ionic strengths: methanol (80%), 1,4 dioxane (60%), DMSO (60%), ethanol (60%), ethylene glycol (60%), DMF (60%), THF (60%) and acetonitrile (50%). The instrument because of the compatibility of the electrodes supports these solvents. In addition, the electrode behaviour in each of the solvents is known and incorporated into the instrument software accordingly. The advantage is that using organic solvents help in determination ionization constants of poorly soluble compounds.

As per the manufacturers indications the functions of the instruments include:

1. pK_a `s measured from 2 to 12
2. Log P measurements from –2 to +8
3. Overlapping and multiple pK_a `s routinely measured
4. Easily handles protogenic counter ions
5. Sparingly soluble compounds titrated in eight possible supported cosolvents (aqueous pKa extrapolated)
6. Typical sample concentrations of 0.25 to 0.5 mM (1-2 mg of 400 MW compound in 10 ml)
7. Fast (typical titration = 25 minutes)
8. Accurate and precise.

In spectrophotometric method of determination, at a given pH, if the ion concentrations are determined using Beers Law one can calculate the approximate pK_a for a drug. For example, if the drug is a free acid [HA] in equilibrium with its base [A^-], then

$$pK_a = pH + \log [HA]/[A^-]$$

when [HA]=[A^-], as determined by their respective absorbances in the spectrophotometric determination, pK_a =pH.

Solubility Analysis

Solubility analysis of a new chemical entity is essential for further processing of a compound. The routine practice is to determine the saturation solubility of a compound in different solvents in different pH conditions. The factors that would affect the solubility of a new chemical entity are pH, temperature, ionic strength, and buffer concentrations. For equilibrium solubility determination, different methods are employed. To determine the aqueous solubility, the drug is solubilized in which it is highly soluble and this solution is slowly added to the distilled water and agitated. At the end of agitation, the suspension is filtered to obtain a filtrate that is then assayed using techniques like spectrophotometry and high-pressure liquid chromatography. In this regard, temperature also plays a role some time. Usually, the solubility of drugs is more in high temperature conditions. This principle can be used to saturate the aqueous suspension containing a drug. Subsequently at the end of the equilibration period (usually 24 hours), it is slowly cooled down. The compound that is not soluble is precipitated out. This is filtered and submitted for analysis to determine the solubility of a drug substance. The simplest technique that is routinely used is to add excess of drug to water and this is then agitated overnight to obtain maximum solubility of the drug in the media and then filtered and assayed to obtain the desired aqueous solubility.

Similar is the case with the solubility of a new chemical entity in other organic solvents. The technique of solubility determination can be tailored according to the convenience depending on the drug. It is some times very wrong to consider the solubility studies as trivial esp. for highly water-soluble drugs. However, initial investigations and determinations would be very essential for further formulation developments.

The other aspect of solubility is dissolution. To determine the solubility of a poorly soluble compound in water, generally 24 hours equilibration time is given. During this time the drug slowly dissolves in water. It is a similar phenomenon with the dissolution of a drug in gastric fluid or dissolution media from a solid powder or a capsule or from a tablet dosage form. The drug is slowly dissolved and the drug dispersed by agitation to form a uniform solution. It is then analyzed to obtain the concentration of the drug in the dissolution medium. Drugs with limited solubility ($< 1\%$) in the fluids of the gastrointestinal tract often exhibit poor or erratic absorption unless dosage forms are specifically tailored for the drug. However, solubility profiles are not predictors of biologic performance, but do provide rationale for more extensive *in vivo* studies and formulation development prior to drug evaluation in humans.

Partition Coefficient

Octanol-water partition coefficient is the ratio of the concentration of a chemical in octanol and in water at equilibrium and at a specified temperature. Octanol is an organic solvent that is used as a surrogate for natural organic matter. The octanol-water partition coefficient has been correlated to water solubility; therefore, the water solubility of a substance can be used to estimate its octanol-water partition coefficient.

As mentioned previously, the octanol/water partition coefficient (K_{ow})1 is defined as the ratio of a chemical's concentration in the octanol phase to its concentration in the aqueous phase of a two-phase octanol/water system.

K_{ow} = Concentration in octanol phase / Concentration in aqueous phase (I – 1)

Values of K_{ow} are thus unitless. The parameter is measured using low solute concentrations, where K_{ow} is a very weak function of solute concentration. Values of K_{ow} are usually measured at room temperature (20 or 25'C). The effect of temperature on K_{ow} is not great - usually on the order of 0.001 to 0.01 log K_{ow} units per degree - and may be either positive or negative. Measured values of K_{ow} for organic chemicals have been found as low as 10^{-3} and as high as 10^{7}, thus encompassing a range of ten orders of magnitude. In terms of $\log K_{ow}$, this range is from -3 to 7. It is frequently possible to estimate $\log K_{ow}$ with an uncertainty (i.e., method error) of no more than 10.1-0.2 $\log K_{ow}$ units.

The octanol/water partition coefficient is not the same as the ratio of a chemical's solubility in octanol to its solubility in water, because the organic and aqueous phases of the binary octanol/water system are not pure octanol and pure water. At equilibrium, the organic phase contains 2.3 mol/L of water, and the aqueous phase contains 4.5 X 10^{-8} mol/L of octanol. Moreover, K_{ow} is often found to be a function of solute concentration. The chemical in question is added to a mixture of octanol and water whose volume ratio is adjusted according to the expected value of K_{ow}. Very pure octanol and water must be used, and the concentration of the solute in the system should be less than 0.01 mol/L. The system is shaken gently until equilibrium is achieved (15 min to I hr). Centrifugation is generally required to separate the two phases, especially if an emulsion has formed. An appropriate analytical technique is then used to determine the solute concentration in each phase. A rapid laboratory estimate of K_{ow} may be obtained by measuring the retention time in a high-pressure liquid chromatography system; the logarithm of the retention time and the logarithm of K_{ow} have been found to be linearly correlated. Conversely, chemicals with high K_{ow} values (e.g., greater than 10^4) are very hydrophobic.

Dissolution Rate

Dissolution rate is the predictable measure of time required for a given drug or active ingredient in an oral solid dosage form to go into solution under a specified set of conditions. Since absorption and physiological availability of any nutritional supplement is largely dependent upon having it in a dissolved state, a suitable dissolution rate is crucial. Calculating intrinsic dissolution rate makes comparison of the dissolution of individual drug substances and the affect of different conditions on drug dissolution. The intrinsic dissolution rate is generally defined as the dissolution rate of a pure drug substance under the condition of constant surface area. The true intrinsic dissolution rate may be better described as the rate of mass transfer from the solid surface to the liquid phase. Intrinsic dissolution is generally determined by measuring the dissolution of a non-disintegrating disk made by compressing pure powdered drug substance under high pressure using a specially constructed punch and die system. The test material is compressed with a bench-top tablet press for 1 minute at the minimum compression pressure necessary to form a non-disintegrating compacted tablet. Compression for 1 minute at 250MPa (~36000 pounds/in^2) is sufficient for many organic crystalline compounds, but alternative compression conditions that achieve the desired degree of compaction may be required. Because changes in the crystal form may occur during compression, confirmation of the solid form should be verified by powder X-ray diffraction or another similar technique. Compression pressure plays an important role in the test. If it is too low, a non-disintegrating tablet may not be obtained, and if it is too high, it may change the crystal form. Compression pressure should be high enough to produce a translucent pellet with no powder or flakes on the surface. It is important to study the effect of the compression pressure on intrinsic dissolution rates as it has been observed for several drug substances that the intrinsic dissolution rate varies with changes in compression pressure.

Dissolution rate determines the availability of the drug for absorption. When slower than absorption, dissolution becomes the rate-limiting step. Overall selection of an appropriate formulation can control absorption. For example, reducing the particle size increases the drug's surface area, thus increasing the rate and extent of GI absorption of a drug whose absorption is normally limited by slow dissolution. Dissolution rate is affected by whether the drug is in salt, crystal, or hydrate form. The Na salts of weak acids (eg, barbiturates, salicylates) dissolve faster than their corresponding free acids regardless of the pH of the medium. Certain drugs are polymorphic, existing in amorphous or various crystalline forms. Chloramphenicol palmitate has two forms, but only one sufficiently dissolves and is absorbed to be clinically useful. A hydrate is formed when one or more water molecules combine with a drug molecule in crystal form. The solubility of such a solvate may markedly differ from the nonsolvated form; eg, anhydrous ampicillin has a greater rate of dissolution and absorption than its corresponding trihydrate.

Solid State Stability

The very important operation in drug discovery is the solid-state stability. This involves stability of the drug substance as a solid and stability of a drug substance in a solid dosage form. Drug instability in pharmaceutical formulations may be detected in some instances by a change in the physical appearance, color, odor, taste or texture of the formulation whereas as the chemical stability of a drug substance is determined by the chemical analysis. The second study is termed reaction kinetics. Altogether, these two instabilities appear in both the drug substance and in a formulation. A kinetic study on a drug substance is examined by subjecting an NCE in several physical and chemical and stressed conditions. The samples are withdrawn at periodic times and assayed for the drug content using a HPLC or other analytical techniques. Then the active chemicals and degradants are mathematically dissected to obtain chemical kinetics of the drug substance. These reaction kinetics could be zero-order, first-order, second-order and sometimes inverse reaction kinetics. Inverse kinetics are determined when there is a transition of one impurity to the other or one degradant to the drug, which may help in long run in the formulation movement predictions and during storage. These kinds of methodologies are generally one of the first investigations with an NCE. Subsequently, formulations are developed. Intuitive development of formulations prior to the determination of physical stability is not a valid methodology. As a standard stability protocol, the utilization of exaggerated conditions such as high temperature, high light intensity and high humidity are investigated for the stability determination. Once upon a time when these conditions were not available, high temperature was generally investigated. Accelerated temperature stability studies, for example, may be conducted for six months at 40°C with 75% relative humidity. If a significant change occurs in the drug/drug product under these conditions, lesser temperature and humidity may be used, such as 30°C and 60% relative humidity. Product containers, closures, and other packaging features are also to be considered in stability testing during this stage. The data that is obtained is useful in the prediction of stability of a drug in the formulations and also to investigate the stability kinetics of the individual impurities or degradation products.

Solution State Stability

Solution state stability of a drug is valid for stability testing of liquid formulations and for HPLC method developments. To determine solution state stability, the NCE is generally mixed in aqueous media at different pH conditions. The samples are withdrawn at regular time intervals and are submitted for analysis. Once the data is obtained, the active amount present is mathematically fitted to obtain the reaction kinetics in the solution state. Different pH conditions, different humidity conditions and different temperature conditions, different packaging conditions can be used in the solution state stability determinations. The use of the solution state stability data will be in proper selection of liquid dosage form for preclinical testing or market formulation testing. In addition, stability in different organic media as well as in different cosolvents could be determined at this stage. The reaction kinetics is the same and is zero-order, first-order, second-order, multi-order and inverse kinetics. The data is similar to that fitted for solid-state stability.

Regulatory Considerations

The current guidelines of The Food and Drug Administration's Current Good Manufacturing Practice regulations include protocols for the determination of stability and stability testing of pharmaceutical components and finished products. The following regulations regarding stability protocols for a new chemical entity were discussed in one of the recent International Conference on Harmonization (ICH) meeting. These are currently valid guidelines and regulatory considerations for the stability determination of new chemical entities (NCEs). These include "Stability Testing of New Drug Substances and Products", "Quality of Biotechnology Products: Stability Testing of Biotechnology/Biological Drug Products", "Photostability Testing of New Drug Substances and Products", and

"Stability Testing of New Dosage Forms". In solid-state characterization apart from the stability, impurity, polymorphs, racemates etc are determined as a first step in the physical characterization of a new chemical entity. The following discussions reveal the requirement for physical characterization as per the regulatory agencies.

1. Enantiomers and Racemates

Stereoisomers are molecules that have the same constitution (i.e., molecular formula and chemical connectivity), but differ in the spatial orientation of the atoms. When two stereoisomers are mirror images, but are not superimposable upon each other (like left and right hands), they are referred to as enantiomers. Enantiomeric molecules are identical in all physical and chemical properties, except in an environment that is also chiral (characterized by handedness). Polarized light is such an environment, and pairs of enantiomers rotate the plane of polarization by equal amounts in opposite directions. Enantiomers may be either right-handed (dextro-rotary) S(+)-isomers or left-handed (levo-rotary) R(-)-isomers. Racemates are equimolar mixtures of enantiomers of the same molecule. Frequently, both enantiomers found in a racemate will have similar desirable pharmacological activity. In other cases, one member of a pair of enantiomers is pharmacologically active and the other inactive or nearly inactive, as in baclofen where the R(-)-isomer is a muscle relaxant and antispastic, and the S(+)-isomer is essentially inactive. In other racemates, the enantiomers show significantly different pharmacological activity. For example, both isomers of sotalol have similar antiarrhythmic effects, but only the R(-)-isomer has significant beta-blocking activity. There are also instances where only one member of a pair of enantiomers has shown significant toxicity; an example of this may be found with thalidomide, where it is generally believed that most, if not all, of the teratogenicity associated with the drug is attributable to the R(-)-isomer.

In the past, the usual practice in the pharmaceutical industry has been to develop either a racemate or an enantiomer without fully characterizing or studying its respective properties. When separation of enantiomers was difficult, the question of which stereoisomeric form should be developed was largely an academic one. However, in many cases, current technology permits production of pure enantiomers on a commercial scale. Improved pharmacologic study of enantiomers has been permitted by developments in analytical technology that frequently enable detection of one enantiomer in the presence of the other at concentrations found in biological fluids.

The Stereoisomeric Drug Policy provides general recommendations for conducting and reviewing studies of the safety and effectiveness of drug products whose active ingredient is an enantiomer, a racemate, or a nonracemic mixture of enantiomers. Although the Stereoisomeric Drug Policy does not address issues of marketing exclusivity, it does contain the agency's thinking on the approval of stereoisomeric drug products.

2. Impurities

Impurities in new drug substances are addressed from two perspectives:

1. Chemistry aspects include classification and identification of impurities, report generation, listing of impurities in specifications, and a brief discussion of analytical procedures
2. Safety aspects include specific guidance for qualifying those impurities that were not present, or were present at substantially lower levels, in batches of a new drug substance used in safety and clinical studies.

   The studies conducted to characterize the structure of actual impurities present in a new drug substance at a level greater than 1% the identification threshold (e.g., calculated using the response factor of the drug substance). Note that any impurity at a level greater than 1% (>) the identification threshold in any batch manufactured by the proposed commercial process should be identified. In addition, any degradation product observed in stability studies at recommended storage conditions at a level greater than 1% (>) the identification threshold should be identified. When identification of an impurity is not feasible, a summary of the laboratory studies demonstrating the unsuccessful effort should be included in the application. Where attempts have been made to identify impurities present at levels of not more than 1%the identification thresholds, it is useful also to report the results of these studies. Identification of impurities present at an apparent level of not more than 1% the identification threshold is generally not considered necessary. However, analytical procedures should be developed for those potential impurities that are expected to be unusually potent, producing toxic or pharmacological effects at a level not more than 1% the identification threshold.

3. Polymorphs

Many pharmaceutical solids can exist in different physical forms. Polymorphism is often characterized as the ability of a drug substance to exist as two or more crystalline phases that have different arrangements and/or conformations of the molecules in the crystal lattice. Amorphous solids consist of disordered arrangements of molecules and do not possess a distinguishable crystal lattice. Solvates are crystalline solid adducts containing either stoichiometric or nonstoichiometric amounts of a solvent incorporated within the crystal structure. If the incorporated solvent is water, the solvates are also commonly known as hydrates. Polymorphism refers to the occurrence of different crystalline forms of the same drug substance. Polymorphism in this commentary is defined as in the International Conference on Harmonization (ICH) Guideline Q6A (2), to include solvation products and amorphous forms.

Polymorphs and solvates of a pharmaceutical solid can have different chemical and physical properties such as melting point, chemical reactivity, apparent solubility, dissolution rate, optical and electrical properties, vapor pressure, and density. These properties can have a direct impact on the processability of drug substances and the quality/performance of drug products, such as stability, dissolution, and bioavailability. A metastable pharmaceutical solid form can change crystalline structure or solvate/desolvate in response to changes in environmental conditions, processing, or over time.

Several regulatory documents and literature reports address issues relevant to the regulation of polymorphism. The concepts and principles outlined in these are applicable for “A New Drug Application (ANDA)”. However, certain additional considerations may be applicable in case of ANDAs. Often, at the time FDA receives an ANDA a monograph defining certain key attributes of the drug substance and drug product may be available in the Unites States Pharmacopoeia (USP). These public standards play a significant role in the ANDA regulatory review process and in case of polymorphism, when some differences are noted, lead to additional requirements and considerations. This commentary is intended to provide a perspective on polymorphism in pharmaceutical solid in the context of ANDAs. It highlights major considerations for monitoring and controlling drug substance polymorphs and describes a framework for regulatory decisions regarding drug substance "sameness" considering the role and impact of polymorphism in pharmaceutical solids.

Conclusions

The first step in the physical state determinations and consideration of new chemical entities is to procure the drug from synthetic chemists in as pure as possible chemical state. The enantiomers and polymorphic states are determined using several physico-chemical methods. Subsequently, solid-state stability is determined. In case of multiple polymorphs or racemic mixtures, the most stable and safer chemical state is selected. All these steps can be done in tandem with the formulation, toxicological and clinical trial methods. However, keeping in view the enormous price the industry has to be pay at the end of determination of a candidate is not of that important for further development, in every likely, a thorough physical characterization in the earlier stages would be essential. On the other hand, keeping in view the regulatory requirements, it is better advised to fully characterize the physical state of an NCE and further only investigate the very ideal or also called utopian molecule for further development.

Questions for Practice and Exercise

1. Why is it important to know the physical properties of early development candidates?
2. What is an exploratory compound? Why is its formulation development essential?
3. List the physico-chemical properties of early development candidates.
4. Define "Specific Surface Area of early development drug leads".
5. Define "Hygroscopicity of early development drug candidates" for an ideal new drug substance.
6. Define "bulk density and flow properties of early development drug candidate".
7. Describe "Crystallization".
8. Explain the physicochemical properties of early development candidates.

References

1. Wang X, Cui F, Yonezawa Y, Sunada H. Preparation and evaluation of high drug content particles, Drug Dev Ind Pharm. 2003 Nov;29(10):1109-18.

Bibliography

1. The Theory and Practice of Industrial Pharmacy, Third Edition, Edited by Leon Lachman, Herbert A. Lieberman, and Joseph L. Kanig, Lea & Febiger Publications, 1986.
2. Physical Characterization of Pharmaceutical Solids (Drugs and the Pharmaceutical Sciences: a Series of Textbooks and Monographs), First Edition, Edited by Harry G. Brittain, Marcel Dekker Inc., 1995.
3. New Drug Development: Regulatory Paradigms for Clinical Pharmacology and Biopharmaceutics (Drugs and the Pharmaceutical Sciences: a Series of Textbooks and Monographs), First Edition, Edited by Chandrahas G. Sahajwalla, Marcel Dekker Inc., 2004.

4. The Practice of Medicinal Chemistry, Second Edition, Edited by Camille Georges Wermuth, Elsevier Publications, 2003.
5. Foye`s Principles of Medicinal Chemistry, Fifth Edition, David A. Williams and Thomas L. Lemke, Lippincott Williams & Wilkins, 2002.
6. Physical Pharmacy: Physical Chemical Principles in the Pharmaceutical Sciences, Third Edition, Alfred Martin, James Swarbrick and Arthur Cammarata, Lea & Febiger Publications, 1983.
7. Pharmaceutical Dosage Forms and Drug Delivery Systems, Seventh Edition, Howard C. Ansel, Loyd V. Allen, Jr., and Nicholas G. Popovich, Lippincott Williams & Wilkins, 1999.

CHAPTER 4

COMPLEMENTARY TECHNIQUES FOR SOLID STATE DRUG ANALYSIS

- **Introduction**
- **Techniques**
  - Physical Property Evaluations and Thermal Methods
    - Purity and Melting Point
    - Water Content
    - Differential Thermal Analysis
    - Differential scanning calorimetry
    - Thermogravimetric Analysis
  - Microscopy
  - Molecular Modeling
  - Infra-Red Spectroscopy
  - X-ray Diffraction
  - Solid-state Nuclear Magnetic
    - Resonance Spectrophotometry (NMR)
- **Conclusions**

Introduction

Many drugs are administered as solids. The characterization of these solid drugs is critical for formulation development and quality assurance. To begin with, an NCE could exist in different polymorphic forms with variable therapeutic and physico-chemical properties. In addition, any changes in NCE during processing or storage would lead to changes in its therapeutic and physico-chemical properties. Thus, characterization of these molecules is necessary for the development of ideal formulations. Techniques currently used to characterize the solid state of a drug substance include microscopy, IR, X-ray diffraction, NMR, DSC, TGA, molecular modeling etc. This chapter discusses the fundamentals of these instruments with specific examples of characterization of drugs.

Techniques

Characterization techniques could include physical property evaluation and thermal methods, microscopy, molecular modeling, infrared spectroscopy, x-ray diffraction and nuclear magnetic resonance spectroscopy.

Physical Property Evaluations and Thermal Methods

The polymorphic and solvate state determinations of new chemical entities are the first investigations with regard to their solid-state assessments. These behaviours could be very simply predicted with very simple determinations like melting point, water content determination, density, stability and solubility etc. These were the changes in the physical properties that were noticed in the initial ages of drug discovery. These properties were very commonly used in organic chemistry and thus were adopted into pharmaceutical chemistry. However, with the increase in the sophistication of the techniques available and the generation of several new chemical entities, modern techniques were developed and applied. This not only resulted in the increase in the productivity in solid-state characterization, but also resulted in increased output. With the very simple tools like melting point determinations, the conclusions may be sometimes very laborious and may result in several repetitions of the experiments. However, when it comes to thermal methods of characterization, the simple physical property evaluations along with several modified and complicated technical methodologies are routinely investigated. Technological advances in these simple thermal property measurements in different forms of instrumentation are currently in the market and are very routinely applied. However, complicated and modern these technological advances are, some times very simple physical property determinations, at least for some new chemical entities are worth investigating in a very thorough manner. The other aspect to be considered is the instrumentation used in the thermal analysis of a drug substance. In one way or other most solids are “thermally active” and can therefore be profitably studied by calorimetry. The heat evolved or absorbed in different processes is then measured and can be related to both physical and chemical properties of compounds. Thermal analysis instruments are calorimeters for which the temperature is changed during the analysis. Three different kinds of instruments are available in this regard. These include thermal analysis instruments (DTA), differential scanning calorimetry (DSC) and thermogravimetric analysis (TGA).

Purity and Melting Point

The core aspect of these methods of solid-state characterization of drug substances is to determine their purity. Purity is important because it affects several physico-chemical, biochemical and pharmacological properties of drug substances. Thus, these studies are the first priority in solid-state characterization of drugs. The concept of pure substances is very complicated despite its fundamental role in chemistry. While spectroscopic detection of known instances is routine work, pure substances do not reveal any simple physical or chemical characteristics to distinguish them from ‘impures’. Nor do we have any theoretical account about the content of impurity in a pure substance. Instead it is only what we call ‘purification processing’, that allows us both to make pure substances and to give a general definition in operational terms.

The basic means of purification are, at least by the final step; various thermal processes all including one or the other phase transition, such as distillation, crystallization, sublimation, etc. Although there are several separation methods to determine the purity of a drug substance, the classical thermal methods have still methodological priority. Chromatography is the routine test in chemistry laboratories which some time do not work as a general and independent pureness test. Chromatographic fractions of an unknown sample cannot claim the purity because in the initial stages it is not known whether the initially chosen pairs of effective chromatographic phases are appropriate to the mixture separated. That is to say, that chromatography works in practice only if there is some background information about what is going to be separated. Thus it does not provide a general criterion of pureness.

A material is usually regarded as a pure substance, if the temperature or any other material property remains constant in the course of further phase transition. But such a sophisticated property does not work as blind operational criterion, since it turns out that, for instance, azeotropic and enantiomer mixtures, though showing constant transition temperatures, can nonetheless be separated further under modified conditions. Mixtures like those are handled either by modifying thermodynamic conditions or by performing other appropriate separation steps before. But finally, at least whenever we want to be sure and do not have enough background information, the sample has to pass the thermal purification test. These very basic physical tests with regard to the ordinary substance that are obtained after various synthetic steps will be discussed in this context.

The first property that is usually determined is the melting point. This may indicate very preliminarily the physical state of a chemical substance. The simple use could be exemplified by an example melting point of three different crystalline forms of nefidipine. As determined, the melting point of solvate, amorphous A, amorphous B and dihydrate forms of nefidipine are 169, 168, 170 and 165°C, respectively. E2101, a novel antispastic drug, was found to exist in at least two polymorphs, form I and form II, with a single endothermic peak that resulted from the melting at 148.1 ± 0.2 and 139.8 ± 0.4°C, respectively. These results clearly indicate variations in the melting points of different crystalline forms of a drug substance. The two crystals of torasemide I and II, as captured, have melting point ranges from 158-161°C and 155-158°C, respectively. The range may be due to the instrumentation variabilities or judgement problems or due to presence of any impurities.

Most pure solids typically melt at a sharply defined, single temperature value. That is, a pure substance will melt at a single temperature and not over a range of temperature values. Even a small amount of impurity can cause the melting point of a substance to spread out over a range of several degrees. Under these circumstances an impure substance will start the melting process at a temperature that is considerably lower than the melting point of the pure substance and may stop melting at a temperature that is higher than for the pure substance. The greater the amount of contamination in a substance, the wider the range over which it will melt. For this reason the determination of melting point is used by chemists in assessing purity. The melting point of a substance can be used to aid in identifying it. Each pure substance has its own unique melting point. The scientific literature is filled with information about the melting points of different materials. It is very unlikely that two different substances will melt at the exact same temperature. By determining the melting point of a substance and then verifying in literature would give an indication of the purity of a compound.

For an unknown compound the melting point determination has to be accurate. Keeping in view that a very small amount of impurity could result in a range of melting point, as such in the stages of new chemical entities, the accurate determination of melting point with accurate precision is the point. Thus, very proper instrumentation has to be bought by a pharmaceutical company.

Several instruments are available in the market for the purpose of determination of melting points. A very recent instrument in the market will be described. OptiMelt provides a fast and accurate means of automatically determining the melting points and melting ranges of chemical substances. With microprocessor-controlled temperature ramping, a built-in digital camera, and a selling price that is half that of competing models, OptiMelt offers the best value of any commercially available melting point apparatus. OptiMelt is specifically designed for unattended operation. It has a built-in digital camera that continuously captures real-time images of the samples, and it uses digital image processing to determine results. The melting points and melting ranges are prominently displayed on the front panel and automatically recorded into memory for later review. OptiMelt has an intuitive front panel and is very easy to use. Simply select a start temperature, ramp rate, stop temperature, and hit start. Results can be easily seen from across the lab on the large LCD display. Samples can be viewed on the front panel through a removable magnification lens. Up to six individual temperatures can be tagged for each sample. Interactive help is available for all functions and parameters of the instrument. Text and numerical entry keypads are built into the touchscreen interface so that no external keyboard is required. The small, aluminum oven design, along with microprocessor-controlled temperature ramping, provides fast and repeatable warm-up and cool-down cycling. Programmable ramp rates from 0.1°C/min to 20°C/min, in 0.1°C/min increments, provide measurement flexibility. The ability to rapidly preheat the oven to a start temperature slightly below an expected melting point minimizes analysis time. OptiMelt uses a platinum RTD sensor and makes temperature measurements to 400 °C with 0.1°C resolution. It is easily calibrated in the field against certified reference standards and complies with modern Pharmacopeia protocols. The instrument remembers the date of the last calibration that is included in all reports. In addition, the calibration of the instrument is a very important feature for accurate determination of the melting point.

Before performing a **melting point determination** it is advisable to calibrate the thermometer being used. This will make sure that the thermometer is recording temperatures properly, or if it is not, then it will be possible to know how big a correction factor to use. To calibrate the thermometer it is suspended in a beaker of boiling water for several minutes. The thermometer's temperature is then compared with the actual known temperature of boiling water for that day. If the thermometer's value differs from the known boiling point of water, then the thermometer must be corrected to the proper temperature by adding or subtracting the number. Thus, accurate determination of melting points is possible.

Hygroscopicity or Water Content Determination

Drying of a drug substance is typically the last step in its production prior to formulation. In some instances, the drying step can become the critical step in production from either a quality or time cycle perspective. This is certainly true for drug substances exhibiting several hydrate forms. Maintaining an intermediate hydrate form of a drug substance can be challenging. Therefore, in-line monitoring of drying processes can assist in both the development and optimization of the drying process as well as the production of quality bulk drug substance. In this context and for several reasons mentioned previously estimation of moisture is a very crucial step.

The presence of moisture is important for the physical and chemical properties of pharmaceutical solids. Properties such as flow, compaction, disintegration, dissolution, hardness and chemical stability are all influenced by moisture. The amount of water present, where it is located and in what state it is associated with the solid are all important issues to address to be able to predict and control the behaviour of a solid powder during processing. Water sorption can be measured both by gravimetric methods and by volumetric methods. In addition, drug substances possess different hydration states that would result in different water contents, sometimes may result in increased hydrolysis of a drug substance perse.

Conventional methods for water determination in pharmaceutical drug products are based on weight loss on drying and Karl Fischer titration. Other methods such as gas chromatography are alternative choices that provide comparable results. However, each method has pros and cons in terms of accuracy, speed, ease of operation, and compatibility with certain analytes. For example, Karl Fischer titration is a routine assay in pharmaceutical laboratories, but generally it is labor intensive, time consuming, and often uses toxic reagents. Determining low moisture levels is often difficult requiring control of ambient moisture to achieve reproducible results. In addition, the physical properties of the sample, such as particle size, which affects the dissolution time of solids during Karl Fisher titration, could result in substantial variability in measurement. If large particles are present, it may need a longer time to dissolve entrapped water in the titrator. Above all, all of these techniques are off-line methods that cannot provide real-time water levels during the drying of a drug substance.

Differential Thermal Analysis

As a process of new drug development, the very important aspect is to ascertain whether or not a compound is produced in polymorphic or solvated forms. Solvates, also known as pseudo-polymorphs, are solid forms comprising solvent molecules within their crystalline structure, either in stoichiometric or nonstoichiometric proportions. A hydrate consists of water in a drug compound. Very often water is the determinant factor in the crystalline structure of a hydrate. Since it may increase the hydrolysis of a compound, heating is usually the process of removing the moisture. This may result in a different molecular arrangement. However, sometimes, water removal may not affect the crystalline nature of a drug substance. As mentioned before, polymorphs and pseudo-polymorphs of drug substance display different physical properties (density, melting point, hygroscopicity, stability, and solubility). Since the end result of any pharmaceutical process may lead to variabilities during each of these individual steps, every transition has to be measured very carefully. These transitions are generally accompanied by changes in relative humidity, temperature or pressure and since unwanted modifications cannot be controlled during very early stages of formulation production, critical measurements of these transitions are important. To define the appropriate controls and procedures, the following needs are to be investigated:

1. the extent of dehydration occuring;
2. if, or under which conditions, the anhydrous compound rehydrates; and
3. the conditions for a stable existence of the anhydrous compound.

Most often thermal methods are employed in these identifications. All the methods are accompanied by stress and thus the drug substance is lost during such measurements. One aspect of thermal methods is the techniques and other aspect is the experience. Both are amalgamated to obtain very better characterization of solid state of drug substance. In this regard, several techniques are currently used. Differential thermal analysis is one such technique.

Differential thermal analysis (DTA) measures the difference in temperature between a sample and an inert reference material as a function of temperature and thereby detects changes in heat content. This involves heating or cooling a test sample or a reference sample under identical conditions, while recording any temperature difference between the sample and the reference. This differential temperature is then plotted against time or against temperature. Changes in the sample that leads to the absorption or evolution of heat can be detected relative to the inert reference. Differential temperatures can also arise between two inert samples when their response to the applied heat–treatment is not identical. DTA can therefore be used to study thermal properties and phase changes which do not lead to a change in enthalpy. The baseline of the DTA curve should then exhibit discontinuities at the transition temperatures and the slope of the curve at any point will depend on the microstructural constitution at that temperature. This method is not normally useful for quantitative work, but instead is used to deduce temperatures associated with thermal events. It has been successfully used in the studies of polymorphism determination. The area under a DTA peak can be used to correlate enthalpy change and is not affected by the heat capacity of the sample.

Differential Scanning Calorimetry

The concept of different scanning calorimetry and differential thermal analysis are almost the same, theoretically. Both these techniques measure the heat loss or gain resulting from physical or chemical changes within a sample as a function of temperature. Examples of endothermic processes are fusion, boiling, sublimation, vaporization, desolvation, solid-solid transitions, and chemical degradation. Crystallization and degradation as determined at very high temperatures are usually exothermic processes. Quantitative measurements of these processes have many applications in preformulation studies including purity, polymorphism, solvation, degradation, and excipient compatibility. The sample is placed in a suitable pan and sits upon a constantan disc on a platform in the DSC cell with a chromel wafer immediately underneath. A chromel-alumel thermocouple under the constantan disc measures the sample temperature. An empty reference pan sits on a symmetric platform with its own underlying chromel wafer and chromel-alumel thermocouple. Heat flow is measured by comparing the difference in temperature across the sample and the reference chromel wafers. Temperature can range from -120°C to 725°C, though an inert atmosphere is required above 600°C. The temperature is measured with a repeatability of ±0.1°C. Pans of Al, Cu, and graphite are available and need to be chosen to avoid reactions with samples. A thermogram is produced which can provide T_g, T_m, ΔHm or ΔHc. During initial testing, a variety of atmospheres are tried until the observed thermal process becomes fully understood. For characterizing crystal forms, the heat of fusion, ΔHf, could be obtained from the area-under-the-DSC-curve for the melting endotherm. A sharp symmetric melting endotherm could be used in the identification of relative purity, whereas, broad, asymmetric curves suggest impurities or more than one thermal process. Heating rate affects the kinetics and hence the apparent temperature of solid-solid transitions.

Thermogravimetric Analysis

Thermogravimetric analysis measures changes in sample weight as a function of time (isothermal) or temperature. The principles of thermal kinetics are very much similar to DTA and DSC. Most often the instrument that measures and generates endotherms is used in the measurement of thermogravimetry. Most of the times the data is interpreted based on the results obtained from the two instruments, DSC and TGA. The chance of determination of the transition with the help of these two methods is most of the time more accurate than using only one instrument. Desolvation and decomposition processes are frequently monitored by TGA. The other important application is the determination of dehydration and rehydration processes. Dehydration is essentially a reversible phenomenon, which also produces a change in the crystalline structure (but not of grain morphology) when most water has been lost. Grain morphology could be conveniently determined using microscopy. The instrumentation is very much advanced at this time and this could be very conveniently used in the new drug development process. TGA and DSC analysis could also be used to quantitate the presence of a solvated species within a bulk drug sample. Both these methods are microtechniques and depend on thermal equilibriation within the sample. Significant variables in these methods include sample homogeneity, sample size, particle size, heating rate, sample atmosphere, and sample preparation. Degradation during the heating process may sometimes give erroneous results which could be conveniently identified simultaneously using concurrent HPLC.

Microscopy

Selection of a suitable solid form to be used in the final formulation is a compromise between a number of desirable and undesirable physical properties. Often drugs substances are marketed as crystalline forms. These are more stable and easier to handle. Microscopy has been useful to determine the physical states of drugs and other excipients for quite some time. However, sophisticated microscopes are ever appearing in the market. With the increase in this modernization, it is always advisable to use very appropriate microscope to reduce the costs associated with drug development at the stage of physical characterization. This selection of microscope for use may vary from the type of industry and the special focus. The pharmaceutical sector that is mainly involved in the synthesis and solid-state characterization of new chemical entities definitely needs a very sophisticated microscope. On the other hand, a company that produces generic products may be compromised with less sophisticated microscope, since already some data in this area has been generated and stored in the database. However, no company will rely on one single technique of microscopy. The other area is the solid-state characterization of controlled delivery systems. In this section, a brief overview with a case study of a recent drug candidate will be presented.

Generally in an optical microscope experiment, the crystals are viewed at magnifications ranging from 100 X to 400 X under either polarization or non-polarized light. The refractive indices are determined using oil immersion. Several vendors of optical microscopes include Rolyn optics company, CA; Unitron Inc.

NY; Chroma Inc. CA; Sun-Tec corp; Prior Scientific Inc. MA; and Olympus America Inc. NY. Etc. A case study for the enlightenment of a student and a researcher to better know about the solid state will be presented here.

A brief description of an experiment conducted by Cantera et al., (2002) with regard to the solid state characeterization of tenoxicam, an anti-inflammatory agent, indicates what investigations and results a solid-state pharmaceutical scientist expects using an optical microscope. Tenoxicam is a sparingly soluble molecule belonging to the class of non-steroidal anti-inflammatory agent intended for use against inflammatory disorders along with several other very potent anti-inflammatory agents. Prior to Canerra group's investigation it was found that this compound exists as five different physical forms (three polymorphic forms, one amorphous form and an acetonitrile solvate). This group identified a fourth new crystal form, two new solvates obtained using DMF and dioxane, and three different solvates obtained using acetone, isopropyl alcohol and ethyl acetate and investigated their solid-state. One technique that was used is the optical microscopy. An Olympus BH2S polarizing light microscope was used in their study. As per these investigations, UV light provided a very useful and convenient method for differentiating tenoxicam polymorphs and solvates. Tenoxicam polymorphs and solvates show different coloration under UV light; this property known as phototropism is commonly associated with the existence of intramolecular hydrogen bondings and charge transfer complexes. Under solar lighting, the tenoxicam polymorphs and solvates displayed yellow-orange coloration, with the exception of the greenish tinge showed by form-1 under cross polarization. Form-I had fluorescent hue, form-IV was lemon-yellow, and form-II was grayish-yellow. Polymorph-I was composed of small crystals of irregular shape with a tendency to agglomerate; their size is generally less than 25 μm. Polymorph-II was composed of very thin needles, less than 3μm in length, or as grains of undefined shape with a tendency to agglomerate, of a dark yellow color similar to polymorph-IV. Polymorphic form-III and IV demonstrated prismatic of bright orange color and polymorphic-IV composed of flat tubular crystals, with first order straight edges and a tendency to aggregate into hemispheric druses that yielded fan-like bundles of crystals when ground. The amorphous phase is composed of loose irregular grains less than 3μm. Acetonitrile solvate was composed of long transparent flat needles, bright yellow in color, and observable to the naked eye. Dioxane solvate is composed of very small granules (> 2μm) with first order, a tendency to aggregate, and a color comparable to that of form-I. NN-DMF solvate closely resembled dioxane solvate.

Molecular Modeling

The physical structure of a new chemical entity could be determined using *in silico* methods or simply molecular modeling techniques. Molecular modeling is used in pharmaceutical research for a variety of purposes ranging from investigations of the influence of crystal packing on molecular structures to the determination of thermodynamic and dynamic properties of crystals. Recently, this has been used in the polymorph prediction, morphology modification, crystal engineering, and more recently to the solution of crystal structures from powder patterns. These *in silico* methods have an advantage over the usual techniques. With the emergence of simple software packages such as "Cerius", these predictions have become easy and convenient. The good news with these modeling techniques compared to other methods is that the interaction energy and its variation with structure could be investigated at the atomic and molecular levels.

Drugs such as celecoxib and a 5-α reductase inhibitor along with several similar examples were investigated using molecular modeling techniques and the physical structures concluded and reported, recently. Zhu and Sachetti (2004) investigated the solid state of a 5-α reductase inhibitor using several techniques including microscopy and molecular modeling. This molecule is useful for the treatment of androgenetic alopecia. A polymorph screening was conducted using suspension equilibration and solution recrystallization methods. Single crystals of this compound were obtained using pyridine/water. Crystals of suitable size were mounted on a glass fiber. The crystal measurements were made on a diffractometer with Cu Kα radiation and a graphite monochromator. The structures are solved by other direct methods. Hydrogen bonds, three-dimensional coordinates, and cell parameters were identified. The lattice energies of these bonds were calculated using software techniques. Several vendors of software are available in the market. In this study, "Cerius" software, release 1.6, program version 2.2 (Molecular Simulation, CA) running on commercial workstations: Silicon Graphics, Personal Iris 4D/20, Power series 2 X R 3000, and Indigo R 4000 was used. Minimization and maximization techniques using this software are used in the determination of crystal structure of the molecule. The crystal structure was determined using a Bruker Smart diffractometer. Single structure crystals were imported into Cerius 2 (Accelyrs Inc., Sandiago, CA), v. 4.2 and Accelyrs Inc. Sandiago, CA was used to provide visualization of the crystal structure and calculation of the simulated XRPD patterns. Simulated vaccum based crystal morphology (habit) was calculated using various equations to determine the crystal structure. The same principles were recently used in the identification and verification of crystal structures of chiral drugs. These included comparison of ephedrine derivatives with other chiral drugs. These techniques thus help in identification of the best suitable crystal for a particular use.

Near-Infrared Spectroscopy

Near-infrared (IR) spectroscopy is a rapid, very sensitive and nondestructive analytical method for the determination of hydration states and polymorphic compositions of bulk powder drug and excipient substances as well as hydration states of drugs in finished solid dosage forms. This is a technique that could be used without sample preparation requirements. In this technique, significant local spectral changes in the near-IR region as observed with the exposure of a bulk powder or a solid dosage form are used in the determination of hydration and polymorphic states. The effects of bound (hydrogen-bonded) and unbound (physically absorbed) water in a bulk powder are used in the identification of the hydration states of drugs. Corresponding local structural changes are used in the identification of polymorphic forms such as solvates etc. In this context, the importance of this technique will be illustrated with the investigation of hydrate forms of a drug. Several such examples are found in current literature with regard to the identification of polymorphic forms.

In one example presented by Higgins et al., (2003), the effect of humidity and temperature on the hydration state and absorption of moisture of an example drug was determined using bulk drug exposed to a wide range of humidity conditions (1-96% RH, at 25 and 40°C) in a glove box. The near-IR spectra were acquired simultaneously *in situ*. More details of infra-red spectroscopy would be essential to better appreciate this technique. Spectra were obtained at 40°C. Large spectral changes were seen in the –OH combination vibrational band near 1950 nm as a function of increasing humidity to which the sample is exposed. A detrend-corrected absorbance maximum of the water combination band in the region of 1930-1950 nm was plotted as a function of RH. The data from the near-IR spectra form four unique absorption intensity levels as a function of humidity. Comparison of the humidity conditions under which the individual spectra are obtained reveals that each unique grouping corresponds to the anhydrate, hemihydrate, tetrahydrate, and pentahydrate forms of the bulk drug. The assignment of individual spectra to specific hydration forms is based on moisture uptake studies combined with X-ray powder diffraction data.

Second-derivative spectra of infrared spectrum indicate the strength of the hydrogen bonding. In this study, three prominent peaks corresponding to H_2O molecules with zero (1420-1426nm), one (1444-1462nm), and two hydrogen bonds (1476nm) were observed in the second derivative spectra. The shift of the absorption maximum was scaled to the peak position of the anhydrate obtained by using X-ray powder diffraction data and moisture uptake studies as mentioned before. Significant red shifts were observed as the sample transformed from anhydrate ⟶ hemihydrate ⟶ dihydrate ⟶ tetrahydrate form. This suggests an increase in hydrogen bonding consistent with additional water molecules incorporating into the crystal lattice. The near-IR spectra reveal that the water in the hemihydrate, dihydrate, and tetrahydrate forms is bound and associated to the drug molecules and to each other. The additional water added upon conversion to the pentahydrate resides in an environment within the drug crystal that is not in direct association with the four other water molecules already present in the tetrahydrate state. In addition to the quantitative data on hydration state obtained from the near-IR spectra, the peak positions in the spectra provide detailed information on the microscopic environment of the absorbed water molecules probed by the near-IR radiation. The details are beyond the scope of this textbook and interested readers could refer other books.

X-ray Diffraction

According to Lachman (1991), an important technique for establishing the batch-to-batch reproducibility of a crystalline form is x-ray powder diffraction. As dispersing visible light using a ruled grating produces “vibgyor”, crystals to produce “x-ray diffraction pattern” diffract x-rays. The reason for this phenomenon is that the x-rays have wavelengths of about the same magnitude as the distance between the atoms or molecules of crystals. The random orientation of a crystal lattice in a powder sample causes the x-rays to scatter in a reproducible pattern of peak intensities at distinct angles relative to the incident beam. Each diffraction pattern is characteristic of a specific crystalline lattice for a given compound. This pattern is photographed on a sensitive plate arranged behind the crystal to be used for further investigations. An amorphous form does not produce a pattern.

A mixture of crystalline forms of a drug could be investigated by determining various plane diffraction patterns. A reflectance pattern from the atomic planes of the crystal is used to determine the distance of various planes of the crystal lattice. This aids in the determination of the distance of various planes of the crystal lattice. In this way, mixture of crystalline forms can be analyzed. However, single-crystal x-ray analysis helps in precise identification and description of a crystalline substance. Unit cell dimensions and angles conclusively establish the crystal lattice system. This will provide specific differences between crystalline forms of a given compound. One important classic older example in which x-ray diffraction was useful was in the total synthesis of penicillin. Penicillin is an antibiotic obtained by fermentation. It was available to a chemist long before its chemical structure was determined. X-ray diffraction technique was used to identify its chemical structure. In this study, the electron density map of crystalline potassium benzylpenicillin was determined using x-ray diffraction. The electron density and, accordingly, the position of the atoms in complex structures, such as penicillin were determined from a mathematical study of the data obtained from x-ray diffraction.

A recent example (Foppoli et al., 2003) that illustrates the use of x-ray diffraction is the identification of the polymorphic forms of NCX-4016, an NO releasing derivative of acetylsalicylic acid. Recently, a new family of nonsteroidal anti-inflammatory drugs was developed by addition of a nitric oxide (NO)-releasing moiety to conventional nonsteroidal anti-inflammatory drug molecules. These molecules were synthesized as a method to exploit the role of NO on the maintenance of the intensity of gastro-intestinal damage. NCX-4016 belongs to this class of drugs. At the time of publication, there was no information on the solid-state characterization of this new chemical entity. Extensive investigations suggested that this is a very promising molecule in terms of pharmacological properties as well as formulation properties. Since there was no solid-state data, obtaining this information was a priority. Identification of a polymorphic form is a critical step in the process of drug development of a new chemical entity before a study proceeds to the phase of clinical trials. The hypothetical termination of the molecule could occur in the earlier stages before the clinical trials are culminated if the solid-state is not properly characterized. The first step in such investigations is the procurement of various crystals of the drug substance isolated using various solvents. These crystals are further subjected to structural determinations using x-ray diffractions.

In this study, crystals of NCX- 4016 were obtained using a variety of solvents. Crystals of higher melting point obtained as thin colorless plates isolated using isopropyl alcohol were used for x-ray diffraction studies. Two different crystals form I and form II were obtained. Repeated recrystallization trials were performed to obtain single crystals of each polymorphic form of suitable amount for structure determination. Because of very low amounts of crystal form II, the x-ray diffraction of this form was not investigated. Crystals of form I were generally very thin (< 0.05mm) plates, but a specimen with sufficient volume was isolated and the X-ray structure was successfully determined. A single crystal was mounted on a Nonnius Kappa CCD diffractometer and irradiated with MoK X-rays. Data was collected using COLLECT 2000 program. Program DENZO-SMN was used for cell refinement and data reduction. The crystal structure was solved by direct methods using program SHELXS 86 and refined by full-matrix least-squares with program SHELXL 97. The structure indicated that this crystal is orthorhombic with lack of hydrogen bonding or other predominant intermolecular interactions and the molecule possessed eight torsional degrees of freedom suggested that the compound is an obvious candidate for conformational polymorphism. Crystal cohesion was affected basically by Vander Waals interaction. As mentioned before, only one technique fully cannot categorize the solid-state of a new chemical entity. In addition, judicious selection of the vendors of the instruments is also a key issue. However, X-ray diffraction is one of the key techniques in determining the crystal structure of an API.

Nuclear Magnetic Resonance Spectroscopy

A nuclear magnetic resonance (NMR) spectrogram is generated from the interaction of electromagnetic radiation from the radio-wave region of the spectrum with the spin of nuclei in a magnetic field. It is a well-known concept that the nuclei consist of electrons and protons. These nuclei have charge attributed to their protons and in addition, possess a spin about their nuclear axis. Spinning charges generate magnetic field and thus have magnetic moments. Some nuclei like carbon and oxygen emit the magnetic moments as NMR signals. The electrons nearby to this nucleus produce shielding to the NMR signals. When such atoms are exposed to large external magnetic field, the shielding is multiplied. When a reference material is also exposed to the material of interest, the differences in the shielding result in a chemical shift. This chemical shift of a nucleus provides information about its local magnetic environment and therefore can "type" a nuclear species. This typing results in an NMR spectrum.

NMR is a versatile tool in pharmaceutical research. Spectra could provide powerful evidence for a particular molecular conformation of a drug, including the distinction between closely related isomeric structures. These identifications are normally based on the relative position of chemical shifts as well as peak multiplicity and other parameters associated with spin coupling. These interpretations and examinations in the subtle changes and deletions in the spectra are used in pharmaceutical research for various purposes. Crystallographic effects such as polymorphism, multimolecules per asymmetric unit cell, disorder, intra- and inter-molecular hydrogen bonding, tautomerism, and solvation were all investigated by solid-state NMR spectroscopy.

NMR provides a complimentary data and thus the solid state of a new chemical entity is entirely determined using several techniques including solid-state NMR spectroscopy, the basics of which are the same as liquid NMR. Hydroquinone was the first compound to be investigated by solid-state NMR. Several compounds were later investigated for their solid-state characteristics. These compounds include N-desmethylnefopam hydrochloride, patellin, erythromycin A hydrate, ursodeoxycholic acid, gramicidin and amiodarone hydrochloride. In particular many drugs and excipients undergo amorphous transformation or polymorphic transformations towards metastable state upon milling. The integral of NMR signal could be correlated to the number of 13C atoms involved and used in the determination of polymorphic content of a new chemical entity. In another example with a drug substance, the potential for polymorphism in anhydrous theophylline was examined by theoretical structure calculations using X-ray powder diffraction data and *ab initio* calculations of NMR shielding tensors. The hydrogen bonding in theophylline was determined by 13C and 15N NMR spectroscopy. The results from this study eliminated one of the two possible hydrogen-bonding configurations, and the remaining structure was similar to the crystal structure of anhydrous theophylline. This is one example and similar examples of drug substance characterization could be seen in literature.

Lefort et al., (2004) investigated the amount of amorphous content of trehalose in a mixture of crystalline-amorphous mixture of trehalose using a 13C solid-state NMR. During the milling process crystalline trehalose is transformed into a glassy state. The requirement is to obtain a complete amorphous state from crystalline state. Amorphous trehalose was prepared by mechanical milling. Samples with different amorphous fractions were prepared by physical mixing of purely amorphous and purely crystalline powders. NMR signals of these mixtures were determined. The ratio of the areas of NMR signal provided the extent of conversion of crystalline form to amorphous form. The NMR method is then used to determine the evolution of the amorphous fraction in a trehalose powder, during a milling procedure that ultimately leads to a fully amorphous state.

Conclusions

Several analytical methods to characterize the solid state of a drug substance are discussed in this chapter. Generally, 1mg of drug substance is used for microscopy studies, 1mg of drug substance is used for fusion methods (hot stage microscopy), 2-5mg of drug substance is used for differential scanning calorimetry (DSC/DTA), 2-20 mg of drug substance is used for infrared spectroscopy, 500mg of drug substance is used for X-ray powder diffraction, 2mg of drug substance is required for scanning electron microscopy, 10mg of drug substance is required for thermogravimetric analysis and mg to gm drug substance is required for dissolution/solubility analysis. Currently, most of the techniques are in very advanced stages of drug and formulation discovery and routinely used. Concurrently, several techniques and the data from these techniques with proper interpretation are required for FDA submissions as a part of solid-state characterization for NDA filing.

Questions for Practice and Exercise

1. Describe any one or two integrated methodologies that could be successfully used in a conclusive solid-state analysis of new drug substances.
2. Mention clearly and conclusively the requirements of the drug quantities for various methods of solid-state characterization of new drug substances currently in pharmaceutical practice. Specify the advantages and disadvantages associated with each technique mentioning the best stage of its utility in drug discovery process.

References

1. Cantera RG, Leza MG, Bachiller CM. Solid phases of tenoxicam. J Pharm Sci. 2002 Oct; 91(10):2240-51.
2. Zhu HJ, Sacchetti M. Solubilization and solid-state characterization of a poorly soluble 5-alpha reductase inhibitor. Drug Dev Ind Pharm. 2004 Jul; 30(6):573-80.
3. Higgins JP, Arrivo SM, Reed RA. Approach to the determination of hydrate form conversions of drug compounds and solid dosage forms by near-infrared spectroscopy, J Pharm Sci. 2003 Nov; 92(11):2303-16.
4. Foppoli A, Sangalli ME, Maroni A, Gazzaniga A, Caira MR, Giordano F. Polymorphism of NCX4016, an NO-releasing derivative of acetylsalicylic acid, J Pharm Sci. 2004 Mar;93(3):521-31.
5. Lefort R, De Gusseme A, Willart JF, Danede F, Descamps M., Solid state NMR and DSC methods for quantifying the amorphous content in solid dosage forms: an application to ball-milling of trehalose. Int J Pharm. 2004 Aug 6; 280 (1-2):209-19.

Bibliography

1. The Theory and Practice of Industrial Pharmacy, Third Edition, Edited by Leon Lachman, Herbert A. Lieberman, and Joseph L. Kanig, Lea & Febiger Publications, 1986.
2. Physical Characterization of Pharmaceutical Solids (Drugs and the Pharmaceutical Sciences: a Series of Textbooks and Monographs), First Edition, Edited by Harry G. Brittain, Marcel Dekker Inc., 1995.
3. New Drug Development: Regulatory Paradigms for Clinical Pharmacology and Biopharmaceutics (Drugs and the Pharmaceutical Sciences: a Series of Textbooks and Monographs), First Edition, Edited by Chandrahas G. Sahajwalla, Marcel Dekker Inc., 2004.

4. The Practice of Medicinal Chemistry, Second Edition, Edited by Camille Georges Wermuth, Elsevier Publications, 2003.
5. Foye`s Principles of Medicinal Chemistry, Fifth Edition, David A. Williams and Thomas L. Lemke, Lippincott Williams & Wilkins, 2002.
6. Physical Pharmacy: Physical Chemical Principles in the Pharmaceutical Sciences, Third Edition, Alfred Martin, James Swarbrick and Arthur Cammarata, Lea & Febiger Publications, 1983.
7. Pharmaceutical Dosage Forms and Drug Delivery Systems, Seventh Edition, Howard C. Ansel, Loyd V. Allen, Jr., and Nicholas G. Popovich, Lippincott Williams & Wilkins, 1999.

CHAPTER 5

GASTRO INTESTINAL TRACT MEMBRANE: DRUG TRANSPORT AND BIOPHARMACEUTICS

- **Introduction**
- **Intestinal Tract: Anatomy and Physiology**
- **Membrane Transport**
- **Common Pathways of Drugs Reaching Systemic Circulation from Gastro-Intestinal Tract**
    - Intestinal Absorption
    - Sublingual/Buccal Transport of Drugs
    - Lymphatic Transport of Drugs
    - Persorption
- **Intestinal Metabolism**
- **Factors Influencing Drug Absorption Across Gastro Intestinal Tract**
- **Drug Absorption through Various Regions of GastroIntestinal Tract**

- **Solutes**
    - Classification Based on Mechanism of Transport
    - Classification Based on Chemical Nature
    - BCS Classification
- **Delivery Systems that Influence Drug Absorption**
- **Conclusions**

Introduction

The food that is consumed by mouth travels all the way from mouth and reaches the intestinal tract. The first portion at which it gets absorbed is the stomach. Here the food is broken down if required prior to absorption into the systemic circulation. Then at subsequent portions of the intestinal tract it is absorbed differently depending on the areas and modes of absorption. During its transit, it is again digested if required in the rest of the intestinal tract into basic components such as amino acids, glucose, vitamins etc. The situation could be similarly extrapolated to the neutraceuticals and drugs administered by the oral route. Thus, not all drugs reach the systemic circulation from a particular location of the gastro-intestinal tract. Thus, the study of drug absorption across the gastro-intestinal tract should be complex and should be very carefully reviewed. In addition, most of the studies conducted use animal models, which may make things more complicated. Extrapolations are drawn from animal data to human absorption parameters. However, there is always an inter species difference. In addition, subject-to-subject variation even among human beings could lead to a wide range of differences in the absorption paterns of new drug substances. Thus, genetics also may play a major role. Conclusions should be carefully drawn. Keeping these in view this chapter very comprehensively discusses the transport across the gastrointestinal tract.

For convenience, gastro intestinal tract could be dissected into several localized units of the membrane with different physiological, pharmacological and biochemical environment. Some drugs reach the systemic circulation after passing through the membrane over the entire gastro intestinal tract while others reach from within a particular site. Thus, this aspect of drug absorption investigation and study into each of these segments would be essential in understanding the drug absorption through the gastrointestinal tract. A drug has to reach its target cell or tissue in appropriate concentrations to elicit desired therapeutic action. It has to overcome several barriers to reach the target tissue. Gastro intestinal membrane is the critical barrier a drug has to overcome to reach the systemic circulation after oral administration. The mechanism of transport may be either paracellular or transcellular. Paracellular pathway involves transport through the gaps within each cell. Transcellular pathway involves the transport of molecules through the membrane of the cells. Transcellular pathway could be again active pathway or passive pathway.

The general mechanism by which a molecule passes across the gastrointestinal tract is the passive diffusion. For a molecule that is transported by passive diffusion, the rate of diffusion across a homogenous membrane is governed by Fick's law, that states,

$$dA/dt = D_c P_c S \, dc/dx$$

where D_c is the diffusion coefficient of the drug through the membrane; P_c is the partition coefficient between the membrane and the donor medium containing the drug, S is the membrane surface area, dC is the concentration differential across the membrane, and dX is the membrane thickness. Fick's law of diffusion is a perfect fit for lipophilic molecules. However, hydrophilic or charged molecules are generally transported across the membrane by specialized transport mechanisms. These mechanisms are several fold and could be conveniently clubbed into active transport mechanisms and thus involve transport proteins, termed carrier proteins. The most notable features of carrier-mediated transport are substrate specificity, saturability and regional variability. Substrate specificity is limited to only a few molecules. The existence of aminoacid transporters and glucose transporters on the intestinal membranes is very well known. This substrate specificity prevents several molecules from entering into the intestines. In addition, the bioavailability of some drug substances is limited to more of the similar types of molecules that are substrates to the carrier proteins. Examples include the transport of oligopeptides with the help of oligopeptide transporter; examples of drugs include beta-lactam antibiotics and ACE inhibitors; nucleoside and phosphate analogs are transported using nucleoside transporters. The other recent investigations in the intestinal membrane transport suggested active efflux of some molecules from systemic circulation into the gastrointestinal tract. The presence of these types of transporters is very crucial as related to the toxic substances. Most of the drug metabolites or xenobiotics re-enter into the gastrointestinal tract before being eliminated. It was hypothesized for over several years that transporters that facilitate the efflux of these types of molecules are present on the gastrointestinal tract and could dump the molecules back into the gastrointestinal tract. However, it was recently, for over a decade the proof for the existence of these kinds of transport proteins in the gastrointestinal tract was obtained. These are called efflux transporters. In addition, the presence of efflux transporters on the apical side of the membrane is found to reduce the bioavailability of a molecule that is a substrate for an efflux transporter. Molecules like vincristine and indomethacin are substrates for efflux transporters like p-glycoprotein and multi-drug resistance associated proteins that may limit the bioavailability of the substrates of these transporters.

Solubility of a drug in the intestinal fluids is the first important factor for a drug to reach the systemic circulation and elicit its action. Deviations include the drugs very highly soluble in the biological membranes or drugs that are encapsulated in particulates so as to translocate across the membranes to reach the systemic circulation. From a dosage form a drug has to dissolve to get absorbed. This is a different situation with very poorly soluble drugs. As the solubilities of these molecules are poor in the intestines special techniques are to be used to dissolve these compounds. In these situations, development of nanoparticulate systems, liposomes or microparticulates would be helpful. These particulates upon entering into the intestinal tract slowly release drugs which are absorbed into the membranes to be transported to reach the systemic circulation. The other path is that the particulates are endocytosized or phagocytosized across the membranes and then reach the systemic circulation. Surface area of drug particles is another parameter that influences drug dissociation, and in turn, drug absorption. Particle size is a determinant of surface area. Smaller particles with greater surface area dissolve more rapidly than larger particles, even though both have the same intrinsic solubility. As increasing number of newly developed drugs are sparingly soluble in water and are often also insoluble in organic solvents, the formulation of these drugs is a major obstacle to their clinical application. Because of their extremely low solubility, these drugs usually also possess poor bioavailability. One way of overcoming this problem is to increase the surface area of drug particles with the development of nanosuspensions. Nanosuspensions consist of the drugs that are broken into crystals in the nanometer range by high-pressure homogenization and then stabilized by surfactants. As a result of the reduction in the size and the increase in the dissolution velocity, bioavailability is generally increased. Apart from these issues there are several factors that are to be considered during a presentation of a drug absorption process. A thorough understanding of these factors, the mechanisms of transport and the anatomy and the physiology of the gastrointestinal tract as related to new drugs and the delivery systems is very essential; rather than blindly develop bioavailability models for new drug substances. Keeping in view the enormous amount a pharmaceutical company invests on one promising drug substance; definitely it is worth understanding all these factors before further processing a new drug substance.

Intestinal Tract: Anatomy and Physiology

Five different regions of the gastrointestinal tract are composed of the absorption sites for drugs. Although very parallel in terms of anatomy and physiology, they have a variety of repercussional and interrelated functions. Repercussion means the motion. Each of these is always in motion like a pendulum. The motion is both lateral and longitudinal. Lateral motion helps in the chewing and longitudinal motion helps in the further movement and finally the deification.

The mouth is the first place and also plays a key role in the digestive system, but it does much more than get digestion started. Generally mouth and nose are described together. A schematic diagram of mouth is shown in the Figure 1 for convenience. The oral and nasal cavities lie near the body midline, inferior and medial to the orbital cavities, anterior to the pharynx and medial to the infratemporal fossa. They are separated from one another by the palate. Each cavity has an entrance and an exit. The oral cavity opens at the mouth and is bounded at its sides by teeth and cheeks. It is bounded posteriorly by two pairs of folds of mucous membrane. It is lined with mucuous membrane that may be sometimes responsible for drug absorption. The mucosal membranes lead drugs to the systemic circulation very quickly and some time this is utilized in the need of very quick action. This pathway is utilized for the need of rapid action of drugs. For instance, oral sprays have a non-toxic aerosol (spray) pump which delivers the purest form of vitamins, minerals, herbs and other nutritional supplements directly into the bloodstream. When sprayed into the mouth, micro-sized beads or droplets are immediately absorbed into the tissue through the capillaries, which lie close to the surface of the lining in the mouth. This process allows the nutrients to be absorbed within seconds without causing any extra stress to the organs. The hardest substances in the body, the teeth are also necessary for chewing (or mastication) - the process by which we tear, cut, and grind food in preparation for swallowing. Chewing allows enzymes and lubricants released in the mouth to further digest, or break down, food.

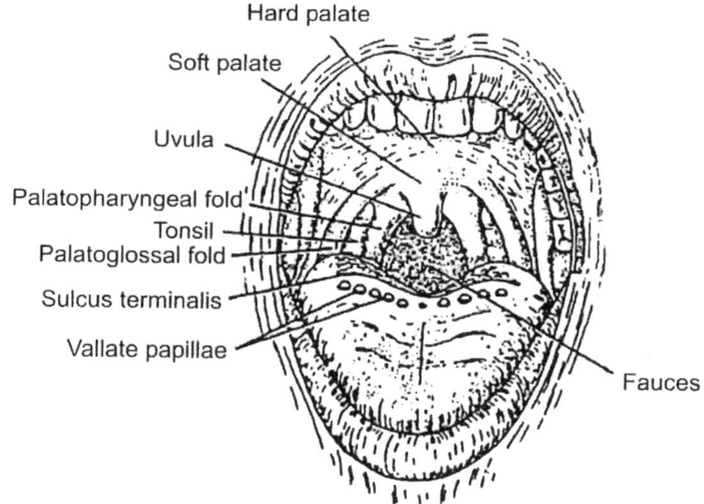

Figure 5.1 A scheme of the oral cavity that includes various parts that encompass the boundaries and the cavity for the intake of food, water, medicines, etc. (Courtesy: Internet site: anatomy of the mouth, USA atlas).

Seldom does the dosage form remain in this cavity long enough for drug absorption to take place, unless the drug is administered buccally or sublingually. The absorption mechanism under the tongue is different than that in the GI tract. Materials absorb directly into the circulatory system under the tongue; they do not pass to the liver and then out into systemic circulation. The mucosal membranes of the oral cavity can be divided into five regions: the floor of the mouth (sublingual), the buccal mucosa (cheeks), the gums (gingiva), the palatal mucosa, and the lining of the lips. These oral mucosal regions are different from each other in terms of anatomy, permeability to drug, and their ability to retain a system for a desired length of time. Although the buccal mucosa is less permeable than the sublingual mucosa, it does not yield a rapid onset of action as seen with sublingual delivery. Mucosa of the buccal area has an expanse of smooth and relatively immobile surface, which is suitable for placement of a retentive system. These characteristics make the buccal mucosa a more appropriate site for prolonged systemic delivery of drugs. It has been shown that buccal route offers excellent opportunities for systemic delivery of drugs. In general, drug delivery through this route has the advantages of preventing the drug from degradation in the gastrointestinal tract, avoiding first-pass effect, and bypassing gastrointestinal absorption.

The next portion a drug enters is the stomach. Human stomachs are vessels with .5-1 liter capacity. The contents of the stomach include hydrochloric acid, pepsinogen, and mucus. The pH of the stomach in a normal, healthy human is in the 1-3 range. There are many purposes for the high acidity found in the stomach including the destruction of bacteria that are ingested. Few bacteria can survive in an environment with a pH of 1 to 3. Some do, though, because of an impenetrable outer coat that can resist acid breakdown. Another purpose for such a low pH is that high acidity is required to activate pepsinogen. Pepsinogen is the enzyme that initiates the digestion and breakdown of proteins that are ingested. The other major component of gastric fluid is mucus. Mucus provides protection to the stomach lining from the high acid content. Gastric pH varies from time to time. Gastric acid is secreted in anticipation of a meal, to prepare for digestion. Gastric pH decreases as a result of acid secretion, and, after a heavy meal, blood pH correspondingly increases, particularly in those segments of the circulatory system associated with supplying the gastrointestinal tract. This increase in blood pH is known as the "alkaline tide", and is caused by bicarbonate ions that are secreted into extracellular fluid of the stomach, then into venous blood. Sometimes external agents can also contribute to this. Very few drugs enter the systemic circulation from stomach.

Further down the alimentary canal is the small intestine, the first part of which is the duodenum. The pH of the duodenum is 6 to 6.5. The majority of nutrients, vitamins, and drugs are absorbed in this 6 inch area of the gastrointestinal tract. In addition to water, mucus, and electrolytes, secretions from the liver and pancreas join secretions from the intestinal mucosa to facilitate digestion and absorption. Intestines are the best paths for drugs to follow. These are the middle paths of a gastrointestinal tract. A drug may not change its original form during its stay at this middle portion because this part of the intestinal tract is free from the relative metabolisms.

Bile tree is the first area that needs to be described at this juncture as it was the first area that interested the early scientists. In addition, here comes the relevance of metabolism of drugs as the bile and the associated organ liver are important as metabolism is discussed. The anatomy of the biliary tree is a little complicated, but it is important to understand. The liver's cells (hepatocytes) excrete bile into canaliculi, which are intercellular spaces between the liver cells. These drain into the right and left hepatic ducts, after which bile travels via the common hepatic and cystic ducts to the gallbladder. The gall bladder, which has a capacity of 50 milliliters (about 5 tablespoons), concentrates the bile 10-fold by removing water and stores it until a person eats. At this time, bile is discharged from the gallbladder via the cystic duct into the common bile duct and then into the duodenum (the first part of the small intestine), where it begins to dissolve the fat in ingested food. The liver secrets approximately 500 to 1000 milliliters (50 to 100 tablespoons) of bile each day. Most (95%) of the bile that has entered the intestines is resorbed in the last part of the small intestine (known as the terminal ileum), and returned to the liver for reuse. Cholesterol and other associated chemicals follow this pathway of transport into the intestinal tract. Each portion of the human gastrointestinal tract typically has a different pH. In the major absorptive part of small intestine duodenum, pH 6.0 - 6.5 favoring absorption of weak base drugs. The lining of the small intestines is composed of many villi, or finger like projections, which extend even more as projections called the brush border. The area is highly perfused with blood. These factors contribute to a very high surface area, increasing the likelihood of drug absorption taking place, if the ionization criterion is met. The pH can reach 7 to 8 in this area.

Further along the small intestine, beyond the duodenum, lies the jejunum and ileum. These sections of the small intestine lack the high surface area of the duodenum and only small amounts of absorption across the lipid membranes occur in this section of the small intestine. As we get further away from the stomach, the pH rises to about 7.5 in this region. And the final organ of the digestive tract is the large intestine, which includes the colon and rectum. The large intestine is the site for water resorption and the production of feces. Seldom does drug absorption take place in this region. The pH of the large intestine is 5.5-7, and like the buccal area, blood that drains the rectum is not first transported to the liver. So, absorption that takes place in the rectum (from rectal suppositories and enemas) goes into the systemic circulation without biotransformation that takes place due to liver enzymes.

Membrane Transport

As drug transport is related, the first thing that should comes into the mind is the pathways by which drugs move within or in/out a cell. Nutrients and other substances should reach inside a cell from within outside. Not all the nutrients are of similar nature. As mentioned in the introduction there is a special status for some chemicals and inferior status for other chemicals. This has to be always kept in the mind. Otherwise the comprehension of common cellular pathways is not complete. In this regard, several cellular pathways that could be mentioned include diffusion, active transport, pinocytosis and phagocytosis. Most of the substances pass through the cell membrane by diffusion and active transport. Diffusion means the very simple random movement of molecules through the membrane pores with aqueous molecules and with lipid soluble molecules through the lipid matrix of the membrane. Active transport involves the very confidential means of carrying of a substance through the membrane by a physical protein structure that penetrates all the way through the membrane. Very special or macromolecules traverse using this type of mechanism of transport. One of the most important factors that determine how rapidly a substance diffuses through the lipid bilayer is the lipid solubility of the substance. For instance, the lipid solubilities of oxygen, nitrogen, carbon dioxide, and alcohols are high, so that all these can dissolve directly in the lipid bilayer and diffuse through the cell membrane in the same manner that diffusion of solutes occurs in a watery solution. The rate of diffusion of these substances through the membrane is directly proportional to their lipid solubility. On the other hand, facilitated diffusion requires the interaction of a carrier protein with the molecules or ions. The carrier protein aids passage of the molecules or ions through the membrane by binding chemically with them and shuttling them through the membrane in this form.

Very large particles travel across the membrane through the endocytic processes. Endocytic process could be either pinocytic or phagocytic. Pinocytosis occurs continually at the membranes of most cells but especially rapidly in some cells. This pathway involves the help of pinocytic vesicles. These are very small vesicles of the particle sizes between 100 to 200 nanometers in diameter. The particles suspended or the macromolecules solubilized in the solution form are slowly pinched into the small pinocytic vesicles. The cells then engulf these pinocytic vesicles. Depending on the requirement, the vesicle can release the drug within the cell or it can take the vesicle to the other side of the cell and dump the molecule or the particle onto the other side. It is found that several factors influence the pinocytic activity of a cell. Of which the two important factors are ATP and calcium ions. The other mode of cellular transport is phagocytosis. This is very much similar to pinocytosis but involves the transport of larger particles. Mostly tissue macrophages or some of the white blood cells are involved in phagocytic activity. This process is initiated when a particle such as a bacterium, a dead cell, or tissue debris binds with receptors on the surface of the phagocyte. In the case of bacteria, each bacterium usually is already attached to a specific antibody, and it is the antibody that attaches to the phagocyte receptors, dragging the bacterium along with it. Drug delivery systems such as nanoparticles and microparticles are likely to enter a cell using phagocytosis.

Common Transporters

Any cell has to maintain its balance in terms of the concentration of the ions inside and outside the cell. In this regard, the first balance is provided by the electrochemical gradient. This is according to the concentration gradient of the ions within and outside the cells. However, this is generally maintained by either passive diffusion or transport through the pores as mentioned before. Similar is the case with the drug substances. However, not all the times either the concentration or the electrochemical gradient facilitates the diffusion of molecules across a cell and definitely across a gastrointestinal tract. However, the balance of the ionic gradients has to be maintained. These situations are facilitated by active transport mechanisms that involve transporters. Several types of transporters exist on the membranes. Several transporters have been discovered for over some time specifically for a particular class of drugs. However, the focus of this discussion is not to talk about drug transporters. Here the focus is only the very common cellular transporters that help maintain the homeostasis (balance) of a cellular physiology. Some of the common transporters utilized either for the transport of nutrients or maintenance of ion gradients can also be utilized by drugs for their transport into the systemic circulation.

Active transport

Active transport is the pumping of molecules or ions through a membrane against their concentration gradient. It requires: a transmembrane protein (usually a complex of them) called a transporter and energy. The source of this energy is ATP. The energy of ATP may be used directly or indirectly.

Direct active transport: Some transporters bind ATP directly and use the energy of its hydrolysis to drive active transport.

Indirect active transport: Other transporters use the energy already stored in the gradient of a directly-pumped ion. Direct active transport of the ion establishes a concentration gradient. When this is relieved by facilitated diffusion, the energy released can be harnessed to the pumping of some other ion or molecule. Some of these transporters are henceforth discussed.

Direct active transport

This type of transport involves transporters, which utilizes energy to transport the molecules.

The Na^+/K^+ ATPase: The **cytosol** of animal cells contains a concentration of potassium ions (K^+) as much as 20 times higher than that in the extracellular fluid. Conversely, the extracellular fluid contains a concentration of sodium ions (Na^+) as much as 10 times greater than that within the cell. These concentration gradients are established by the active transport of both ions. And, in fact, the same transporter, called the Na^+/K^+ ATPase, does both jobs. It uses the energy from the hydrolysis of ATP to actively transport 3 Na^+ ions out of the cell, for each 2 K^+ ions pumped into the cell. This accomplishes several vital functions: It helps establish a net charge across the plasma membrane with the interior of the cell being negatively charged with respect to the exterior. This **resting potential** prepares nerve and muscle cells for the propagation of action potentials leading to nerve impulses and muscle contraction. The accumulation of sodium ions outside of the cell draws water out of the cell and thus enables it to maintain **osmotic balance** (otherwise it would swell and burst from the inward diffusion of water). The gradient of sodium ions is harnessed to provide the energy to run several types of **indirect pumps**. The crucial roles of the Na^+/K^+ ATPase are reflected in the fact that almost one-third of all the energy generated by the mitochondria in animal cells is used just to run this pump.

The H^+/K^+ ATPase: The parietal cells of the stomach use this pump to secrete gastric juice. These cells transport protons (H^+) from a concentration of about 4 x 10^{-8} M within the cell to a concentration of about 0.15 M in the gastric juice (giving it a pH close to 1). Small wonder is that parietal cells are stuffed with mitochondria and uses huge amounts of energy as they carry out this three-million fold concentration of protons.

The Ca^{2+} ATPases: In resting skeletal muscle, there is a much higher concentration of calcium ions (Ca^{2+}) in the sarcoplasmic reticulum than in the cytosol. Activation of the muscle fiber allows some of this Ca^{2+} to pass by facilitated diffusion into the cytosol where it triggers contraction. After contraction, this Ca^{2+} is pumped back into the sarcoplasmic reticulum. This is done by a Ca^{2+} ATPase that uses the energy from each molecule of ATP to pump 2 Ca^{2+} ions. A Ca^{2+} ATPase is also located in the plasma membrane of all eukaryotic cells. It pumps Ca^{2+} out of the cell helping to maintain the ~10,000-fold concentration gradient of Ca^{2+} between the cytosol (~ 10^{-7}M) and the ECF (~ 10^{-3}M). Pumps 1. - 3. are designated P-type ion transporters because they use the same basic mechanism: a conformational change in the proteins as they are reversibly phosphorylated by ATP. And all three pumps can be made to run backward. That is, if the pumped ions are allowed to diffuse back through the membrane complex, ATP can be synthesized from ADP and inorganic phosphate. Some of the smooth muscle relaxants in the intestines or cardiotonic agents could practically act at the level of these transporters.

ABC transporters: ABC ("ATP-Binding Cassette") transporters are transmembrane proteins that expose a ligand-binding domain at one surface and a ATP-binding domain at the other surface. The ligand-binding domain is usually restricted to a single type of molecule. The ATP bound to its domain provides the energy to pump the ligand across the membrane. The human genome contains 48 genes for ABC transporters. Some examples: CFTR — the cystic fibrosis transmembrane conductance regulator TAP, the transporter associated with antigen processing, the transporter that liver cells use to pump the salts of bile acids out into the bile, and ABC transporters that pump chemotherapeutic drugs out of cancer cells thus reducing their effectiveness. ABC transporters must have evolved early in the history of life. The ATP-binding domains in archaea, eubacteria, and eukaryotes all share a homologous structure, the ATP-binding "cassette".

Indirect active transport

Indirect active transport uses the downhill flow of an ion to pump some other molecule or ion against its gradient. The driving ion is usually sodium (Na^+) with its gradient established by the Na^+/K^+ ATPase.

Symport pumps: In this type of indirect active transport, the driving ion (Na^+) and the pumped molecule pass through the membrane pump in the same direction. Examples: The Na^+/glucose transporter. This transmembrane protein allows sodium ions and glucose to enter the cell together. The sodium ions flow down their concentration gradient while the glucose molecules are pumped up theirs. Later the sodium is pumped back out of the cell by the Na^+/K^+ ATPase. The Na^+/glucose transporter is used to actively transport glucose out of the intestine and also out of the kidney tubules and back into the blood. All the amino acids can be actively transported, for example out of the kidney tubules and into the blood eg. the reuptake of Glu from the synapse back into the presynaptic neuron by sodium-driven symport pumps.

The Na^+/iodide transporter: This symporter pumps iodide ions into the cells of the thyroid gland (for the manufacture of thyroxine) and also into the cells of the mammary gland (to supply the baby's need for iodide).

Antiport pumps: In antiport pumps, the driving ion (again, usually sodium) diffuses through the pump in one direction providing the energy for the active transport of some other molecule or ion in the opposite direction. Example: Ca^{2+} ions are pumped out of cells by a sodium-driven antiport pump An antiport pump in the vacuole of some plants harnesses the outward facilitated diffusion of protons (themselves pumped into the vacuole by a H^+ ATPase) to the active inward transport of sodium ions. This sodium/proton antiport pump enables the plant to sequester sodium ions in its vacuole.

Paracellular Transport

Paracellular transport refers to transport in between cells. It is now well recognized that paracellular transport is a major route for vectorial transport of solutes and water. This transport modality is currently being learnt more than previously as it has been proved that this pathway is involved in several severe disease conditions. The rate-limiting step in paracellular transport (the paracellular "barrier") is constituted by the tight junction, which is the most apical of the intercellular junctions. Tight junctions consist of large complexes of multiple different proteins. Tight junctions constitute the main barrier to paracellular diffusion. The diameters of the tight junction pores are approximately 4-8 Å and 10-15 Å in humans and animals, respectively. Because in humans the paracellular route will not allow the passage of molecules with diameters greater than ~8 Å, this route is unlikely to play an important role in the absorption of most compounds of pharmaceutical interest. In addition to the narrow diameter of the tight junctions, this pathway is of little importance for most drugs because of the small surface area of the tight junctions, which accounts for 0.01% of the total surface area i.e. cell membrane plus tight junctions. However, evidence has shown that the diameter of tight junctions can be increased by cellular regulatory processes, thus efforts to increase the paracellular permeability of poorly absorbed compounds through co-administration of agents that open up tight junctions has been affected. At present, the potential application of this approach is limited by safety concerns with a few possible exceptions. Apart from tight junctions there are other junctions in the human epithelium. Epithelia is a layer of cells joined together with the help of several junctions; most of the times these junctions talk to each other and thereby promotes and facilitates the transcellular movement of molecules through the cell layer apart from offering several other functional roles. The other main function of these proteins is its ability to act as a barrier between the outside and inside world that definitely depends on the integrity of these junctions. Any movement of molecules from within the pores of the cells is termed paracellular transport that definitely depends on the size of the pores.

Several proteins are involved in the formation of the joints to the cells controlling various aspects. The different types of junctions are gap junctions, desmosomes and tight junctions (Figure 5.2).

Gap junctions are hexagonal array of cylindrical tubules that connect adjacent cells and allow the passage of small molecules for cell-to-cell communication. Gap junctions are intercellular channels some 1.5–2 nm in diameter. These permit the free passage between the cells of ions and small molecules (up to a molecular weight of about 1000 daltons). They are constructed from 4 (sometimes 6) copies of one of a family of transmembrane proteins called connexins. Because ions can flow through them, gap junctions permit changes in membrane potential to pass from cell to cell.

Desmosomes are of two types: spot desmosomes and belt desmosomes. Spot desmosomes (macula adherens) are the connections at punctuate locations. They offer great resistance as a barrier. These are very prominent in tissues like stratified squamous epithelia that are subject to great mechanical stress. On the other hand, belt desmosomes (intermediate junctions or zonula adherens) are bandlike areas exactly in the middle most of the times and these areas encompass the cells. Actin-containing filaments attach to these desmosomes and, by contracting in response to ATP, calcium and magnesium, give the cell membrane active movement and thus these bands like junctions are very important junctions that interconnect the cells. The third class of junctions is tight junctions, also called limiting junctions or zonula occludens, attaching each cell to its neighbor by encircling them completely. These are basically near the apices of the cells. These junctions seal off the space between the cells completely and thus act as a passive diffusion barrier. Along with the cell membranes, the tight junction allows the development of osmotic gradients between the lumen and the interstitial space of the organ. Tight junctions seal adjacent epithelial cells in a narrow band just beneath their apical surface. Tight junctions perform two vital functions: They prevent the passage of molecules and ions through the space between cells. So materials must actually enter the cells (by diffusion or active transport) in order to pass through the tissue. This pathway provides control over what substances are allowed through. They block the movement of integral membrane proteins between the apical and basolateral surfaces of the cell. Thus the special functions of each surface, for example receptor-mediated endocytosis at the apical surface exocytosis at the basolateral surface can be preserved. One of the important contributors of paracellular barrier, tight junctions alters the movement of water, solutes, and immune cells between both epithelial and endothelial cells. In addition, tight junctions have other more roles. Paracellular barriers vary among epithelia in electrical resistance and behave as if they are lined with pores that have charge and size selectivity. Most epithelial membranes have tight junctions (less than 1 nm in diameter; 1 nm=10A) between the cells, so that paracellular transport of drugs or ligands (particular those with molecular weights greater than about 200) through epithelial junctions is next to impossible. In these epithelial cell layers, the drugs have to pass through only transcellularly as mentioned before. This paracellular route is only for hydrophilic drugs and the absorption also depends on the width of the tight junctions at a given site of the gastrointestinal tract. The tight junction width in jejunum is 8-12 A, in ileum it is 4-5 A, in colon it is 2-2.5 A. The narrower tight junctions in colon suggest that the paracellular drug transport will be less significant, which helps to explain the lower ratio of colon: jejunal permeability of hydrophilic drugs in colon. As mentioned previously, the paracellular route of transport of drugs across gastrointestinal tract is very minute. Previously it was thought that the drugs atenolol (Mwt 266) and terbutaline (Mwt: 180) transport across gastrointestinal tract by paracellular passive transport. However, recently it was found that they are bigger for passive paracellular transport.

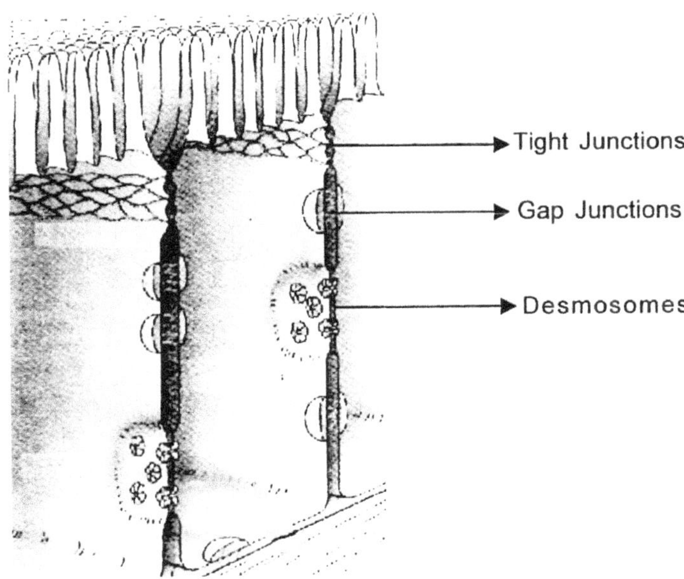

Figure 5.2 Junctions Between Cells.

Transcellular Transport

Transcellular transport of molecules is the movement of molecules through the cells and not within the gaps between the cells. Figure 5.3 demonstrates different pathways across cell membranes. Thus transcellular pathway involves either carrier mediated transport or passive diffusion or a combination of the two. Transcellular transport involves luminal and basolateral steps. This has to be always kept in the mind. In addition to passive and active transport, transcellular route also supports other miscellaneous transport mechanisms such as endocytosis, phagocytosis and transcytosis.

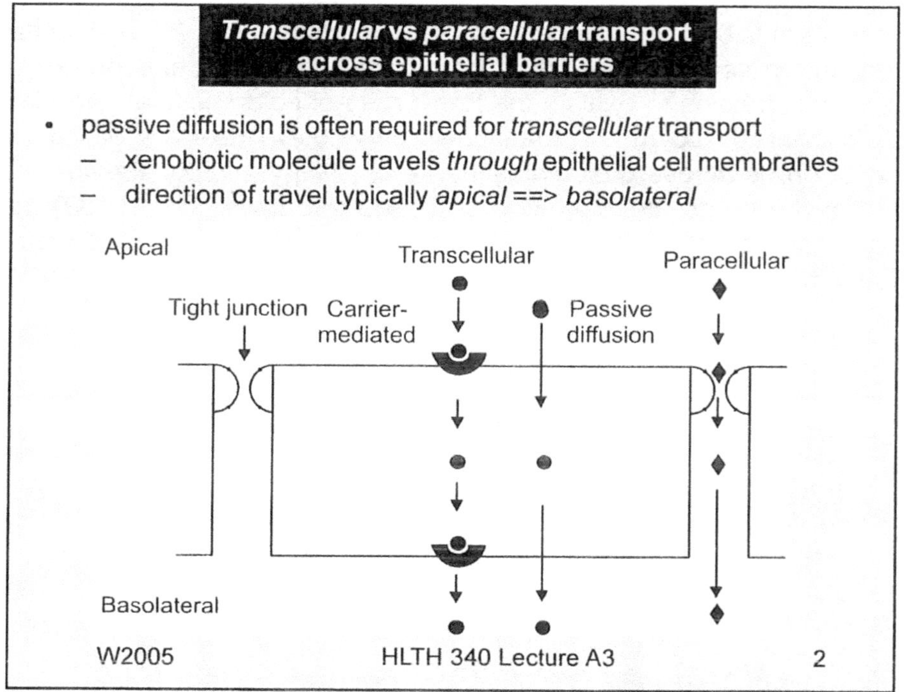

(Courtesy: Internet site: http://www.ahs.uwaterloo.ca/~hlth340/LectA3.ppt)

Figure 5.3 Transport modalities across epithelial barriers.

Passive Transport

A passive transport process does not involve energy. Passive transport of molecules can be observed with both transcellular and paracellular routes. However, for paracellular route this process can be very insignificant that passive transport can be conveniently discussed in the transcellular route. Transcellular transport generally has a higher permeation rate than paracellular transport due to the smaller surface area in paracellular pathway (<1000 fold). Passive transport properties are of utmost importance for pharmacological and biopharmaceutical effectiveness of drug substances. Diffusion within different compartments and the transport between the compartments are rate-determining steps for the distribution in the body and mostly depend on passive transport properties. The intestinal transport investigations as related to the passive permeability are complicated because of different pH values that exist in the entire gastrointestinal tract. That is one reason why *in vitro* studies or other models are generally used. These things could conveniently outlaw the number of factors that effect *in vivo* and would thus help understand the process of transport. Further decimation of drug substances by metabolism at this stage is a likely cause for the reduced bioavailability of these drugs. It is generally assumed that small (<200 Dalton) water-soluble drugs having P (partition coefficient) values less than 2 pass through cell monolayers only by passive paracellular diffusion through aqueous pores. On the other hand the transcellular movement of the unionized fraction of drug increases with increasing logP (increasing lipophilicity) values up to 2.5-3.5 and declines thereafter. For more hydrophobic drugs paracellular transport is negligible and transcellular permeability is strongly dependent on lipophilicity.

Active Transport

A drug has to reach its target site for its action to be elicited. In this regard, oral route is the most preferred route. This is because of the convenience this route provides. However, drugs have to be solubilized in the intestinal tract before reaching the systemic circulation. Most of the times once a drug is solubilized it reaches the systemic circulation and this extent of reaching the systemic circulation depends on the concentration and the electrochemical gradient. However, not all the times the concentration or electrochemical gradient facilitates the diffusion of molecules across the gastrointestinal tract. Special mechanisms are required. These mechanisms are termed active transport mechanisms and are influenced by the presence of various transporters. Several types of transporters exist on the membrane. The absorption of drugs from the gastrointestinal tract is one of the important determinants for oral bioavailability. It has long been considered that intestinal absorption of drugs after oral administration is mediated by a simple diffusion process, which depends on the physicochemical properties of drugs such as hydrophobicity and ionizing state. However, there have been numerous drugs exhibiting higher absorption rates after oral administration than expected from their physicochemical properties. Active transporters have been identified for such observations. Several transporters have been discovered over some time specifically for a particular class of drugs. The use of various biochemical techniques further facilitated the process. Several types of transporters are present and again within several transporters there is further classification. Thus, the major groups are called transporter families. The major transporter families involved in the absorption and disposition include ABC transporter, peptide transporter, monocarboxylic acid transporter, organic anion transporter, organic ion transporter and nucleoside transporter.

ABC transporter family include MDR family (MDR1 etc.) and MRP family (MRP2, MRP3 etc.). MDR famility carries hydrophobic compounds, anticancer agents, digoxin and immunosuppressants where as MRP famility transports anionic conjugates, anticancer agents, methotrexate and pravastatin. PEPT1 and

PEPT2 are peptide transporters and the substrates for these transporters include di/tripeptides, β-lactam antibiotics, bestatin, and valacyclovir. MCT family belongs to monocarboxylic acid transporter and the very common substrates are lactic acid, salicylic acid etc. OATP/oatp family are organic anion transporters and the substrates include taurocholic acid, estradiol 17β-glucuronide, sulfobromophthalein, thyroxin, pravastatin etc. OAT family, OCT family and OCTN families are organic ion transporters and the substrates include p-aminohippuric acid, β-lactam antibiotics, estrone e-sulfate, methotrexate, cimetidine tetraethylammonium, choline, dopamine, 1-methyl-4-phenylpyridinium, cimetidine L-carnitine, tetraethylammonium. CNT and ENT (NT stands for nucleoside transporter; C and E are different subclasses of nucleoside transporters) families belong to nucleoside transporter and the substrates are purine/pyrimidine nucleoside and nucleoside derivatives. This is a very short summary of various transporters in the intestines. Understanding of the mechanisms underlying the regulation of drug transporters will help in the predictions of the intra- and inter-individual variability of oral bioavailability. In addition, the bioavailability of a series of compounds can be increased by appropriate modifications to make the compounds better substrates to transporters and thereby leading to an increase in the substrate bioavailability. This issue is discussed later in this chapter in drug transport section.

Miscellaneous Transport Systems

Apart from the above two mechanisms of transport i.e., active transport and passive transport, several other types of transport systems also exist to export molecules into the systemic circulation from the gastrointestinal tract via transcellular route. These are especially applicable in the export of particulate systems, macromolecules, vaccine systems, gene therapeutics etc. The investigations of such types of transport systems instigated several scientists eversince research into the gastrointestinal tract absorption was initiated. The amazing thing is the curiousity about the transport of iron, zinc, gold etc. into the systemic circulation after oral administration. This metal therapeutics existed in treatment in several civilizations including Africa, Europa, Egypt, Babylonia, etc. Thus, when first anatomists of modern era erupted, they were very curious about the investigations into the translocation of these large metal particles. Thus, the concept of several transport systems including active transport, passive transport and other miscellaneous transport systems has evolved. However, because of the great adversities to study the miscellaneous sytems and with the introduction of synthetic chemistry at the same time, passive transport investigations and active transport mechanisms were very actively studied. However, the curiosity remained despite their lagging behind. This is mainly because of the role of these metals in several biochemical pathways. As a result several theories were hypothesized. Eventually a day has come when sustained release systems in the form of liposomes, nanoparticles and microparticles were introduced into modern formulation systems. Although the sustained release of drugs was hypothesized to be the key for the efficacy of these particle systems, trace amounts of particles always appeared in the systemic ciruculation. At the same time confocal microscopy and other advanced microscopic techniques were introduced into the scientific investigations. Now there was a definite proof that particles did move into the systemic circulation keeping their structure intact, however, with very minute morphological changes. In addition, a very clear outline of the anatomy of the gastrointestinal tract including different cell layers, their sizes, the compositions etc. began to evolve. These factors led to the further growth in the research on these miscellaneous transport systems. The result is the introduction of the terms endocytosis, pinocytosis, phagocytosis and transcytosis. These terms could be very conveniently described using the techniques associated with the transcellular transport of proteins and other macromolecules. These pathways of transport of particulates are via the cell membranes unlike persorption which is described later.

Endocytosis {Endo (within) cytosis (cell)} is a process in which a substance gains entry into a cell without passing through the cell membrane. This process is subdivided into three different types: pinocytosis, phagocytosis, receptor-mediated endocytosis. In the process of pinocytosis the plasma membrane forms an invagination. What ever substance is found within the area of invagination is brought into the cell. In general this material will be dissolved in water and thus this process is also refered to as "cellular drinking" to indicate that liquids and material dissolved in liquids are ingested by the cell. This is opposed to the ingestion of large particulate material like bacteria or other cells or cell debris. Phagocytosis is a form of endocytosis. In the process of phagocytosis the cell changes shape by sending out projections which are called pseudpodia (false feet). The phagocytic cell such as a macrophage may be attracted to a particle like a bacteria or virus by chemical attractant. This process is called chemotaxis (movement toward a source of chemical attractant). The phagocytic cell sends out membrane projections that make contact with some particle. Some sort of receptor ligand interaction occurs between the phagocytic cell surface and the particle that will be ingested. The pseudopodia then surround the particle and when the plasma membrane of the projections meet, membrane fusion occurs. This results in the formation of an intracellular vesicle. Receptor mediated endocytosis is an endocytotic mechanism in which specific molecules are ingested into the cell. The specificity results from a receptor-ligand interaction. Receptors on the plasma membrane of the target tissue will specifically bind to ligands on the outside of the cell. An endocytotic process occurs and the ligand is ingested. Transcytosis is involved in the internalization of proteins and ligands at one surface and their transport to another. The apical and basolateral borders of epithelial cells are distinguished by their different protein and lipid components.

The sorting of newly synthesized membrane constituents to the appropriate region of the cell is accomplished either in the trans-Golgi network or by transcytosis, the selected transport of proteins to the appropriate surface. These are some of the miscallaneous transport mechanisms in which transcellular route is involved in.

Common Pathways of Drugs Reaching the Systemic Circulation from the GastroIntestinal Tract

A cell has to live and a cell has to grow to perform its everyday activities. Apart from these there are several other functions a cell has to deliver. These include transport, reproduction and metabolism. Thus in physiology the first concept that has to be investigated is the cellular functions. Drugs reach systemic circulation after oral administration via various pathways from various anatomical sites of the gastrointestinal tract. The common pathway is to transport across the membranes present starting from the sites in the stomach and reach the circulation. However, sublingual/buccal transport, lymphatic transport and persorption are other pathways that can be utilized for the drug delivery to systemic circulation after oral administration.

Intestinal Absorption

It is always better to get intestinal absorption process understood based on a simple schematic diagram of different layers involved in the transport. Figure 5.4 is such an example. Lumen is a passage for a drug in which different absorption processes takes place. A drug particle administered as a tablet gets dissolved in the intestinal fluids. Once it is in the form of a solution, it slowly passes across the various layers from first layer to the bottom layer and finally gets absorbed into the blood most of the times and into the lymphatics some times. Blood vessels are generally embedded in this membrane in the bottom layers. The first layer is the mucous layer followed by the epithelium layer. The small intestine has the paradoxical dual function of being a digestive/absorptive organ as well as a barrier to the penetration of toxic compounds and macromolecules. The mucosal membranes accomplish this barrier function through a combination of intestinal immune function and mechanical exclusion. The mucosa: is the innermost layer and consists of three sublayers, beginning from the innermost, they are: an epithelial cell lining, lamina propria: a supportive connective tissue, muscularis mucosa: a thin smooth muscle layer which produces local movements The submucosa: is a loose connective tissue-supporting layer which contains large blood vessels, lymphatic vessels and nerves (e.g. the myenteric plexi). The muscularis: is a functional muscle layer involved in the movement of ingesta through the gastrointestinal tract (peristalsis). It is divided into two layers an inner, circular layer, an outer longitudinal layer, oriented at a 90 degree angle to the circular layer The adventitia/serosa: is the outer layer containing the major vessels and nerves; the outer portion of this layer, the portion exposed to the abdominal cavity is lined by epithelial cells, collectively referred to as the mesothelium. This is the major barrier to the drug transport.

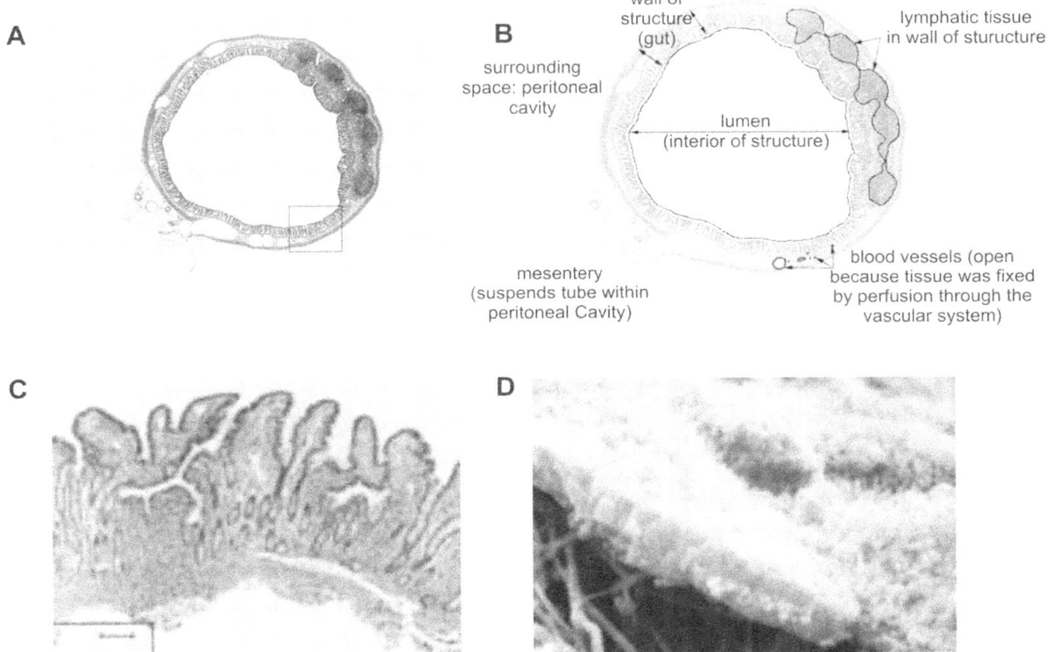

Figure 5.4 Various illustrations of the gastrointestinal tract. A. histological picture of rat gut, B. labeled histological picture of rat gut, C. histological picture of pig mucosa, and D. SEM picture of a CACO-2 cell monolayer. Description in the figure is from top of the paper to the bottom of the paper (Courtesy: UNMC libraries, USA).

Transport

A detailed study of transport of a molecule from the intestinal tract into the systemic circulation is very essential not only in the perspective of drug transport, but also in the point of view of various pathologies. Figure 5.5 shows a typical picture of the transport of drugs.

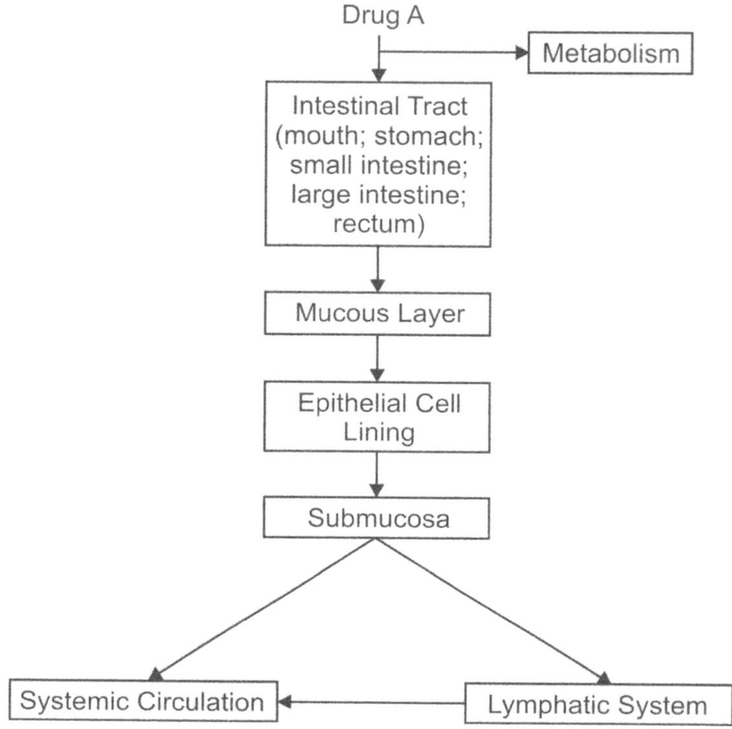

Figure 5.5 A schematic diagram of pathway of a Typical Molecule from the mouth to the intestinal tract to the systemic circulation. This picture deals with all the pathways associated with the molecular movement from the mouth to the systemic circulation. All through the chapter the description of the molecular pathways is presented.

The mucosa followed by submucosa is the important transport limiting layer of the gastrointestinal tract. There are several compositions and several cell types layered or embedded in these two layers. The epithelium, lamina propria and muscularis mucosae form the mucosa and the submucosa consists of loose connective tissues in which large blood vessels, lymph vessels, and nerves are embedded. The mucosa is thrown into longitudinal folds (*gastric folds or rugae*), which disappear when the stomach is fully distended. A network of shallow grooves divides the mucosa into gastric areas (1-5 mm). On the mucosal surface we see small, funnel-shaped depressions (*gastric pits*). Simple, tubular gastric glands that open into the bottom of the gastric pits occupy almost the entire mucosa. The structure and cellular composition of the surface epithelium (simple, tall columnar) does not change throughout the stomach. It contains mucus-producing cells, which form a *secretory sheath* (glandular epithelium). The mucus is alkaline and adheres to the epithelium. The mucus forms a ~ 1 mm thick layer, which protects the mucosa from the acidic contents of the stomach. The surface epithelium is renewed approximately every third day. The source of the new cells is the isthmus, i.e. the upper part of the neck, of the gastric glands, where cells divide and then migrate towards the surface epithelium and differentiate into mature epithelial cells. In contrast to the surface epithelium, cellular composition and function of the gastric glands are specialized in the different parts of the stomach. The different cell types of the mucosa are surface epithelium (simple, tall columnar), cardiac glands, principle glands (chief cells, parietal cells, mucous neck cells and endocrine cells), pyloric glands (endocrine cells, parietal cells). The lamina propria is formed by a very cell-rich loose connective tissue (fibroblasts, lymphocytes, plasma cells, macrophages, eosinophilic leukocytes and mast cells). The muscularis mucosae of the stomach contain both circular and longitudinal layers of muscle cells. Its organization is somewhat variable depending on the location of the stomach. Chief cells produce pepsinogen, which is a precursor of the proteolytic enzyme pepsin. Parietal cells secrete hydrochloric acid and intrinsic factor. Hydrochloric acid is important in activating the pepsinogen and also sterilizes the contents of the stomach. Intrinsic factor is necessary for the resorption of vitamin B12. Mucous neck cells and endocrine cells are useful in the stimulation of the secretion of acid and pepsinogen. The entire intestinal mucosa forms intestinal villi (about 1 mm long), which increase the surface area by a factor of ~10. The surface of the villi is formed by a simple columnar epithelium. Each absorptive cell or enterocyte of the epithelium form number microvilli. Microvilli increase the surface area by a factor of ~20. Apart from these several other cells with a variety of functions also exist in the mucosa. The other important cells that needs to be described as related to the phagocytic process is the Peyers Patches. These are present in the lamina propria. The lamina propria is, similar to the lamina propria of the stomach, unusually cell rich. Lymphocytes often invade the epithelium or form solitary lymphoid nodules in the lamina propria. Lymph nodules may form longitudinal aggregations of 30-50 nodules in the lamina propria of the ileum. These large aggregates are called Peyers Patches. It is widely known that these patches are responsible for phagocytosis of microparticles, nanoparticles and macromolecules. Different individual functionalities are henceforth described.

Mucous layer

Understanding the mucous that protects the intestinal lining is definitely an important aspect as related to the transport of molecules across the gastrointestinal tract. Mucous is made of mucins. Mucins are naturally produced in the intestinal tract of all mammals. They have the same effect as the wax we use on our floors or cars. They protect the intestinal cells from allergens and from reacting to our own friendly flora. Whether it's the eyes, sinuses, throat, chest or intestinal tract, mucin (from colixen) provides a first line of defense. Mucin is a protein that forms a protective gel layer over all mucous membranes of the body. In the intestinal tract, mucins protect the intestinal lining from the hostile environment of bacteria, viruses and toxins. Elaborate immunological and mechanical processes for excluding harmful dietary antigens, bacterial products and viable microbial organisms are present at the mucosal level. The abundant carbohydrates on mucin molecules bind to bacteria, which aids in preventing epithelial colonization and, by causing aggregation, accelerates clearance. Diffusion of hydrophilic molecules is considerably lower in mucus than in aqueous solution, which is thought to retard diffusion of a variety of damaging chemicals, including gastric acid, to the epithelial surface. In addition to being coated with a mucus layer, gastric and duodenal epithelial cells secrete bicarbonate ion on their apical faces. This serves to maintain a neutral pH along the epithelial plasma membrane, even though highly acidic conditions exist in the lumen.

The high molecular weight mucins are responsible for the viscoelastic properties of the mucous barrier. They are widely expressed in epithelial tissues and are characterised by variable number tandem repeat peptide sequences rich in serine, threonine, and proline which carry large numbers of *O*-linked oligosaccharide chains. Secreted and membrane associated forms have been found based on their function as extracellular viscous secretions or viscoelastic polymer gels or location as membrane anchored molecules in the glycocalyx. Two clusters have been reported, the secretory mucin genes MUC2, MUC5AC, MUC5B, and MUC6 on chromosome 11p15.5, and MUC3, MUC11, and MUC12 on on chromosome 7q22. However, these genetic mapping is definitely not important at this stage. Normal stomach mucosa is characterised by expression of MUC1, MUC5AC, and MUC6. High levels of MUC2 and MUC3 appear in IM. The complete form (type I) demonstrates only MUC2 in goblet cells. In contrast, incomplete forms (types II and III) exhibit MUC1 and MUC5AC in both goblet and absorptive cells, MUC2 in goblet cells only, and MUC6 in over 60% of cases. This represents two phenotypes, a small intestinal/colonic pattern and a typical gastric pattern with MUC2. MUC3 and MUC4 have not been examined.

Epithelial layer

Epithelial layer constitutes the important barrier to the drug transport. This layer has been widely investigated by various scientists with multiple interests for over several years. Detailed picture of these cell layers could be obtained from various literature sources. The importance of this cell layer would be depicted with the help of the Figure 5.6.

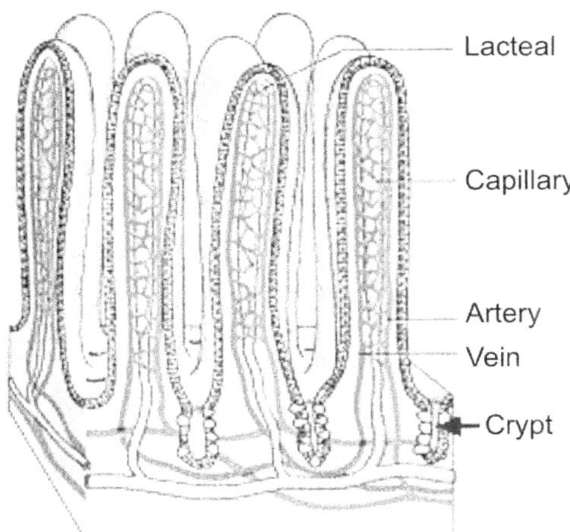

Figure 5.6 The epithelial layer is the top most layer of the villi in the figure (Courtesy: Atlas of the anatomy, picture: intestinal epithelium; right side shows the labels).

The alimentary canal is lined by sheets of epithelial cells that form the defining structure of the mucosa. With few exceptions, epithelial cells in the stomach and intestines are circumferentially tied to one another by tight junctions, which seal the paracellular spaces and thereby establish the basic gastrointestinal barrier. Throughout the digestive tube, maintenance of an intact epithelium is thus critical to the integrity of the barrier. In general, toxins and microorganisms that are able to breach the single layer of epithelial cells have unimpeded access to the systemic circulation. As might be anticipated, there is diversity among different types of epithelial cells in specific barrier functions. For example, the apical plasma membranes of gastric parietal and chief cells have atypically low permeability to protons, which aids in preventing damage due to back diffusion of acid into the cells. Small intestinal epithelial cells lack this specialized ability and thus are much more susceptible to acid-induced damage. Tight junctions encircling gastrointestinal epithelial cells are a critical component of the intrinsic barrier. These structures used to be viewed as passive structures akin to welds, but recent studies indicate that they are much more dynamic than previously thought, and their permeability may be regulated by a number of factors that affect the epithelial cells. The gastrointestinal epithelium is populated by a variety of functionally-mature cells derived from proliferation of stem cells. Most of the mature epithelial cells, including mucous cells in the stomach and absorptive cells in the small intestine, show rapid turnover rates, and die within only a few days after their formation. Maintenance of epithelial integrity thus requires a precise balance between cell proliferation and cell death. Stem cells that support continual replenishment of gastrointestinal epithelium reside in the middle of the gastric pits and within the crypts of the small and large intestine. Epithelial cell dynamics of the small intestine have been particularly well studied. These stem cells proliferate continually to supply cells that then differentiate into absorptive enterocytes, mucus-secreting goblet cells, enteroendocrine cells and Paneth cells. Except for Paneth cells, which remain in the crypts, the other cells differentiate into their mature forms as they migrate up from the crypts to replace cells extruded from the tips of the villi. This migration takes approximately 3 to 6 days.

Submucosa

The tunica submucosa is the region of connective tissue immediately outside the muscularis mucosae. It has fair numbers of blood vessels and lymphatics in it, too, and if it is carefully looked at several localized collections of neuronal cell bodies could be distinguished. Drugs get transported across various layers and reach the blood vessels and then gets distributed thoughout the body.

The elements of the submucosal plexus were discovered by George Meissner (1829-1905), a German histologist. This plexus, together with another one located in the tunica muscularis helps to coordinate the movements of the intestine and facilitate the passage of food through its lumen. Two major nerve plexus are found in this area. These help control the movements of the stomach and the intestine. The neural elements include neurons and their attendant satellite cells plus nerve fibers that connect the neurons from each other. They bring in sensations, and carry motor commands to effector cells. It has collections of neuron cell bodies (which, by definition, are ganglia) linked together by nerve fibers. Some of the motor fibers from these nodal points control the muscles of the muscularis mucosae; others are routed to the strands of smooth muscle that run through the cores of the villi. The submucosal plexus primarily controls the contractions of the muscularis mucosae and the villi. The pulsatile contraction of the innermost part of the mucosa, and the movements of the villi, are important in digestion, because they cause mixing and overturn of the food, and emptying of the mucosal crypts. Nervous signals running through the submucosal plexus are coordinated with the signals sent out from the myenteric plexus, which controls the larger movements of the gut wall, and peristalsis. The submucosal and myenteric plexuses together constitute an autonomous "enteric division" of the nervous system with its own sensory and motor arcs and feedback loops. The submucosa of the duodenum also has true glandular elements, called Brunner's glands (Johann C. Brunner (1653-1727), a Swiss anatomist). These submucosal glands are specifically a feature of the duodenum, and are typically found in the first portion of it. They aren't present in the jejunum or the ileum. The submucosal glands produce an alkaline secretion which helps to neutralize the very acidic (pH 2.0-3.0) material entering the duodenum from the pyloric region of the stomach. Blood vessels and lymphatics are very widely distributed in this area. For most of the layers from the lumen to the blood vessels, the drug transport is not rate-limiting, exception being the epithelial layer. Thus, once a drug passes through the epithelial layer it quickly gets transported across the other layer before reaching the blood vessels. Most of the times the endothelium of the blood vessels is also not a rate-limiting membrane. Similar is the case with the lymphatic vessels. Thus, the submucosa of the intestinal tract helps in the transport of molecules from lumen into the systemic circulations and also aids in the neuronal control of the gastrointestinal tract.

Miscellaneous cells

Apart from the epithelial cells, there are several other cells in the intestinal tract that may be helpful in the process of transport of various foreign and indigenous chemicals. Foreign chemicals could include those that are friendly to the system and those that are unfriendly or could be called toxic to the human system. The transport of these molecules into the systemic circulation for further processing or for the rejection of these molecules to the excretion takes place because of these variegated roles of these variegated cells. Not only understanding the system is important but also understanding the chemicals that might enter into the body is important. In this regard the utmost importance could be given not only to the epithelial or to the mucosal lining but also this importance could be given to a variety of the cells located in the intestinal tract. For instance, the very common transport processes that could better describe the role of these cells involve the transport of pathogens.

A pathogen could enter the intestinal tract by oral route. This slowly travels from mouth to the respective location. Once a pathogen penetrates the surface epithelium, the process of immune activation begins. The pathogen is transported across the intestinal epithelium by M cells and presented to the underlying lymphocytes in Peyer's patches by MHCII positive enterocytes. At the same time, intraepithelial lymphocytes are activated and secrete interferon tau that increases the ability of enterocytes to present antigen. Simultaneously, intraepithelial lymphocytes may also cytolyse pathogens. In Peyer's patches, T-lymphocytes in parafollicular areas interact with antigen presenting cells and antigenic peptides to become activated. B-lymphocytes in follicular areas are also initially activated by the interaction of antigen and their surface Ig. Helper T-lymphocytes increases B-lymphocyte activation so that B-lymphocytes begin to proliferate in germinal centres. Most B-lymphocytes at this stage are surface IgA positive whether induced by T-switch cells or by isotype specific T-lymphocytes. At the same time activated T-suppressor cells and contrasuppressors regulate the immune response to maintain it at an optimum level. All these lymphocytes then leave Peyer's patches via blood vessels to mesenteric lymph nodes and the spleen where further cellular activation occurs. Thereafter, activated lymphocytes return to the intestine either directly or via the peripheral circulation. Those that reach the intestine directly differentiate into effector cells and enter the lamina propria. In the lamina propria, plasma cells and cytotoxic T-lymphocytes destroy pathogens by secreting specific Ig and by cytotoxicity, respectively. Activated helper T-lymphocytes in the lamina propria probably help in local responses by acting on the few resting B-lymphocytes present there. T-suppressor lymphocytes enter the epithelium to become intraepithelial lymphocytes and regulate responses by suppressor and contrasuppressor activities. Intraepithelial lymphocytes are also cytotoxic for luminal pathogens. Activated lymphocytes which do not return to the intestine directly enter the thoracic duct and thereby the general circulation. In this way a local gut response is converted into a systemic one and memory lymphocytes are disseminated throughout the body. In addition, suppressor and contrasuppressor T-lymphocytes also become available for peripheral effects. Large number of these lymphocytes remain in circulation, while others return to the intestine to provide local protection. Thus, in this game of the transport of this pathogen several cells such as intraepithelial lymphocytes, M cells, lymphocytes in the Peyers Patches, T-lymphocytes, B-lymphocytes, etc. are involved. Similarly, food proteins, commensal bacteria, nanoparticles, microparticles etc. could be transported using the same pathway.

Sublingual/buccal Transport of Drugs

The oral cavity as a site for drug delivery also has reached commercial status with several drugs, including nitroglycerin as sublingual tablets for angina and fentanyl as a transmucosal buccal device (Actiq,Abbott Laboratories, Abbott Park, IL) for breakthrough cancer pain. Furthermore, oral transmucosal drug delivery bypasses first-pass effects in the GI tract and liver and avoids GI side effects. Drug delivery via the oral cavity is highly acceptable by patients. The mucosa is relatively permeable, has a rich blood supply, is robust, and shows short recovery times after stress or damage.Within the oral cavity the two common regions for drug delivery are the sublingual mucosa (area beneath the tongue) and the buccal mucosa (inner lining of the cheeks). Selecting one over the other is mainly based on anatomical and permeability properties of the vari ous oral mucosal sites, the desired residence time, and the desired effects of the drug. Via these routes drugs can be travelled either by paracellular route or transcellular route.

Three different categories of drug delivery fall within the oral cavity: sublingual, buccal, and local. The sublingual mucosa is relatively permeable, giving rapid absorption and acceptable bioavailabilities of many drugs, and is convenient, accessible, and generally well accepted. The sublingual route is by far the most widely studied of these routes. Sublingual dosage forms are most often one of two designs: those composed of rapidly disintegrating tablets and those consisting of soft gelatin capsules filled with liquid drug. Such systems create a very high drug concentration in the sublingual region before they are systemically absorbed across the mucosa. The buccal mucosa is considerably less permeable than the sublingual area, and is generally not able to provide the rapid absorption and good bioavailabilities seen with sublingual administration. Even though the sublingual mucosa is relatively more permeable than the buccal mucosa, it is not suitable for a retentive oral transmucosal delivery system. The sublingual region lacks an expanse of smooth and immobile mucosa and is constantly washed by a considerable amount of saliva, making device placement difficult. Because of the high permeability and the rich blood supply, transport via the sublingual route results in a rapid onset of action, making it appropriate for highly permeable drugs with short delivery period requirements and an infrequent dosing regimen. However, the preferred site for retentive oral transmucosal delivery systems and for sustained- and controlled-release delivery devices is the buccal mucosa, mainly because of the differences in permeability characteristics between the two regions and the buccal mucosa's expanse of smooth and relatively immobile mucosa.

Lymphatic Transport of Drugs

Intestinal lymphatic transport is another absorptive pathway following oral administration. This route is particularly applicable to lipids and an increasing number of lipophilic drugs. These compounds once absorbed, diffuse across the intestinal enterocyte and while in transit associate with secretable enterocyte lipoproteins. The chylomicron-associated drug will be then secreted from the enterocyte into the lymphatic circulation, rather than the portal circulation, thus avoiding the metabolically-active liver, but still ultimately returning to the systemic circulation. Because of this parallel and potentially alternative absorptive pathway, first-pass metabolism can be reduced while increasing lymphatic drug exposure, which opens the potential for novel therapeutic methodologies and allows the implementation of lipid-based drug delivery systems.

The lymphatic system consists of a network of lymphatic vessels which drain most regions of the body. The system is structured such that fluid, i.e. lymph, drained from the interstitial space is returned via the lymphatics into the blood system. The nature and size of the lymphatic vessels vary along the route.

Among the lymphatic vessels there are numerous lymph nodes through which the lymph is filtered. Anatomical and physiological differences exist between blood and lymphatic capillaries. At the cellular level in blood capillaries tight intercellular junctions exist, in contrast, the basement membrane of lymphatic capillaries is much less well organised and the junctions between the endothelial cells are much leakier. Macromolecules and colloidal particles such as chylomicrons are selectively taken up from the interstitial space via the lymphatics. This molecular Sieving mechanism may be potentially exploited for drug delivery. The anatomy and physiology of the lymphatic system varies in different regions of the body. The lymphatics of the small intestine are characterised by the presence of a centrally located lacteal in each villi. The lacteals join a plexus of lymphatic capillaries and drain, via the mesenteric lymph vessel, into the cisterna chyli. Lymph from the cisterna chyli is drained by the thoracic duct which empties directly into the general circulation at the junction of the left internal jugular and left subclavian veins. This unique physiology potentially enables orally administered drugs to bypass the liver and thus avoid first pass metabolism. As a result of lipid digestion and absorption lipoproteins, such as chylomicrons, are synthesized within the intestinal enterocytes. The chylomicrons are excreted from the enterocyte and as they are too large to enter the blood capillaries they are taken up exclusively by the lymphatics. These lipoproteins formed by the intestinal enterocytes play a fundamental role in the transport of orally administered lipophilic compounds. Different strategies are used to enhance lymphatic drug transport after oral administration.

Different strategies to enhance lymphatic drug transport, depending on the route of administration, have been explored to varying degrees of success. In general the two main approaches used involve increasing lipophilicity and increasing molecular size. Since the rate of lymph *flow* in the intestine is approximately 500 times less than that of blood flow in the portal vein, unless selective uptake into the lymphatics occurs, most drugs will be transported almost exclusively by the portal circulation. However, it is known that certain highly lipophilic compounds, i.e. with high partition coefficients and significant solubilities in a triglyceride lipid, are transported to a certain extent via the lymphatic route. In addition, the transport of these compounds may be enhanced by coadministration of specific types of lipid vehicles. The mechanisms of the enhanced lymphatic transport are complex and not completely understood. However, it has been suggested that the stimulation of lipoprotein synthesis by the enterocyte and the subsequent association of the drug with the chylomicrons is fundamental to the process. Compounds including DDT, probucol, cyclosporin A and halofantrine are known to be incorporated into the lipid vehicles and then transported into lymph and then systemic circulation avoiding first pass metabolism. The prodrug approach has also been examined in an attempt to achieve significant lymphatic transport following oral administration. The aim was to synthesis promoieties with enhanced lipophilicity, which are metabolically and chemically stable during the absorption and transport phases of delivery to the lymph, and which undergo conversion selectively at sites other than the liver. Limited success has been achieved with the simple ester/ether approaches. In contrast, monoglyceride, triglyceride or phospholipid mimics have shown more potential. Other approaches to lymphatic transport not dependent on lipoprotein formation have been investigated. For example in the case of macromolecules and microparticles the anatomical characteristics of the lymphatic system, i.e. the relatively open structure of the lymphatic endothelium, are the major features responsible for the lymphatic transport. In the case of macromolecules work has been done to examine the molecular weight-dependent lymph/plasma level ratio of exogenous macromolecules. Lymphotropic delivery systems, where the drug is complexed with a high molecular weight carrier, e.g. dextran sulphate, have been used in the presence of absorption enhancers to potentiate the selective lymphatic delivery of anticancer drugs. Many studies have reported uptake of particles following oral administration, however, the mechanism and extent of uptake remains controversial. Several mechanisms have been proposed including uptake by the M cells in the Peyer's patches, and distribution via the mesenteric lymph towards the lymph nodes. Microparticles have been successfully used as antigen delivery systems for oral immunization. This is due to the fact that Peyer's patches are the sites of induction for the secretory immune response and are also the sites for maximum uptake. In addition, systemic immune responses are also induced as particles are transferred to mesenteric lymph nodes.

Lymphatic transport has also been utilized via various other routes and not only after oral administration. As the focus of this book is only oral administration, these are not discussed here.

Persorption

The uptake of particulates into systemic circulation from gastrointestinal tract was observed for the first time in 1844 and subsequently confirmed on several occasions. However, it was not considered credible and little notice was taken of it. This phenomenon of the enteral translocation of solid microparticles was termed as persorption and the question of where persorbed particles end was investigated in detail between 1959 and 1967 in the laboratories for experimental gastroenterology of the 1st Medical Clinic (Charité) of the Humboldt University, Berlin. *Herbst* gave a starch infusion to a female dog and three hours later found starch-granules in the chyle and in the blood. *Oesterlen* demonstrated some of the charcoal particles fed to chicken and rabbits in their blood. Recently this route of administration of drugs has gained prominence because it has several advantages. Nanoparticles and microparticles are found to reach the systemic circulation after oral administration. General cellular translocation and persorption were the mechanisms proposed. If drugs such as proteins, peptides, antisensense oligonucleotides, genes etc. are encapsulated in nanoparticles and microparticles and administered orally, with the suitable mechanism they can be taken into the systemic circulation and eventually released slowly. Later investigations were carried out for such a model of drug absorption for vaccines. The gastrointestinal uptake of micro- and nanoparticles has been the subject of recent efforts to develop effective carriers that enhance the oral uptake of drugs and vaccines. This group used correlative instrumental neutron activation analysis and electron microscopy to quantitatively and qualitatively study the gastrointestinal uptake and subsequent tissue/organ distribution of 4, 10, 28, and 58 nm diameter metallic colloidal gold particles following oral administration to mice. In their quantitative studies they found that colloidal gold uptake is dependent on particle size: smaller particles cross the gastrointestinal tract more readily. Electron microscopic studies showed that particle uptake occurred in the small intestine by persorption through single, degrading enterocytes in the process of being extruded from a villus. Basically, when something enteres the systemic circulation by persorption after oral administration, the transport is through the gaps created by extruding enterocytes.

Intestinal Metabolism

Metabolism of drugs is the first defence mechanism against the foreign invasion. Drug metabolism or biotransformation refers to the process of modifying or altering the chemical composition of the drug. The pharmacological activity of the drug is usually removed by metabolism. Metabolites (products of metabolism) are produced which are more polar and less lipid-soluble than the original drug, which ultimately promotes their excretion from the body. Most drug metabolism occurs in the liver, where hepatic enzymes catalyze various biochemical reactions. Metabolism of drugs may also occur in the kidneys, intestinal mucosa, lungs, plasma and placenta. Sometimes the metabolism in the intestines also occurs due to the intestinal flora. Although this may not be very significant for several drugs, this could have major impact on the treatment with some drugs. Drugs administered orally are absorbed from the gastrointestinal tract, carried via the hepatic portal vein to the liver, and then undergo some metabolism by the liver before the drug has even had the opportunity to work. This removal of a drug by the liver, before the drug has become available for use, is called the first pass effect. Some drugs, when swallowed and absorbed, will be almost totally inactivated by the first pass effect eg. glyceryl trinitrate. The first pass effect can, however, be avoided if the drug is given by another route. Thus, glyceryl trinitrate, when administered sublingually or transdermally, avoids first pass metabolism by the liver and is able to cause a therapeutic effect. In addition, the actions of these types of substances are often times very rapid with such administrations. Before moving further it is worth mentioning about the movement of molecules within the system for a clearer illustration (Figure 5.7). Blood leaving the GI tract does not return directly to the heart but first passes to the liver via the hepatic portal vein and then returns to the general circulation via the hepatic vein. This ensures that all digestive products as well as other materials absorbed from the GI tract first reach the liver. The liver removes large quantities of nutrients from the blood; these are used to synthesize essential metabolic products such as the plasma proteins and liver glycogen. The liver also removes from the portal blood, potentially dangerous materials such as pathogens (viruses, bacteria, toxins, drugs, alcohol etc), which have been absorbed from the GI tract, thus limiting their access to other vulnerable organs such as the brain, heart and kidneys. However, on several occasions metabolism occurs in the intestinal tract thereby reducing the bioavailability of drugs.

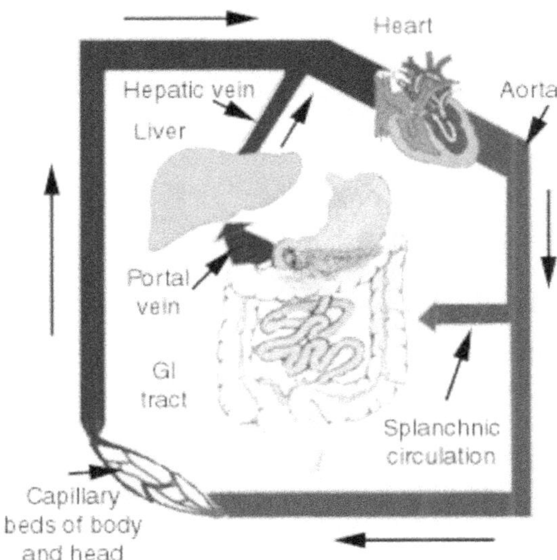

Figure 5.7 The simple movement of molecules from within the system: through the gastrointestinal tract to the target capillary beds of the body and target tissue.

Metabolism also plays a major factor in several other situations. The distal intestine contains numerous dietary and bacterial products with toxic properties, including actual bacterial cell wall polymers, chemotactic peptides, bacterial antigens capable of inducing antibodies that cross-react with host antigens, and bacterial and dietary antigens that can form systemic immune complexes. Normal human bacterial microflora in the small and large intestine maintain a delicate balance. Their metabolic and enzymatic activity is critical in the metabolism/bio-transformation and absorption of nutrients. These nutrients include all compounds taken orally and all substances entering the intestine via the biliary tract or by direct secretion into the lumen. When the microflora balance is disturbed (dysbiosis) these metabolic and enzymatic activities can be severely compromised. Dysbiosis is a state where imbalances in intestinal flora cause changes to normal gastrointestinal processes, manifesting in clinical and pre-clinical conditions, which can lead to varying degrees of 'unwellness'. The symptoms of dysbiosis can vary significantly between individuals, however, the causes can be placed into four major categories namely, putrefaction, fermentation, deficiency and sensitisation. Infection by viruses, bacteria, fungi and parasites and chemical attack (intoxication) by xenobiotics and therapeutic agents (drugs, etc.) can also be implicated. Dysbiosis can lead to the breakdown of mucosal integrity ('leaky gut') contributing to increased absorption and compromised liver function.

As related to the gastrointestinal tract metabolism, different case scenarios could be presented in the sequential order.

1. Extensive intestinal metabolism contributing to the overall first-pass effect.
2. Metabolism by the intestinal flora.
3. Metabolism by the gastric pH.
4. Metabolism by the digestive enzymes.
5. Metabolism by the intestinal wall enzymes.

Extensive intestinal metabolism-contributing to overall first-pass effect

Some orally administered drugs (e.g., clonazepam, chlorpromazine) are more extensively metabolized in the intestine than in the liver. This effect is very often termed first-pass effect. Thus, intestinal metabolism may contribute to the overall first-pass effect. Although the liver plays the major role in drug metabolism [e.g. by oxidative cytochrome P-450 (CYP)-dependent phase I and conjugation or phase II reactions], drug metabolising enzymes are also present at other sites. Depending on the particular drug and enzymes involved, these extrahepatic organs and/or tissues can contribute to the elimination of drugs and, thus, should be considered in any discussion of drug disposition. By the use of relatively new techniques in molecular biology, e.g. immunoblotting with antibodies directed to various CYP isoenzymes, the tissue and organ distribution of these drug metabolising enzymes can be determined. In addition, microsomal and cytosolic enzyme activity and capacity can be directly assessed *in vitro* by incubation of the enzymes with the drugs of interest. Both approaches have demonstrated the presence of 3 CYP families at different extrahepatic sites, such as the mucosa of the gastrointestinal tract, kidney, lung, brain or skin. Examples of such enzymes include epoxide hydrolases, hydrolysing enzymes, glutathione S-transferases, UDP-glucuronosyltransferases, sulphotransferases, N-acetyltransferases, and methyltransferases. Indirect evidence of extrahepatic drug metabolism can be generated from pharmacokinetic studies whenever total body clearance exceeds liver blood flow, or when severe liver dysfunction or anhepatic conditions do not affect metabolic clearance. Indeed, extrahepatic metabolism has been demonstrated for numerous drugs. Cytochrome P-450 (CYP) 3A is the dominant CYP in the human small intestine and accounts for the majority of total microsomal P-450 found in the mucosal epithelium of the small intestine. CYP3A is also a major CYP in the rat small intestine. In literature, several examples of drugs degrading in the intestines can be found.

Metabolism by the intestinal flora

The indigenous intestinal microflora is involved in a variety of processes within the human body, and is important for maintaining host health. As such, interindividual differences in the ability to harbor certain intestinal bacteria might be associated with interindividual differences in health and/or disease susceptibility. The actual number of bacteria in the human colon is unknown, but it has been estimated that there are more than 400 species. In some instances, as an alternative to physically isolating and identifying the bacteria, host phenotypes that result from the metabolic functions of certain bacteria can be used to indicate their presence in the intestines. For example, breath levels of methane indicate the presence of methanogenic bacteria. Similarly, breath levels of [^{13}C] labeled carbon dioxide (produced by bacterial breakdown of administered [^{13}C] labeled urea) indicate the presence of *Helicobacter pylori*. Several candidate bacteria have been found to be involved in the drug metabolism. These include *Clostridium* sp., *Eubacterium ramulus*, *Bifidobacterium*, *Escherichia coli*, *Bacteroides ovatus*, *Ruminococcus productus*, and *Streptococcus intermedius*. In addition, the intestinal microflora can metabolize a wide variety of pharmacological agents resulting in production of metabolites required for the physiological activity of these agents or conversely in the inactivation of these agents. The conversion of specific substrates such as, rutin, digoxin, cycasin, azulfidine, isoflavones, lignans and cyclamate is found to take place in the intestines utilizing microbial flora.

Metabolism by the gastric pH

In several diseased situations, metabolism or degradation due to the changes in the gastric pH is also affected that may lead to altered drug bioavailability which may be of significant importance. The metabolic activity of the abundantly present intestinal lactobacilli can also affect the enteral drug absorption in patients with short small bowel as this result in the production of lactic acid, gaseous CO_2, ethanol and an increased bile acid deconjugation. The likely reason would be the alteration in the gastric pH. The bioavailability generally decreases with drugs unstable in the gastric pH. Examples of such drugs include benzylpenicillin, salicylazosulfonilic acid, didanosine, etc. The other example worth mentioning is ketoconazole. Orally administered ketoconazole requires an acidic medium to dissolve adequately and therefore should not be given simultaneously with antacids, anticholinergic drugs, H_2 blockers, or acid (proton) pump inhibitors (eg, omeprazole). If needed, such drugs should be given at least 2 h after ketoconazole. Thus, it is very likely that the bioavailability is altered with the alterations in the intestinal pH.

Metabolism by the digestive enzymes

Metabolism conversion involves the use of enzymes to chemically convert substances to different substances that may be less active and, in any case, are more easily carried in blood to the kidneys for excretion. The original substances are called 'substrates' of the enzymes; after conversion they are called 'metabolites'. For example, an enzyme called 'aromatase' converts the substance testosterone into estradiol. Testosterone is a substrate of the aromatase enzyme; estradiol is a metabolite of testosterone. Although estradiol is by itself an important hormone in the body, it also serves as an excretable form of testosterone. Other enzymes convert estradiol into even more easily excreted forms, such as estriol. Similarly the drug insulin is digested with the help of the enzymes in the gastrointestinal tract thereby leading to its reduced oral bioavailability. Such investigations with new drug substances are very important.

Metabolism by the intestinal wall enzymes

The small intestinal wall enzymes finish the job begun by the pancreatic enzymes, the oligopeptides, dipeptides and disaccharides are all digested (hydrolyzed) to monomers. Many of these enzymes are not secreted into the small intestine, but remain attached to the cells that produce them. These enzymes are sometimes responsible for drug metabolism. Examples of drugs metabolized using these enzymes are sympathomimetic catecholamines. The other interesting aspect with these enzymes is that some of the food substances are found to inhibit these enzymes thereby resulting in the increased bioavailability of certain drugs. Grapefruit juice has the ability to potentiate the effects of certain drugs, simply by inhibiting certain intestinal-wall enzymes that normally break them down and reduce their influence. Levels of these intestinal enzymes vary from patient to patient, making it difficult to predict the degree of reaction. On the other hand, the effects of a daily dose of grapefruit juice increase over time. Thus, the very recent investigations that instigated many scientists were on these lines.

Factors Affecting Drug Absorption Across the Gastro Intestinal Tract

Since gastro intestinal tract is a medley of anatomical, physiological, pharmacological and functional system, it is more complicated than the other routes of administration of drugs in terms of drug absorption. However, since this is the very convenient route of administration, very wide investigations have been done long time ago. The factor that affects drug absorption can be conveniently grouped into physical and physiological. Physical factors can include solubility, dissolution rate, molecular size, partition coefficient, chemical degradation and delivery system. Physiological factors could include binding or complexation, regional pH, intestinal permeability, metabolism (luminal and hepatic) and gastric and intestinal transit.

Physical Factors

Solubility of a drug substance is the first important physical factor. The general observation would be the greater the solubility the greater the bioavailability. This can be visioned from the food products. For instance the absorption of water-soluble food components is more compared to the oil soluble vitamins. Specialized transport mechanisms or solubility methods are needed to increase the bioavailability of these compounds. Similarly, the same principle can be extrapolated to drugs of interest. A water-soluble drug is likely to have more bioavailability compared to its water insoluble drug counterpart. Similarly this may also lead to the differences in the bioavailabilities. A water insoluble drug can attach itself indiscreetly and thereby lead to the variabilities in the bioavaialbility with each dosing. Thus, the first factor that definitely needs to be controlled in the solubility of the drug substance is the intestinal media. Several means are available for this purpose. Examples include dispersable tablets, microencapsulated drugs, solid dispersions etc. The next similar physical factor that can be discussed is the dissolution rate. Solubility doesnot always result in maximum bioavailability. For instance if a drug has mouth as its absorption site and it is released in the soluble form in the lower gastrointestinal tract, definitely there would not be any absorption. It is worthless to investigate such a kind of mechanims of absorption. Similarly the case is the same with drugs absorbed at a particular site. Thus, dissolution rate is a very important aspect. The rate of dissolution is the speed at which a drug dissolves in the intestinal environment. The greater the dissolution rate the rapid is the achievement of a solution form of this drug. These are the very fundamentals of drug therapy. The next physical factors molecular size and partition coefficient could be clubbed under one discussion as related functionalities of factors affecting the drug absorption.

Biological membranes are porous and definitely are lipid in nature. Molecular size of the drug would result in the more bioavailability if its size is lower than the size of the membrane and similarly the more lipophilic a molecule is the more is its general bioavaialability. However, there should be always a balance. Since the biological membrane is made up of both water and lipid, an optimum lipophilicity indicates an optimum bioavailability. In a similar way the molecular size could be discussed. The next physical factors that could be clubbed are chemical degradation and delivery system. More stable drug in the intestinal tract means longer it stays and if all the properties are positive then it is definitely a possibility that it is absorbed more compared to its counter part drug substance with less stability. Thus, stability is definitely a very key issue. This is the reflective of the property of the chemical substance. Delivery system is another similar factor. The better the delivery system the better is the therapy with a new drug substance. Unfortunately, most of the times new delivery systems are not well characterized before these enter into the market. Say for instance, if a drug is safe and it is put into a toxic or uncharacterized delivery sytem and administered for human use without complete study designs and output, it would definitely lead to deleterious affects as noticed by several scientists. Thus, it has to be always kept in mind that delivery system is a very key issue to be considered. Other times it is the control release requirement. For drugs that are needed to slowly release into the systemic circulation, a controlled release system is a worth. Sustained release system consumes several volumes of discussion and some of these issues are discussed in the chapter on Novel Drug Delivery Systems.

Physiological Factors

The next factors that govern the drug absorption are the physiological factors. The gastrointestinal tract is an important barrier and interface for a drug's absorption and transport. The dissolution rate of poorly soluble drugs can be limited due to volume and pH of the intestinal fluid available at that time. Bile salts can increase the solubility of lipophilic drugs, and presence of food can also have significant impact on GI dissolution and membrane permeability into the mucosa and therefore alter the absorption and bioavailability. In addition, gastric emptying and GI transit time play an important role in the fate of drugs in the body. Many drugs get ionized within the physiological pH range, which impacts their aqueous solubility. The drug can have increased solubility or may even precipitate already solubilized drug. The impact is more complicated due to variation in time, regions of GIT and surfactants concentration, and time profile. The distal region of the stomach (antrum) is the potential site of mixing and acts as a pump to facilitate the gastric emptying process. Gastric emptying occurs both during fasting and fed states, but the pattern varies.

The liver is the primary site for metabolism. Liver contains the necessary enzymes for metabolism of drugs and other xenobiotics. These enzymes induce two metabolism pathways: Phase I (functionalization reactions) and Phase II (biosynthetic reactions) metabolism. Some typical examples of Phase I metabolism include oxidation and hydrolysis. The enzymes involved in Phase I reactions are primarily located in the endoplasmic reticulum of the liver cell, they are called microsomal enzymes. Phase II metabolism involves the introduction of a hydrophilic endogenous species, such as glucuronic acid or sulfate, to the drug molecule. Enzymes involved in phase II reactions are mainly located in the cytosol, except glucuronidation enzyme, which is also a microsomal enzyme. Drugs are usually lipophilic substances (Oil-like) so they can pass plasma membranes and reach the site of action. Drug metabolism is basically a process that introduces hydrophilic functionalities onto the drug molecule to facilitate excretion. When the drug molecule is oxidized, hydrolyzed, or covalently attached to a hydrophilic species, the whole molecule becomes more hydrophilic, and is excreted more easily. Drugs often undergo both Phase I and II reactions before excretion. The Phase I reaction introduces a functional group such as a hydroxyl group onto the molecule, or exposes a preexisting functional group, and Phase II reaction connects this functional group to the endogenous species such as a glucuronic acid. The modified drug molecule may then be hydrophilic enough to be excreted. Although liver is the primary site for metabolism, virtually all tissue cells have some metabolic activities. Other organs having significant metabolic activities include the gastrointestinal tract, kidneys, and lungs. When a drug is administrated orally, it undergoes metabolism in the GI track and the liver before reaching the systemic circulation. This process is called first-pass metabolism. First-pass metabolism limits the oral bioavailability of drugs, sometimes significantly.

Drug Absorption through Various Regions of Gastrointestinal Tract

The first section that an oral dosage form comes in touch is the mouth and the esophagus. The next section is the stomach. These two are not that much important in the angle of oral drug absorption excepting for sublingual/buccal delivery. Absorption from the mouth is some times possible. That is one reason for the development of mucoadhesive patches for mouth delivery. Because absorption from the stomach is negligible for most drugs, due to the small surface area and time that is available for absorption, until it is recognized that significant absorption is achieved through stomach, in every likely it is possible to develop a dosage form that can stay in the stomach for longer period of time leading to sustained release of the drug, thereby enhancing the bioavailability.

Small intestine is the next section that a drug enters. Small intestine is described as a tube with a total length of approximately 250 cm in 70 kg male and linearly decreasing radius ranging from 1.65 cm to approximately 0.90 cm at the distal end. This can be further divided into the duodenum (19 cm length), the jejunum (102 cm length), and the ileum (153 cm length). The average pH of intestinal fluids in each area are as follow: duodenum: 5.0 to 6.0; jejunum: 6.0 to 7.0; ileum: 7.5. Since pH is very important controlling factor in allowing the drug stature that decides the drug absorption, this would be an important factor. The other major factor that may some time contribute is the composition of the fluids in each individual location. The inner surface of the small intestine that is in contact with the luminal fluid is largely increased due to the three structural elements: the folds, villi and microvilli. The large folds are typically found from the lower half of the duodenum to about mid-ileum. The villi become smaller and their density becomes lower as we move further in the small intestine. Villi are cylindrical membrane pouches that incorporate blood vessels inside, outside and along them. Since they extend through out the small intestine as cylindrical tubes, the effective surface area for drug absorption would be equivalent to a tennis court. Thus, because of this enormous surface area, in ideal conditions drug absorption through small intestines is the highest.

And the final organ of the digestive tract is the large intestine, which includes the colon and rectum. The large intestine is the site for water resorption and the production of feces. Seldom does drug absorption take place in this region. The pH of the large intestine is 5.5-7, and like the buccal area, blood that drains the rectum is not first transported to the liver. Absorption that takes place in the rectum (from rectal suppositories and enemas) goes into the systemic circulation without biotransformation that takes place due to liver enzymes. Colon is the final stage of drug absorption. Previously this section was not considered as important in drug absorption. However, of late it has been recognized for peptide and protein drugs that this is a fine target for drug delivery. The main reason for such investigations is the less presence of degradation enzymes and microbial flora that is normally present in the small intestine. Although folds and villi are absent in the colonic mucosa and, thus, the effective surface area is much smaller compared to the small intestine, the longer time of exposure can result in a high extent of absorption, comparable in some cases to absorption in the small intestine. Colon could be conveniently described as of length 1.5 m and a diameter of 7 cm. As a first approximation, the effective surface area is identical to the cylindrical area of the segment.

Solutes

Solutes as related to drug transport could be classified in several ways. In the older days these substances were purely classified into organic and inorganic. With further progress the classification became more of therapeutic or could be called pharmacological classification. This was when many of these candidates were synthesized and were entering into the arena of potential clinical investigations. In addition, classification based on the lead structure was also prominent. Later water soluble or water insoluble compounds was prominent. The other way of classifying the drugs was based on the transport properties which include transcellular drugs, paracellular drugs, active drugs, passive drugs etc. The current trend is to classify the drugs based on biopharmaceutical concepts. Biopharmaceutical concepts of drug substances such as formulation benefits, dissolution attitudes, absorption properties etc. are recognized to be important to understand drug transport. High-throughput screening and sophisticated tools in new drug discovery research further facilitated this process. This type of classification is called Biopharmaceutical Classification System or simply BCS classification.

Classification based on Mechanism of Transport

Based on the transport properties drugs could be classified into passive transcellular, passive paracellular, and carrier-mediated molecules. The overlapping of these properties is very common. However, most often the majority of molecules have definitely one typical transport property. In the case of a molecule having multiple mechanisms of transport it is always the predominant mechanism that governs the bioavailability of this molecule. The variability in the bioavailability that could be seen is most often because of these multiple transport properties of this particular molecule. In this situation, if the molecule is very potent then several means of avoiding the variability in the bioavailability can be investigated as the first means for a transport scientist. At this juncture of combinatorial chemistry this is as well important. The advent of combinatorial chemistry and high-throughput screening technologies has resulted in a large increase in the number of potential drug candidates being identified for development. Selecting the best compound to take forward into the drug development process is further complicated by development time frames that continue to shrink. Together, these factors have increased the need for an intelligent lead compound selection process that is based not only on biological activities but also on the pharmacological and chemical characteristics of the potential lead compounds. Failure to consider any of these characteristics could lead to significant and costly development problems, delays in getting the product to market, or the failure of the development project altogether. A better scientist should be able to predict the possible clinical and market outcome of a new drug substance by knowing the preliminary safety, pharmacology and toxicity and definitely amalgamating those properties with the transport properties. As the number of new drug substances coming out from medicinal chemistry groups is increasing, the outlook of transport scientists should also be parallel to these developments. Thus, discussing this section on these lines is justified at this juncture of drug development. In this regard understanding the basic and current concepts of transport and the corresponding investigations is always helpful.

Cellular permeability is one drug characteristic that is now being considered much earlier in the drug discovery process. Permeability assays using the CACO-2 colon carcinoma cell line are being used throughout the pharmaceutical industry to estimate the ability of potential drug compounds to cross the intestinal epithelium. Traditional permeability assays are very labor-intensive and have a throughput of fewer than 10 compounds per week. Fortunately, however, automation of permeability assays is possible. The Tecan Genesis workstation is ideal for automating permeability assays because it can perform all of these tasks. Unique to this workstation is a robotic manipulator arm (ROMA) that can pick up and move plates, lids, or permeability inserts to and from various locations within its work space. The workstation also includes software that dynamically schedules multiwell plate processing and automatically adjusts the schedule to account for process time variation. Together, the software, liquid handler, and robotic manipulator of the system allow the workstation to perform the entire CACO-2 permeability assay without manual intervention. Similarly there are several workstations in several companies that are routinely performing these assays, atleast in big pharmaceutical companies of developed countries.

Paracellular Drugs

Paracellular drugs are most of the times not popular among new drug leads or new drug substances. This is mostly because of their generally low permeability. First of all, it is well-known that hydrophilic macromolecular compounds, such as endogenous peptides and peptidomimetic drugs, will merely be transported paracellularly via the tight junctions. Tight junctions are the main barriers involved in the paracellular route of transport of drugs. The approximate diameter of paracellular pores is 4-8 A° and 10-15 A° in humans and animals, respectively. Because in humans the paracellular route will not allow the passage of molecules with diameters greater than ~8 Å, this route is unlikely to play an important role in the absorption of most compounds of pharmaceutical interest.

Paracellular capillary circulating macromolecules, such as albumin, by an unknown mechanism, modulate permeability thought to involve the intra-endothelial cell Ca^{2+} concentration. However, there are several other means of modulating tight junctions. A particular thing to be mentioned here is the transport across myocardial endothelium. As the majority of drug molecules are relatively small and lipophilic, capillary uptake in those regions with a continuous endothelium, such as the heart, has generally been regarded as taking place by flow-limited transcellular capillary transport. Little attention has been paid to myocardial paracellular capillary transport of hydrophilic drugs, despite efficient transport of hydrophilic solutes, such as sucrose, inulin and EDTA, by this route. Paracellular transport increases in capillary inflammation. Therefore, if there is a significant paracellular transport of hydrophilic drugs, an increase in uptake of such drugs in areas of inflamed myocardium associated with acute myocardial infarction would be expected to result. Studies in perfused rat heart have shown that capillary permeability of quinidine does not vary when perfusate pH is varied from 7.0-8.0, suggesting that capillary transport involves the ionized as well as unionized moiety. Addition of albumin to the perfusion medium reduced quinidine capillary permeability, which is consistent with paracellular transport of quinidine ions. This suggests that pore size is very important for paracellular transport.

As a support, a recent investigation with the use of SYBYL software would be helpful. The aim of one of the research areas conducted by Rudrakash Sharan during 2001 AD is to model the effect of methylation on hydrogen bonding ability, surface area, polar surface area, volume, lipophilicity, charge, and cross-sectional diameters of a series of mono-, di-, and tri- methyl substituted analogs of arginine-glycine-aspartic acid (RGD) and compare these parameters to *in vitro* transport properties across Caco-2 monolayers. Molecular modeling was used to investigate the structural parameters that may influence the transport properties of RGD and its methyl analogs at pH 7.4. Log P was experimentally determined using a potentiometric method and compared to cLogP. Transport studies were carried out using CACO-2 cell monolayers. Parameters such as polar and total surface area, volume, and Log P were found to vary with both the number and the sites of methyl substitution on the RGD molecule. The calculated as well as the experimental Log P values were found to be less than minus 2. The calculated maximum cross-sectional diameters ranged from 9 to 12 Å. No detectable transport was noted. Results of their study indicated that in the design considerations for the development of new peptidomimetic RGD analogs with enhanced oral bioavailability, an important parameter to consider is the three dimensional conformation of the peptides which influences their hydrogen bonding ability, polarity and molecular geometry. The variation in molecular surface area was both a function of the site as well as the number of methyl substitution, ranging between 340 $Å^2$ and 416 $Å^2$. The molecular volume varied between 358 Å and 416 Å. An increase in the number of methyl substitutions was accompanied by an increase in molecular volume. No correlation was observed between the molecular weight of the peptide and the molecular surface area, however in general an increase in molecular weight with successive methylations resulted in an increase in molecular volume. The maximum and minimum cross-sectional diameters were determined using SYBYL. Maximum cross-sectional diameter varied between 9.2 Å and 11.8 Å, which was greater than the value of 8 Å obtained by the equivalent pore theory for the paracellular space, therefore supporting the prediction of low transepithelial transport of the analogs. Some reports indicate that this minimum cut-off pore size is 15 Å. Thus, in such discussions this has to be always kept in the mind. The minimum cross-sectional diameter varied between 4.9 Å to 7.9 Å. This study clearly suggests that the molecular size is an important aspect that governs the paracellular permeability. However, this pore size definitely varies with the type of the membrane. There is a big difference between endothelial barrier and epithelial barrier. This could be conveniently explained in terms of their architecture. The molecular architecture of tight junctions and adherens junctions is moderately well defined in terms of molecular species, and there are differences at both sites between the endothelial and epithelial spectra of protein expression. However, definition of the size-restricting pore remains elusive and may require structural biology approaches to the spatial arrangements and interactions of the membrane molecular complexes surrounding the endothelial paracellular clefts, suggesting that pore size always varies depending on the type of the barrier for paracellular transport. Although the paracellular route is not advisable, on several occasions, paracellular route is the only means of transport of molecules across the gastrointestinal tract. However, because of the low pore size and the only mechanism that is involved for the molecules to move across is the passive diffusion, in every likely the absorption of these types of molecules could be achieved by increasing the paracellular pore size. Ever since this route has been actively identified to be important for some types of compounds, the paracellular permeability enhancers came into vogue among research circles. In addition, use of this route also avoids cellular metabolism. The other aspect to be mentioned is the use of nanoparticles to facilitate the paracellular transport of molecules. Nanoparticles offer the advantage of protecting incorporated peptides from enzymatic degradation and they can cross over the mucosal barrier through either Peyers patches or the paracellular route. After having reached the systemic circulation the particles are biodegraded and releasing the incorporated peptide. However, the focus with this route has always been the permeation modulation. Thus, the current literature in this area is vast and definitely needs to be mentioned in an understanding way in this section.

Attempts to reduce the absorption barrier are mainly based on the use of permeation enhancers as auxiliary agents in the oral drug delivery system. Due to their low molecular size, however, many permeation enhancers such as sodium salicylate and medium-chain glycerides are absorbed across the gut more rapidly than the drug itself causing systemic toxicity. Interaction of absorption enhancers with membrane lipids or proteins, which leads to membrane perturbation, is followed by an increase in permeability. This could be demonstrated using mixed micelles, middle chain fatty acids, salicylic acids and

Acylcarnitine. These are called low molecular weight (LMM) absorption enhancers. The maximum permeable molecular radius of drugs was evaluated to be 3 nm and the diameter of an epithelial cell is approximately 10 μm. First the area of the cell surface was calculated according to the circle equations. Thereafter, the cell diameter and the tight junctional diameter were added up to reach a total diameter of cell plus tight junction. This new diameter was used for a second circle area equation. The total tight junctional area was reached by subtracting the area of the cell from the total area. According to this consideration the tight junctional area is limited to approximately 0.2% of the whole intestinal absorption area. In one study, chelation between enhancer and calcium/ magnesium ions around tight junctions by the use of EDTA resulted in a decrease in the extracellular Ca level leading to an opening of the tight junctions. The mechanism of sodium caprate opening the tight junctions was demonstrated to be dependent on increasing the intracellular calcium level through interaction with phospholipase C leading to activation of junctional actomyosin contraction. A new way of opening the tight junctions is to administer Zonula occludens toxin (Zot) elaborated by *Vibrio cholerae*. Zot appears to activate a complex intracellular cascade of events that regulate membrane permeability. Several innovations are currently in place in this area. However, the toxicity issues are always the important determinants.

Another class of permeation enhancers that has received lot of attention are high molecular mass polymers such as chitosan and polyacrylates. They display some advantages in comparison to LMM enhancers like additional mucoadhesive properties which allow them to remain concentrated at the area of drug absorption. In general the polymers can be divided into cationic and anionic polymers. Representative for cationic polymers is the widely used chitosan. The permeation enhancing effect of this polymer can be demonstrated via various studies on CACO-2 monolayers and *in vivo* rat models. The underlying mechanism of opening of tight junctions by chitosan is attributed to the interaction of the positively charged amino groups with the negatively charged sialic groups of membrane-bound glycoproteins. Furthermore, anionic polymers such as polycarbophil or carboxymethylcellulose also demonstrated permeation enhancing properties. In contrast to the direct interaction of chitosan to the mucosal surface, these two polymers are shown to express a high Ca-binding ability that is similar to the Ca-binding mechanism of the LMM enhancer EDTA. The depletion of Ca-ions from the extracellular cell medium has been shown to increase the permeation of sodium-fluorescein, bacitracin, a vasopressin analogue and insulin. High molecular mass polymers will not be absorbed from the mucosal barriers, therefore systemic side effects can be excluded. Similarly there are several paracellular permeation enhancers in the market or in the clinical investigations.

Very often paracellular drugs are converted to drugs that are transported by transcellular route or substrates for active transporters, which can enhance their permeability. As an innovation, this conversion took place long time ago in the form of prodrugs, when the innovators of new synthetic leads, which beat the older and traditional plant medicines, recognized that some group of compounds always are troublesome in the *in vivo* situation, although they were found to be very potent in *in vitro* pharmacological assays. However, later on several investigations and rules were developed to avoid this competition to further facilitate the development of drug discovery both as paracellular and transcellular drugs. Now, books are written over these types of drug molecules suggesting that route is not a big issue. However, rules have to be followed.

Let's look at a practical example. DB75 [2.5-bis(4-amidinophenyl)furan] is a promising antimicrobial agent although it has poor oral potency. In contrast, its novel prodrug, 2,5-bis(4-amidinophenyl)furan-bis-O-methylamidoxime (DB289) has excellent oral potency. The mechanisms of transport of DB289 and DB75 across intestinal epithelium have been investigated in these studies to understand differences in their oral potency. CACO-2 cell monolayers were used as an *in vitro* model to examine the mechanisms of transport of DB289 and DB75. Samples collected from the transport studies were quantified using high-performance liquid chromatography with ultraviolet and fluorescence detection. A low permeability coefficient (3.8 x 10(-7) cm/s for transport in apical [AP] to basolateral [BL] direction) and high sensitivity to extracellular Ca^{2+} suggest that AP to BL transport of DB75 across CACO-2 cell monolayers occurs predominantly via a paracellular route. DB289 has an 85-fold higher transport rate (322.0 x 10^{-7}) cm/s for transport in the AP to BL direction) across CACO-2 monolayers than that of DB75. This, with its insensitivity to extracellular Ca^{2+} indicates that AP to BL transport of DB289 across CACO-2 cell monolayers occurs predominantly via a transcellular route. DB75 is transported across CACO-2 cell monolayers predominantly via paracellular pathways, whereas the prodrug DB289 is transported via transcellular pathways. This could account for the much higher oral activity of DB289 over DB75.

To differentiate the basic difference that is found in the paracellular and transcellular compounds a simple illustration is always helpful. A recent case study presented by Umetrics AB is as follows:

The effective permeability (P_{eff}) of 22 drugs in human jejunum was measured in living patients. The 22 compounds selected for the study are transported across the intestinal membrane by different mechanisms. 15 compounds are transported by transcellular passive diffusion (PD), five use a carrier-mediated active transport mechanism (AT) and two are transported through a paracellular route. In order to characterise the properties of the 22 compounds multivariately, a set of 18 experimentally determined and theoretically derived molecular descriptors compiled. The biological activity (BA) was the permeability, log Peff. The general observation was "the passively diffused compounds are found to have high values of LogP and molecular weight". The actively transported drugs have high levels of hydrogen bonding (HBA, HBD, HB) and polar surface area (PSA). The paracellular compounds have low MW and high H and E-LUMO. Although these predictions and rules are there, they definitely do not fall in place for all the types of drugs.

Transcellular Drugs

Transcellular drugs are those candidates that move from one side of the cell to the other side through the cell membranes and the transporter proteins that are present on the membranes. Thus, these drugs pass through all the cell organelles. Since the other side of the intestinal tract (systemic circulation) is always in sink, these are the preferred molecules for pharmaceutical investigations because of their rapid movement across the membranes. Both passive transport and active transport with the help of carrier proteins on the membrane could be included in this section. This barrier, which extends even to the control of water and ion movement, is crucial for the normal functioning of the intestine. Without control over water and ion movement, diarrhoea can result, as observed in a number of intestinal pathologies in which barrier properties have been compromised. It is said that passive diffusion across intestinal epithelial cells occurs through nonspecific permeability pathways. However, further research needs to be accomplished to define these nonspecific permeability pathways. The passive transport definitely involves the intracellular cytoskeleton and the mechanisms of transport. In this regard, it is worthwhile knowing about these structures and mechanisms. Apart from the membrane structures, which are described in detail in this chapter in the initial sections, cytoskeletal structure is also important. These drugs at the highest levels could occupy the entire cell including the membranes and cytoskeleton. Since cellular cytoskeletons are very flexible, statistically speaking there are generally more fluctuations in the transport with the agents associated or conditions associated with the transport of these drugs. A simple example of transport of drug molecules across neuron would be very decent at this stage, to know about how to understand intracellular transport. Simple diffusion is always common. However, in bigger cells simple diffusion could be very slow. Thus, these cells have developed definite cellular functionalities as related to the intracellular transport. Neuronal cells are generally long and thus, this particular motility would be best cited with this example. Motor proteins interact with the filamentous structural proteins of the cytoskeleton to generate the forces required for cell locomotion and intracellular transport. Together, motors and the cytoskeleton function as a complex protein machine. Without this machine, the elaborate organization of the eukaryotic cell interior would not occur. The cytoskeleton, composed of f-actin, microtubules, and intermediate filaments, penetrates the entire volume of the cytosol and is by any standard the largest and one of the most complex intracellular structures. It is not a static structure as the name implies, and its dynamic self-assembly and reorganization is the heart of the cellular processes as diverse and fundamental as mitosis, locomotion, neuronal growth cone extension and guidance, membrane trafficking, and cell adhesion. In this area several questions are yet to be answered. [These questions may include: How do motor proteins couple ATP hydrolysis to generation of force and movement? How is transport within the cell targeted and regulated? How is the structural organization of the cytoskeleton generated, maintained, and altered in response to external or internal events? These broad questions will occupy the field for some time to come. At present most activity in the field is still focused on simply identifying the proteins involved in cytoskeletal and motor function and generating some information on what roles they play. Several other important questions in this arena could include: How are single kinesin molecules able to move micron-scale distances on microtubules (termed processive movement)? What is the relationship between the motor parameters (velocity, force, processivity) and the *in vivo* function of a motor protein? And, what is the intracellular distribution of particular kinesins, and what are the fluxes due to diffusion, binding interactions, and active movement that give rise to this distribution? This kind of information on properties, distributions, and fluxes of particular protein molecules will be required to arrive at a complete, systems-level description of the cytoskeleton.] The answering of these questions could further elucidate the role of the cytoskeletal proteins and cytoskeleton in the passive transcellular movement of molecules. However, at this stage this field is still considered to be in the beginning.

The general guidelines for the intestinal transport and absorption of a drug include:

1. Small amphipathic drugs move efficiently through the transcellular route by partitioning into and out of lipid bilayers
2. Small hydrophilic drugs are restricted to the paracellular route, or to aqueous routes that normally absorb nutrients, vitamins or cofactors
3. Peptides and proteins are poorly absorbed intact and require the application of enhancing agents or special uptake mechanisms
4. In general, the permeability of drugs decreases along the intestine, but this is obviously very dependent upon the drug and the route of transport.

Paracellular diffusion is different from the facilitated transport, which occurs through specific membrane-associated channels or transporters. The importance of specific structural groups and their involvement in altering the solubility and partition coefficient in the passive diffusion of small molecules and peptides has been discussed at several places. Furthermore, the coefficient of drug partitioning between an organic phase (representing the intestinal lumen, epithelial cytosol and interstitial spaces) and aqueous phase (blood) has been used to predict passive diffusion. Small molecule drugs that are too hydrophilic cannot enter the lipid bilayer, and those that are too lipophilic tend not to leave it. Transport of peptides across epithelia cannot be predicted by this index, but rather by the number of hydrogen bonds that must be broken for the molecule to traverse the membrane. In some cases, prodrugs modified to mask charged hydrophilic regions show sufficiently improved passive diffusion to warrant this modification.

As related to the active transporter or the facilitated diffusion, several transporters are present on the intestinal membranes. Several scientists visioned the presence of transporters for drugs very early on when they found that the transporters export the common food substrates such as glucose. Unfortunately, during these stages the orientation was more rapid generation of the molecules, which could be used, for clinical investigations. In addition, most of these were accidental discoveries. However, with time several transporters for drugs have been recognized. Some of these transporters are very well characterized by now. The major transporters include peptide transporter, monocarboxylic acid transporter, organic anion transporter, organic ion transporter, and nucleoside transporter. Peptide transporters mediate hydrogen ion coupled active transport of di- or tripeptides across the brush-border membranes of the small intestine and the renal promimal tubules. These are important and there is always an exchange in this regard. The acidic luminal pH generated by the Na^+/H^+ exchanger (NHE3) expressed in the brush-border membrane serves as the driving force for the transport of small peptides. Several examples of peptide drugs include b-lactam antibiotics, anticancer agent bestatin, angiotensin converting enzyme inhibitors, rennin inhibitors and thrombin inhibitors. PEPT1 and PEPT2 can be considered examples of peptide transporters. PEPT1 is the most widely studied transporter. Several scientists were involved in the investigations and characterizations associated with the transporter PEPT1. The most general substrates for PEPT1 are di- or tripeptides. Several di- and tri-peptides are currently under pharmacological investigations and thus it would be of research interest to site these transporters and their specific functions. In addition, several drugs are also substrates for PEPT1 transporter. PEPT2 is functionally active and localized on the apical membrane of rat choroid plexus epithelial cells. However, little is known about the transport mechanisms of endogenous neuropeptides in choroid plexus, and the role of PEPT2 in this process. This transporter mediates the cellular uptake of di- and tripeptides and selected drugs by proton-substrate cotransport across the plasma membrane. PEPT2 was functionally identified initially in the apical membrane of renal tubular cells but was later shown to be expressed in other tissues also.

In general, peptide transporters have broad substrate requirements and tolerate diverse chemical modification. In addition to the endogenous peptides, various therapeutic drugs, including nonpeptidyl drugs, can be recognized as substrates by peptide transporters. β-lactam antibiotics, ACE inhibitors, renin inhibitors, and bestatin are well-known substrates for peptide transporters and possess peptide-like chemical structures with a peptide bond, an N-terminal α-amino group, and a C-terminal carboxyl group. Substitution of an N-terminal α-amino group or a C-terminal carboxyl group of the peptidyl substrates may significantly reduce their affinity for the peptide transport system, but these groups are still recognized as substrates of peptide transporters. For example, without having an N-terminal α-amino group, peptidyl prodrugs (eg, α-methyldopa-L-phenylalanine), β-lactam antibiotics (eg, cefixime or cefdinir), and ACE inhibitors (eg,captopril, enalapril, quinapril, or benazepril) have been shown to be transported via the intestinal peptide transport system. Also, thyrotropin-releasing hormone and some renin inhibitors lacking a free C-terminal carboxyl group are reported as the substrates of peptide transporters. Therefore, an N-terminal α-amino group and a C-terminal carboxyl group do not appear to be critical requirements for the peptide transporters, although modification of these groups generally diminishes the substrate affinity to the transporters.

Several current investigations in this area indicate that the intestinal and renal peptide transporters are stereoselective. Peptidomimetic drugs as well as peptides containing L-amino acids interact with peptide transporters with greater affinity than do those containing D-amino acids. In addition, a D-amino acid at the N-terminal end of a peptide may have a greater effect on transport than one at the carboxyl terminal end. Until recently, the presence of a peptide bond in the substrate has been considered a prerequisite for recognition by peptide transporters. However, recent findings on the nonpeptidyl substrates of peptide transporters such as arpharmenine A, 4-aminophenylacetic acid, and amino acid ester prodrugs of acyclovir and zidovudine (AZT) strongly challenge the obligatory need for a peptide bond. Arphamenine A, an Arg-Phe analogue without a peptide bond, appeared to be the substrate of peptide transporters in CACO-2 cells, as well as renal brush border membrane vesicles. This study suggests that these peptide transporters can be conveniently used to develop new drug substances. As the entire summary at this time indicates, it can be concluded that PEPT1 is widely studied and several substrates have been found and it is definitely not specific to only di- or tri-peptides and several molecules other than peptide substrates have been found to be its substrates. Fortunately or unfortunately, these transporters are not expressed in all the tissues and since these are found in the intestinal tract, further investigations in this area are mandatory keeping in view their high substrate specificity and speed of uptake into intestinal epithelium.

The next groups of transporters that are worth mentioning are organic cationic and anionic transporters. These are expressed in the kidney, small intestine and liver. They are of similar type and possess similar substrate specificity. However, when it comes to the disposition characteristics, they can be differentiated. Another transporter that can be clubbed in this group is monocarboxylic acid transporter, MCT family (MCT1 etc.). Organic cation transporter 1 (OCT1) is the first member of the OCT family cloned from rat kidney in 1994. Subsequently, members of a family of organic cation transporters (OCT1-3), as well as the more distantly related proteins that transport carnitine and organic cation (OCTN1-3) and organic anion transporters (OAT1-4), have been cloned and characterized. Due to their significant homology, these transporters turned out to be members of the organic ion transporter super family (SLC 22). It is likely that OCT1 and OCT3 are expressed in the small intestine. It is not only the biochemical character that is important to investigate drug transport but also the substrate specificity. The other important transporter protein family is OAT family that includes OAT1, OAT3, etc. These transporters are found to be expressed in several tissues including blood-brain barrier and kidneys. They may be similar outwardly. However, the real picture is that definitely there is a difference within each other.

The OCT transporters belong to a superfamily that includes multidrug-resistance proteins, facilitative diffusion systems, and proton antiporters. They mediate electrogenic transport of small organic cations with different molecular structures, independen of sodium and proton gradients. The current knowledge of the distribution and functional properties of cloned cation transport systems and of cation transport measured in intact plasma membranes is used to postulate identical or homologous transporters in intestine, liver, kidney, and brain. Thus, this transporter might play a major role in the drug transport across the intestines. These are expressed in the brush-border of the intestines along with being expressed at several other tissues. Mammalian kidney and liver are critical in maintaining physiological ionic environment. Kidney specializes in removing toxins, drugs, and other organic cations from the blood by a process called "renal secretion". Organic solutes must enter the cell (influx) via the basolateral membrane, move inside the cells, and then be transported into the lumen across the apical membrane (efflux).

Functional studies have identified two distinct categories of organic cation transporters (OCTs): a system driven by transmembrane potential difference that governs the influx of cations, whereas the H^+-gradient-dependent transport system may mediate the efflux of cations. Several multispecific, potential-sensitive transporters (OCT3) and H^+-dependent transporters (OCTN1-3) have been cloned and characterized from various tissues.

OCT superfamily of proteins shares high degree of sequence homology; display 12 transmembrane domains with cytoplasmic N- and C-terminus. OCT1 (rat/mouse 556 aa, ~95% homology; human 554 aa, ~78% homology with rat OCT1) is expressed primarily in the kidney, liver, and intestine. Rat OCT1 has been localized to the basolateral membrane of small intestinal enterocytes, hepatocytes, and S1 segment of the proximal renal tubules. OCT1 mediated uptake of tetraethylammonium (TEA) was pH and Na^{+}-independent and was reduced when membrane potential decreased. OCT1 also transported NMN, choline, MPP, dopamine, thiamine, noradrenaline, histamine, and spermine but not putrescine. Rat OCT2 was initially cloned from kidney by homology screening. OCT2 (rat 593 aa, mouse 553 aa, human 555 aa) shares ~70% homology with OCT1. In rat, it is expressed primarily in kidney, and traces were found in colon stomach, and brain. Rat OCT2 has been localized to the basolateral membrane of S2 and S3 segments of proximal tubules. In contrast, OCT2 was localized to the luminal membranes of distal tubule. OCT2 mediates uptake of a variety of cations. OCT3 (rat/mouse 551 aa; human 556 aa) share 30% homology with OCT1 and 51% with OCT2. It is most abundant in rat placenta, and moderate in the intestine, heart, and brain. OCT3 expression is very low in kidney and lung and is undetectable in the liver. OCT3 recognized TEA and guanidine along with other cations including neurotoxin (MPP), neurotransmitter dopamine, and steroids. OCT3 has been identified as extraneuronal monoamine transporter (uptake2). The substrates for organic cation transporters include p-aminohippuric acid, β-lactam antibiotics, estrone-3-sulfate, methotrexate, cimetidine, tetraethylammonium, choline, dopamine chloride, 1-methyl-4-phenylpyridiuium, cimetidine hydrochlorie, L-carnitine, tetraethylammonium etc.

Classification based on chemical nature

Although BCS classification is very often helpful, it may not dissect the investigations as related to the drug transport across the gastrointestinal tract. Keeping in view this type of orientations this book is based on, the drugs can be classified into nonionizable solutes, ionizable solutes, solutes with low membrane affinity and solutes substrates for active uptake or efflux transporters. Although this classification may not deal with the permeability, it would help dissect if any, experimental discrepancies with the solubility and permeability studies that may be helpful to place the drugs into the above BCS classification.

Nonionizable Drugs

Drugs that do not ionize at any pH could be termed as nonionizable drugs. Most of the times these drugs do not have ionizable functionalities. Thus, the typical properties that influence their transport across the gastrointestinal tract are most often those factors that are discussed in the section "Intestinal Absorption". Provided there is no metabolism of this drug in the intestinal tract, these drugs transport across the biological membranes using filtration, passive diffusion, and carrier mediated process. In lay mans terms there is no hindrance for the transport of these molecules across the biological membrane especially in terms of fraction absorbed. At equilibrium, the concentrations of unionized molecules on both sides of a membrane are equal. Since the systemic circulation acts as a sink, there is always unimpeded movement of such molecules across the gastrointestinal tract. As a non-ionizable compound, ethanol is not influenced by the low pH of the stomach and is, therefore, primarily absorbed from this region of the gastrointestinal tract, although it is absorbed from the gastrointestinal tract. Theophylline, caffeine, cyclosporin A and diphylline are the three examples of nonionizable drugs. The surface area property of the gastrointestinal tract should always be kept in mind when the transport of non-ionizable drugs is discussed. While many factors influence the absorption of drugs across the gastrointestinal tract, the surface area is the most important factor. For example, based on pH-pK_a considerations, one would anticipate that salicylate would be most extensively absorbed in the stomach. As a weak acid, it will be mostly unionized in the acidic environment of the stomach, which should favor its absorption. In the small intestine, where the pH is ~6, the drug will be largely ionized and, therefore, in an environment unfavorable for absorption. In reality, however, salicylate is absorbed much more extensively from the small intestine than from the stomach, as an applied example. This is because the surface area of the small intestine is several orders of magnitude greater than the stomach. This is similarly the case with nonionizable drugs. The greater the surface area the greater is the absorption.

Ionizable Drugs

Although the BCS classification includes the term solubility when the transport across the gastrointestinal tract is discussed and for further approving generic compounds, it may not be valid for some compounds, especially ionizable drugs. Since this has not taken into consideration, the ionic component of a drug, which may demonstrate significant difference from nonionic form in terms of drug absorption, this factor has to be clearly dealt at this time since this BCS classification is the very latest theory in terms of drug absorption predictions. Thus, classifying drugs as ionizable and nonionizable forms is always beneficial. In many cases, transfer of a drug through a trancellular pathway only occurs efficiently for the fraction of the drug that is non-charged, since the compound needs to cross the lipid barrier. Charged forms of the drug (whether positively or negatively), do not significantly partake in the distribution equilibrium across the membrane. This will affect drug uptake, distribution, and elimination. Not only in terms of absorption this issue is important, this issue is also important in pathological situations. Very often pH is affected in the diseased states, which may definitely lead to the altered drug absorption across the gastrointestinal tract. Clearly, protonation can change the character of a compound either from charged to non-charged, or vice versa. In the former case, the drug will be designated here as "acid" (since this situation is exemplified by carboxyl-groups). In the latter, as "basic" (amines are the most common instance of this situation). Polar molecules and all ionized compounds partition poorly into lipids, and are not able to pass through membranes, or do so at a much lower rate. With molecules that are ionizable, there are always two fractions; one ionized and the other unionized. Thus, the permeability of these molecules is not easy to predict whatever their transport properties are.

The total flux (J_{tot}) of a permeant through the gastrointestinal tract is a composite term, which can be attributed to transport of both the ionized and unionized moieties. The tranport properties could be described by the permeabilities of the ionized and unionized species and the respective K_{pion}, K_{punion}, C_{ion}, and C_{union}. Thus, $J_{tot} = K_{punion}*C_{union} + K_{pion}*C_{ion}$. The ambient pH and the pK_a of the permeant will give the relative amounts of ionized and unionized species. For a base, the fraction of the permeant that is ionized (f_{ion}) is given by the well-described equation: fion = $100/ [1+10^{(pH - pKa)}]$. For any given pH, pKa and total applied concentration it is therefore possible to calculate the amounts of C_{union} and C_{ion}. Different methods to determine the K_{punion} and K_{pion} can be obtained from the literature. This may be some times complicated. The value will be considerably less than that for the unionized species but it must be remembered that the overall flux is a composite term that includes the concentration of the species. The solubility of the ionized species will be considerably higher than that for the unionized species. It may therefore be possible that, given a set pH or permeant concentration, the amounts of drug permeating is dominated by the diffusion of the ionized moieties. Examples of such drugs include ibuprofen and lignocaine. Some of the salient features with regard to the transport of ionizable drugs across the gastrointestinal tract are:

1. The interaction of ionizable solutes with lipid bilayers decreases with increasing ionic strength of the aqueous buffer. The type of buffer also influences positively charged drug partitioning into the lipid bilayers. The interaction of positively charged drugs with charged lipid bilayer membranes is selectively influenced by the pK_a of the drug.
2. For ionizable molecules, pH plays a crucial role. The charge state that the molecule exhibits at a particular pH is characterized by the ionization constant (pKa) of the molecule. Buffers effect pH gradients in the unstirred water layer which can dramatically affect both permeability and dissolution of ionizable drugs.

3. The diffusion of weak acids or bases across planar lipid bilayer membranes results in aqueous boundary layer pH gradients. If not properly taken into account, such pH gradients will lead to errors in estimated membrane permeability coefficients, Pm.
4. A positive correlation between the absorption rate and the lipophilic drugs was observed with a variety of drugs. The absorption of ionizable compounds was poor in the ionized form. Some times these issues lead to lag time in the absorption of drugs that have to be carefully dissected to properly evaluate the mechanism of a new drug substance.
5. Sialic acid residues on the mucin molecules may affect the transport of charged drug substances. This may be the major barrier to the drug transport, especially in difficult situations, especially with the charged drug substances.

Drugs with Low Membrane Affinity

The physical association between the pharmaceutical compounds and membranes is crucial for absorption and its passage across the gastrointestinal tract. The accumulation of a drug at membrane surface may counter pharmacological efficacy by lowering the effective concentration of the drug and reducing its bioavailability. As mentioned previously the physico-chemical properties of the membranes and the drug association may have a profound impact on the drug transport. This is the basic factor that governs the association and dissociation of therapeutic agents with the cellular membranes. Access of drugs to the cells is established by their physico-chemical properties (lipophilicity, charge, and molecular size). The pharmacological behaviour of drugs is very often related to their distribution or non-specific binding in or to the membranes. Transport and distribution of most drugs are considered to mainly result from passive diffusion, which depends mainly on the lipophilicity of the molecule. The major strength of knowing the drugs lipophilicity, however, is that it directly influences the degree of membrane partitioning and hence passive membrane transport of solutes. In fact, from a definition viewpoint, the term lipophilicity is used to indicate the physicochemical property of a molecule which governs its partitioning into the non-aqueous partner of an immiscible or partially immiscible solvent pair. The biological importance of this parameter justifies that the want for lipophilicity data in studies of biologically interesting compounds can be traced back at least to the turn of the nineteenth century. For instance, the partition of drug across n-octanol|water junctions is commonly employed as a criterion for drug distribution in biological membranes. Therefore, the logarithm of partition coefficient (log P) found an extensive use in the conception of drugs and pesticides. However, this rule is not applicable for the drugs that bind profoundly to the membranes and definitely the transport of these molecules is affected and there is a deviation with the partition hypothesis. Thus, the data from transport studies have to be carefully dissected very early on with new drug substances. The binding affinity to the membrane in particular media conditions could be determined by simple determination of apparent partition coefficient and then fitting it appropriately to determine the binding component.

Drugs Substrates for Efflux or Active Uptake

Studies attempting to increase the bioavailability of orally administered drugs have been performed in mice and humans with several anticancer drugs (e.g. the taxanes and topoisomerase I inhibitors) and also with noncytotoxic drugs such as protease inhibitors. Protease inhibitors are important drugs in the treatment of HIV-1 infection. The taxanes, paclitaxel, and docetaxel, have proven anticancer activity in several tumor types (e.g. breast, ovarian, head and neck cancer, and non-small cell lung cancer). Currently these drugs are administered intravenously at different dosage schedules. In this respect discussions associated with their efflux into the gastrointestinal tract is very important. In general, the oral administration of drugs is convenient and practical. An increasing number of oral formulations of anticancer drugs have been developed in the past few years. The availability of an oral anticancer drug analogue is important when treatment must be applied chronically to be optimally effective. In addition, oral drugs could be administered on an outpatient basis or at home, increasing convenience and patient quality of life, and possibly decreasing the costs by reducing hospital admissions. In this regard, as most of these agents have to be administered by intravenous route, development of oral dosage forms is always the priority. However, the aim would be to increase oral bioavailability of these drugs. Fortunately most of these drugs are substrates for efflux proteins found in the gastrointestinal tract. Two important efflux proteins are to be discussed at this stage. These are found to be expressed in the intestinal tract. These proteins are P-glycoprotein and MDR-Associated Proteins. In the beginning they were discovered in cancer cells. However, it was found that these are expressed in various cellular membranes limiting their absorption. P-glycoprotein (P-gp, mdr1, ABCB1) is a member of the ATP binding cassette (ABC) superfamily of drug transporters discovered long time ago. Apart from several anticancer molecules, a wide range of drugs with varying physicochemical characteristics and pharmacological activity, such as verapamil, quinidine, and cyclosporin A (CsA) and the new blockers GF 120918 (elacridar), LY335979 (zosuquidar), and R101933, were tested in clinical studies to modulate the drug resistence. Thus, when these drugs are administered along with the efflux modulators, it is very likely that the bioavailability of these drugs can be enhanced. In this regard, the latest trend is the improvement of oral drug treatment by temporary inhibition of drug transporters. A second type of drug efflux pump, the multidrug resistance protein (MRP) was discovered in 1992. Like P-gp, MRPs are members of the ABC drug transporters and have the capacity to mediate transmembrane transport of many (conjugated) drugs and other compounds. The information about the MRP family is expanding rapidly and nine members have been identified. MRP1 (MRP, GSX, ABCC1), which is present in all human tissues, is localized at the basolateral side of the plasma membrane and pumps substrate drugs into the body. MRP functions mainly as a cotransporter of organic anions. It can transport hydrophobic drugs or other compounds that are complexed or conjugated to the anionic tripeptide glutathione (GSH), to glucuronic acid, or to sulphate. Other substrate drugs for MRP1 are mitoxantrone, anthracyclines, camptothecins, epipodophyllotoxines, and vinca alkaloids. Similarly there are several substrates in the literature for this efflux transporter. Thus, these two efflux transporters could be inhibited so as to increase the bioavaialability of drugs by co-administering with these substrates.

The other interesting aspect is with the drugs substrates for active transport. There are a number of important mechanisms that can explain the variable and/or low oral bioavaialability, such as high affinity for drug transporters in the gastrointestinal tract, which limits absorption, and high extraction of the drug by extensive metabolism in the intestine and/or liver (first-pass effect). In addition, despite the adsorption to the transporter problem, the other problem that is associated with drugs that are substrates for transporters is the variable bioavailability with different dosage administrations. A drug given orally in solution is subjected to numerous GI secretions and, to be absorbed, must survive encounters with low pH and potentially degrading enzymes. Usually, even if a drug is stable in the enteral environment, little of it remains to pass into the large intestine. Drugs with low lipophilicity (ie, low membrane permeability), such as aminoglycosides, are absorbed slowly from solution in the stomach and small intestine; for such drugs, absorption in the large intestine is expected to be even slower because the surface area is smaller. Consequently, these drugs are not candidates for controlled release. In addition, in this regard drugs substrates for transporter should be essentially discussed at this juncture. Drug absorption that occurs by active transport is usually more rapid than that which occurs by passive diffusion.

A large amount of absorptive intestinal membrane transporters play an important part in absorption and distribution of several nutrients, drugs and prodrugs. A number of absorptive intestinal transporters are described in terms of gene and protein classification, driving forces, substrate specificities and cellular localization. When targeting absorptive large capacity membrane transporters in the small intestine in order to increase oral bioavailabilities of drug or prodrug, the major influence on *in vivo* pharmacokinetics is suggested to be dose-dependent increase in bioavailability as well as prolonged blood circulation due to large capacity facilitated absorption, and renal re-absorption. In contrast, when targeting low-capacity transporters such as vitamin transporters, dose independent saturable absorption kinetics is suggested. Several groups thus believe that targeting drug substrates for absorptive intestinal membrane transporters can be a feasible strategy for optimizing drug bioavailability and distribution.

Protein and Peptide Drugs

Proteins are one of the earliest living molecules discovered. Active research has been persued on proteins and now as molecules associated with living matter, there is an ample literature. However, they failed miserably at the pharmaceutical or drug point of view. This is especially because of their three dimensional structure and the size. Although they are very active in the *in vitro* assays, there is always delivery issue. However, after several years of research on these lines, several protein drugs definitely came upto the clinical trials and were stuck up at that stage. Although they sound to be very potent molecules, further amenities of their delivery and their applications have to be investigated. Similar is the situation with peptides and peptide drugs. Though both proteins and peptides may fall at the same place in the classification of drugs, there is a vast difference. The earlier scientists, who investigated, thought that this area is very promising and thus have spent a lot of time on the research associated with these molecules. There was not much progress as far as their therapeutic benefit is concerned. However, areas like proteins and peptide drugs, should never be taken into the corner because of their natural existence and their compatibility with the body tissues. Thus, in this regard, a brief overview of the size and the structure would be of immense help at this stage. This will be followed by drug delivery issues of these molecules. That way the biopharmaceutics of protein and peptide drugs would be better appreciated.

Proteins are polymers of amino acids joined together by peptide bonds. There are 20 different amino acids that make up essentially all proteins on earth. Each of these amino acids has a fundamental design composed of a central carbon (also called the alpha carbon) bonded to:

- a hydrogen
- a carboxyl group
- an amino group
- a unique side chain or R-group

Thus, the characteristic that distinguishes one amino acid from another is its unique side chain, and it is the side chain that dictates an amino acids chemical properties. With rare exceptions, all of the amino acids in proteins are L amino acids. The unique side chains confer unique chemical properties on amino acids, and dictate how each amino acid interacts with the others in a protein. Amino acids can thus be classified as being *hydrophobic versus hydrophilic*, and *uncharged versus positively-charged versus negatively-charged*. Ultimately, the three dimensional conformation of a protein - and its activity - is determined by complex interactions among side chains. Some aspects of protein structure can be deduced by examining the properties of clusters of amino acids.

Peptides and Proteins

Amino acids are covalently bonded together in chains by peptide bonds. If the chain length is short (say less than 30 amino acids) it is called a peptide; longer chains are called polypeptides or proteins. Peptide bonds are formed between the carboxyl group of one amino acid and the amino group of the next amino acid. Peptide bond formation occurs in a condensation reaction involving loss of a molecule of water.

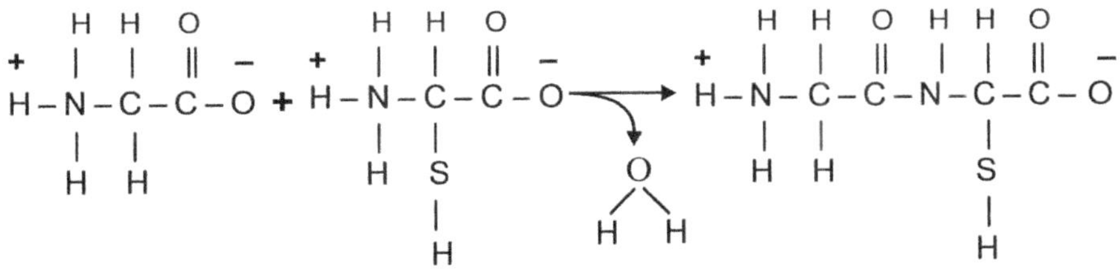

```
    H H  O            H H  O                  H H  O  H H  O
+   | |  ||  -    +   | |  ||  -          +   | |  || | |  ||   -
H-N-C-C-O  +  H-N-C-C-O  ------>  H-N-C-C-N-C-C-O
    | |               | |         |             | |       |
    H H               H S         O             H H       S
                        |        / \                      |
                        H       H   H                     H
```

Figure 5.8 A model reaction between two amino acids to form a peptide bond and thence peptides and proteins which are not so easily amenable to hydrolysis under normal conditions and thus form the building blocks of the living systems. Several amino acids of different natures gets conjugated to each other by a common amide bond to form a peptide or a protein (Further information could be found in chemistry, pharmacy, biochemistry, biotechnology books).

The head-to-tail arrangment of amino acids in a protein means that there is a amino group on one end (called the *amino-terminus* or *N-terminus*) and a carboxyl group on the other end (*carboxyl-terminus* or *C-terminus*). The carboxy-terminal amino acid corresponds to the last one added to the chain during translation of the messenger RNA.

Levels of Protein Structure

Structural features of proteins are usually described at four levels of complexity:

- *Primary structure*: the linear arrangment of amino acids in a protein and the location of covalent linkages such as disulfide bonds between amino acids.

- *Secondary structure*: areas of folding or coiling within a protein; examples include alpha helices and pleated sheets, which are stabilized by hydrogen bonding.
- *Tertiary structure:* the final three-dimensional structure of a protein, which results from a large number of non-covalent interactions between amino acids.
- *Quaternary structure:* non-covalent interactions that bind multiple polypeptides into a single, larger protein. Hemoglobin has quaternary structure due to association of two alpha globin and two beta globin polyproteins.

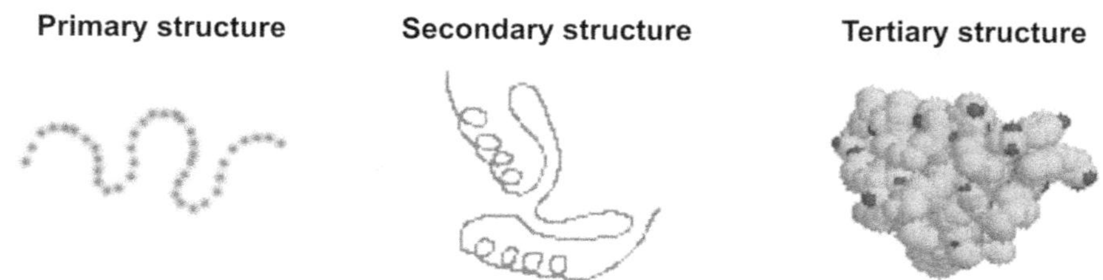

Figure 5.9 The different likely structures of huge peptides (proteins) under different conditions (The first is primary, the next is secondary and finally, tertiary structure; these are very likely the real pictures; although secondary structure may be little more complicated with more medleys).

The primary structure of a protein can readily be deduced from the nucleotide sequence of the corresponding messenger RNA. Based on primary structure, many features of secondary structure can be predicted with the aid of computer programs. However, predicting protein tertiary structure remains a very tough problem, although some progress has been made in this important area. Although the building blocks of peptides and proteins are the same, as a classification as chemicals and drugs, definitely there is a difference. It is worthy to mention the difference at this stage for better appreciation of these both types of drugs as concerned with the drug transport across the gastrointestinal tract.

It becomes imperative to mention more current details about proteins and peptides, their three dimensional unstability for their further understanding of gastrointestinal tract transport of protein drugs. In addition, it is very interesting to note that most of the carrier proteins themselves are proteins embedded in the biological membranes and thus it is definitely worth to delve further on the current investigations in this area. Since the three dimensional structure of the proteins is important in determining their biological functions, this aspect has been investigated by several scientists for over several years. Although lot of efforts were put on in the initial stages on the protein folding problem, the folding kinetics is thus far unclear and thus protein structures are difficult to predict. Probably this would be the case even for the experts in this area who have studied several proteins over several ages. Examples of protein drugs are growth hormone, erythropoietin, interferon (.alpha.,.beta.,.gamma.-type), vaccines, epidermal growth hormone and Factor VIII. Examples of peptide drugs are LHRH analogues, insulin, somatostatin, calcitonin, vasopressin and its derivatives.

GastroIntestinal Transport of Protein and Peptide Drugs

Proteins and peptides are metabolized quite extensively in the kidney, liver, and the gastrointestinal tract via the enzymatic hydrolysis of the peptide bond. Metabolism can also occur in nasal mucosa, the lung, and in the blood. Because large proteins can assume complex tertiary structures, which thus better shields or hides internal peptide bonds, they are often metabolized slower, or less completely than smaller proteins and polypeptides. The enzymes involved in peptide bond hydrolysis, and thus the degradation of peptides and proteins, are known as peptidases and can be found in the blood, in the vascular bed, in the interstitial fluid, on cell membranes and within the cells. These include carboxypeptidases (cleaves C-terminal residues), dipeptidyl carboxypeptidases (cleaves dipeptides from the C-terminus), aminopeptidases (cleaves N-terminal residues), and amidases (cleaves internal peptide bonds). The oral administration of protein or peptide drugs generally results in very extensive metabolism within the GI tract, the loss of biologic activity, and little to no systemic absorption of the original drug. This is due to the prevalence of peptidases within the GI tract, where in the protein or peptide drugs undergo first-pass metabolism. Even if these drugs are administered parenterally they still can undergo extensive metabolism because of their secretion across the intestinal mucosa and from hydrolyzing enzymes found in plasma and the vascular bed.

The fate of orally administered peptide drugs and the action of peptidases in their digestion occur as follows:

As the peptide drugs enter the stomach, where in the gastric juice has a pH of about 2, they are acted upon by pepsin, an enzyme secreted by the gastric mucosa. This enzyme is known as an endopeptidase, which means it can hydrolyze internal peptide bonds at the carbonyl side of aromatic (Tyr, Phe, Trp) and acidic (Asp, Glu) amino acid residues. From the stomach the contents continue on into the small intestine, the pH rises to about 7, and there the peptidases trypsin, chymotrypsin and elastase continue the digestion. These enzymes are endopeptidases secreted by pancreas. Trypsin generally cleaves at the carbonyl side of the basic (Lys, Arg) residues, chymotrypsin at aromatic (Tyr, Phe, Trp) residues, and elastase at small or sterically non-hindered (Ala, Gly, Ser) residues. Finally, the oligopeptides (peptides containing only a few residues) that remains after endopeptidease hydrolysis can be further acted upon by two exopeptidases, namely carboxypeptidase and aminopeptidase. An exopeptidase cleaves at the terminal of peptides. The net result is a thorough breakdown of peptides and protein into single aminoacids and small dipeptides and tripeptides. For the most part, these enzymes are all specific for the natural amino acids of the L-configuration. Proteolysis could be decreased by chemical modification of the protein at planned sites. That way, some times, the bioavailability of the proteins after oral administration can be increased.

Attempts to modify peptides in a way that makes them more resistant to the onslaught of peptidases, thereby enhancing the biologic activity and duration of action, has been pursued by peptide chemists. When metabolism studies indicate a predominant cleavage site, attempts can be made to replace that residue with another that retains the receptor-binding activity of the peptide while yielding enhanced resistance to peptidase activity. Often, this can be accomplished by replacing the offending L-residue with its enatiomer, the D-amino acid or another D-residue. Many peptideases cannot cleave peptide bonds consisting of a fraudulent D-amino acid, and peptides containing such changes can have enhanced biologic activity because of an increase in their half-life. Such successes have been documented. Also, the replacement of an L-amino acid with L-proline or N-methylation of the amide nitrogen, offers the possibility of generating a peptide that is more resistant to enzymatic hydrolysis. The introduction of pseudo peptide bonds and the design of retro-in-verso peptides are two examples of strategies that can afford more peptidase-resistant peptides.

As one might imagine from the foregoing discussion, a major barrier to the use of peptides as clinically useful drugs has to do with their poor delivery properties. This is because proteolytic enzymes present at most routes of administration are able to quickly metabolize most peptides. Peptides and proteins are, for the most part, hydrophilic in nature and for this reason do not readily penetrate lipophilic biomembranes. In addition, they have short biological half-lives because of rapid metabolism and clearance, all of which detracts from their efficient use in drug therepay. It is for these reasons that alternate drug delivery methods for peptides and proteins are an area of particular interest to the pharmaceutical industry. To appreciate the problems of drug absorption via different routes one has to look at the table below. This table compares the percent of dose that is absorbed for two important peptides, insulin and an analog of gonadotropin-releasing hormone, leuprolide, when administered by the oral, nasal,buccal, rectal, vaginal, and subcutaneous ISC) routes. Note the poor bioavailability when the drugs are adminisertered by the oral, nasal, buccal, rectal, vaginal and subcutaneous routes. Note the poor bioavailability when the drugs are administered orally.

Dose of Insulin and Leuprolide Absorbed (%) Via Different Routes of Administration

Route	% Dose Absorbed	
	Insulin	**Leuprolide**
Oral	0.05	0.05
Nasal	30	2-3
Buccal	0.5	–
Rectal	2.5	8
Vaginal	18	38
Subcutaneous	80	65

Antisense and Gene Therapeutics

A brief clue about the synthesis of proteins would be essential to understand the therapeutics associated with genes and antisense oligonucleotides. There are two steps in the protein synthesis that occur inside a cell: transcription and translation. Genes are present inside the nucleus and several proteins responsible for the steps of protein synthesis are both inside the nucleus and in the cytoplasm. A gene is transcribed to mRNA and then this is converted to the protein. Thus, the majority of genes are expressed as the proteins they encode. Thus, inhibition of any of the steps in the process would stop the production or reduction of the production of protein of interest. The process as mentioned before occurs in two steps:

1. Transcription = DNA → RNA and
2. Translation = RNA → protein. Taken together, they make up the "central dogma" of biology: DNA → RNA → protein. Here is an overview.

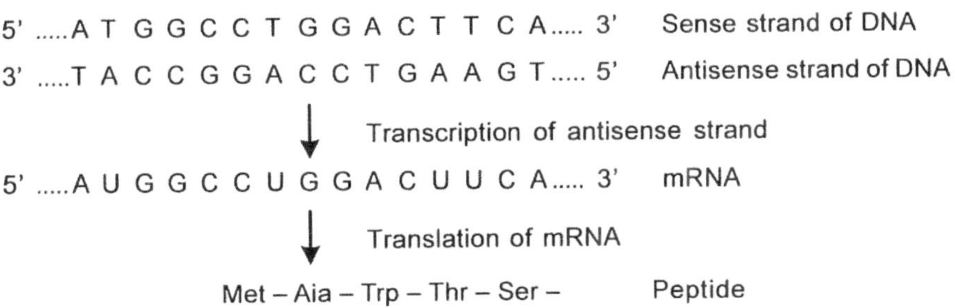

Figure 5.10 Current pathways of the formation of a peptide from a DNA.

Step 1. Gene transcription: DNA → RNA

DNA serves as the template for the synthesis of RNA much as it does for its own replication. The steps involved in the gene transcription are:

1. Some 50 different protein transcription factors bind to promoter sites, usually on the 5′ side of the gene to be transcribed.
2. An enzyme, an RNA polymerase, binds to the complex of transcription factors.
3. Working together, they open the DNA double helix.
4. The RNA polymerase proceeds down one strand moving in the 3′ → 5′ direction.
5. In eukaryotes, this requires — at least for protein-encoding genes — that the nucleosomes in front of the advancing RNA polymerase (RNAP II) be removed. A complex of proteins is responsible for this. The same complex replaces the nucleosomes after the DNA has been transcribed and RNAP II has moved on.
6. As the RNA polymerase travels along the DNA strand, it assembles ribonucleotides (supplied as triphosphates, e.g., ATP) into a strand of RNA.
7. Each ribonucleotide is inserted into the growing RNA strand following the rules of base pairing. Thus, for each C encountered on the DNA strand, a G is inserted in the RNA; for each G, a C; and for each T, an A. However, each A on the DNA guides the insertion of the pyrimidine uracil (**U**, from uridine triphosphate, UTP). There is no T in RNA.
8. Synthesis of the RNA proceeds in the 5′ → 3′ direction.
9. As each nucleoside triphosphate is brought in to add to the 3′ end of the growing strand, the two terminal phosphates are removed.
10. When transcription is complete, the transcript is released from the polymerase and, shortly thereafter, the polymerase is released from the DNA.

Step 2. Gene translation

The steps involved in gene translation are initiation, elongation and termination, respectively in the consecutive order.

1. Initiation

In the first step in protein synthesis, the small 30S subunit of the ribosome binds to the mRNA molecule: this contains triplet codon (AUG, or GUG) at which protein synthesis starts. In bacteria, the first AA-tRNA to initiate translation is always a formyl derivative of methionine called FMet-tRNA. The ribosome is able to discriminate between an AUG within an RNA sequence and at the beginning of mRNA. When this codon appears in the middle of messenger RNA, a normal methionine is incorporated. In eukaryotes, synthesis is started by a special initiation Met-tRNA, but the methionine is not formylated. However, the initial methionine is usually split off from the finished polypeptide. The start of translation requires three protein factors, and the binding of an initiator Fmet-tRNA (or Met) to the first AUG codon found on mRNA.

2. Elongation

Binding of the bigger subunit of the ribosome to the small one, to form the complete 70S ribosome. Then the second AA-tRNA arrives in the Aminoacyl site (acceptor site), and binds to the complex. The reaction between the first amino acid and the second one leads to the formation of a peptide bond. A molecule of water is released (it is a condensation reaction). This only happens after hydrolysis of a GTP into GDP that allows the elongation factor to leave. This delay allows for proof reading, as a wrong tRNA would leave before the reaction takes place. Now, The second tRNA has now moved into place and the now free tRNA has been released. Translocation can take place: it is the transfer of the newly formed dipeptide into the peptidyl site (the first one, also called donor site) when the ribosome shifts 3 nucleotides. The third AA (R)-tRNA can then bind to the mRNA / ribosome complex, and a new peptide bond is formed. This step is a repeat of step two, to show that once the process starts, it is fast, and repetitive.

3. Termination

Termination of the polypeptide occurs when the ribosome reaches a "Stop" Codon. Chain termination leads to the release of a polypeptide, and tRNA, and the dissociation of the ribosome into 30S and 50S subunits. Stop codons are triplets that are not recognized by any tRNA (UAA, UAG, UGA), but by two proteins: the releasing factors (R), (R1 recognizes UAG and UAA, R2 recognizes UAA and UGA). The polypeptide released will be processed in different parts of the cell, depending on its role, and destination. All the processing involved depends on the polypeptide sequence, therefore on the mRNA sequence (and therefore on the original DNA base sequence). Thus, a protein or a polypeptide is formed.

Antisense and Gene Therapeutics

Antisense and gene therapeutics are based on nucleosides and nucleotides. These are the building blocks of DNA and RNA. Antisense oligonucleotides could be called shortforms of the DNA. However, they are very unstable outside and also inside and thus several modifications were in place for some time. Some of these antisense oligonucleotides are currently in clinical investigations. Similar is the situation with the gene therapy. The aim of the antisense therapy is to interface with gene expression by preventing the translation of proteins from mRNA. The mechanisms of mRNA interactions include: sterical blocking of mRNA by antisense binding and destruction of antisense mRNA hybrids by RNaseH enzyme; formation of triple helix between genomic double-stranded DNA and oligonucleotides and the cleavage of target RNA by ribozymes.

Gene therapy involves the method for treatment or prevention of genetic disorders based on delivery of repaired or the replacement of incorrect genes and aimed at treating or eliminating the cause of the disease. The most preferable route is the oral route for the delivery of drugs and could be conveniently extrapolated to the antisense and gene therapies. However, as with protein delivery, oral route cannot be used with antisense and gene therapies due to both the degradation of these molecules within the intestine and their low uptake across the intestinal wall. One possible solution for the delivery of similar types of agents is the incorporation of these substances within biodegradable nanoparticles. Apart from these, these drugs could be incorporated into microspheres and liposomes for their oral delivery. The incorporation of these agents into biodegradable nanoparticles has advantages of protecting the pharmaceuticals from proteolysis within the intestine, or amplifying the uptake capacity of the oral delivery system. To increase antisense stability, to improve cell penetration and also to avoid non-specific aptameric effects (leading to non-specific binding of antisense oligonucleotides) the use of particulate carrier such as nanoparticles, has been considered (the size of nanoparticles is 350 $\pm$ 100 nm). These are used to delivery antisense oligonucleotides for oral route of administration. Nanotechnology in gene therapy would be able to replace the currently used viral vectors by potentially less immunogenic nanosize gene carriers. Vector based on nanoparticles (50 to 500 nm in size) were developed to transport plasmid DNA. Nanoparticles, microparticles and liposomes reach systemic circulation after oral administration by any of the means including phagocytosis, endocytosis or pinocytosis. The other important aspect that has to be mentioned as related to the oral drug therapy is the role of delivery systems for the oral transport of these antisense oligonucleotides and genes. Both these are highly susceptible to hydrolysis and metabolism by various enzymes. Although several modifications to the backbone of the antisensense and gene therapies are always in place, these are synthetic techniques and very often associated with failures as related to the oral delivery of these agents. Several volumes itself are written on these lines and can be found among several literature circles. However, the problem with these chemical modifications is that, although they help in the intestinal transport of the molecules, most of the times they are not helpful in the localization of these classes of drugs at the target locations. The best alternative in this situation is the use of homing devices such as liposomes, nanoparticles and microparticles which both serve to increase their oral bioavailability and further help release the drug at the target tissue. In addition, these systems are also helpful as delivery systems for other classes of compounds.

BCS Classification

Recognizing a need to demonstrate the bioequivalence of drug substances in immediate release (IR) dosage forms, without performing the traditional bioequivalence study, the United States Food and Drug Administration (FDA) has issued a set of guidelines outlining what is now known as the Biopharmaceutical Classification System (BCS). The BCS sets the criteria for allowing a drug substance, in an immediate release form, to circumvent a Bioequivalence study. To be considered for a Biowaiver, the drug substance must be classified as being highly soluble, highly permeable, and having a new formulation with a similar dissolution profile to the original. The FDA will be accepting *in vitro* data for the solubility and permeability components of the BCS. Saving pharmaceutical companies the time and man-power to set up a GLP laboratory dedicated to the BCS, Absorption Systems has taken the necessary steps to provide a profiling service which is in accordance with the FDA's guidelines. Performed under the required GLP conditions, Absorption Systems performs the solubility and permeability components of the BCS for its clients.

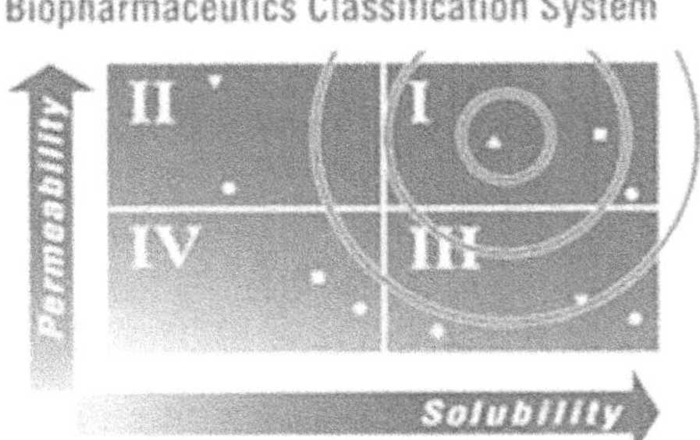

Figure 5.11 Biopharmaceutical classification of drugs (latest introduction in the drug classification supported by the FDA, USA, a very informative classification as concerned to the current new drug substance marking, 2005).

According to BCS, drug substances are classified as (Figure 5.11)

Class I : High Solubility – High Permeability

Class II : Low Solubility – High Permeability

Class III: High Solubility – Low Permeability

Class IV: Low Solubility – Low Permeability

Combined with the dissolution, the BCS takes into account the three major factors governing bioavailability viz. dissolution, solubility and permeability. This classification is associated with drug dissolution and absorption model, which identifies the key parameters controlling drug absorption as a set of dimensionless numbers viz. Absorption number, defined as the ratio of the mean residence time to mean absorption time; Dissolution number, defined as the ratio of mean residence time to mean dissolution time; Dose number, defined as the mass divided by the product of uptake volume (250 ml) and solubility of drug.

Class I drugs exhibit a high absorption number and a high dissolution number. The rate-limiting step is drug dissolution and if dissolution is very rapid then gastric emptying rate becomes the rate-determining step. e.g. Metoprolol, Diltiazem, Verapamil, Propranolol. Class II drugs have a high absorption number but a low dissolution number. *In vivo* drug dissolution is then a rate-limiting step for absorption except at a very high dose number. The absorption for class II drugs is usually slower than class II and occurs over a longer period of time. *In vitro - In vivo* correlation (IVIVC) is usually excepted for class I and class II drugs. e.g. Phenytoin, Danazol, Ketoconazole, Mefenamic acid, Nifedinpine. For Class III drugs, permeability is rate-limiting step for drug absorption. These drugs exhibit a high variation in the rate and extent of drug absorption. Since the dissolution is rapid, the variation is attributable to alteration of physiology and membrane permeability rather than the dosage form factors. e.g. Cimetidine, Acyclovir, Neomycin B, Captopril. Class IV drugs exhibit a lot of problems for effective oral administration. Fortunately, extreme examples of class IV compounds are the exception rather than the rule and are rarely developed and reach the market. Nevertheless a number of class IV drugs do exist. e.g. Taxol.

Delivery Systems that Influence the Drug Absorption

Delivery systems that influence the drug absorption can be classified into those that can affect at the level of absorption (absorption modulators/ alterors/ enhancers) or those that influence the outcome of the absorption (bioavailability improvers, solubility promoters, etc.). Examples of the first class could include prodrugs, chewing gums, wafers, and mucoadhesives. Examples of the second class could include prodrugs, nanoparticles, liposomes, etc. Prodrugs are the first type of delivery systems that can modulate the drug absorption.

Prodrugs are drug conjugates. Upon conjugation with a carrier the drug property can be tailored as per the needs. The conjugate is generally non-toxic and definitely the drug is also non-toxic. Most of the time investigations of prodrugs come when the need arises. When it is thought that the project is not expensive and it can yield tremendous profits, it is taken up. Most of the times the drug is potent. The fortunate prodrug comes into the market after extensive research is performed on it. These investigations are most of the times very time-consuming. In addition, the regulatory authorities consider this delivery system as a new drug. Thus, major pharma companies are only interested when the outcome of the drug product is thought to be beneficial. Thus, this compound is a new drug substance and the entire filings etc. have to be very properly considered. Several kinds of prodrugs are currently in existence. They can alter the absorption of the drug by altering the mode of transport of this drug. Since this reaction is not reversible, most of the times, a prodrug is cleaved at its active site. However, the prodrugs that modulate drug absorption can be either those that increases the absorption or those that are metabolized in the gastrointestinal tract (for formulation benefits), or those that activate the cell membrane permeability (permeability modifying linkers). The next delivery systems that can be discussed include suspensions and nanosuspensions.

According to Lachman (1976) in "The Theory and Practice of Industrial Pharmacy" 3rd Edition", "an important factor affecting drug absorption from an intramuscular parenteral suspension is that of body movement (stirring) at the injection site. Thus, Robinson administered an intramuscular injection of procaine penicillin G suspension in which small drug particles were suspended in peanut oil with 2% aluminium monostearate (Robinson, 1949). She showed that active ambulatory patients had serum penicillin levels that were initially higher than those of sedentary patients. She believes this was due to increased massage of the injection site, which released penicillin into the blood stream earlier. Other workers have confirmed that the degree of body movement influences the onset and duration of benzathine penicillin G depot preparation". This was one of the early successful pharmaceutical formulations. The popularity of suspensions continued. Very early on in the formulation development programs, either oral or parenteral, it was believed and worked on that suspension are the key in the formulation development. However, several disadvantages were realized with the general suspension formulations. One problem is the formation of fibrous tissue after parenteral administration and scratches on the GIT after oral administration. One way by which this can be avoided is by the reduction of the size of the particles. Agitation is the commonly used unit process in the formulation development. This was very early on identified to be the main factor that may influence the final particle size in the suspension and thereby reduce the disadvantages associated with the suspension formulations. Several physical factors were associated in such unit processes. So when it comes to making the final formulation, several other factors have to be considered. The main factors include the mixing rate, the dimension of the container, the flow of fluids, the mixing speeds of the ingredients. Oral formulations manufactured in this way were very promising formulations. However, several factors have to be considered as regarding the improvement of oral bioavailability of the drugs using these formulations. A good physical suspension does not mean that the drug absorption is good. In addition, the mixing, the appropriate selection of the volume of the containers, its glowing size etc. would not help in a nice suspension for all the suspension formulations of all the drugs. Thus, it is anticipated that further requirements are needed to improve the development of suspension formulations.

New drug substances were synthesized at a higher rate compared to the older drug discovery programs. In these situations, there was a dire and rapid need of the suspension formulations for initial toxic and pharmacological activity testing. The maturity in this area continued. It was soon realized that not only the size and the mixing speed matter, but also the use of the impellers, the type of the impellers, the speed of the impellers, etc. all mattered. It was realized that the smaller the size of the vessel, the greater the shear produced with appropriate containers. The aim now of the scientists working in the suspension technology was to reduce the particle size, for a variety of reasons. The older techniques did not help the formulation scientists any more. However, some of the accidental discoveries led to the notice of the preparation of finer suspensions. Some groups were successful and some groups were unsuccessful. However, there was a light at the end of the tunnel. More labs in the Universities and Companies started to investigate on these finer suspensions. These were termed microsuspensions. These formulations were very promising in terms of increasing the drug absorption after oral administration. However, in the earlier techniques used to produce these formulations the generated heat was some times very degrading to the drug as well as the formulation. Several new techniques were actively investigated and introduced into the suspension technology. In this regard, a new term called micronization was used. **Micronizing** is breaking something up to particles that are only a few micrometres in diameter.

The latest focus in this area is nanoparticles. With the formulation development of nanoparticles the first thing that has to come in mind is the simple mixer. Several mixers are available in the market. In the initial stages, the prepartion could be accomplished in a laboratory with the help of a beaker. In this situation, to accomplish better mixing, mixers such as lab sizer homogenizer, ultrasonicator, etc. could be conveniently used. The shear they produce should be enough to obtain very appropriate nanoparticle formulation. However, the pilot scale batches can be prepared using a mixer such as Remi Mixer. In these situations, the manufacturing process should be optimized. Dispersing means may be provided by any of the standard mixing equipment known in the art and may be, for example a turbine or static mixer. If the process is to be carried out under aseptic conditions, it is preferable to use a static mixer. Static mixers suitable for use, e.g. any of those mixers known for use in fluid-fluid mixing. The specifications of suitable static mixers, e.g. length, diameter and number of baffles will depend upon a number of factors including the flow rate and viscosity of the fluids passing through the mixer and may be determined by routine experimentation by a skilled addressee having regard to the foregoing discussion. Thus, the preparation of a nanosuspension of drugs requires lot of skill.

The basic principle of nanoparticles improving drug bioavailability is by increasing the dissolution, saturation solubility and thereby the bioavailability. On most of the occasions these nanoparticles are not taken up into the gastrointestinal tract or their aim is not to get them entered into the systemic circulation. In any aspect it is the solubility and dissolution that is also important with these nanoparticles and not only the bioavailability. The increase in the solubility of particles in the nanometer range can be explained by the Kelvin equation:

$$\ln \frac{P_r}{P_\infty} = \frac{2\gamma M_r}{r RT\rho}$$

where P_r is the dissolution pressure of a particle with the radius r, P_∞ is the dissolution pressure of an infinitely large particle, γ is the surface tension, R is the gas constant, T is the absolute temperature, r is the radius of the particle, M_r is the molecular weight and ρ is the density of the particle. According to this equation, size reduction leads to an increase in the dissolution pressure. However, this effect alone cannot explain the increased solubility and dissolution velocity of particles in the nanometer range. Another important factor is the diffusional distance h_D, which, as a part of the hydrodynamic boundary layer h_H, is also strongly dependent on the particle size, as the Prandtl-equation shows:

$$h_H = \dot{k}(L^{1/2} / V^{1/2})$$

where h_H is the hydrodynamic boundary layer, k denotes a constant, L is the length of the particle surface and V is the relative velocity of the flowing liquid surrounding the particle.

According to the Noyes-Whitney-equation, the dissolution velocity increases with a reduction in the diffusional distance h_D:

$$\frac{dm}{dt} = \frac{DA}{h_D}(C_s - C_t)$$

where *dm/dt* is the dissolution velocity (mass change), *D* is the diffusion coefficient, *A* is the surface area, h_D is the diffusional distance, c_s is the saturation solubility and c_t is the concentration around the particles. Therefore, a reduction in the drug particle size in the nanometer range leads to an increase in solubility as well as the dissolution velocity. Both are very important factors with regard to the aim of improving the bioavailability of poorly soluble drugs. Major advantages of nanosuspensions are their simplicity, fast and cost-effective production method by high-pressure homogenization, the use of physiologically accepted excipients (which is a major advantage in view of regulatory issues) and the broad coverage of potential application fields such as dispersions, lyophilizates, tablets, granules or creams.

Table 2

RBx11082 Formulation Development for PK Studies

- Objective
  - To develop a nanoparticulate suspension formulation for dog PK studies
- Rationale
  - To reduce observed variability in systemic exposure by enhancing the rate of drug dissolution *in-vivo*
- Formulation Development Strategy
  - Wet Bead Milling
- Formulation Requirement
  - Median particle size (D_{50}) < 1 μm
  - Stability (after milling)
    - No solid-state transition
    - No increase in drug-related impurities
    - Suspension homogeneity

R&D RANBAXY

Nanosuspensions are produced by the use of high-pressure homogenization. One method of nanosuspension is presented in the Table 2. Liposome is another class of delivery systems that could enhance the effectiveness of oral therapy of drugs.

The applications for oral delivery of liposomes include enhancement of the rate and the extent of dissolution, enhancement of the permeation of water-soluble and water-insoluble molecules and protection of drug molecules from acidic and enzymatic degradation. Several groups investigated the pharmacokinetic efficacy of drugs in rats after encapsulating in a novel lipid formulation and administering it orally. The AUC and C_{max} with the lipid formulations was more compared to the control formulations. In addition, the transport of drugs across the CACO-2 cell monolayer was also increased. Several charged and uncharged liposomes were tested for drug transport after encapsulating in the liposomes. These liposomes were found to be more effective compared to the control systems in the transport studies. Similarly cumulative amount of the drug transported to the other side of the membrane was more with the formulation compared to the solution form of the drug. Similarly the dissolution of the drug was found to be more in the formulations compared to the solution form. Some of the drugs tested in liposomes were halofantine, gliburide, famotidine, testosterone. The basic use of liposomes for oral delivery would be to enhance the oral bioavailability of compounds either by increasing the permeation or sustaining the release of the drug.

Recently, various bioadhesive mucosal dosage forms including adhesive tablets, gels, and, very recently, films have been developed. Several other novel drug delivery systems are also manufactured using mucoadhesive polymers. This mucoadhesive technology offers several advantages and at the same time currently there are several limitations associated with the delivery systems using mucoadhesive polymers. The main limitation is that it is not known whether these systems are beneficial or deleterious at this time. Toxicity is still a major issue with these systems. Investigations are on their way. The preamble of the use of mucoadhesives came from the highly viscous polymers that were in use for some period. These polymers can include PEG, Acacia, and Tragacanth etc. Mucoadhesive delivery systems have been developed both for the local and the systemic administration of drugs through different mucosal routes: buccal, nasal, and vaginal. Mucoadhesive delivery systems are developed to extend drug residence time at the administration site, and to reduce dosing frequency and the amount of drug administered. Further, to name a few the different mucoadhesive polymers could include carbopol 971, carbomer 940, polycarbophil, methocel K4M, methocel K15M, HPMC, chitosan, its related polymers and carboxymethylcellulose sodium (NaCMC). Appropriate selection of suitable polymers tailored accordingly is very essential and some times needs lot of focus.

Desirable properties for a mucoadhesives can include (i) good adhesive and cohesive strength in moist environments, (ii) elasticity and flexibility, and (iii) tissue biocompatibility, including microporosity that permits gas/nutrient exchange and perhaps allows cell infiltration. While none of the existing commercial products provides a good combination of these attributes, the work is always towards identifying a very ideal bioadhesive polymer. A bioadhesive polymer once administered orally in the form of a tablet along with the drug slowly reaches the site of absorption, where it gets bioadhered. The mechanisms of bioadhesions may be several, depending on the polymer. Slowly the intestinal fluids from the cell layer hydrates the tablet, the tablet swells further and gets attached more stiffly. Slowly small pores are formed in the bioadhesive. Contacts between the lipids of the membrane and the bioadhesive are formed. Generally, the membrane pore sizes are smaller at lipid sites for drug absorption to occur, however, this aids in the binding mechanism. In the paracellular spaces, the pore sizes are large. The biological membrane in the first situation occurs as a membrane and in the second case it is definitely not the rate-limiting step. The tiny pores of the bioadhesives develop osmotic gradients and thereby will push the drug from within the membrane pores to the biological membrane. Because of this osmotic gradient, the drug slowly gets diffused from within the membrane into the cell. This is called dialysis and since the pores are very small such a mechanistic movement could be called microdialysis. This *in situ* device that forms between the polymer and biological membrane can be conveniently called *in situ* microdialysis device. This device can be used to increase drug absorption after any route of administration. Although this might be the predominant mechanism, most of the times the retention time of the system in the device and thereby increasing the concentration at the site of absorption could be the main mechanism of increase in the bioavailability of the drug into the system using bioadhesive delivery systems. Several drug molecules were incorporated into the bioadhesive polymers and these products were tested both *in vitro* and *in vivo* for their efficacy.

Thomas Adams discovered chewing gum long time ago in 1870s. Although his aim was different, he ended up with a very successful and happy discovery i.e., a chewing gum. However, the popularity of chewing gums did not crop up till Second World War. Before this war chewing gum was given routinely among specialized circles. The other form of chewing gum that was widely used was a chicle around the world. He had first tried to make chicle (the sap from the sapodilla tree) into car tyres, toys, masks, and rain boots but every experiment failed. One day, he popped a piece in his mouth and liked the taste. Chewing away, he had the idea to add flavouring to the chicle. Shortly after, he opened the world's first chewing gum factory. In February 1871, Adams New York Gum went on sale in drug stores for a penny apiece, and in 1876 he founded Adams Sons and Company. This has been a very successful business. Clorets, the first heavy-duty breath freshener, was introduced in 1951. New developments in chemical research provide more powerful formulas to fight bad breath. It is interesting to note that altogether the normal chewing gums and drugged chewing gums are totally different. Chewing gums are to be chewed and then after enjoyment to be thrown off. Unlike milk products like candies and wafers these do not enter into the stomach as a whole. Only, a small component of the chewing gum reaches the intestinal tract and then into the blood. Most of the times it is only the mouth that is the site of absorption. The buccal cavity also plays an important role in the absorption process, the formulations utilizing this aspect would have rapid absorption, which is most of the times required for drugs like nitroglycerin. Currently, several chewing gum products are in the pharmaceutical and clinical investigations, and chewing gum products such as chewing gum to prevent ear infection, analgesic chewing gum, nicotine chewing, etc. are already in the market. The complexity associated with the chewing gum is that several uncontrollable factors may play a major role. These factors include temperature, chewing frequency, chewing times, volume of the saliva, distance between the jaws and the twisting angle of the versatility plays a major role.

A small thin crisp cake, biscuit or a candy is a wafer. Although the aim of a wafer was different, it ended up with a very successful and happy discovery i.e., a medicated wafer. However, the popularity of medicated wafers did not crop up till very recently. Before this time wafer was given routinely as a food product. KLONOPIN® WAFERS is approved by the U.S. Food and Drug Administration (FDA) for the treatment of panic disorder with or without agoraphobia in adults. Panic disorder affects more than three million adults in the U.S. at some time in their lives. Today, Metamucin Apple Crisp Fiber Wafer continues to be the pioneer laxative wafers throughout the world. The wafer formulations would have rapid absorption, which is most of the times required for several drugs. Currently, several wafer products are in the pharmaceutical and clinical investigations not for oral route of administration and for local delivery such as brain. The complexity associated with the wafers is that several uncontrollable factors may play a major role. These are the same factors associated with chewing gums.

Apart from the above-mentioned delivery systems there are several potentially useful formulation that could influence drug transport across the gastrointestinal tract. These may include chewable tablets, controlled release syrups, rapid dissolving systems, syrups, suspensions, gelling liquids, etc. may either influence drug transport or extent of drug penetration into the systemic circulation. All these systems can be clubbed together. The disadvantage is that since they are liquid in nature, the drug is not stable most of the times. Included in this apart from the above-discussed formulations are the effervescent tablets. The best example for an effervescent tablet is Aspirin effervescent tablets. Suspensions and syrups increase the residence time of soluble drug in the intestinal tract, thereby enhances the extent of drug absorbed into the system. Chewable tablets are very much similar to the chewing gums in terms of their use as dosage forms. However, their make-up is totally different. Some times they are very valuable. However, most of the times, these products are not in the market because of their expensive nature as related to the new oral drug formulations, although these are very attractive. Similar extrapolations can be made to sustained release syrups.

These formulations generally incorporate viscous vehicles, which have several linkers all over the place, thereby promoting a solution form as well as possessing a viscous background. This viscous background helps in the sustained release of the drug.

The other delivery systems that are worth mentioning at this juncture are gastroretentive drug delivery systems (GRDDS). Gastric emptying of dosage forms is an extremely variable process and ability to prolong and control the emptying time is a valuable asset for dosage forms, which reside in the stomach for a longer period of time than conventional dosage forms. Several difficulties are faced in designing controlled release systems for better absorption and enhanced bioavailability. One of such difficulties is the inability to confine the dosage form in the desired area of the gastrointestinal tract. It is widely acknowledged that the extent of gastrointestinal tract drug absorption is related to contact time with the small intestinal mucosa. Thus, small intestinal transit time is an important parameter for drugs that are incompletely absorbed. Gastro retentive systems can remain in the gastric region for several hours and hence significantly prolong the gastric residence time of drugs. Prolonged gastric retention improves bioavailability, reduces drug waste, and improves solubility for drugs that are less soluble in a high pH environment. It has applications also for local drug delivery to the stomach and proximal small intestines. Gastro retention helps to provide better availability of new products with new therapeutic possibilities and substantial benefits for patients.

Conclusions

The need of the hour for a pharmaceutical industry is to put a better drug into the market. In this regard several chemical, pharmacological, pharmaceutical principles have to be applied. For a pharmaceutical scientist, the comprehension of drug transport across the membranes as one of the major areas is essential. Additionally as the more important membrane is gastrointestinal membrane, the transport across this membrane is important. In this regard, some of the basics of this science oriented towards a pharmaceutical scientist are presented.

Questions for Practice and Exercise

1. Briefly describe the anatomy and physiology of the gastrointestinal tract.
2. Briefly describe the following factors that affect drug absorption across the gastro-intestinal tract:
    1. physical factors,
    2. physiological factors.

3. Mention about the various cellular layers a drug has to cross before reaching the systemic circulation from the gastrointestinal tract.
4. Describe elaborately about BCS classification of drugs.
5. Classify and discuss drugs as nonionizable drugs, ionizable drugs, drugs with low membrane affinity, and drugs substrates for efflux or active uptake in terms of gastrointestinal tract membrane transport.
6. Describe briefly paracellular drugs. What are the common pathways of transport of drugs across the GIT tract?
7. Why is the size of the molecule important for drug transport investigations? Elaborate specifically focusing on different pore sizes and the proteins involved in the transport processes. Why is the pore size important parameter for investigations? Pull out from literature if the pore size varies during disease states. How would this affect the bioavailability of drugs across the gastrointestinal tract membrane?
8. Discuss and detail the importance of the rank order in the paracellular drugs when drug transport is discussed. Describe the paracellular transport of endogenous peptides and peptidomimetic drugs.
9. What are the different methods that could be used to increase the paracellular transport of endogenous peptides and peptidomimetic drugs?
10. Discuss high through put permeability assays.
11. Describe briefly transcellular drugs.
12. How are the investigations associated with the cytoskeleton important for comprehending drug transport mechanisms? Describe briefly the cytoskeleton?
13. What are the general guidelines for the intestinal transport and absorption of a drug?
14. Describe about:
    (a) Transport of drugs across cell membranes
    (b) Lymphatic transport of drugs
    (c) Persorption
    (d) Buccal delivery
    (e) Sublinqual delivery
15. Write about the types of efflux transporters and their role in drug delivery.

16. Write about:
    (a) Cell junctions-structure and role in drug absorption
    (b) Mucus-structure and function
    (c) Permeation enhancers – classes and their mode of action
17. Explain the role of peptide transport in the drug transport across the gastrointestinal tract membrane.
18. Explain the role of organic cationic transporters in the drug transport across the gastrointestinal tract membrane.
19. Explain the role of organic anion transporters in the drug transport across the gastrointestinal tract membrane.
20. Explain nanosuspensions and nanoparticles.
21. Explain liposomes.
22. Explain mucoadhesives and bioadhesives.
23. Explain Chewing gums.
24. Explain Wafers. Dissect and pinpoint from this chapter the various salient features about wafers as delivery systems to increase drug transport across the gastrointestinal tract. Extrapolate and elaborate.

References

1. Sharan R, Rubas W, Kolling W, Ghandehari H. Molecular Modeling of Arginine-Glycine-Aspartic Acid (RGD) Analogs: Relevance to Transepithelial Transport. J Pharm Pharmaceut Sci (www.ualberta.ca/~csps) 4(1):32-41, 2001.
2. http://www.umetrics.com/pdfs/applicationnotes/Case__Drug_Permeability_2.pdf.
3. Ennis RD, Borden L, Lee WA. The effects of permeation enhancers on the surface morphology of the rat nasal mucosa: a scanning electron microscopy study. Pharm Res. 1990 May;7(5):468-75.
4. B J Aungst, and N J Rogers, “Comparison of the Effects of Various Transmucosal Absorption Promoters on Buccal Insulin Delivery”, Int. J. Pharm., 53 (1989), pp. 227–235.

Bibliography

1. The Practice of Medicinal Chemistry, Second Edition, Edited by Camille Georges Wermuth, Elsevier Publications, 2003.
2. Pharmaceutical Salts: Properties, Selection, and Use, First Edition, Edited by P. Heinrich Stahl and Camille G. Wermuth, Wiley VCH, 2002.
3. Membrane Transport: A Practical Approach, First Edition, Edited by Stephen A. Baldwin, Oxford University Press, 2000.
4. Elementary kinetics of membrane carrier transport, by K. D Neame, Wiley, 1972.
5. Gastrointestinal Transport (Current Topics in Membranes, Volume 50) (Current Topics in Membranes), First Edition, Edited by Kim E. Barrett, and Mark Donowitz, Academic Press, 2000.
6. Membrane Structure and Function: Membrane Transport of Nonelectrolytes: Membrane Transport of Electrolytes (Pretest Key Concepts, Vol 1), Edited by John R. Thornborough, McGraw-Hill Publishing Company, 1995.
7. Transport Processes in Pharmaceutical Systems (Drugs and the Pharmaceutical Sciences: a Series of Textbooks and Monographs), First Edition, Edited by Gordon L. Amidon, Ping I. Lee, Elizabeth M. Topp, Marcel Dekker, 2000.
8. Membrane Transporters as Drug Targets (Pharmaceutical Biotechnology), First Edition, Edited by Gordon L. Amidon and Wolfgang Sadée, Plenum US, 2000.
9. Cell Culture Models of Biological Barriers: In vitro Test Systems for Drug Absorption and Delivery, First Edition, Edited by Claus-Michael Lehr, CRC Press, 2002.

CHAPTER 6

DRUG ABSORPTION ASSESSMENT

- **Introduction**
- **Chemical Parameters that Influence Drug Absorption**
- **Predictions**
  - Theoretical Predictions
  - *In silico* Models and Artificial Membranes
  - Neural Networks
- **Cell Culture Models**
- **Animal Models**
  - *In vitro* Models
  - *In situ* Models
  - *In vivo* Models
- **Human Models**
- **Permeability Determination**
- **Conclusions**
- **References**
- **Bibliograpy**

Introduction

With the introduction of new high through put screening methods, the number of drugs reaching the market place is increasing. The average time of discovery process has decreased and the investment of a pharmaceutical company has increased. Thus, in view of the huge investment, an ideal discovery process should curtail the expenditure. Effective drug absorption study models aid in the reduction of the cost of the drug in the early stages of drug development when the possibility of the compound reaching the market place is not yet finalized. These models can be classified into predictions, animal models and human models. These absorption models help in the understanding of the absorption processes and the prediction of absorption across the gastro intestinal tract. Drug absorption through the gastrointestinal tract is the process of getting a drug from its dosage form into the systemic circulation after oral administration. The gastric, superior mesenteric and inferior mesenteric veins of the gastro intestinal tract drain drugs into the liver via the hepatic portal vein and then the drugs are carried to the systemic circulation.

Different *in vitro* models, *in situ* and *in vivo* animal models and human models are generally used to determine the drug absorption. Several techniques were developed and used for over some time. Mathematical principles to calculate the absorption parameters are currently in place. A huge chemical database has been generated over several years. Using the database, several prediction theories were developed or lately being investigated. Such predictions help to curtail the cost of drug discovery in its early stages. In earlier times, the prediction of drug absorption was made by simple physico-chemical measurements such as solubility, and octanol-water partition coefficients. However, these were very simple methods and often tended to the oversimplification of the real values. With the introduction of new technologies and increased database of the absorption parameters, these predictions became sophisticated. Several new parameters and detailed investigations of the older parameters are reported and are currently applied to new chemical moieties. The basic goal of absorption screening of new chemical moieties or compounds either using prediction models or live tissues is to break down to reach a commonality of determining absorption to reduce the cost of drug discovery. Before delving further into this topic, an introduction to Lipinski`s rule of five would be essential to further make understand the absorption study models.

In modern drug discovery process, before a molecule is screened for its activity, ideally a chemist should register the compound in its database. To take the molecule further, the “rule of five” as proposed by Lipinsky is applied to the compound. According to this rule, poor absorption or permeation are likely when there are more than five-hydrogen bond donors in a molecule, the molecular weight of the compound is over 500, Clogp is over 5 (Mlogp is over 4.15) and the sums of n's and o's is over 10. Generally, the compounds that do not fall in this range i.e., poorly absorbed compounds are eliminated. Compound classes that are substrates for transporters and prodrugs may also be eliminated from this rule. Most of the parameters used by Lipinsky to come to his theory along with other important parameters are used in the current practice of oral drug absorption predictions as related to new drug discovery. Since drug discovery process is costly, the most poorly behaved compounds in this area of research are weeded out during this one of the early stages of discovery. As a support to the Lipinsky rule, the majority of compounds that are currently administered orally have molecular weights less than 500 and polar surface areas smaller than 120 A^{o2}.

Chemical Parameters that Influence Drug Absorption

Although absorption, either transcellular or paracellular, play an important role in the membrane transport, the basic phenomenon is a physicochemical process. Thus, transport depends on the physical and chemical parameters termed as absorption parameters. The parameters that influence the absorption include molecular descriptors, solubility, dissociation coefficient (pKa), partition coefficients, and the capacity factor.

Molecular Descriptors

Molecular descriptors that affect intestinal absorption include molecular size, polar surface area and hydrogen bonding. Each of these parameters is interdependent and also co-influential. The correlation between the above factors and the intestinal absorption as studied may not be applicable for all the chemical compounds of a particular series. However, studies indicate that definitely these three molecular descriptors affect the intestinal absorption of a molecule. The simplest molecular descriptor that could be used is the number of atoms. The general trend would show that the lower the atomic number, the higher is the permeability. Such a simple correlation would generate a scattered relationship with membrane permeability, and more fine-tuned descriptors such as molecular size, polar surface area and hydrogen bonding are generally used. The most convenient way to define molecular size is the use of molecular weight. However, this is not sufficient because molecular weight does not give information on the three dimensional structure and the polarity of a molecule. However, experiments indicated that the higher the molecular weight, the lower is the intestinal absorption. Studies with lipid bilayers indicated rapid drop in the permeation with increasing molecular weight compared to the permeation in the aqueous media (Cohen and Bangham, 1972).

Palm et al., (1996) attempted to correlate the dynamic surface area properties of drug molecules with drug absorption. A homologous series of β-adrenoreceptor blocking agents was picked for investigations. The drug absorption for these compounds was not predictable with simple properties like logD. In addition, their oral absorption and lipophilicity displayed a wide variability. Also, the molecular weight and Ka values were similar thereby shielding the influence of these parameters on the results. In that situation, perfect inverse linear correlations between the dynamic polar surface area of these compounds and permeability coefficients in monolayers of human intestinal epithelial CACO-2 cells and excised rat intestine were obtained indicating that the dynamic polar surface area is the most important factor in passive transcellular transport across membranes. Palm et al., (1997) with a series of 20 structurally diverse compounds with percent absorption ranging from 0.3 to 100% investigated theoretical methods for the prediction of drug absorption. In their study, an excellent sigmoidal relationship was established between fraction absorbed and the dynamic polar surface area. Orally administered drugs with large polar surface area (>120 to 140 A°) are hardly absorbed (<10%) by passive diffusion where as drugs/molecules with a smaller surface area are absorbed completely (<60 A°2). In Palm et al., (1996) study, it was found that the high probability of formation of intramolecular hydrogen bonding capacity in oxprenolol would reduce the dynamic polar surface area thereby reducing the absorption. However, interestingly pindolol, metoprolol and oxprenolol, which have the same hydrogen bond formation capacity, had significantly different permeability coefficients, indicating that the theoretical calculation of hydrogen bonding capacity is not applicable to the β-receptor antagonists. They concluded that probably this simple method do not consider the three-dimensional shape of the molecule. The affect of molecular descriptors on drug absorption also comes from the investigations into the databases of the already existing compounds. As per Lipinski, (2000), (J. Pharmacol. Toxicol. Methods), there are 10,000 drugs like compounds recorded. The physico-chemical properties of these compounds were introduced into various *in-silico* software programs and investigated. Based on the results generated from these studies, rule of 5 as mentioned before has been proposed. The molecular weight and polar surface area as hydrogen bond descriptors are key molecular predictors in the rule of 5.

Solubility

Solubility of a molecule is an important parameter used in the description of absorption of a new chemical entity. Once a medicinal chemistry group synthesizes a compound, the first thing that this group could do is to send this molecule to identify its chemical structure. Once the structure is confirmed, using several softwares available in the market several physico-chemical properties, including solubilities can be determined. A list of the solubility properties or the solubility data associated with new chemical substances that a software can give its customer include:

- pH-dependent solubility at different pH values
- intrinsic solubility (of the neutral form)
- solubility of the compound in pure (unbuffered) water
- the solubility in g/l or mol/l units
- solubility calculations even without the melting point and aggregate state data and
- allowing users to limit the calculation time per compound to speed up processing of large volumes of data.

The methods that are described above are software generated. However, very routinely before even the structure of a compound is determined, the solubility can be determined using simple laboratory experiments. In a laboratory, the solubility is determined by dissolving the drug in the desired medium. The end point of the solubility is when a clear solution is obtained. Several techniques are in place to obtain this end point. However, agitation is very commonly used. When a scientist makes sure that the compound is soluble in a particular solvent then filtration is performed, the filtrate is assayed to have an estimate of the drug in the solvent. The technique of solubility determination could be tailored according to the convenience depending on the drug. It is some times very ignorance to consider the solubility studies as trivial esp. for highly water-soluble drugs. However, initial investigations and determinations would be very essential for further formulation developments. The other aspect of solubility is dissolution. To determine the solubility of a poorly soluble compound in water, generally 24 hours equilibration time is given. During this time the drug slowly dissolves in water. It is a similar phenomenon with the dissolution of a drug in gastric fluid or dissolution media from a solid powder or a capsule or from a tablet dosage form. The drug is slowly dissolved and the drug dispersed by agitation to form a uniform solution. It is then analyzed to obtain the concentration of the drug in the dissolution medium. Drugs with limited solubility (<1%) in the fluids of the gastrointestinal tract often exhibit poor or erratic absorption unless dosage forms are specially tailored for the drug. However, solubility profiles are not predictors of biologic performance, but do provide rationale for more extensive *in vivo* studies and formulation development prior to drug evaluation in humans.

Dissociation Coefficient (pKa)

Dissociation constant is one of the most important characteristics of a pharmaceutical compound in terms of new drug discovery as well as to understand and predict the absorption of molecules across the gastro intestinal tract. Thus, understanding the importance of the dissociation constant and its calculation is a very important consideration in new drug development. Lists of some drugs that are weak acids or bases are in the Table 1. In addition, several drugs are weak acids or weak bases and like acetic acid or like ammonia, they react with water to form conjugate pairs. The mathematic expression of the extent of dissociation is called the dissociation constant.

Weak Acid Drug + Water <=> H_3O^+ + Weak Base Drug Anion$^-$
acid base conjugate acid conjugate base

Weak Base Drug + Water <=> OH^- + H^+Weak Base Drug
base acid conjugate base conjugate acid

Proton transfer exists not only with water, but occurs for all electrolytes that are in solution. Because water is the very common solvent used, most of the derivations and equations are generally in aqueous medium. Dissociation constant is sometimes called the acidity constant or the ionization constant. It is a numeric representative of the relative proton transfer for that substance, or the likelihood of that compound donating a proton. It is calculated in the same fashion as the equilibrium constant. Drug pharmaceutics and the determination of useful dosage forms and regimens for drugs depend upon an understanding of drug dissociation and the extent of dissociation that will occur in the systems of the body. Dissociation constant is one of the most important characteristics of a pharmaceutical compound. It is important to understand both how it is calculated, and its significance.

Let's take a look at our equation for the protolysis of water by an acidic drug.

$$HA + H_2O \Longleftrightarrow H_3O^+ + A^-$$

At equilibrium, the velocity of the reaction proceeding to the ionized components (k_1) is equal to the velocity of the reaction resulting in the unionized HA and H_2O (k_2).

$$(k_1) = [HA][H_2O]$$

$$(k_2) = [H_3O^+][A^-]$$

Most drugs are weak acids and bases. They ionize only slightly in the presence of water. That being the case, the concentration of water in the above equation may be taken as a constant, allowing us to rearrange the equation to yield:

$$k_a = k_2(55.53)/k_1 = [A^-][H3O^+]/[HA]$$

where 55.53 is the number of moles of water per liter at 25°C.

This value, k_a, gives us numeric value to express the degree to which a compound ionizes, or dissociates, in aqueous solution. This dissociation constant is an important characteristic of drug molecules, and provides a tool to anticipate some of the "behaviors" of that compound. Dissociation constants are determined by experimental data, and are unique to each molecule. Conductivity, freezing point depression, pH of solution, and spectrophotometric data may be used to determine a compound's dissociation constant.

Table 1

Acidic Drugs: **$HA + H_2O \Longleftrightarrow H_3O^+ + A^-$**	**Ka**	**kb***	**Pka**	**pkb***
Penicillin V	$2.0\text{x}10^{-3}$	$5.4\text{x}10^{-12}$	2.7	11.3
Acetylsalicylic Acid (Aspirin)	$3.3\text{x}10^{-4}$	$3.1\text{x}10^{-11}$	3.5	10.5
Ascorbic Acid (vitamin C)	$5.0\text{x}10^{-5}$	$2.0\text{x}10^{-10}$	4.3	9.7
Phenobarbital	$3.9\text{x}10^{-8}$	$2.6\text{x}10^{-7}$	7.4	6.6
Phenytoin (Dilantin®)	$7.9\text{x}10^{-9}$	$1.3\text{x}10^{-6}$	8.1	5.9
Boric Acid	$5.8\text{x}10^{-10}$	$1.7\text{x}10^{-5}$	9.2	4.8
Zidovudine (AZT, Retrovir®)	$2.0\text{x}10^{-10}$	$5.0\text{x}10^{-5}$	9.7	4.3
Basic Drugs: $A + H_2O \Longleftrightarrow HA^+ + OH^-$				
Caffeine	$2.5\text{x}10^{-4}$	$4.0\text{x}10^{-11}$	3.6	10.4
Zalcitabine (ddC, Hivid®)	$6.3\text{x}10^{-5}$	$1.6\text{x}10\text{-}^{-10}$	4.2	9.8
Theophylline (Theo-Dur®)	$3.4\text{x}10^{-6}$	$1.6\text{x}10^{-9}$	5.2	8.8
Morphine	$7.4\text{x}10^{-7}$	$7.4\text{x}10^{-7}$	7.9	6.1
Erythromycin	$2.0\text{x}10^{-9}$	$6.3\text{x}10^{-6}$	8.8	5.2
Amphetamine	$1.6\text{x}10^{-10}$	$6.3\text{x}10^{-5}$	9.8	4.2

The numeric value of dissociation constant gives an indication of the degree to which the electrolyte will dissociate, that way acids with large ionization constants (ka) are more likely to ionize in aqueous solution. Conversely, acids with smaller dissociation constants are less likely to ionize. The order of magnitude is a good predictor of acid strength. Acetaminophen is an acidic drug with a ka of $1.2\text{x}10^{-10}$, and is thus much less likely to ionize in aqueous solution than aspirin (acetyl salicylic acid) that has a ka of $3.27\text{x}10^{-4}$. In these situations, numerical value is far less than the exponential value. Often, it is cumbersome to deal with exponential forms, and thus another expression of a compound's acid strength is generally used. The pka may be used to describe the tendency of a weak acid to ionize. The following equation should be used to calculate the pka of a substance.

$$pka = -\log [A^-][H3O^+]/[HA]$$

It is interesting to note the relationship between the pKa and acid strength: The smaller the pKa, the stronger the acid. It is just the opposite of the relationship to the ka. Another point that should be made is that acids and bases have both ka and kb, pka and pkb values. It is clear by these examples that acidic and basic drugs may have pka values within the same range. This is often quite confusing. It might help to remember that the ka and pka represent the likelihood of a substance to ionize, not whether or not hydrogen ions will be liberated when it does. The pH, however, represents the hydronium concentration in solution when the compound ionizes. This is how someone could identify an acid or a base.

In the current situations, several software programs have been developed to determine several physico-chemical properties of new chemical moieties. Dissociation constant is one of the physico-chemical constant of a compound that is determined using a software program. One such example of a software program is ACD/pKa Batch. ACD/pK_a Batch is a program that allows rapid and automatic calculation of acid-base ionization constants (pK_a values) for large sets of compounds at once. This package is available for Microsoft® Windows, SUN, and SGI platforms. ACD/pK_a Batch has the same powerful and fast structure-fragment algorithm as ACD/pK_a DB, but it is stream-lined for large-scale users who require pK_a values for thousands of compounds at a time. For each compound, ACD/pK_a Batch calculates the apparent pK_a values (those that are measured in aqueous solution at 25°C and at zero ionic strength) and single pK_a values (those that are measured for all possible dissociation centers when the rest of the molecule is considered neutral) at the specified pH range. Although it has several limitations as of today, it definitely serves several fold in the physico-chemical parameter determination of new chemical substances.

Features of ACD/pKa Software

With ACD/pK_a Batch the following can be calculated:

- Calculates apparent or single pK_a values
- Specifies the pH range of interest
- Calculates the most basic and most acidic pK_a values
- Calculations could be speeded up by defining amides or sulfonic/sulfuric groups
- Labels the ionized groups and corresponding pK_a values (OH, NH group, etc.) and
- Limits the calculation time per structure to makesure high throughput output.

Something to remember:

- A weak acid or a weak base drug, in water, will disassociate to some extent. The pH of the drug solution will depend upon the pK_a.

Partition Coefficients

In the current high-through put synthetic methods, one of the first parameters that needs to be investigated is the partition coefficient. Since partition coefficient reflects the ability of a drug to cross the cell membranes that is important for oral absorption, it is one of the first properties of a new chemical entity to be investigated. In the determination of partition coefficient either a system like octanol/water or chloroform/water are used. Different ratios of the solvents are prepared and mixed to obtain thorough equilibrium of solvents within each other. Then the compound of interest is added to the mixture, shaked thoroughly and subsequently allowed to equilibriate before the drug is estimated in each of the solvent and the partition coefficient calculated using the formula

$$Po/w = \frac{C_{oil}}{C_{water}}$$

For series of compounds, the partition coefficient could provide an empirical handling in screening for some biological properties. For drug delivery, the lipophilic/hydrophilic balance has been shown to be a contributing factor for the rate and extent of drug absorption. Although partition coefficient data alone does not provide understanding of *in vivo* absorption, it does provide a means of characterizing the lipophilic/hydrophilic nature of the drug. Similar to other physico-chemical parameters, partition coefficient can be determined by various softwares available in the market.

Capacity Factor (K_{IAM})

Capacity factor is a recent introduction in the physico-chemical parameter evaluations of new chemical moieties. Since this is a new parameter, it needs further elaboration. Several studies demonstrated the superiority of the capacity factor in the determination and prediction of oral drug absorption over other physico-chemical properties. Chromatography is normally used in the determination of this parameter. The columns are made out of immobilized artificial membranes (IAMs). The lipophilicity in these situations is expressed as the chromatographic capacity factor (log kIAM) determined by high-performance liquid chromatography on an immobilized artificial membrane (IAM) column. One recent study mainly focused on the potentialities and limitations of IAMs as a predictive tool in comparison to the convential methods based on octanol/water partitioning and octadecylsilane (ODS)-HPLC. IAM-and ODS-HPLC capacity factors were determined in order to derive the hydrophobic indices log kIAM and log kW for two sets of compounds ranging from very lipid soluble (steroids) to more hydrophilic agents (biogenic amines). The uptake of the compounds across the *in vivo* BBB expressed as brain uptake index (BUI) has been correlated with these HPLC capacity factors as well as octanol/ water partition (ClogP) and distribution coefficients (log D7.4). The results suggested that for both test groups log kIAM correlates significantly with the respective log BUI of the drug ($r2 = 0.729$ and 0.747, $p < 0.05$), whereas with log kW, log D7.4 and ClogP there is only a correlation for the group of steroids ($r2 = 0.789$, 0.659 and 0.809, $p < 0.05$) but not for the group of biogenic amines. There was a good correlation between log kIAM and log kW. ClogP or log D7.4 for the group of steroids ($r2 = 0.945.0867$ and 0.974, $p < 0.01$) but not for the biogenic amines. Thus, this study indicated that all the physico-chemical descriptors examined in this study equally well describe brain uptake of lipophilic compounds, while log kIAM is superior over log D7.4, ClogP and log kW when polar and ionizable compounds are included. The predictive value of IAMs, combined with the power of HPLC thus holds great promise for the selection process of drug candidates with high brain penetration. Another example for the betterment of the readers is also presented.

A quantitative structure-activity relationship (QSAR) analysis of a series of arylpropionic acid non-steroidal anti-inflammatory drugs (NSAIDs) has been performed to determine which physicochemical properties of these compounds are involved in their diffusion into the cerebrospinal fluid (CSF). The penetration of eight arylpropionic acid derivatives into CSF was studied in male Wistar rats. After intraperitoneal administration of each compound (5 mg/kg), blood and CSF samples were collected at different times (0.5, 1, 3 and 6 hours). The fraction unbound to plasma protein was determined using ultrafiltration. The areas under the curve of the free plasma (AUCF) and CSF (AUCCSF) concentrations were calculated according to the trapezoidal rule. The overall drug transit into CSF was estimated by the ratio RAUC (AUCCSF: AUCF). The lipophilicity was expressed as the chromatographic capacity factor (log kIAM) determined by high-performance liquid chromatography on an immobilized artificial membrane (IAM) column. A significant parabolic relationship was sought between lipophilicity (log kIAM) and the capacity of diffusion across the blood-brain barrier (log RAUC) ($r = 0.928$; $P < 0.01$). The arylpropionic acid NSAIDs exhibiting a lipophilicity value between 1.1 and 1.7 entered the CSF easily ($RAUC > 1$). Molecular weight (MW) was included in this parabolic relationship by means of a multiple regression analysis. This physicochemical parameter improved the correlation ($r = 0.976$; $P < 0.005$). Based on the findings of this study, diffusion of arylpropionic acid NSAIDs into CSF appears to depend primarily on their lipophilicity and MW.

Predictions

Drug absorption prediction is an important factor in new drug discovery process. Several methods are in vogue as mentioned in the introductory section. However, any of these techniques require cell cultures, animal models or human system. These are either very simple or too complex. In any situation, they may also lead to a lot of errors. Depending on the experimental conditions, the nature of the selected tissues and other natural errors, the results may fluctuate. Some times several of the parameters may affect these results. Instead, prediction using any of the *in silico* techniques, that may be some times costly, may be used in such predictions. In addition, several software networking techniques could be included as new techniques in this area of prediction of absorption of new chemical substances. One such kind of the new techniques that is described in detail in this section is the neural networks. This review is not to elaborate these concepts in detail but to give a brief introduction to each of the important techniques.

Theoretical Predictions

Clinical development of new drugs is often terminated because of unfavourable pharmacokinetic properties such as poor intestinal absorption after oral administration. Intestinal permeability and solubility are two of the most important factors that determine the absorption properties of a compound. Efficient and reliable computational models that predict these properties as early as possible in drug discovery and development are therefore desirable. Eversince new compounds (synthetic compounds) have been generated and investigated for the use of diseases afflicting human beings, the idea of prediction of their behaviours has been important. In this regard, research in this area progressed with a common series of compounds. To be applicable in a drug discovery or development setting, any model for permeability and solubility predictions have to be accurate, since a high level of false negative predictions would lead to compounds with the potential of becoming good drugs being discarded, whereas a high level of false positive predictions would lead to significant investment of time and money into compounds that subsequently turned out to be useless.

The first step in the development of a model that predicts membrane permeability is to construct a description of the drug molecule. In its simplest form, this description may be the number of atoms in the drug molecule (the general trend would show that the lower the atom number, the higher the permeability). Such a simple descriptor, however, would generate a scattered relationship with membrane permeabitliy, and more fine-tuned descriptions are often required. These descriptors are either based on two-dimensional representations, three dimensional representations and wave functions. Molecules can be represented by their two dimensional structure or by their Simplified Molecular Input Line Entry Specification (SMILES) line notation code. Such representations identify atom types and functional groups, and this information can be used to rapidly calculate the physico-chemical properties like hydrogen bonding capacity, lipophilicity and charge. A number of topological descriptors can also be derived from the two-dimensional structure. Two-dimensional representations provide incomplete information about a molecule, and three-dimensional structures may be required. Further, using the three dimensional structure of the molecule allows several different spatial arrangements that are not accounted for in the two-dimensional representation to be distinguished. The two-dimensional and three-dimensional structures do not generally provide an accurate description of the electron distribution of the molecules. The electron distribution determines the valence properties of the molecules, and the molecules must be represented by wave functions in order to obtain information about the electron distribution. Wave functions are generated by quantum mechanics calculations. Whether simple or complex, the descriptors outlined in this section and several other descriptors may be related to membrane permeability by appropriate statistical methods, and in this way provides predictive models of intestinal membrane permeability.

In silico Models and Artificial Membranes

Quantitative structure-transport relationship models allow the estimation of complex transport-related phenomena from relatively simple calculated descriptors. Such models could be used for the design of structural analogs of bioactive compounds with improved transport properties, evaluation of excretion kinetics, estimation of approximate rates of metabolic conversion for prodrugs or soft drug candidate7s, and assessment of potential toxic effects of novel compounds. Several groups have developed computational algorithms for assessment of the general probability of transport mechanisms for drug like compounds and for prediction of absorption constants for these compounds based on the above properties. These are termed *in silico* models. *In silico* models such as GASTROPLUS 3.1.0 and iDEA 2.0, etc. are helpful in the prediction of ADME. In GASTROPLUS software, the advance compartmental absorption and transit model (ACAT) is used. Predictions in these systems are generally assessed with different kind of input data such as

(i) pure *in silico* input,
(ii) thermodynamic solubility and *in silico* permeability,
(iii) thermodynamic solubility and human colon carcinoma cell line (CACO-2) permeability.

Currently, neural networks have also proved to be helpful in the determinations of drug absorption. The theory behind the use of this software is very complex. However, a brief introduction to this concept of the use of software would be essential at this stage and is discussed in the next section.

It is widely recognized that preclinical drug discovery could be improved via the parallel assessment of bioactivity, absorption, distribution, metabolism, excretion and toxicity properties of molecules. High-throughput computational methods may enable such assessment at the earliest, least expensive discovery stages, such as during screening compound libraries and the hit-to-lead process. As an attempt to predict drug metabolism and toxicity, an approach for evaluation of the rate of N-dealkylation mediated by two of the most important human cytochrome P450s (P450), namely CYP3A4 and CYP2D6 was recently attempted. A novel approach by using descriptors generated for the whole molecule, the reaction centroid, and the leaving group, and then the data was used by various computer techniques to determine QSAR relationships. To clean the input data for their subsequent use in QSAR modeling, Konstantin V. Balakin et al., (2004) performed an initial analysis of the initial training data set obtained from the Meta Drug database. The analysis is based on Sammon nonlinear mapping (NLM) of the initial substrates property space. NLM is an advanced multivariate statistical technique that approximates local geometric relationships on a two- or three-dimensional plot. Sammon maps have previously been used for the visualization of protein sequence relationships in two dimensions and comparisons between large compound collections, represented by a set of molecular descriptors. In this work, this group used NLM for analysis of heterogeneity of the initial data set of N-dealkylation reaction substrates. Five molecular descriptors, molecular weight, logarithm of 1-octanol/water partition coefficient (log P), the number of H-bond donors and acceptors, and the number of rotatable bonds were calculated for the entire initial data set of CYP3A4 and CYP2D6 substrates. These descriptors encode the most significant molecular features, such as molecular size, lipophilicity, H-bonding capacity, and flexibility, and are commonly associated with molecular properties determining drug-likeness of small molecule compounds. The Sammon NLM procedure allows the creation of a 2-D image of the studied five-dimensional property space.

The sammon map generation was conducted using a program developed internally at Chemical Diversity Labs as part of the ChemoSoft software suite (Chemical Diversity Labs, Inc. San Diego, CA.). The nonlinear map was built based on the following parameters: maximal number of iterations 300, optimization step 0.3; Euclidean distance was used as a similarity measure. After the outliers were removed with this technique, they obtained two sets of metabolic N-dealkylation reactions mediated by CYP3A4 and CYP2D6 enzymes. Twenty one molecules were common between these two enzymes, but are characterized with different log V_{max} values.

Artificial membrane techniques are useful in categorizing compounds into low and high permeability groups. These models are not ideal in the identification of transporter mechanisms because of the lack of transporters in these membranes. PAMPA models are commercially available models routinely being used in determining passive diffusion across biological membranes. In these models, a phospholipid bilayer is coated on to a filter and the transport of molecules is studied across the phospholipid bilayer. Currently, these models are available in the market as high-throughput screening techniques. pION has been developing PAMPA systems for the past 6 years. As claimed by pION, so far their scientists investigated 50 different membrane models and have perfected systems that mimic gastrointestinal absorption. Little more than 40 drugs screened using these models have been published in the literature. With the introduction of new high-throughput screening techniques in medicinal chemistry lot of new drugs would be introduced into the market. Further innovations and modifications in the older methods would definitely enhance the productivity of the screening techniques and would further take these models into the next step of absorption screening.

Neural Networks

There are a number of reasons why it would be useful to be able to predict the permeability of molecules across the gastrointestinal tract. Some of the reasons are mentioned in the previous sections and in the entirety of this textbook. Currently, one of the most precise ways of the prediction of absorption of molecules across the gastrointestinal tract involves the use of neural networks. The use of computers for the prediction of transport properties with the help of several softwares has been in vogue for long time. However, neural network concept is somewhat a different concept. It is like a human brain. After several rotes of a statement, a person will be able to repeat it without even looking at it when he is a child. However, comprehension slowly develops. He will be able to understand this statement. Subsequently, after repeated exposures of similar types of statements, a day will come when this child will be able to understand this statement without the help of any person. As he grows, the sophistication increases. Neural network concept is similar to this phenomenon. It is more sophisticated than the routine softwares, which rely on various statistical and regression models. In computer vocabulary and technological usage, neural networks could be simply compared to artificial intelligence. Neural network modeling has been used in the pharmaceutical arena for long time. The first report of neural network modeling in QSPR was the work of Bodor and co-workers on the estimation of the aqueous solubility in 1991. Since then, neural network modeling has been applied to most physicochemical properties, for which suitable experimental data can be found in the literature.

The basic neural network method involves a feed-forward neural network containing three layers: the input layer, one hidden layer and the output layer with one node. Occassionally, network configurations with more than one output have been used. Variability of the networks has been taken into account by training an ensemble networks and averaging predictions. There are several neural network programs currently available in the market. Examples include NeuroSolution 4.0, The ANN program Pythia, etc. Neural networks are used to detect hidden relationships in a set of patterns and Pythia uses back propagation networks to achieve this. It is similar to diagnostics in computer aided car diagnosis and testing. The network parameters (weights) are initially set to random values. During the training phase, the actual output of the network is compared with the desired output and the error propagated back toward the input of the network. A special feature of the program is the evolutionary optimizer. This module of the software automatically generates suitable networks for a given training data set. The best network model was developed using the optimizer and the ANN that achieved the lowest square deviations. A neural network has two phases, commonly, referred to as the "training phase" and the "reproduction phase". During the training phase, sample data containing both-inputs and desired outputs-are processed to optimize the networks output, meaning to minimize the deviations $(\text{OutputData-OutputNet})^2$. OutputData is the output value in the training data; OutputNet is the output value provided by reproducing the input data with the network. During the "reproduction phase,", the networks parameters are not changed anymore and the network is used for the reproduction of input data in order to "predict" suitable output data. Similar is the case with backpropagation networks. In backpropagation networks, each neuron has one output and as many inputs as neurons in the previous level. Each network input is connected to every neuron in the first level. Each neuron output is connected to every neuron in the next level. The networks output is the output of the last levels neurons. The network is processed from the left to the right.

In one study by Degim et al., (2002), Pythia was used to construct an appropriate ANN. The optimizer function in the program was used with MW, log Koct, and charge values were used as inputs and the literature log Kp values as the output. The aim of this study was to predict skin penetration using artificial neural network modeling. The most successful ANN created contained five neurons at level 1, four neurons at level 2, two neurons at level 3, and one neuron at level 4. Other configurations were also studied but none gave superior results. The optimization of the model (number of hidden layers and hidden units) was performed automatically and the lowest value of square deviation was obtained with this model (for instance, square deviations were 0.001131 for model ANN-5421, 0.001231 for model ANN-5431, 0.003403 for model ANN-541, and 0.011583 for model ANN-5221). Therefore, the model ANN-5421 was used for further calculations. It is also interesting to note that an ANN model was attempted using inputs of logKoct and MW (the two parameters) from the well-established Potts and Guy equation. It was not possible to build an adequate ANN from these two simple inputs.

The computer program trained itself (program parameters set as follows: trained until: repetition=100,000, deviationsquare < 0.000170, time passed = 300; use learn rate = 0.5, automatically adjust; finally: reproduce pattern set and show results in native form). Other parameters such as transfer function, etc. were selected as default. The program trained itself until the square deviations were less then 0.00017 (0.000167 is the lowest value that the program could achieve). A relationship between the theoretically calculated logKp values and experimental results using the ANN model was obtained. The interpretation of effects of each descriptor is difficult because the model is multivariate and nonlinear. However, some insight into the degree of nonlinear behavior of descriptors has been assessed with a functional dependence to understand relationships. The value of input variables was varied through its range, whereas others were held constant. The network output was plotted against two input descriptors to generate a functional dependence surface. This gives an idea and indication of how the network output alters in response to two selected input variables. The descriptors were shown to be functionally dependent. Nonlinearity of the inputs was clearly evident, suggesting a very complex relationship. This demonstrates and indicates that the quality of the data has a very important role in modeling; this is particularly important in neural computing.

In the study by Balakin et al. (2004), the aim of using neural networks was to establish a quantitative structure-metabolism relationship modeling of metabolic N-dealkylation reaction rates. The NeuroSolution 4.0 program (NeuroDimension, Inc. Gainesville, FL.) was used for all neural network operations. The modular neural networks were generated, basically with two hidden layers. Modular feed-forward networks with two hidden layers were generated. Modular feed-forward networks are a special class of multiplayer perceptrons. These networks process their input using several parallel multiplayer perceptrons, and then the results are combined. This action tends to create some structure within the topology, which will foster specialization of function in each submodule. Using modular networks, one needs a smaller number of weights for the same size network (i.e., the same number of input variables). This tends to speed up training times and reduce the number of required training examples. The training was performed over 1000 iterations. All the computers actions were performed using a personal computer workstation with the Pentium 1.8 GHz processor on a Windows 2000 platform. Molecular descriptors were calculated for the three structural types A to C using the Crius and ChemoSoft software tools. A wide range of molecular descriptors of different types were calculated for all initial substrates, including electronic, topological, spatial, structural, and thermodynamic descriptors. Electronic descriptors included polarizability and dipole moment. Topological descriptors included Wiener and Zagreb indices, Kier and Hall molecular connectivity indices, Kiers shape indices, the molecular flexibility index and Balaban indices. Several other spatial, thermodynamic and structural descriptors were generated using the software. A feed-forward back-propagated neural network was generated and trained using the entire training set (31 objects) and 121 input variables, which included 120 calculated descriptors and one phantom variable. After the neural network had been trained, a sensitivity measure per feature was obtained, and the procedure was repeated three times. These sensitivities were then combined as the average of three runs to obtain the final sensitivity value for each feature. The sensitivities were then sorted in ascending order and all features with sensitivities smaller than or similar to the random phantom variable were dropped. This elimination process was done in successive iterations for feature reduction stages, constructing a new model based on the new reduced feature set. After the relevant descriptors were found, an optimal learning algorithm was identified. Several different neural networks were testing using the cross-validation LOO procedure. Among the neural networks tested, modular neural networks with 2 hidden layers provided the best predictive ability. This learning algorithm was used in all further experiments. The results indicated that neural networks could be conveniently and sophisticatedly used in such predictions with more accuracy than the routinely used marketed softwares.

Cell Culture Models

In drug transport or solute transport investigations it is the membrane transport that is generally discussed. There are several techniques currently in place to study membrane transport. However, the most common method is to isolate membranes from the live tissues, place it between two chambers and then add the buffer on one side and buffer containing a solute of interest on the other side. The transport of the solute of interest to other side during a particular time is determined by obtaining the sample and then analyzing the solute using a variety of approaches. Several mathematical equations are then used to determine the parameters of the transport across the membranes for this particular molecule. On the other hand, cell culture models as well as single cell transport studies are also routinely investigated. In any case the most common and convenient models currently available are cell culture models. The other current contemporary techniques are tissue culture and organ culture models. Keeping in view their importance and use, these cell culture models are further discussed.

Several techniques, sometimes, totally unrelated, are currently used in cellular or drug transport investigations. These could be termed tissue culture methods or cell culture methods. The comprehension of these separate methods and their respective applications would be very essential for a person attempting to step into this, sometimes, complicated arena.

Tissue culture was first devised at the beginning of this century as a method for studying the behaviour of animal cells free of systematic variations that might arise in the animal both during normal homeostasis and under the stress of an experiment. The study is basically in the undisaggregated fragments of tissues. The disadvantage with such technique is that the study is within a group of cells. Eventually it was realized that cells of only particular type should be used for further processing and studying. The attempt culminated into primary cultures. In this model the tissue is disintegrated into individual cells. The particular cell type of interest is placed, cultured in the media and then is allowed to grow. With proper nourishment and supplies it was found that a single cell growth was possible, thereby allowing the study using only one cell type. This is similar to weeding out technologies in the agricultural investigations. In addition, this technology could also be used for culturing human cells. The cultivation of human cells received a further stimulus when a number of different serum-free selective media were developed for specific cell types such as epidermal keratinocytes, bronchial epithelium, and vascular endothelium. If the primary culture is maintained for more than a few hours, a further selection step will occur. Cells that are capable of proliferation will increase and finally end up occupying the entire surface. This stage is termed confluency. Growth of the cells sensitive to the available surface will stop here and further the other types of cells mainly fibroblasts continue. However, most of the studies with primary cultures are performed during confluency. After the first subculture, or passage, the primary culture becomes known as a cell line and may be propogated and subcultured several times (3-4 generations). Thus, this cell line is not continuous and the cells retain their properties during these generations. However, most of the currently used cell lines in the drug transport across the gastrointestinal tract are continuous cell lines. This situation arises only with a very few cell lines. The ability of a cell line to grow continuously probably reflects its capacity for genetic variation, allowing subsequent selection. Genetic variation most of the times has a deletion or mutation of the p53 gene, which would normally arrest cell cycle progression, if DNA were to become mutated, and over expression of the telomerase gene. This phenomenon is termed *in vitro* transformation or more specifically immortalization. These cell lines now have infinite life span.

The major requirement that distinguishes tissue culture from most other laboratory techniques is the need to maintain asepsis. Although a large surface area for such as laboratory is always not essential, it is essential that the tissue culture laboratory should be dust free and have no through traffic. The introduction of laminar-flow hoods has greatly simplified the problem and allows the utilization of unspecialized laboratory accommodation, provided that the location satisfies the aforementioned requirements. Several consultancies are currently in place for the development of sterile areas. This has facilitated the further development of the utilization of cell cultures to investigate drug transport across the gastrointestinal tract. In addition, several supports of several cultures with a variety of uses have been recently introduced. Thus, the further applications of the use of cell cultures in pharmaceutical industry have increased. Attachment and growth could be done either in glass containers or disposable plastic containers. Most of the cultures are grown as monolayers in t-25, t-75 or t-150 plastic containers. Subsequently, the monolayers are transferred to appropriate systems for further studies. These systems could include permeable supports, filter wells, hollow fibers, treated surfaces, matrix coating, feed layers, three-dimensional matrices, alternative artificial substrates, microcarriers, metallic substrates, nonadhesive substrates, liquid-gel or liquid-liquid interfaces etc. Apart from these requirements, there are several fold media preferences and requirements that have to be investigated or used for drug related cell culture studies.

In any case it is definitely a daunting task to develop models for a particular system. For instance, to study the transport across retinal pigment epithelial cells, the first thing is to isolate the cells of interest from the tissue of interest. The tissue of interest here is the posterior segment of the eye. Once this tissue is obtained, using specialized digestive media, the retinal pigment epithelial cells can be isolated. These are further allowed to grow to form monolayers that subsequently could be utilized for a variety of purposes. This may take several trials before perfectly simulated retinal pigment epithelial cells *in vitro* are obtained and used for investigating several concepts, including targeting, pharmacological efficacy, disease models, gene delivery, etc. Thus things are complicated at this stage. However, if things go well definitely a model that could save lot of time and money could be utilized for any number of investigations if an immortal cell line of these cells is developed. One such cell line already present in the market is a ARPE-19 cell. Currently, there are definitely several cell types that are used to investigate the gastrointestinal transport of drugs. These include CACO-2 cells, HT29-H cells, CACO-2/HT29-MTX cells, TC-7 cells, MDCK cells, IEC cells and REI cells. To understand the transport of drugs across the gastrointestinal tract, either single cell studies or monolayer studies are used. Before describing further a protocol that can be conveniently used in the drug transport studies with the help of a tissue culture model will be presented.

A protocol to Demonstrate and Conduct the Transport Assays using Monolayers

The following describes a protocol for performing 10-day drug transport assays using Caco-2 cells cultured in the 96-well MultiScreen Caco-2 plate. Monolayer integrity was tested by Lucifer yellow (LY) rejection for 10- and 21-day cultures grown using a 96-well MultiScreen Caco-2 plate, a 96-well plate, and a 24-well plate. Comparing manual to automated drug transport protocols was also conducted.

Methods

Caco-2 cells (obtained from ATCC) were cultured in DMEM with 10% serum. Cells were grown to 80 to 90% confluency before setting up the drug transport experiment. Cells were seeded in 75µL volumes at 35,000 cells/well and 12,500 cells/well for the 10- and 21-day experiments, respectively. Cells were fed basolaterally and apically with 250µL and 75µL of fresh medium every other day, and were incubated at 37°C, 5% CO_2 for 10 or 21 days. LY Rejection Method: Monolayer integrity was measured by LY diffusion. 75µL (100µg/mL) of LY (Sigma) in HBSS buffer, pH 7.4, was added to the filter well with 250µL HBSS in the bottom well. The cells were incubated with shaking (60rpm) for two hours at room temperature. LY fluorescence (RFU) was measured at 485/535nm. Percent rejection of LY was calculated using: % Rejection = 100 x (1 - [RFU (LY passing through monolayer)/RFU starting solution]) Results indicate that MultiScreen Caco-2 plates gave similar % LY rejection values as the other plates.

Atenolol and propanolol (10µM) were added apically or basolaterally. Volumes for the drug transport were 75µL in the filter well, and 250µL in the transport analysis plate wells. Plates were assembled and the transport was allowed to occur with shaking for two hours at 25°C. P*app* (APÆBL) and P_{app} (BLÆAP) were measured in both directions using Multiscreen CACO-2 cells. Tecan Automation Method: The automated experiment was performed on a Tecan Genesis RSP 150 (with RoMa) workstation. 400µL and 90µL of growth medium were aspired basolaterally and apically. 300µL and 90µL of HBSS buffer, pH 7.4, were added basolaterally and apically using low-volume Teflon-coated tips. Washing sequence was carried out two times in three-position carrier I. The Caco-2 plate was then incubated in a four-position incubator for 30 minutes at 37°C. The buffer was aspirated off basolaterally (400µL) and apically (90µL). The Caco-2 plate was then moved to the transport analysis plate in three-position carrier I. Drug addition was performed in three-position carrier II from V-bottom plates containing prediluted drugs. 250µL or 75µL of drugs were added basolaterally or apically. The Caco-2 plate was then incubated in a four-position incubator for two hours at 37°C at a speed of 5Hz to allow for drug transport.

Drug samples were analyzed by liquid chromatography/mass spectrometry (LC/MS). Papps were finally calculated. Study results demonstrate that MultiScreen Caco-2 plates can be used successfully in automated HTS protocols to determine apparent drug permeability rates. Using ATCC Caco-2 cells, seeding at densities of 3.2 x $10^6/cm^2$ for 10 days gave optimal drug transport results. LY rejection method results were comparable for 96-well MultiScreen Caco-2 plates and 24-well plates for 10- and 21-day cultures, supporting the use of 10-day cultures for drug transport studies. And manual Caco-2 protocol was successfully transferred to the Tecan workstation. These workstations are helpful in the high-throughput screening of drug transport studies.

Transport using Single Cell Systems

Microelectrodes are small probes that can be inserted into tissues to measure the electrical potential difference between the probe tip and an external reference point, usually another electrode placed in the external solution bathing the tissue. The measuring microelectrode can be placed on the surface of the tissues or directly inserted into single cells. The microelectrode is the interface between the circuitry, for measuring the potential difference, and the tissue material. This electrical contact occurs at the surface of a metal and aqueous solution, with the actual measurement of a membrane potential requiring the movement of charge at the boundary. The chief requirement for a good electrical contact is that the properties of this interface are stable and do not change significantly during a recording. For intracellular measurements the probe is commonly a glass micropipette that has been back-filled with a salt-solution and has a tip diameter suitable for insertion into a cell. The tip diameter of this micropipette is selected to give a size that will not destroy the cell and allows the membrane to seal around the tip once inserted into a cell to record a stable membrane potential. The glass micropipette tip is commonly called a microelectrode, this provides a salt solution bridge between the back-filling solution and the metal circuit contact in the base of the micropipette holder.

One of the benefits of microelectrode measurements is that they can be used to study transport and metabolism in single cells. The way cells modify metabolism in response to changes in the environment is usually studied by molecular and biochemical analysis of whole tissue samples. Microelectrode measurements can be used to report the response of a single cell to a particular treatment. Several techniques to investigate these responses are available. Microelectrodes can also be used to determine the membrane transport properties of the cell. Ion-selective microelectrodes actually respond to changes in activity and this parameter is more relevant biologically than the more familiar concentration (Miller, 1995).

Inorganic nutrient ions can be divided into two types according to whether or not they are substrates for metabolic assimilation within the cell. Ions such as Ca^{2+}, K^{+}, Na^{+}, and Cl^{-} are considered as essential for growth because they are cofactors for life processes, but are not directly incorporated into organic molecules. In contrast, the 'metabolite ions' inorganic phosphate (Pi), NH_4^{-}, NO_3, and SO_4^{2-} are assimilated by cells. The intracellular concentrations of these ions can be indicators of the metabolic activity of a cell. Changes in the cytosolic pools of a primary substrate can indicate the metabolic activity of a cell. Furthermore, the transport of a primary substrate into a cell provides entry into the metabolic pool, so the presence of a particular type of membrane transporter can indicate the activity of a particular assimilatory pathway. These are the very basics of the transport investigations of drug in single cell systems.

Transport across Monolayers

Although single cell systems are not very often used currently because of the lack of technological advances in this area, these are the first methods for investigating cellular transport mechanisms, especially drug transport. However, these would not indicate drug transport across a barrier that is made of a medley of monolayers of cells in the gastrointestinal tract. Currently, these methods are in very advanced stages compared to single cell systems and are very routinely used in high-throughput screening of drug transport across the gastrointestinal tract. The functionalities of single cell transport methods and monolayer transport methods are totally different and sometimes the utility of both these technologies in dissecting drug transport mechanisms would be important. Monolayers can also be used to determine the mechanims when the substrate uptake or accumulation studies are done. In these situations, although the cells are definitely grown as monolayers, they have only one side for the study because the other side is generally a glass or plastic barrier which is most of the times useless. All the transporters and other proteins that may be grown in the apical or basolateral side will come up and thus the uptake and accumulation mechanisms are because of these variegated cell structures. However, these kinds of studies are very preliminary. These studies do not indicate whether the transporter for a particular substrate is located on the apical side or the basolateral side. In addition, things are more complicated because of the most likely overlap, if exists, in the substrates for transporters. Thus, these studies are not generally suggested to make a perfect conclusion in the beginning stages. On the other hand, when transport studies are performed, both the apical and basolateral sides are intact. This is because the monolayers are grown on a totally permeable barrier. However, these techniques are most of the times expensive. In labs with short supplies, the best studies with intelligent planning are the uptake and accumulation studies.

The intestinal mucosa is characterised by the presence of villi that constitute the anatomical and functional unit for nutrient and drug absorption. The presence of villi and microvilli provides a massive surface area for absorption (approximately 250m^2 in a human). The mucosa consists of the epithelial layer, the lamina propria (collagen matrix containing blood and lymphatic vessels) and the muscularis mucosa. Therefore, any xenobiotic entering the bloodstream has to pass through the epithelial layer, part of the lamina propria, and the wall of the respective vessel. It is crucial to select an appropriate model for understanding the rate-limiting step in the absorption process. It is generally the epithelial monolayer that is important for gastrointestinal drug transport and thus very often used in such investigations.

The CACO-2 cell culture model was introduced in the early 1990s, and has become a widely used tool for the determination of the intestinal transport characteristics of drug candidates. CACO-2 cells differentiate spontaneously under standard culturing conditions to form confluent monolayers; although they are derived from a colon cancer, they acquire many features of absorptive intestinal cells during culture. Several reports have demonstrated the possibility to predict the oral absorption of drugs in humans based on their permeability observed in CACO-2 monolayers. CACO-2 cells have been widely used as *invitro* models to evaluate the transport of drug candidates across the intestinal epithelial barrier. Traditionally the assay is performed on 21-day cultures in a 24-well format. Millipore researchers have specifically developed the 96-well MultiScreen CACO-2 filter plate for CACO-2 drug candidate transport to increase throughput and automation compatibility. These plates are quality control released. The design facilitates use with various robotics, and ports provide contamination-free access to cells and medium.

The other important rate-limiting membrane for gastrointestinal transport is the mucus layer on the epithelial barrier. Although the cellular barrier and the unstirred water layer/aqueous boundary layer have been thoroughly studied as barriers to drug absorption, the mucus layer has received less attention. The mucus layer forms an adherent gel layer on the intestinal cell surface where it acts as a lubricant and a protective barrier against harmful agents, such as hydrogen ions and pepsin. It has also been suggested that the epithelial cells are protected from gastric acid by the hydrophobic lining of surface-active phospholipids present in the gastric mucus layer. The mucus layer may act as a barrier to drug absorption by stabilizing the unstirred water layer and by an interaction between the diffusing molecules and the components of mucus. The influence of the mucus layer on drug absorption has been investigated in *in vivo* studies of intestinal perfusion, *in vitro* everted gut studies, and diffusion studies in two or three compartment models. These studies confirmed that mucus is a barrier to the diffusion and absorption of drug molecules. Studies using the mucus-producing HT29-H cell line have demonstrated that the mucus layer is a barrier to absorption of the lipophilic molecule testesterone but not to that of the hydrophilic molecule mannitol. However, a large variability in monolayer permeability and mucus layer thickness over time was apparent in the HT29-H cell line. To reduce one problem associated with CACO-2 cells i.e., lack of mucus HT29-H cells are the best substitutes. HT29 is relatively a new mucus-secreting *in vitro* drug absorption model based on monolayers of goblet cell like sub-clones of the human colon carcinoma cell line HT29. These cells have been shown (a) to form monolayers of mature goblet cells under standard cell culture conditions, (b) to secrete mucin molecules, (c) to produce a mucus layer that covers the apical cell surface, and (d) that this mucus layer is a significant barrier to the absorption of the lipophilic drug testosterone.

Despite the proven usefulness of the model, there are still different shortcomings intrinsic to the model, which have to be taken into consideration when using the CACO-2 model as a screening tool, including the absence of mucus, the lack of cytochrome P450 enzymes, and the inability to study regional intestinal differences in oral absorption. Different approaches have been proposed to overcome these intrinsic shortcomings, such as the use of mucus-producing cell lines (e.g., HT29-H) or cocultures (e.g., CACO-2 /HT29-MTX). To allow the concurrent study of transport and metabolism, models that express higher levels of CYP3A4 have also been developed, including transfected CACO-2 cells and cells in which the CYP3A4 expression is upregulated by adding 1α ,25-dihydroxy vitamin-D_3 to the growth medium. The main drawback associated with the use of transfected cells is the unstability of the vector (half-life of about 4 weeks). The major disadvantages in the use of upregulated CACO-2 cells are their cost (for inducer and coated inserts) and the high variability in the level of expression of CYP3A4. Also, the levels of enzymes obtained by both methods do not always reach the activity observed *in vivo*. The inability to study regional intestinal differences in oral absorption may be overcome by using other techniques such as intestinal tissues mounted in modified Ussing chambers or perfused intestinal segments. These techniques permit studying site-dependent carrier-mediated absorption and metabolism of drug compounds.

The TC-7 **cell line** is a subclone isolated from the CACO-2 cells. Based on a comparion between the TC-7 subclone and the parent CACO-2 cells by Gres *et al.*, 1998, it was found that characteristics between both **cell** lines are strongly comparable, although TEER (Transepithelial Electrical Resistance) values appeared to be much higher in the TC-7 clone. Permeability values of passively absorbed drugs obtained in the TC-7 clone correlated equally well as in parental CACO-2 cells to the extent of absorption in humans. Further investigation demonstrated that the TC-7 clone displayed CYP 3A5 activity. Because CYP 3A5 is an important CYP form in the human colon, the TC-7 **cell line** may be useful for colonic drug transport and metabolism. Raessi et al., 1997, also demonstrated the presence of CYP3A4 mRNA in the TC-7 clone, whereas this could not be found in the native CACO-2 cultures.

MDCK is a non-intestinal cell system that is sometimes used to investigate gastrointestinal transport of New Drug Substances (NDSs). Madin Darby canine kidney (MDCK) cells were isolated from a dog kidney by Madin & Darby. These are currently used to study the regulation of cell growth, drug metabolism, toxicity and transport at the distal renal tubule epithelial level. MDCK cells have been shown to differentiate into columnar epithelial cells, and to form tight junctions when cultured on semi-permeable membranes. The use of these cells as a cellular barrier model for assessing intestinal epithelial drug transport was discussed by Cho et al, 1989. The results suggested that MDCK cells, like CACO-2 cells, are suitable for molecular-permeability screening studies. Interestingly, these cells do not need 3 weeks in culture before they can be used and, unlike CACO-2 cells, they do not express P-gp. Cell lines such as IEC (Intestinal Epithelium Cell Line) and RIE (Rat Intestinal Epithelium Cell Line) have been isolated after the repeated cloning of epithelial cells from neonatal rat small intestines. These cell lines show morphological and functional characteristics that suggest that they are derived from crypt cells. The IEC line was specifically employed to analyze the role of growth factors in epithelial cell physiology, and for studies on the specific functions of intestinal cells (for example, involving amino acids, glucose and nucleotide transport, or cholesterol synthesis), as well as to perform fundamental studies. In contrast, only few studies have dealt with test compounds.

In vitro **cell culture models** of the intestinal epithelial cell barrier have evolved to become widely used experimental devices. Among them, Caco-2 (colon carcinoma) cell line, has been used as industry standard to model human intestine absorption. Though derived from large intestine, Caco-2 cells demonstrate differentiation into polarized monolayer with the characteristics of small intestine, developing microvilli structure in apical membrane of epithelia, and expressing multiple absorptive transporters and several efflux transporters. But this cell line lacks the most prevalent isoform of cytochrome P450 in intestine epithelia, CYP3A4, which also contributes to the first pass effect. A novel *in vitro* model for concurrent transport and metabolism would be needed. CYP3A4-transfected Caco-2 cells can express high level CYP3A4 when induced by sodium butyrate, phorbol ester 12-o-tetradecanoylphorbol-13acetate along or in combination without sacrifice of the expression of transporters. At the subcellular level, multiple proteins function to affect the level of bioavailability of oral administered drugs. P-glycoprotein (P-gp), an efflux transporter, present in apical membrane of intestine epithelia, defending against potential toxic substances, actively transports xenobiotics, including drugs, out of intestine epithelial cells.

CYP3A4 can metabolize the parent drugs from active form to inactive metabolite. The considerable overlap of substrates and cellular localization imply that P-gp and CYP3A4 could pair to act as a coordinated absorption barrier against drugs. Moreover, both P-gp and CYP3A4 can be induced and inhibited by the same compounds. Recently, it has been confirmed at gene regulation level that they are coordinately regulated by nuclear receptor SXR. From one hand, the enzyme metabolism might be sufficient to alter the net absorption across the intestine epithelia. On the other hand, P-gp not only decreases the drug absorption by efflux mechanism, but also could prolong the intracellular residence of the drugs while increasing the access of drugs to CYP3A4 by repeated cycles of absorption and efflux. Initial experiment results have confirmed the existence of this process.

Animal Models

Although several predictions help in the initial assessment of absorption parameters as related to the new drug candidates, when it comes to real time picture, the predictions may entirely go wrong. This is particularly true with the drug candidates with active transport or other types of transport mechanisms. In addition, when more than two drugs are administered at one time, it is definitely not possible, at this time to predict the absorption of one molecule as interacted with the absorption of the other using any of the software technologies.Dissecting individual absorption processes play a major role. Definitely predictions do not help in this scenario. On the other hand, animal models definitely would be helpful in this regard. In addition, human models could also be investigated based on the pharmacodynamic or therapeutic observations apart from the use of several novel techniques currently in vogue in the literature and practice, respectfully. A very brief outline of some of these techniques will be presented in this section. The animal models currently used and published include *in vitro* models, *in situ* models and *in vivo* models.

In Vitro Models

Transport across isolated membranes or cell monolayers are routinely used in studying drug transport. These models are commonly used in the identification and characterization of active transport or site-specific absorption and allow the evaluation of transport of drug modifications or transport alterations. The advantage of such models is that these models determine the permeability across individual membranes without being interfered by other factors such as blood flow, transit, etc. These models could also be used in the determination of *in vivo* drug transport in humans with appropriate correlations. As a whole, different types of *in vitro* models that have been studied include, everted sacs, intestinal sacs and isolated tissues. Otherwise not stated, these models are currently routinely used in the investigations of intestinal drug absorption. Very complicated and tailored models to suit for a particular use for a particular variety of situation and for a particular disease are also in practice. Some of these models are very briefly discussed henceforth.

The very old model of the investigation of intestinal transport with the help of isolated tissue studies is **Everted Sac (Everted gut sacs)** method. This was first introduced by Wison and Wiseman in 1954. In everted intestinal rings the musculature is intact because whole intestinal segments are used. This is a very important method of estimation of intestinal permeability. It is different from cell culture studies. It is the most important method in the intestinal absorption: this involves the sacrifice of an animal. Briefly, intestinal segments are quickly excised, usually from rats, and flushed with saline solution. The segment is tied at one end and by placing on glass rod it is carefully everted and cut into small rings. Transport across the rings is then studied. Everted Sac method predicts how the physiological status of the tissue outlines major absorption prediction. Take, for instance, the drugs with transporter mechanisms of absorption, the transporter may be viable for only limited time after isolation. The drugs with passive transport may not be affected, but the use of everted sac will definitely impact the predictions involving drugs with active transport mechanisms, if the study is not performed on time. It will either make the predictions better with the viability of the tissue or worsen the results, as time is crucial. Not only the absorption, but also the permeability rates can also be measured with the use of these techniques. These results are definitely closer to the studies in the human beings in these stages when properly extrapolated and correlated.

Advantages:

- Method is relatively simple and quick
- Method is fast and inexpensive
- Regional differences in drug absorption can be studied
- Each animal acts as its own control as many rings can be prepared from each segment of the intestine isolated
- Mechanism of drug absorption can be studied by changing the experimental conditions

Disadvantages: Extreme care is needed to maintain the viability of the tissue through out the experiment.

Intestinal rings, isolated cell suspensions and membrane vesicles have all been employed with varying degrees of success. A very brief mention of membrane vesicles was described in the artificial membrane section. Of these, Porter et al. (1998), have found that both mucosal cells and intestinal rings are capable of absorbing a variety of drugs, with rings giving slightly less variability than cell suspensions. Stewart et al. (1986), have also demonstrated the utility of this method for evaluation of the uptake of prodrugs. Since transport rate constants cannot be obtained from these systems, uptake rates are generally reported. It is impossible, however, to define a rate-limiting barrier to absorption since enterocytes, connective tissue and muscle layers are all exposed to the drug solution.

The other very commonly used technique of studying drug transport is the use of **isolated tissues**. In the study of ion transport across frog skin, Ussing and Zrahn (1951) introduced the use of a short circuit current technique, i.e., voltage clamping, to distinguish between active and passive ion movement. For intestine, the tissue is separated from the accompanying muscle layers, mounted between two half-cells, and bathed in warmed oxygenated buffer solutions. This technique has been commonly used in the examination of GI pharmacology, but until the last decade, only little utilized in the examination of intestinal transport of drug substances. The method of Ussing and Zrahn (Ussing and Zrahn, 1951; Koefed-Johnson et al., 1952; Uchiyama et al., 1998) in an unclamped state has found increasing use in the investigation of drug absorption. Several shortcomings of the application of this apparatus for permeability studies have led to the development of newer diffusion chamber systems, but the general technique is similar. Modifications to these devices have also included the use of cultured cells grown on permeable supports.

Advantages of isolated tissue studies:

- Permeability across different regions can be determined and thus regional differences in intestinal absorption can be studied.
- Determination of permeability in different animal models can be performing by using different animal tissue. Thus, species differences with respect to intestinal absorption characteristics can be determined.
- Transepithelial drug transport can be investigated in combination of intestinal metabolism.
- Amount of drug needed is relatively small (mg quantities).
- Samples are analytically clean/pure.

Disadvantages:

- The viability of intestinal tissue mounted in Ussing Chamber is quite controversial.
- Dissection of epithelial tissue is quite difficult and serosal muscle layer can be partially removed.

In Situ Models (Perfusion Models)

Most of the times predictions based on *in silico* methods and *in vitro* transport studies should suffice for initial compound screening and taking a molecule into further toxicological investigations. However, if found very efficacious in terms of dose, toxicity and pharmacodynamic effects, a chemist is generally given a project to further develop this series of compounds. During this stage of development, transport studies, mostly *in situ* models, would be of immense help in further elucidating structure-transport relationships. The disadvantages with *in vitro* models are several fold as mentioned in the previous section. These disadvantages can be conveniently eliminated using *in situ* models. In these models, the animals are generally live and functional. However, the gut tissue is eviscerated, several catheters placed to investigate the absorption phenomenon.

Two types of models are used: in situ perfusion and vascular perfused intestine. In in situ perfusion, measurement of drug disappearance from either closed or open loop perfusate of segments of intestine is studied. In the second case, measurement of drug disappearance from perfusate and its appearance in blood is studied. During the study, several transporter modifiers could be added to further investigate the transport. The transport of multiple drugs can also be investigated. Provided proper washout period is given, the same model can be used for investigating several kinds of molecules. The unfortunate thing with these systems is that the animal is generally under anaesthesia and some times the interaction between the anaesthesia and the drug could complicate the transport investigations. Transport across a particular area of the intestinal tract could be measured one upon other. This flexibility is not available with any of the *in vitro* techniques. Compared to whole animal studies, these models also provide a comparitive advantage. A primary problem with whole animal studies is the inability to correlate all of the factors of a specific animal species to human, *in situ* studies provide the advantage of isolating the comparison to the level of the intestine. In addition, these models effectively remove complications such as GI transit and dosage form performance from the experiment. In situ models also enables the study of intestinal events in isolation without complication of billiary excretion and enterohepatic circulation. Both drug disappearance from the intestines and the drug transport across the intestines is generally used in these models. The main disadvantage with these models is that surgery is required for such investigations. Among various absorption models, in situ perfustion of intestinal segments in anaesthetized rats most closely mimics in vivo rat absorption.

Several modifications of the in situ absorption have been developed. In case o open loop method, dilute drug solution will be passed slowly through the intestine. Drug concentration of the solution in the inlet and outlet is determined. The permeability is then determined. In case of close loop method, dilute drug solution is added to the section of intestine and intestine is closed. The intestine is then excised and drug content in luminal solution is analyzed at specific intervals. This method has the same disadvantage as everted intestinal rings as the drug content measurement requires tissue disruption. Also by this approach it is not always practical to determine the steady state disappearance rate of drug from the lumen. As the disappearance rate from the lumen is used for calculating the absorption rate constant, it is important to confirm that the drug is not degraded in the intestines.

In Situ models are based on the assumption that disappearance of drug from the intestinal lumen correctly reflects drug absorption in the portal circulation. Thus, this approach may overestimate the absorption in case of drugs undergoing extensive metabolism and drugs having significant accumulation in the intestine. This short coming can be overcome by collecting the samples from mesenteric vein, which is draining the blood from the perfused intestinal segment. These models are also first calibrated with standard drugs.

In vivo models

It has been an early goal of drug development to evaluate the potential oral absorption of a candidate compound. Classically, these studies have been performed in animals. The results of these studies depend upon the species selected, and little consistency is observed in the study of specific compound in different species. No single laboratory species has been defined as a reliable model of human drug absorption, so that species selection for early studies often results from such physiologically irrelevant characteristics as ease of handling and cost. Whole animal studies are also not suitable to the large numbers of screening studies that must be conducted in the drug discovery process. Each animal must be dosed and plasma samples taken and analyzed. It is difficult to imagine this technique easily adapted to the requirement of screening hundreds or thousands of compounds. Some times controversial reports have been demonstrated for a molecule compared to human beings over animal models although several correlations are possible. The general problem with whole animal studies could be described as follows: when one selects an animal species for *in vivo* bioavailability studies, one selects all of the characteristics of that animal and tries to correlate them summarily to humans. For example, when selecting dogs, one attempt to force a correlation for all the characteristics of GI transit, pH, bile secretion, enzyme systems, etc., from dogs to humans.

Human Models

To study solute and drug absorption across human intestines, several techniques have been developed and used for the last 40 years. It is difficult to study *in vivo* drug or solute absorption in human beings; however, most of the techniques developed were single-pass perfusion. The absorption is calculated from the disappearance rate of the drug from the perfused segment. The fundamental principle in these experiments is that the absorption is calculated from the disappearance rate of the drug from the perfused segment. Techniques including:1. a triple lumen tube including a mixing segment, 2. a multilumen tube with a proximal occluding balloon, and 3. a multilumen tube with two balloons occluding a 10 cm long intestinal segment were investigated. The first and the most common technique that was used is the triple lumen tube with a mixing segment. An example of such a technique is Loc-I-Gut technique. The Loc-I-Gut is a multichannel tube system with a proximal and a distal balloon. It is a perfusate technique, which gives insight into human permeability. The balloons are 100 mm apart. Thus, isolates a 100 mm long intestinal segment to be perfused. As soon as proximal balloon passes the ligament of Treitz, both balloons are filled with air. This separates the luminal contents of isolated segment of intestine from the rest of the luminal contents of the intestine. The proper working of the balloons is checked using a non-absorbable marker. The passage of distal balloon down the GI tract is enhanced by attaching tungsten weights. The use of high frequency capsule has also been tried to study absorption. The transit of high frequency capsule through gastrointestinal tract is followed by X-ray fluoroscopy. As soon as capsule reaches its intended site, the drug release is initiated by high frequency signal, which leaded to rupturing of the latex balloon, which is loaded with the drug.

Relatively newer models are being developed as aids in drug discovery or formulation developed. These are generally third party tools. One such tool is termed as Enterion Capsule offered by Pharmaceutical profiles Ltd. Results from these studies provide an early warning of challenging compounds and simultaneously provide a route map for their development. These drug absorption studies are called as human drug absorption studies (HAD studies). The concept behind an HDA study is simple. Essentially, the drug is targeted at key sites in the human gastrointestinal (GI) tract and the relative bioavailability determined by measuring the resulting plasma concentration – time curves in the normal way. All that is needed is a reliable method of delivering the drug in a variety of pharmaceutical or physical forms where and when the scientist requires. The Enterion™ capsule (Phaeton Research, Nottingham, UK) was designed for exactly this purpose. Enterion™ is the latest advance in the arena of remote-controlled, 'clever capsule' technologies.3 It is an electromechanical device 32mm in length and 11mm in diameter, with a drug reservoir of approximately 1ml in volume located within the main body (see *Figure 1*). To track capsule location within the GI tract, a radioactive marker is sealed inside a separate compartment. This allows the position of the capsule to be followed in realtime using GS. When the capsule arrives at the target site, a radiofrequency generator (situated externally) is used to generate an electromagnetic field over the subject's abdomen for just a few seconds. The field is picked up by a receiving coil embedded inside the capsule wall, causing induction of a tiny electric current. This electric current operates a latch mechanism, releasing a spring-driven piston that then actively expels the capsule contents in a rapid, bolus fashion. This delivery mechanism makes the technology extremely versatile and fully effective in delivering a wide variety of formulations, including solutions, viscous suspensions, particulates, pellets and minitablets. Once the capsule has activated, the induced current is diverted to a transmitter coil that generates a radio signal. Detection of this signal confirms that the drug has been delivered and is used to initiate the blood sampling protocol.

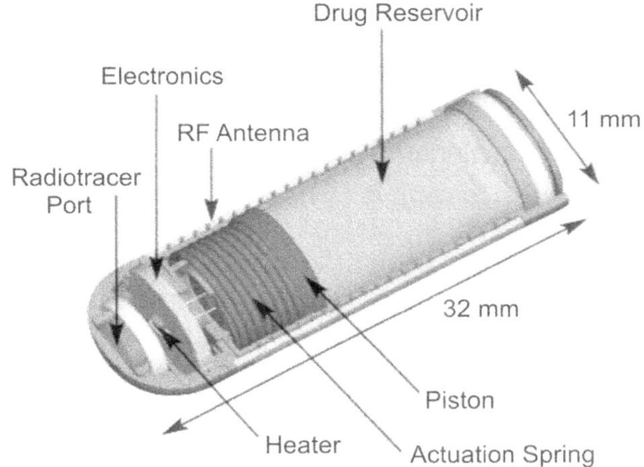

Figure 6.1 The Enterion Capsule.

Permeability Determination

The investigation of gastrointestinal absorption of new drugs is always exciting. Several techniques as mentioned in the chapter titled "Drug absorption study models" can be employed to evaluate the drug absorption properties of the new entities. In any of these techniques either *permeability coefficient* or *apparent permeability coefficient* are used to describe the transport properties of the molecules. In such evaluations, the simple assumption is that "the membrane is a homogenous layer in which a drug transports across in a dynamic equilibrium state between the membrane". Based on this hypothesis, the movement of a molecule through a membrane is mathematically derived using Ficks law of diffusion. However, on practical occasions, the hypothesis of a free movement of molecule across membranes is not observed. When molecules travel using transport mechanisms like active transport or facilitated diffusion such assumptions are no more valid. The same is true when molecules travel through several layers rather than one single monolayer. In these situations, apparent permeability coefficient could closely define the transport properties of NDSs. Several modifications to such experimentations would help dissect the transport properties of the molecules. In addition, presently several mathematical modifications to the apparent permeability value could be found in the literature. Thus, either of these, i.e., permeability value or apparent permeability value could describe the movement of molecules across the gastrointestinal tract. Similarly either permeability coefficient or apparent permeability coefficient could describe the transport properties of microparticles, nanoparticles, and other larger molecules across the gastrointestinal tract. In these conditions the substrates are traveled with transport mechanisms like phagocytosis, pinocytosis and receptor-medicated endocytosis. Some of the equations associated with permeability through any of the GIT models are described in this section. These equations and evaluations are also applicable to transport of new chemicals, particles, etc., across blood-brain barrier, blood-CSF barrier, vagina (human ecto-cervical tissue), maternal-fetal transplacental passage, etc.

In the evaluation of the transport of new drug substances (NDSs) across the gastrointestinal tract by diffusion, plasma is generally the receiving compartment and the gut is the donor compartment. The movement of a molecule from within the donor compartment to the receiving compartment is described by diffusivity in the intestinal membrane. After a drug is administered by oral route, the plasma is collected at specific time intervals and the drug extracted and assayed. Theoretically, the profiles obtained from plasma data are fit into plasmaconcentration-time profiles and the permeability coefficients are determined. However, this is always complicated because of several interfering factors in animal models or human studies. Thus, most of the times the permeabilities are determined using isolated tissues or cell culture monolayers mounted on diffusion chambers. Thus, several of the interefering factors are eliminated. The best possible permeability coefficients are obtained. Subsequently, absorption patterns are evaluated. However, there are several constraints. In one instance, if NDS1 and NDS2 (Figure 6.2) show similar permeability coefficient ranges in transport properties they could be clubbed under the molecules having the same mechanisms of transport, whether active or passive. However such a determination is not conclusive. Same ranges of permeability coefficients do not always mean that the molecules have the same mechanisms of transport. If concentration dependency is investigated one would show passive transport and the other active transport.

Previously apparent permeability of an NDS was calculated and reported. The equation to calculate apparent permeability coefficient was based on Ficks law of diffusion. Using this approach passive permeability was well discussed. However, the same equation was used in evaluating the mechanism of transport to differentiate different types of transport mechanisms. The studies are conducted in a variety of conditions to properly draw a conclusion. The permeability values obtained from the con-comitant use of metabolic inhibitors, low-temperature studies, concentration dependency, paracellular and transcellular transport inhibitors, cytoskeleton modulators, transporter inhibitors etc. were used in differentiating the transport mechanisms of NDSs. Peripherally, these studies and conclusions are fine. However, there were several constraints. For instance, hydrophilic compounds are mostly transported via the paracellular route. However, permeation of more hydrophilic compounds that typically use the paracellular route is often underestimated compared to the *in vivo* absorption characteristics because of several factors such as more resistance offered to these compounds by the mucus layer and the tightness of the membrane. For example, one scientist body reported significantly lower transport of the hydrophilic drugs terbutaline and atenolol across CACO-2 monolayers compared to the human jejenum, which may be sometimes more complicated than anticipated. This could be explained by the fact that tight junctions in CACO-2 monolayers are more tighter compared to the tight junctions of normal small intestinal epithelium *in vivo*. Additionally, there could be more complicated transport models. The current trend is to use permeability coefficients straightly obtained from the equations either derived separately or derived using apparent permeability coefficient values. Some of these issues and equations will be presented in this section.

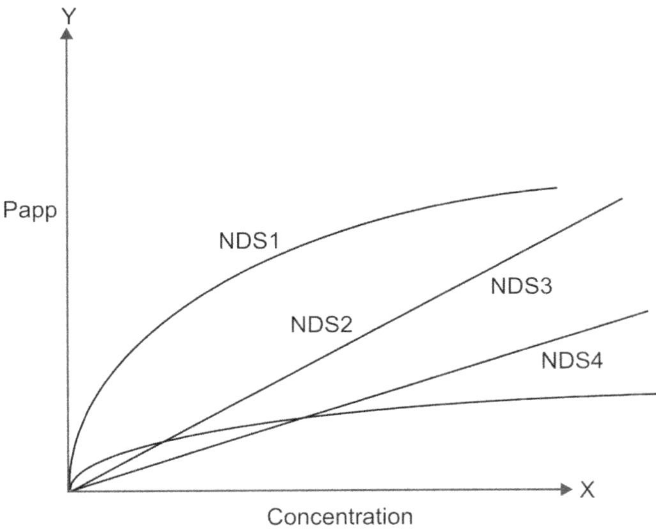

Figure 6.2 Possible profiles of active and passive transport of new drug substances through the membranes. These plots help in dissecting the mechanisms and orders of transport and the role of the transporters (NDS stands for new drug substance).

Mathematics

Knowledge of the permeability coefficient for new drugs is useful for estimating the fraction absorbed across the gastrointestinal tract. The commonly used approximate formula for the permeability coefficient (used to determine the apparent permeability coefficient) is based on the initial rate of permeation across cell monolayers, requires measurement during the linear phase of permeation, and is not applicable when there is significant backflux of compound or mass balance problem. Thus, very perfect equations and evaluations are required in such assessment of passive permeability coefficient for new drugs. In addition, things are very complex when the permeability coefficients are determined for multilayered systems or when the membranes have transporters and the molecules are transported using active transport mechanisms. For instance both the passively and actively transported compounds may be affected by the so-called 'unstirred water layer' (UWL), which lines the apical surface of the monolayer. Diffusion across the UWL may become rate-limiting for the transport of rapidly absorbed compounds. Stirring the apical and basolateral media during transport experiments with lipophilic compounds is recommended to reduce the effect of the UWL. In such situations the apparent coefficient determinations and interpretations have more meaning rather than evaluating the passive permeability coefficient.

Apparent Permeability Coefficients: Determinations, Extrapolations, Applications

Single monolayer passive permeability coefficient determination

Permeability coefficient determinations for therapeutic agents are in place for over some time. However, because of the new drug discovery, several molecules are coming into the hands of a researcher. Thus, the understanding of the transport properties would take longer periods before a proper molecule with proper transport properties is picked up. However, currently high-through put screening techniques are in place for this purpose. In high-throughput discovery drug screening studies, there will be low (<10 nm/s) and high (>300 nm/s) permeability compounds run at the same time, while the test compounds must be balanced with the analytical detection. Likewise mass balance problems are not usually predictable. Most of the times the currently used equations may not be valid to determine the permeability in the entire range of the transport. The instance would be the inappropriate use of drug transport curve during the first 10% transport for highly permeable molecules. In addition, there are generally many mass balance problems that could take a lot of effort to dissect the problems associated with the mass balance and come out with proper prediction of permeability of new drug substances. Thus, several scientists have devised new equations to predict such permeabilities. Most of these equations are generally applicable to monolayer systems that are definitely suitable for high-througput screening purposes. A very recently devised and practically applicable equation published by Tran et al., (2004) is mentioned in the Table 1. Last but not the least that could be mentioned is the use of bilayer of lipids for estimating the passive transport. These are called PAMPA models (Parallel Artificial Membrane Permeability Assay). However, these systems donot exactly simulate the internal system. Thus, monolayers or similar models are the most convenient forms of tools to predict the permeability.

Two barrier models for passive transport are much more complex. If intracellular concentrations can be measured or estimated, then two barrier models could be used to assess differences in apical and basolateral passive permeabilities. When the cell monolayer is treated as a single permeability barrier and it is static, that is, unchanging in time, then the passive permeability coefficient will be the same in both directions regardless of the inner structure of the barrier, provided that the volume of a static passive permeability barrier times the partition coefficient of the drug into the barrier, is negligible compared with the donor and receiver chamber volumes. In these cases flux is symmetric because it depends only on the concentration gradient across the barrier. This is the first scenario.

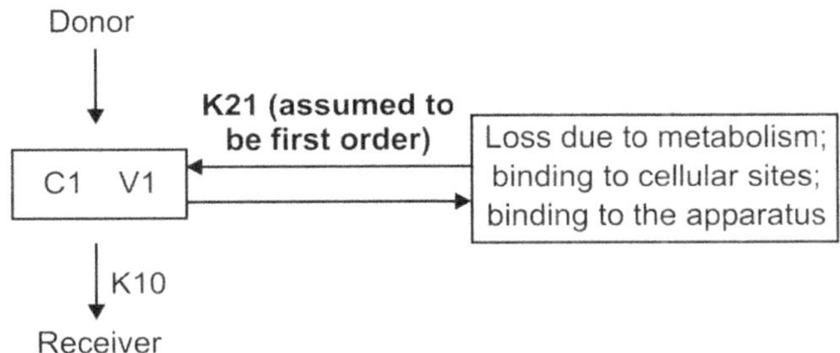

Figure 6.3 A schematic representation of drug transport study in diffusion chambers (Donor may contain a simple solution, a suspension, a suspension of nanoparticles, liposomes or microparticles).

Figure 6.3 depicts a passive permeability model with first order drug loss due to metabolism, binding to the cellular sites and binding to the apparatus. This is the second scenario of passive permeability coefficients. The equations related to these two scenario are presented in the box below. Their derivations and further references with several layer passive permeability values could be obtained from the literature.

Table 2

Passive Permeability Coefficient Determinations

P_{apx} = $(V_R C_R (t_i))/ (At_i C_D(0))$ 2

P_{apx} =- $(V_R V_D)*\ln \{1-(C_R(t_i))/ C(t))\}/ (V_R+V_D)/ (At_i)$............3

The first equation is the classical approximate solution for the initial passive permeability for a single barrier while the second equation is the the exact equation for passive permeation through a single barrier when there is no loss of drug or drug loss is first order, in the second equation, the following equations are used to calculate C(t);

C(t) $= (V_D C_D (t) + V_R C_R (t))/ (V_D + V_R)$....................4
C(t) $= (V_D C_D (0))*\exp \{-kvt)/ (V_D + V_R)$.....................5

Where V_D and V_R are the donor and receiver chamber volumes, A is the area of permeability barrier, t is the time of measurement, C_R (t) and C_D (t) denote the drug concentrations in the receiver and the donor chambers at the measuring time

Permeability Coefficient Determination Through the Gastrointestinal Tract

A general model used for the absorption of a drug through the mucosal membrane of the small intestine consists of several parallel biological layers including the rate limiting and the mucus layer. The aqueous boundary layer is in series with the biomembrane, which is composed of lipid regions and aqueous pores in parallel. The final reservoir is a sink consisting of the blood. The flux of a drug permeating the mucosal membrane is

$$J = P_{app}(C_b - C_{blood})$$

Or, since the blood reservoir is a sink, $C_{blood} \sim 0$;

$$J = P_{app}C_b$$

In which P_{app} is the apparent permeability coefficient (cm/sec) and C_b is the total drug concentration in bulk solution in the lumen of the intestine.

The apparent permeability coefficient is given by

$$P_{app} = \frac{1}{(1/P_{aq} + 1/P_m)}$$

in which P_{aq} is the permeability coefficient of the drug in the aqueous boundary layer (cm/sec), and P_m is the effective permeability coefficient for the drug in the lipoidal and polar aqueous regions of the membrane (cm/sec).

The flux may be written in terms of drug concentration C_b in the intestinal lumen by combining with it a term for the volume, or

$$J = -(dC_b/dt)*V/S$$

In which S is the surface area and V is the volume of the intestinal segment. The first-order disappearance rate, K_u (Second inverse) of the drug in the intestine is found in the expression,

$$DC_b/dt = -K_uC_b$$

Combining the previous two equations gives,

$$J = (V/S)*K_uC_b$$

Combining the previous two equations gives,

$$P_{app} = \frac{1}{(1/P_{aq} + 1/P_m)} = V^*K_u / S$$

Consideration of two cases, (1) aqueous boundary layer control and (2) membrane control, results in simplification of above equations.

1. When the permeability coefficient of the intestinal membrane (i.e., the velocity of drug passage through the membrane in cm/sec) is much greater than that of the aqueous layer, the aqueous layer will cause a slower passage of the drug and becomes a rate-limiting barrier (The slower passage is always the rate-determining process). Therefore, P_{aq}/P_m will be much less than unity, and equation reduces to

   $$K_{u,max} = (S/V)P_{aq}$$

   K_u is now written as $K_{u,max}$ because the maximum possible diffusional rate constant is determined by passage across the aqueous boundary layer.

2. If, on the other hand, the permeability of the aqueous boundary layer is much greater than that of the membrane, P_{aq}/P_m will become larger than unity, and the equation reduces to:

   $$K_u = (S/V)\, P_m$$

   The rate-determining step for transport of drug across the membrane is now under membrane control. When neither P_{aq} nor P_m is much larger than the other, the process is controlled by the rate of drug passage through both the stationary aqueous layer and the membrane. These permeability determinations are generally complex because of the several fold factors that could affect an experiment.

> Thus, permeability coefficient determinations most of the times are complicated and as a reason a term called apparent permeability coefficient was introduced and is used very commonly in the transport assessments. From this apparent permeability coefficients, several other permeability coefficients as required for further elucidation and discussion are derived.

Derivation of Apparent Permeability Coefficient with the Help of Ficks Law

Ficks law

In biological systems we are dealing with a variety of substances in solutions. The basic solvent is water. The simplest mechanism by which movement can proceed from point A to point B is by diffusion. All molecules possess intrinsic thermal energy, which results in their random movement until they collide with other molecules and transfer the momentum.

Rate of transport per unit area or mathematically

$$J = dn/dt/A$$

Where J = flux, dn/dt = number molecules transported/sec, A = sampling area of the reference plane

In a more practical application of the diffusion process consider now a molecule in solution, for example, sugar. Putting a spoon of sugar into coffee without stirring will result in a very substantial delay in the sweetening of the surface layer. It will occur eventually but will probably take several hours for the sugar to diffuse uniformly throughout the coffee cup. There are several factors which are determining the flux of sugar from the spoonful on the bottom of the cup. Number 1 are the limitations of diffusion as described mathematically by Ficks First Law

$$J = DA(dC/dx) \text{ -(Fick's First Law of Diffusion)}$$

Where D = the diffusion coefficient for a substance usually in water cm^2/sec, dC/dx = the concentration gradient of the diffusing substance, $mole/cm^3/cm$, A = area of the plane through which diffusion is occurring. The self-diffusion constant for water is $2.4x10^{-5}$, sucrose $5.2x10^{-6}$, and hemoglobin $6.0x10^{-7}$.

These differences in diffusion coefficients reflect differences in the ability of molecules to move in solvent under the influence of a driving force (either a concentration gradient and/or an electrical field for ions). The physical size and shape of the molecule will influence its viscous drag and the distribution of charge or polar nature can also produce increased radii of hydration that will alter the mobility of the molecule in solution. The influence of mobility on flux is expressed as

$$J = \text{mobility x concentration x driving force}$$

Extrapolation of ficks law to the permeability of membranes

The mechanics of transition to the membrane phase are still a matter of controversy but in very simple systems a good approximation of the process can be provided using a modification of Fick's First Law. Under steady state conditions where concentrations on both sides of the membrane are not changing, the flux across a membrane under the force of diffusion is described by:

$$J = D_m (Co\text{-}Ci)/x_m$$

Where D_m = diffusion coefficient in the membrane, x_m = thickness of the membrane, C_o = concentration in the receiver and C_i = concentration inside the donor.

Dm is much smaller (two to three orders of magnitude) in the membrane than in water. The flux across a membrane may also be expressed relative to the permeability coefficient that incorporates all the important factors influencing diffusion through a membrane

$$J = P(C_o - C_i)$$

where $$P = D_m/x_m$$

The equations based on diffusion assumptions explain the movement of many small molecules across cell membranes, but there are also many substances which appear to be transported by processes different from simple diffusion. However, a very simple equation for apparent permeability coefficient based upon the Fick's law of diffusion and the above concepts could be derived. Upon combining the above two previous equations, the final equation for apparent permeability coefficient would be

$$P_{app} = (dq/dt)*1/A*Co$$

Where dq/dt is the transport rate (nmol/s), C_0 is the initial concentration (micromolar) in the donor chamber and A is the surface area of the cell monolayer.

Apparent Permeability Coefficient in Non-sink Conditions

The previous equation is very commonly used equation to derive permeabilities across the gastrointestinal tract membrane models. However, the use of the above equation even for very simple conditions could be sometimes very peripheral. Several relevant cases have been discussed and published in the literature. In a simple permeability experiment using diffusion chambers, the assumption is that sink conditions are maintained in the receiver chamber. However, it may not be always the case. Depending on the rate of the movement of a molecule across a membrane, the sink condition could be achieved or not achieved. When it is achieved for a set of molecules in a set of conditions, P_{app} numbers may be very appropriate. However, to identify the sink condition itself would be very tedious and costly. As such the above equation becomes a shorter equation as related to the apparent permeability value determinations. On the other hand several other equations were derived to be used in non-sink conditions. One of such equations is derived as follows:

At "sink" conditions, the apparent permeability coefficients (P_{app}, cm/s) are calculated from:

$$P_{app} = (k.V_R)/(A.60)$$

where k is the transport rate (min^{-1}) defined as the slope obtained by linear regression of the cumulative fraction absorbed as a function of time (min), V_R is the volume in the receiver chamber (ml), and A is the area of the filter (cm^2). The fraction absorbed was defined as the ratio between the concentration on the receiver side (C_R) at the end of an interval and the concentration on the donor side ($C_{D,0}$) at the beginning of that interval. Alfentanil was transported so rapidly at higher pH values that sink conditions could not be maintained. It was therefore necessary to develop a more general method for calculating P_{app}, one also applicable to nonsink conditions. Taking into account the effect of back flux from the receiver compartment, Fick's law gives:

$$dC_R(t)/dt = [P_{app}.A.(C_D(t)-C_R(t))]/V_R$$

where $C_D(t)$ and $C_R(t)$ is the concentration in the donor and receiver compartment, respectively, as a function of time. If the amount of drug in the system (M) is assumed to be constant within each sampling interval, $C_D(t)$ can be expressed as a function of $C_R(t)$. Thus, replacing $C_D(t)$ by this expression in eq. 2 and solving the differential equation for $C_R(t)$ gives:

$$C_R(t) = [M/(V_D+V_R)] + [C_{R,0} - M/(V_D+V_R)].e^{-Papp.A.(1/V_D+1/V_R).t}$$

where V_D is the volume in the donor compartment, $C_{R,0}$ is the drug concentration in the receiver compartment at the beginning of the interval and t is the time from the start of the interval. The sampling procedure necessitates the recalculation of M and $C_{R,0}$ for each succeeding interval according to mass balance. P_{app} values for alfentanil were then determined by nonlinear regression, minimizing the sum of squared residuals ($\Sigma(C_{R,i,obs} - C_{R,i,calc})^2$), where $C_{R,i,obs}$ is the observed receiver concentration at the end of interval i and $C_{R,i,calc}$ is the corresponding concentration calculated according to above equation.

Determination of Various Permeability Coefficients from Apparent Permeability Coefficients

Membrane permeability coefficient

Membrane Permeability Coefficients can be determined based on the two different apparent permeability coefficient determined at two different stirring rates. From these values, the membrane permeability coefficient can be calculated from the slope of the linear relationship V/P_{app} and V as described below.

$$V/P_{app} = 1/K + (1/P_c+1/P_f)*V$$

Where P_m is the membrane permeability coefficient, K is the steady state rate of change in concentration in the receiver chamber (C_t/C_0) versus time (s), P_f is the calculated permeability coefficient of the filter support.

Paracellular permeability coefficient

To determine the paracellular permeability coefficients, transport experiments with new drug substances can be performed to determine the apical-to-basolateral flux at various concentrations. Then kinetic analysis of the data can be fit using various computer softwares to determine whether the process is saturable or non-saturable. To determine if the process is active ATPase inhibitors or metabolic inhibitors can be used concomitantly in the transport studies. Other inhibitors such as paracellular cationic conductance inhibitor 2,4,6-triaminopyridine (TAP), and cytoskeletal inhibitor can also indicate if a new drug substance is transported by paracellular route. Once this is determined, the paracellular permeability can be calculated from the apparent permeability values obtained from concentration-dependency and time-dependency studies. Apparent permeability value is calculated by using the equation given previously. The kinetic parameters for the transport of new drug substances can be calculated by fitting the data to the below equation using nonlinear regression analysis (WINNONLIN Scientific Consulting Inc., Apex, NC)

$$J = \{(J_{max}*S)/ K_{m\ (app)} + S)\} + K_d*S$$

Where J is the flux (J) normalized to unit surface area. $K_{m\ (app)}$ is a constant equivalent to a Michaelis-Menten constant. J_{max} is the maximal flux for the saturable term, K_d is the constant for the nonsaturable term and S is the concentration in the donor compartment.

Permeability coefficients associated with the active transport and facilitated diffusion

The methods to evaluate the active tranport or facilitated diffusion are very much similar to those defined for paracellular transport. Carrier mediated transport is generally determined by using concentration dependency, temperature dependency, inhibition of transport, effect of donor pH etc. studies. If there are both passive and active components in the transport the following equation can be used to determine the flux associated with saturable and linear components representing the saturable (active) and linear (passive) components of the transport by fitting the data to the following equation.

$$J = \{(V_{max}*S)/ K_m + S)\}+ P_{app}*S$$

Where J is the flux (J) normalized to unit surface area. $K_{m\ (app)}$ is a constant equivalent to a Michaelis-Menten constant. V_{max} is the maximal flux for the saturable term, P_{app} is the apparent permability coefficient and S is the concentration in the donor compartment. When there is no active component to transport for a given permeant, its steady-state flux is linear with concentration as defined by Fick's L and the above equation simplifies for both direction to:

$$J = P_{app}*C$$

Thus, the P_{app} of such a permeant across a layer of cells may be readily calculated from the flux divided by the donor concentration.

A simple correlation of the various absorption parameters in the very early stages of drug discovery is definitely an important criteria in new drug discovery process. Although very prominent molecules might have come into the market in the ancient times, the current situation warrants need for more complicated molecules for the treatment of new diseases arising in all parts of the world. This situation is same for several generations and for several histories. The parallel is true for drug discovery and development. In this context, cost also plays a major role. The aim of any discovery process is to curtail the costs. Drug absorption study models are crucial in this regard. This chapter very briefly outlines some of the older techniques, current methods, details several of the new computer aided drug absorption models and finally details permeability assessment.

Questions for Practice and Exercise

1. Explain the application of chemical parameters in assessment of absorption.
2. Explain “rule of five”.

3. Explain how
   (a) the molecular size,
   (b) the polar surface area and
   (c) hydrogen bonding affects the intestinal absorption of a new drug substance.
4. What are the different solubilities that are determined for new drug substances? How is the solubility determined for new drug substances? How is its determination important for new drug development processes?
5. Mention about the significance of dissociation coefficient (pKa) in the new drug development methodologies. Describe the fundamentals involved in the determinations associated with dissociation coefficients?
6. Mention about the significance of partition coefficient in the new drug development methodologies.
7. Explain the various features of ACD/pKa software. How is it helpful in drug development methodologies?
8. Explain in detail about capacity factor?
9. Write a note on the following:
   (a) Theoretical Predictions,
   (b) *In silico* models and artificial membranes and
   (c) Neural Networks.
10. What are the various methods used in the determination of absorption parameters with the help of animal models? Explain in detail about each of them. Mention about the advantages and disadvantages of each of these methods.
11. What are the different drug absorption study models currently used in the development of new drugs? Describe one of them in detail. Explain the advantages and disadvantages associated with this model that you have selected.
12. How are the predictions of drug absorption with new drug substances performed?
13. What are the differences between *in vitro*, *in situ* and *in vivo* animal models used to determine the drug absorption parameters of new drug substances?

14. How are the human models useful in the determination of drug absorption parameters of new drug substances?
15. What are the different parameters that are useful in the prediction and the characterization of absorption of new drug substances through the gastrointestinal tract? Elaborate, extrapolate with suitable examples and then explain.
16. Give a brief idea about the human models used in drug absorption studies. What are the consequences of mishandling at this stage? Is it necessary to use human models in drug absorption studies? Are we tampering the human being? How are these studies different from animal studies? Explain in a nutshell.
17. What are PAMPA models?
18. Define
    1. Product recall and
    2. Dropped out drugs.

    Explain the differences between the two.
19. Why is the study of drug transport across the gastrointestinal tract important in the discovery of new drug substances?
20. Write a brief note on different mechanisms and the associated basics of drug transport across the gastrointestinal tract?
21. What are the important factors that are usually investigated for transport mechanism identification of new drug substances? Explain in brief.
22. Write a brief note on tissue culture and cell culture methods used in drug transport investigations.
23. What are the differences between cell lines and primary cultures?
24. How are the cell lines developed and maintained and how are primary cultures developed and maintained?
25. Mention a protocol to develop single cell systems that are routinely used in biological studies at this time.
26. Describe one study from literature that used single cell systems for transport mechanism investigations. Extrapolate to drug transport mechanism investigations.
27. Write a note on CACO-2 cells. Pull out from literature the several uses of this cell line along with a very precise introduction to the need and utilization of this cell line.

28. Write a basic and very important note on Madin Darby Canine Kidney (MDCK) cells. Pull out from literature the various uses of this cell line in the intestinal drug transport studies with a broad introduction to the need, its source and intestinal drug transport utilization of this cell line.
29. Mention and describe about other cell lines that could be substitutes for CACO-2 cells. How long after the introduction of CACO-2 cells as intestinal membrane substitutes, the other cells came into prominence?
30. What is permeability? Mention briefly the various determinants of permeability?
31. How is permeability calculated from transport studies across the biological membranes or cell monolayers?
32. Mention about the various methods of determining the permeability of molecules across the gastrointestinal tract?
33. Mention about the methods that are used to determine the permeability values of new drug substances across the gastrointestinal tract in vivo?
34. What are the different advantages and disadvantages associated with the various methods of transport studies? Mention very briefly.
35. What are the various interfering factors that are found *in vivo* transport studies that are not found in the monolayer or cell membrane transport studies? How could these be accounted for in the new drug development methodologies?
36. Describe the various methodologies used in the drug transport investigations? How is this very important for new drug discovery? Discuss comprehensively.
37. Mention about the various conditions, inhibitors etc. that coud be used to dissect the transport mechanism of drugs; whether active or passive. Discuss very comprehensively in a precise orientation. How may the structural modifications in a molecule influence the transport? Discuss with one recent example from the literature. Elaborate. How is this very important for new drug discovey?
38. Derive the equation for apparent permeability coefficient with the help of Fick's Law.
39. How is the apparent permeability coefficient usually determined? Describe an experimental protocol that is used in such a determination.

40. How are the different permeability coefficients determined from apparent permeability coefficients? What are the uses of these permeability coefficients? When are they used?
41. What are
    (a) GASTROPLUS 3.1.0,
    (b) idea 2.0 and
    (c) ACAT? Elaborate in detail.

References

1. Cohen BE, Bangham AD. Diffusion of small non-electrolytes across liposome membranes.Nature. 1972 Mar 24;236(5343):173-4.
2. Palm K, Luthman K, Ungell AL, Strandlund G, Artursson P. Correlation of drug absorption with molecular surface properties.J Pharm Sci. 1996 Jan;85(1):32-9.
3. Palm K, Stenberg P, Luthman K, Artursson P. Polar molecular surface properties predict the intestinal absorption of drugs in humans.Pharm Res. 1997 May;14(5):568-71.
4. Lipinski CA. Drug-like properties and the causes of poor solubility and poor permeability. J Pharmacol Toxicol Methods. 2000 Jul-Aug;44(1):235-49. Review.
5. Balakin KV, Ekins S, Bugrim A, Ivanenkov YA, Korolev D, Nikolsky YV, Ivashchenko AA, Savchuk NP, Nikolskaya T. Quantitative structure-metabolism relationship modeling of metabolic N-dealkylation reaction rates.Drug Metab Dispos. 2004 Oct;32(10):1111-20.
6. Degim T, Hadgraft J, Ilbasmis S, Ozkan Y. Prediction of skin penetration using artificial neural network (ANN) modeling. J Pharm Sci. 2003 Mar;92(3):656-64.
7. Balakin KV, Ekins S, Bugrim A, Ivanenkov YA, Korolev D, Nikolsky YV, Ivashchenko AA, Savchuk NP, Nikolskaya T. Quantitative structure-metabolism relationship modeling of metabolic N-dealkylation reaction rates.Drug Metab Dispos. 2004 Oct;32(10):1111-20.
8. Porter J, Robinson J, Pickup R, Edwards C. An evaluation of lectin-mediated magnetic bead cell sorting for the targeted separation of enteric bacteria.J Appl Microbiol. 1998 May;84(5):722-32.
9. Stewart BH, Amidon GL, Brabec RK. Uptake of prodrugs by rat intestinal mucosal cells: mechanism and pharmaceutical implications. J Pharm Sci. 1986 Oct;75(10):940-5.

10. Ussing HH, Zerahn K. Active transport of sodium as the source of electric current in the short-circuited isolated frog skin. Reprinted from Acta. Physiol. Scand. 23: 110-127, 1951.J Am Soc Nephrol. 1999 Sep;10(9):2056-65.

11. Koefoed-Johnsen V, Ussing HH, Zerahn K. The origin of the short-circuit current in the adrenaline stimulated frog skin. Acta Physiol Scand. 1952;27(1):38-48.

12. Ussing HH, Zerahn K. Active transport of sodium as the source of electric current in the short-circuited isolated frog skin. Acta Physiol Scand. 1951 Aug 25;23(2-3):110-27.

13. Uchiyama M, Takeuchi T, Matsuda K. Effects of homologous natriuretic peptides in isolated skin of the bullfrog, Rana catesbeiana. Comp Biochem Physiol C Pharmacol Toxicol Endocrinol. 1998 Jul;120(1):37-42.

14. Van Nijlen T, Brennan K, Van den Mooter G, Blaton N, Kinget R, Augustijns P. Improvement of the dissolution rate of artemisinin by means of supercritical fluid technology and solid dispersions. Int J Pharm. 2003 Mar 26;254(2):173-81.

15. Kondo N, Iwao T, Kikuchi M, Shu H, Yamanouchi K, Yokoyama K, Ohyama K, Ogyu S. Pharmacokinetics of a micronized, poorly water-soluble drug, HO-221, in experimental animals. Biol Pharm Bull. 1993 Aug;16(8):796-800.

16. Fasano A. Regulation of intercellular tight junctions by zonula occludens toxin and its eukaryotic analogue zonulin. Ann N Y Acad Sci. 2000; 915:214-22. Review.

17. Lowes S, Cavet ME, Simmons NL. Evidence for a non-MDR1 component in digoxin secretion by human intestinal Caco-2 epithelial layers. Eur J Pharmacol. 2003 Jan 1;458(1-2):49-56.

18. Miller AJ. Ion-selective microelectrodes for measurement of intracellular ion concentrations. Methods Cell Biol. 1995;49:275-91.

19. Gres MC, Julian B, Bourrie M, Meunier V, Roques C, Berger M, Boulenc X, Berger Y, Fabre G. Correlation between oral drug absorption in humans, and apparent drug permeability in TC-7 cells, a human epithelial intestinal cell line: comparison with the parental Caco-2 cell line. Pharm Res. 1998 May;15(5):726-33.

20. Raessi SD, Guo Z, Dobson GL, Artursson P and Hidalgo IJ (1997) Comparison of CYP3A activities in a subclone of Caco-2 cells (TC7) and human intestine. *Pharm Res* **14:** 1019-1025

21. Cho, M.J., Thompson, D.P., Cramer, C.T., Vidmar, T.J. & Scieszka, J.F (1989). The Madin Darby canine kidney (MDCK) epithelial cell monolayer as a model cellular transport barrier. *Pharmaceutical Research* **6**: 71-77.

22. Tran TT, Mittal A, Gales T, Maleeff B, Aldinger T, Polli JW, Ayrton A, Ellens H, Bentz J. Exact kinetic analysis of passive transport across a polarized confluent MDCK cell monolayer modeled as a single barrier. J Pharm Sci. 2004 Aug;93(8):2108-23.

Bibliography

1. The Practice of Medicinal Chemistry, Second Edition, Edited by Camille Georges Wermuth, Elsevier Publications, 2003.
2. Foye`s Principles of Medicinal Chemistry, Fifth Edition, David A. Williams and Thomas L. Lemke, Lippincott Williams & Wilkins, 2002.
3. Quantitative Chemical Analysis, Sixth Edition, Authored by Daniel C. Harris, W.H. Freeman, 2002.
4. Rowland M, Tozer T, Clinical Pharmacokinetics: Concepts and Application. 3rd ed. Philadelphia: Lea and Febiger, (1994).
5. Physiological Pharmaceuticals: Barriers to Drug Absorption, Second Edition, Authored by Neena Washington, et al, CRC Publication, (2001).
6. Drug Bioavailability: Estimation of Solubility, Permeability, Absorption and Bioavailability (Methods and Principles in Medicinal Chemistry), First Edition, Authored by Han van de Waterbeemd, et al., Wiley-VCH (2003).

CHAPTER 7

DRUG ABSORPTION ENHANCEMENT

Introduction

Oral route is the most preferred route of administration of drugs. However, very often this route is associated with poor bioavailability and erratic absorption. This often results in withdrawl of a molecule from the discovery stages. In addition, any formulation inconsistencies during the production stage would result in ineffectiveness, thereby leading to a product recall. Thorough understanding of absorption processes of a molecule, systematic evaluation of its physico-chemical properties, its pharmacokinetics and judiciously selecting the formulation development process could reduce such drawbacks. Techniques like salt formation, co-administration with absorption and metabolism modulators, prodrugs, size reduction, incorporation of a bioadhesive polymer, fusion with water-soluble polymer and solid-state alterations aid in enhancing the oral bioavailability of a drug and reducing the fluctuations in the plasma levels. Some times a combination of these techniques could be utilized, thereby enhancing the therapy with these molecules.

Need for Drug Absorption Enhancement

Gastro Intestinal Tract Limitations

The requirement for drug absorption improvement for oral pharmaceutical industrial research will be anecdoted using some examples. Recently Bristol-Myers Squibb Pharmacetical Research Institute, New Brunswick, New Jersey, USA investigated the oral absorption of a new chemical entity (NCE), named compound 1. This compound, a weakly basic drug (pKa~ 5.5) had the highest solubility of 0.1 mg/ml at pH 1.5, < 1mcg/ml aqueous solubility between pH 3.5 and 5.5 at 24 ± 1°C, and no detectable solubility (<0.02 mcg/ml) at pH greater than 5.5. The solubility increases with a decrease in the pH, reaching a maximum value of ~ 100 mcg/ml in the region of pH 1.3-1.6. However, below pH 1.3 the solubility decreases due to the *in situ* formation of a hydrochloride salt and the resultant common ion effect with HCl. Unlike in water, the drug is highly soluble in many pharmaceutically acceptable organic solvents. The solubility in PEG 400 is ~110 mg/g at 25°C. Unfortunately, among the attempted salts, only mono-hydrate was isolated as a crystalline material, however, it could not be prepared reproducibly. The absolute bioavailability after administering compound 1 as an oral capsule was only 1.7%. The most likely reason is its poor dissolution in the GIT fluids. Further data suggests that this molecule needs an approach for increasing the oral bioavailability. This has been a common solution that was employed with some of the older molecules. However, this is the very latest molecule that is clubbed to increase the oral bioavailability. Interestingly, the approach of oral solution for this formulation increased the bioavailability to

59.6%. Similar methods of increasing the oral bioavailability of some of the older compounds by a solution form are ample in the literature. A formulation that could dissolve the compound in the intestinal fluids and uniformly disperse it in these fluids would most likely increase its oral bioavailability. That is what was found in this study. Further, this study definitely outlines the need for increase in the bioavailability of poorly soluble compounds. Definitely 1.7% bioavailability is a kind of no availability. An increase to 59.6% is a worthy achievement. If only the first result is considered, this molecule could be a drop out. If its activity were very high, the company could have lost the molecule and would be in a very unfortunate situation.

Several other techniques and examples unveil the importance of solubility and dissolution rate in drug absorption studies. Transition time in the development of tougher and promising molecules would be some times higher and thus this process itself is time consuming in the development of oral formulations for NCE's to increase the bioavailability of poorly bioavailable compounds because of solubility limitations. In another instance, the poorly soluble weak bases, especially the imidazole antifungals, ketoconazole and itraconazole, elevated gastric pH in AIDS patients lead to a reduced rate of drug dissolution and consequently malabsorption. However, the solubility of fluconazole, a weak base with a pKa of 1.5, is sufficiently high (6 mg/ml, dose: solubility ratio about 17 ml) that its administration to patients with elevated gastric pH does not lead to dissolution ratio limited absorption. The other drugs used in the AIDS patients could be dropouts even though they are very potent, only for the same reason.

The aqueous solubility of a drug is a prime determinant of its dissolution rate, and in the case of "poorly soluble" drugs, the aqueous solubility is usually less than 100 mcg/ml. A further parameter that is useful for identifying 'poorly soluble' drugs is the dose:solubility ratio of the drug. *The dose: solubility ratio is defined as the volume of gastrointestinal fluids necessary to dissolve the administered dose.* When this volume exceeds the volume of fluids available, one may anticipate incomplete bioavailability from solid oral dosage forms. Griseofulvin is a classic example of utilization of dose: solubility ratio. Its aqueous solubility is 15 mcg/ml at 37°C and at a dose of 500 mg, its dose: solubility as calculated is 33 l. This combination of poor solubility and high dose is a severe limitation for its oral bioavailability. The solubility of griseofulvin can be increased by several techniques so as to increase its oral bioavailability. For, example in small intestine, drug solubility is sometimes increased with the help of amphiphilic bile components like bile salts, lecithin and monoleins. In a formulation consisting of bile salts at higher concentrations higer than critical micellar concentrations, it is very likely that a drug solubility could be increased 100-fold. Griseofulvin's bioavailability in this study increased by co-administering with bile salts. Other drug formulations with bile salts that demonstrated promise include griseofulvin, glutethimide, digoxin, leucotriene-D4 antagonists and gemfibrozil.

The other case is a drug that might precipitate in the small intestine. A poorly soluble weakly basic drug that may be entirely dissolved in the stomach could precipitate in the small intestine because of the pH dependent solubility phenomenon. However, the drug solution achieves supersaturation before transition from solubility to insolubility occurs. This transition is not easily determined using the very routine dissolution and solubility experiments. Absorption is dependent on the area and it is larger in the small intestine compared to the stomach. In every likely for weakly basic compounds that precipitate in the small intestine, the limited absorption from the stomach and practically no absorption from the small intestine would result in lower bioavailability. The drug eventually passes out unchanged. So, what is the solution under these circumstances? The greater the time this molecule spends in the stomach, the greater is its absorption into the blood, provided it reaches blood from stomach membranes. In these circumstances, one aspect is fed and fasted states. In one *in vitro* study in human beings, the transfer rates varied from 0.5 to 9 ml/min in fasted and fed states, respectively. Thus, this several fold difference would suggest an increase in the stomach residence time and thereby leading to increased absorption and oral bioavailability for this molecule during these two states. If the molecule is not transported across stomach membranes and if it has only intestines as transport means, then several formulations that prevent the precipitation of this drug in the intestines are helpful. Also, gastro retentive drug delivery systems that specifically release the drug at the site of absorption may also be of help. The precipitation may be avoided.

It is very interesting to investigate the precipitation kinetics of NCEs in an *in vitro* set up prior to the initiation of *in vivo* studies. Currently, it is difficult to conduct this experiment in a laboratory because of the complexity of mounting the transition state, very similar to that found in the *in vivo* conditions. As mentioned earlier, the other approach would be to investigate the bioavailability of a molecule routinely in fed and fasted state as a part of comprehensive formulation development process. In this regard, the bioavailability of several molecules including dipyridamole, BIBU 104 XX, BIMT 17 BS were found to be different in these two conditions because of rapid precipitation issues. This would definitely affect the pharmacodynamic results in the pharmacological screening for activity of these molecules. Obviously some times this may lead to the drop out of a new chemical entity. In addition, this drug may show significant gastrointestinal tract toxicity. Thus, precipitation issue is one of the priorities in the investigation of oral bioavailability of new chemical entities. A sustained, controlled and targeted release formulation such as a pellet, a bioadhesive tablet, a nanoparticle, a microparticle or a liposome could sometimes increase the bioavailability of a precipitating drug. These delivery systems may slowly release the drug in the small intestine avoiding precipitation and thus may result in increased bioavailability. That is how an important and potent molecule with the problems of precipitation could be rescued timely if these core concepts are considered.

Target Tissue Requirements

The aim of drug delivery is to see that a drug reaches the target tissue in therapeutic levels. Oral route is a very common and convenient route of administration of drugs. Unfortunately, in many situations a drug may not reach its target after oral administration. The first rate-limiting step is the drug absorption across gastro intestinal tract. The best idea in these situations is to directly inject a drug into the active site. For example, it was found that in several viral pathologies say for example AIDS, the pathogen resides in remote parts like brain or spinal tract. In these situations, after oral administration, intestinal tract is the depot for the drug. The drug slowly reaches the systemic circulation from the gastro intestinal tract. It likely kills the pathogens in the systemic circulation and eventually reaches the remote tissues. However, this is a very ideal situation. In several cases, although the drug is very potent and has tremendous activity, it may not even reach the systemic circulation and thence may not show any therapeutic benefit. Leaving apart the remote location, this drug is not even able to cure the very peripheral pathology. This is one reason for the requirement of drug absorption improvement after oral administration. Directly injecting the drug at the target tissue is one option. However, in many instances target tissue injection is not patient friendly and definitely a drug absorption improvement technique is the priority. In the same case, if a low permeable drug is used to treat patients with a remote target, a higher bioavailability would definitely be a requirement. The drug may reach its target tissue at desired quantities if the drug is well distributed from the systemic circulation. In this context, several methods are available to increase the oral bioavailability of a new chemical entity.

The bioavailability of compound 1 mentioned in the previous section was increased several fold when administered as a solution dosage form compared to a capsule dosage form. This is a very simple example. As mentioned before, in a remote target tissue and severe disease state, very high systemic levels of the drugs are required. If by chance the distribution of the drug from the systemic circulation to the target tissue is not very high, in every likely this disease would not have any significant therapy using this molecule. The bioavailability of this molecule after oral administration needs to be increased several fold using any of the techniques namely physical, chemical or biological. However, when drug targets are diseases such as brain, fetus, cancers, etc. the access of the drug to the target may be very low or the residence of this treatment may not be that significant. In every likely the targeting of the drug to the site of this pathology would be essential. A formulation scientist could conveniently test in sequence physical, chemical and then biological methods for this purpose. Several physical techniques apart from the very simple solution form are currently in active investigation for a variety of reasons for this purpose. Despite efforts to increase the bioavailability fails in the eliciting of therapeutic benefit using a physical method, every likely a chemical system may be helpful. In this regard, a prodrug modification, a salt formation technique or use of permeability enhancers would definitely increase the bioavailability of this molecule and may further help in increasing the drug levels at the target site. Say for instance, if blood-brain barrier has a transporter protein which is very active, and a drug is synthesized into a prodrug with a moiety that could take this molecule at a rapid rate across the BBB because it is a substrate to this transporter and subsequently gets hydrolyzed at the active site to release the drug, it is very likely that the tissue levels of this drug would be of benefit to enhance the therapy with this molecule for this pathology provided it has good bioavailability. If it is a simple disease it should be fine. The body immune system may take care without drug treatment. However, if the pathology is severe such as a cancer or AIDS, definitely spending enough time and resources would benefit the company and society as such. As several complex associated things would take part in the reduction of drugs reaching the target tissue despite ample efforts, then targeting of the drug to the active site is the best option. This could be in the form of sustained release delivery system or just injection of the drug at the active site. In either case the requirement is to achieve therapeutic levels of a drug at the target site.

Methods to Improve Drug Absorption

Physical

Several physical methods are currently being investigated to improve drug absorption. Based on the mechanism of action, these methods can be conveniently clubbed into two broad classes.

1. Methods to increase the saturation solubility of the drug in the intestinal fluids (e.g. complex formation) and
2. Methods to increase the dissolution rate (e.g. particles size reduction).

The first method has been proved to be of limited success as indicated by the number of products in the market. The second method is helpful in the increase in drug absorption by elevation of the dissolution rate of a new chemical entity. This is generally achieved by an increase in the surface area of the drug substance. Some of these techniques are drug particle size reduction, nanosuspension formulations, nanocrystal formulations, nanoparticle formulations, utilization of a surface-active carrier, utilization of self-emulsifying carrier, solid dispersions, complexation, etc. Most of these techniques are dissolution rate enhancement techniques. Despite all the efforts, if the absorption of a new chemical entity is very tough with any of the techniques for whatever reason and however good its pharmacological activity is, the molecule could be a challenge.

Drugs or NCEs can be conveniently classified based on their absorption and solubility patterns into class I: high water-soluble with high absorption; class II: water-insoluble, when dissolved and well absorbed; class III:water soluble with low membrane permeability; and class IV: water insoluble when dissolved and not well absorbed.

Class I: These compounds are generally very well absorbed. Examples include propranolol and metoprolol. These are generally formulated as immediate release products. Their dissolution rate generally exceeds gastric emptying. These are the nicer molecules in terms of drug absorption at the intestinal tract. Nearly 100% absorption is expected if atleast 85% of a product dissolves within 30 min of *in vitro* dissolution in a wide range of pH values.

Class II: The bioavailability of these compounds is dissolution-rate limited. A correlation between *in vivo* bioavailability and *in vitro* dissolution rate (IVIVC) is observed. Examples include piroxicam and naproxen.

Class III: Absorption is permeability-rate limited but dissolution occurs very rapidly. Initially, in physical studies these classes of molecules could be very nice in the hands of the formulation scientist. However, eventually when biological system is exposed, severe drawbacks are foreseen with these classes of molecules. Examples include ranitidine and cimetidine. Sustained release systems are better option for these molecules. For class I drugs, because of the least constraints, *in vivo* bioequivalence data are not necessary to assure product comparibility. As long as the test and the reference formulation do not contain agents that modify drug permeability or GI transit time waiver criteria similar to those associated with class I compounds may be appropriate.

Class IV compounds are very poorly soluble. These are low soluble and low permeable. These compounds tend to be very difficult to formulate and could exhibit very large inter-subject and intra-subject variability (e.g. furosemide).

Generally, appropriate methods of drug bioavailability increase would be investigated conveniently based on the above classification. This would be a very right beginning for a formulation scientist to further investigate formulation strategies for new chemical entities. Some times this development could be very challenging and may require lot of effort and time. Thus, immediately after a molecule reaches the hands of a formulation or biopharmaceutical scientist, the first thing to be done is to investigate the solubility and permeability properties of this NCE. Then classify as per the above properties and conveniently proceed for further promising investigations. Some of these techniques in brief are:

1. **Drug particle size reduction**

   Drug particle size reduction is often the first technique to be attempted to increase drug bioavailability. Since the dissolution rate is directly proportional to the surface area, this would be a very convenient method. Size reduction can be achieved using several techniques. However, the relevant technique for this section is the simple mechanical reduction of drug particle size. Size reduction can be achieved in physical states using techniques such as grinding and pulverization. However, a suspension formulation with reduced drug size can be also conveniently placed in this group, especially when the effective surface area also depends on the ability of the fluid to wet the particle surface.

2. **Solid dispersions**

   Although direct techniques like particle size reduction may increase the oral bioavailability, some times particle size reduction may be either impractical or the desired increase in the bioavailability may not be achieved. One way of dealing with this problem is to develop solid dispersions of drugs using hydrophilic fillers. Solid dispersions are very old dosage forms that were investigated to increase the oral bioavailability and most of the times demonstrated promise in the laboratory set up. These are the systems in which a drug is dispersed in solid water-soluble matrices either molecularly or as fine particles. Since there is an increase in the surface area due to the existence of molecular state, there is obviously an increase in the dissolution rate. To illustrate the application of solid dispersions, a very recent example will be discussed in this section.

   Van Nijlen et al., (2003), investigated the solid dispersions of artemisinin in order to improve the intestinal absorption characteristics. Along with several other techniques, solid dispersions were also investigated for this drug. Solid dispersions of artemisinin with PVPK25 as a carrier were prepared by the solvent method. The dissolution rate of artemesinin with at least 67% of PVPK25 was significantly improved in comparison to untreated and mechanically ground artemisinin. Modulation of the dissolution rate of artemisinin was obtained by the formation of solid dispersions. As a counter part technique, particle size reduction was also investigated. The effect of particle size reduction on the dissolution rate was limited, suggesting that particle size reduction is not helpful in this situation to increase the oral bioavailability and dissolution rate of this molecule. This study suggests that simple mechanical pulverization of a drug some times may not help in increasing the absorption of a drug across gastro intestinal tract. In these situations alternate techniques like solid dispersion will help.

Once prepared, solid dispersions can be administered orally as tablet dosage forms or filled in a capsule and administered as capsules. Although they showed promise in the laboratory set up, their commercial use is however not yet valid because of the manufacturing difficulties and stability problems. Some of these manufacturing difficulties were reduced with the use of surface-active and self-emulsifying agents. Generally, in the preparation process, suitable carriers are melted at elevated temperatures, the drugs are dissolved in molten carriers, and the hot solutions are allowed to cool and then crushed to obtain powders. Alternatively the hot liquid melt can be filled into capsules to obtain plugs. Solid plugs are formed inside capsules at room temperature, and due to the surface activity of the carriers, drugs dissolve and disperse rapidly once the plugs come in contact with the gastro intestinal tract.

3. Micronization

Simple mechanical pulverization may not always help in increasing the dissolution rate of a drug substance. The reason may be either the lack of wetting of the drug or enough surface area for drug dissolution may not be available. One way of achieving this is to further reduce the particle size. Micronization is the technique in which the particle size of the drug particle at the conclusion would be 3-4 microns. Van Nijlen et al., (2003), along with solid dispersion also investigated micronization as means to increase the dissolution rate of artemisinin in order to improve the intestinal absorption characteristics. Micronisation by means of a jet mill and supercritical fluid technology resulted in a significant decrease in the particle size as compared to untreated artemisinin. At the end of production, all the powders appeared to be crystalline. The dissolution rate of the micronised forms improved in comparison to the untreated form in an *in vitro* dissolution testing system, but showed no difference in comparison to the mechanically grounded artemisinin.

In another study by Kondo et al., (1993), the use of micronization to increase the oral bioavailability of an anticancer agent was investigated. HO-221 is a new NCE with anticancer properties with a novel mode of action. This molecule shows poor oral absorption and is only slightly soluble in water

(0.055 micrograms/ml at 37°C). The particle size of the drug was reduced to submicron region (0.453 micrometer, mean by volume) by a wet milling process in a decaglycerin monolaurate aqueous solution in the presence of small glass beads. The wet milling suspension obtained showed improved dissolution rate and oral absorption in rats. A solid dosage form was prepared from this suspension with the addition of sucrose palmitate to prevent aggregation caused by the hydrophobic interaction. The solid dosage form thus obtained showed twice oral absorption in dogs than that of a preparation made by dry milling, suggesting that the control of particle size would be one of the best methods of increasing the oral bioavailability.

4. Nanocrystal technology

The latest technique to increase the dissolution and absorption of a poorly soluble drug is Nanocrystal Technology. According to a recent paper, 40% of the drugs being in the development pipelines are poorly soluble. Upto 60% that come up from direct synthesis are poorly soluble, currently. Oral route of delivery is the first priority of any formulation scientist. In the preformulation step, this is definitely priority followed by the development of an intravenous system. In this context a dosage form that can serve both the purposes at one shot and further take this molecule into a simple oral formulation for clinical and market purpose is quite elegant. Nanocrystal technology serves both the purposes. This technology is still in the investigation stage only. However, further research would be helpful in this regard. Basically this technology is a size reduction technology similar to micronization. Many of the new compounds show such a low solubility that micronization does not lead to a sufficient increase in the bioavailability after oral administration. Therefore the next step is nanonisation. These are drug particles of sizes in typical range from 200-600 nm. Several methods of preparation are currently being developed to obtain solid nanocrystals that could be developed as tablets and capsule dosage forms or suspension dosage forms could be prepared to be injected parenterally. In either case, the generation of the nanocrystals is the same.

Drug nanocrystals can be produced by bottom up techniques (i.e. precipitation) or alternatively by bottom down technique (i.e. disintegration, milling). The bottom up technique is the classical precipitation technique, the drug is dissolved in a solvent which is subsequently added to a nonsolvent to precipitate the crystals. This technique is difficult to handle, the crystal growth needs to be stopped to avoid the formation of microcrystals. Further, this technique is marred by several disadvantages including that it is not applicable to increasing number of drugs; these being poorly soluble in a variety of media. These simple techniques were later modified to industrial scale and currently the different techniques owned by several companies for the manufacture of nanocrystals include:

1. Pearl milling (nanocrystals-elan),
2. Homogenization in water (Nanoedge-Baxter) and
3. Homogenization in nonaqueous media or in water with water miscible liquids (Nanopure-Pharmasol Berlin). The nanocrystals thus formed can be mixed with liquid or solid excipients and filled into capsules or tablets, as per the convenience and administered. This technology is currently in active investigations in the laboratory scale as well as industrial scale. However, the ultimate goal of these investigations is to trace the bad quality of this drug and set it right using these novel technologies.

5. Nanosuspension technology

Nanocrystal technology generates solid drugs, where as its counter part nanosuspension technology is useful in the development of liquid suspensions with the particle size range in nanometers. Use of this technology right from the beginning of the development of a new chemical entity can also help in the development of a dosage form that can be used for targeted delivery such as brain, kidneys, heart and bone marrow and not only for oral or intravenous routes used in the preformulation studies. The advantage is that the generation of particles of nanosize range would be helpful in the development of less toxic intravenous dosage form.

Nanosuspensions consist of drugs broken into crystals in the nanometer range by high-pressure homogenization and then stabilized by surfactants. As a result of the reduced size of the nanocrystals, the saturation solubility and dissolution velocity are increased, which is usually also accompanied by an increase in the bioavailability. An example of a very recent study will be illustrated here. Paclitaxel nanosuspension were developed by Bristol-Myers Squibb and investigated for intravenous administration. The study demonstrated that the LD_{50} of paclitaxel nanosuspension is much lower than that of Taxol (Bristol Myers Suibb, Princeton, USA): nanosuspension shown an LD_{50} value of approximately 100 mg/kg. Thus, these nanosuspensions of drugs can be used both for oral as well as intravenous administration. Using this technology, the production, analysis and processing of formulations containing highly toxic compounds such as cytotoxics, for example Paclitaxel, in the lab scale is possible in a specially designed lab unit. In addition, the same system can be used for controlled and sustained release dosage. Earlier literature demonstrated the advantage of nanoformulations over micronized drugs in improving oral bioavailability. Several successful nanosizing techniques to prepare marketable formulations from drugs such as sirolimus, fenofibrate, aprepitant and megestrol acetate exist. Before considering the application of nanosizing to enhance the oral bioavailability, the biopharmaceutical properties of the drug are to be carefully evaluated. Drugs exhibiting dissolution rate-limited absorption are the best candidates for nanosizing. Nanosizing may attract more pharmabusiness in near future.

6. Use of Cyclodextrins

These starch derivatives are the most widely investigated excipients for enhancing the solubility and dissolution rate of poorly soluble drugs. The interior of these molecules is relatively lipophilic and the exterior relatively hydrophilic. Cyclodextrins and their commercially available derivatives are able to incorporate apolar molecules or parts of molecules inside their hydrophobic cavity resulting in better stability, high water solubility, increased bioavailability or decreased undesirable side effects. The mechanism for the enhanced solubilization is entrenched in the ability of cyclodextrin to form non-covalent dynamic inclusion complexes in solution. Other solubilizing attribute may include the ability to form non-inclusion based complexes, the formation of aggregates and related domains and the ability of cyclodextrins to form and stabilize supersaturated drug solutions. The increase in solubility also can increase dissolution rate and thus improve the oral bioavailability of BCS Class II drugs. The success rate of cyclodextrins for enhancing the dissolution rate of poorly soluble drugs is witnessed by the presence of over 35 marketed drug products in the market. The solubilizing ability of cyclodextrins can be further enhanced by incorporating other water-soluble excipients. The drug-cyclodextrin complexes are prepared by freeze-drying, spray-drying, and co-precipitation of a cyclodextrin/drug solution or simple grinding the slurry of drug and cyclodextrins. The difference in complex formation methodology can affect the dissolution kinetics and subsequently the bioavailability. This may be due to the differences in the extent of complex formation, changes in the particle size and degree of amorphous nature of the resulting material.

7. Self-emulsifying drug delivery systems (SEDDS) and selfmicroemulsifying drug delivery systems (SMEDDS)

Self-emulsifying drug delivery systems (SEDDS) and *selfmicroemulsifying drug delivery systems (SMEDDS)* are isotropic solutions of oil and surfactant which form oil-in-water microemulsions on mild agitation in the presence of water. The poorly soluble drug can be dissolved in a mixture of surfactant and oil which is widely known as preconcentrate. These novel colloidal formulations on oral administration behave like oil-in-water microemulsions. Compared with ready-to-use microemulsions, the SEDDS and SMEDDS have been shown to improve physical stability profile in longterm storage. SEDDS have been reported to enhance the oral bioavailability of paclitaxel, griseofulvin and dexibuprofen. Similarly, SMEDDS were shown to enhance the oral bioavailability of poorly soluble drugs such as simvastatin, acyclovir and exemestane. *Solid SEDDS* are the advanced formulations that can be filled directly into soft or hard gelatin capsules for conventional drug delivery.

8. **Solid lipid nanoparticles**

Solid lipid nanoparticles (SLN) represent an alternative carrier system to traditional colloidal carriers (emulsions, liposomes and polymeric micro- and nanoparticles) in enhancing the oral bioavailability of poorly soluble drugs. These particulate systems contain solid lipids as matrix material which possesses adhesive properties that make them adhere to the gut wall and release the drug exactly where it should be absorbed. In addition, the lipids are known to have properties that promote the oral absorption of lipophilic drugs and drugs in general. Thus, SLN can improve the oral bioavailability of the poorly soluble drugs. Of the available methods, *high-pressure homogenization* and *microemulsion technology* are considered as the most feasible methods for large scale production of SLN. Lipid matrix of solid lipid nanoparticles is made from physiologically tolerated lipid components, which decreases the potential for acute and chronic toxicity. Another significant advantage of SLN formulations is that they have the ability to be stable for 3 years, which is of paramount importance with respect to colloidal drug carriers. There are a number of reports indicating the enhanced oral bioavailability of drugs including praziquantel, quercetin, lovastatin, nitrendipine, vinpocetine and cyclosporine.

9. **Liposomes**

One of the challenges in formulating microemulsions, SEDDS or SMEDDS is the limited availability of formulation components with GRAS status. In this context, liposomal formulations may be preferred over the above colloidal drug delivery systems for solubilizing the drugs and thereby to enhance oral bioavailability. This is because of the GRAS status of phospholipid constituents used in liposomal formulations. *Liposomes* are phospholipid vesicles, comprising a phospholipid bilayer surrounding an aqueous compartment. In the lipid domain of the bilayer membrane, lipophilic drugs can be dissolved. Due to their biphasic characteristic and diversity in design, composition and construction, liposomes offer a dynamic and adaptable technology for enhancing drug solubility. It has been reported that the liposome encapsulation efficiency of lipophilic drugs depends on both the physicochemical properties of the drug, such as its lipophilicity, and on factors including bilayer composition and the method of preparation. Liposomes are shown to be promising carriers for enhancing the bioavailability of poorly soluble drugs such as ibuprofen, amphotericin B, cyclosporine, and griseofulvin. A fenofibrate liposomal formulation was prepared by a dry-film dispersing method coupled with sonication and homogenization using soybean phosphotidylcholine and sodium deoxycholate or cholesterol (Chen et al., 2009). *In vivo* measurements of pharmacokinetics and bioavailability demonstrated higher rates of fenofibrate absorption from the liposomal formulations than micronized fenofibrate.

Chemical

Chemical method of drug absorption increasing includes tagging the molecule with a salt, a chemical moiety (prodrugs) or co-administration with membrane permeation enhancers. A very brief overview with some specific good examples of relevance of each of the above techniques will be discussed in this section.

1. Salt-formation

The very common current technologies investigated to improve the properties of the drug before even a drug is obtained in the pure form to a chemist are the salt-formation techniques. Salt forms of drugs can be developed in tandem with the synthesis of the compounds of specific interest using high-through put screening in a 96-well plate. The different reagents of synthesis along with the reagents involved in the salt formers can be, in tandem, added to the same 96-well plate to obtain the drug as well as its salt forms at the same time. The further advantage using this technique is that the characterization of these salts and the drug along with various crystal forms that could be obtained could be investigated together. Use of hydrochloride salts of drugs to improve the properties of a compound was in practice for over several years. By 1977, nearly 43% of the FDA commercially marketed salts were hydrochlorides. In addition, mesylate salts were also common to alter the properties of drugs. These salts are generally converted back to the active component either in the intestines or at the active site. Several important salt formers that are currently employed include hydrochloric acid, citric acid, pamoic acid, procaine, benzathine, arginine, etc. The prominence of hydrochloric acid is slowly diminishing because of the toxicity associated with the release of hydrogen chloride once the salt is cleaved into the base and the hydrochloric acid. In addition high-throughput synthesis of pharmaceutical salts is also in active state of research, thereby enhancing the importance of salt selection technique in modifying the properties of a new chemical entity. This technique is discussed in length in a different chapter of this textbook. The salient features of a salt selection process include:

(a) Highly soluble and stable salt form of a basic or acidic drug can be synthesized.

(b) High-throughput synthesis techniques to obtain several salt forms of a compound in the early developmental stages can be assessed.

(c) Large number of salt forms synthesized would allow early identification of crystalline forms with desired properties very conveniently.

(d) Based on the practicality and the reality, the appropriate salt form can be either further investigated or discarded.

2. Prodrugs

Prodrugs are the other important forms of drugs and their conjugates that have been investigated for over several years to enhance the permeability of drugs across biological membranes and to increase their stability, apart from several other advantages. Simply a prodrug can be defined as a drug conjugate with improved properties. The drug can be either a small molecule or a macro-molecule. The conjugate could be a small molecule, a macromolecule or a polymer. Prodrugs for paracetamol were synthesized and investigated for over several years to reduce the hepatic toxicity and enhance its bioavailability. Similarly, prodrugs for several small molecules have been synthesized and investigated. The other class of prodrugs called as **"polymeric prodrugs"** can be used for extended or targeted delivery. Generally, a prodrug is cleaved to form the active drug for its action to be elicited. Another class of prodrugs is **"soft drugs"**. Drugs for local delivery such as to the skin, the eyes, or the lungs predominantly belong to the class of soft drugs. A very detailed concept of prodrugs is discussed in the next chapter. However, in this context, the applications of prodrugs with specific examples are briefly presented.

1. **Formulation of water-soluble compounds**

   Diazepam (tranquilizer) has low water solubility but the open-chain amino acid prodrug is very water-soluble. Peptidases (*in vivo*) hydrolyze the prodrug to an intermediate which spontaneously cyclizes to provide the drug.

2. **Prodrugs for improved absorption and distribution**

   Fluocinolone aceteonide and flucinonide are corticosteroid prodrugs that allow dermal absorption by "masking" the hydroxyl groups (that can interact with the skin or binding sites in the keratin) as either esters or acetonides. Once absorbed through the skin, the true drug is revealed by esterases or hydrolysis. Dipivefrin is a prodrug for the antiglaucoma drug epinephrine. The dipivaloyl esters allow for greater corneal permeability which are hydrolyzed by corneal and aqueous humor esterases.

Co-administration with Permeation Enhancers

Some physicochemical properties associated with poor membrane permeability are low octanol/aqueous partitioning, the presence of strongly charged functional groups, high molecular weight, a substantial number of hydrogen-bonding functional groups and high polar surface area. Permeation enhancers are helpful in increasing the bioavialability elevation of molecules with any of the above properties. The typical drugs investigated previously include peptides, peptide analogs, or other polar, high molecular weight drugs, such as heparin. The important factors to be considered in using permeation enhancers are

1. the extent of bioavailability increase achieved,
2. the influence of formulation and physiological variables,
3. toxicity associated with permeation increases and
4. the mechanism of permeation enhancement. Several permeation enhancers are currently being investigated. However, a few very important of the permeation enhancers, currently very active, are discussed in this section. These include:

1. **Surfactants**

   Various nonionic, anionic, and cationic surfactants were previously investigated for permeation enhancement. For nonionic surfactants, the size and structure of both the alkyl chain and the polar group influence absorption-enhancing activity. These permeation enhancers likely increase permeability by solubilizing membrane components. Judicial selection of the permeation increasers is definitely a very important factor accordingly, because of the limited permeation enhancers available with this mechanism. Examples of surfactants include polyoxyehtylene (POE) ethers, POE esters, POE sorbitan esters, nonphenoxypolyoxyethylene derivatives and dodecylmaltoside. Dodecylmaltoside (DM) is a recent addition to this category. Several examples suggest that this molecule increases membrane permeability without elevating membrane protein and phospholipid release. Compounds with enhanced permeability with DM include phenol red in rats (small intestines and colon), adrenocorticotropic hormone (ACTH) in rat (jejunum and colon) and azetirelin in rats (colon) and dogs (oral bioavailability).

2. **Fatty acids**

   Although various fatty acids have been shown to have membrane-permeation-enhancing activity, sodium caprate has been the most thoroughly characterized for use as an absorption-enhancing excipient. In rats the *in situ* absorption of cefmetazole from closed colonic loops was increased approximately 10-fold by sodium caprate, whereas the increases with sodium caprylate and sodium laurate were two-fold and seven fold, respectively. Tissue permeability abruptions, toxicities and tissue death are common with sodium caprate. As a replacement, several fatty acids were investigated with potential promising results. These were found to be as much potent and as much active as sodium caprate. Longer chain fatty acids were found to be effective and currently used in combination with emulsifying agents. As an example, emulsions (w/o/w) containing oleic, linoleic, or linolenic acid were found to be effective in increasing the *in situ* colonic absorption of insulin in rats. Judicious selection of these along with the possible and suitable surfactant, either anionic or cationic could be better opted in this category of penetration enhancers.

3. Medium-Chain Glycerides

The term medium-chain glycerides (MCGs) generally refer to monoglycerides and diglycerides of caprylic and capric acid. These often are supplied as mixtures that may also contain small amounts of triglycerides as well as monoglycerides and diglycerides of shorter and longer chain fatty acids. Medium-chain triglycerides are used as pharmaceutical excipients and as nutritional agents, but these are much less active than monoglycerides and diglycerides as membrane-permeation enhancers. MCGs are lipophilic and poorly water-soluble, they have often been studied in combination with emulsifying or solubilizing agents, accordingly. Very rarely, other glyceride derivatives were investigated. Ex. Monohexanoin was more effective than MCG in increasing oral absorption of dDAVP. A monoolein/sodium taurocholate combination increased colonic absorption of calcitonin, horseradish peroxidase, and polyethylene glycol (PEG) 4000 in rats, while causing no morphologic damage to the colonic environment.

Biological

Several of the techniques of increasing drug permeation across the gastrointestinal tract were previously described. However, a very peculiar situation that would occur is when everything is ideal in terms of dissolution and *in vitro* transport, but the drug absorption would be very poor. The ideality as defined here would be very relevant in the investigation of dissolution and transport properties of a molecule using *in vitro* techniques as the only conclusive and first experiments. These investigations are sometimes very routine studies in early drug discovery processes. This is particularly true when the resources are very limited. Examples of these situations would be investigations in a research laboratory in a University or a very small start-up company. As such the procurement of NCEs in these situations would be after very diligent effort and when this company owner with very limited resources would come to a conclusion that this would be the best way to obtain quick profit with very limited cash flow. The first experiments that would be conducted are simple dissolution experiments and *in vitro* transport studies. The activity of this NCE is already tested, the dissolution experiments and *in vitro* transport studies indicate very rosy picture. However, this formulation administered orally would totally beat the purpose of both the study and the company owner demonstrating no activity or no bioavailability in animal models. Several reasons would be the constraints in this situation. However, most of the times this could be boiled down to simple biological effects. These are elicited only *in vivo* and are not observed in *in vitro* experimental conditions.

The same reasons, which demonstrated negative results in the *in vivo* experiments, can be conveniently modified accordingly to potentially increase the permeation of this molecule. That way this molecule can be proved to be effective *in vitro* and *in vivo* studies. On the other hand, these studies could not go waste. These studies may further help in developing a clinical oriented analog without negative results demonstrated by the earlier molecule. Some of these biological factors along with the modification of the permeability by altering these properties will be discussed in this section. The other situation would be with metabolism-limited approaches. This situation occurs when the bioavailability is determined by metabolism. Say, for instance, 30% of the drug administered is metabolized in the gastrointestinal tract and its net bioavilability is only 40% when metabolism is absent, in every likely the net bioavailability of this molecule in the real situation would be very low. Co-administering with metabolism inhibitors that protect the drug from metabolism could increase this kind of drug absorption. The other instance would be when metabolism needs to be increased. This is a situation with prodrugs that are metabolized in the gastrointestinal tract and subsequently gets transported into the systemic circulation. Metabolism activators would enhance this transport process by activating this molecules intestinal degradation. The other case scenerio is the transporter modification. Membrane transporters could be saturation limited and rate limited. If the bioavailability of a drug is restricted because of the very quick saturation of a transporter, the situation of no absorption reaches very fast. In this condition, the transporter properties could be modified to obtain the desired bioavailability. The compounds that could modify a transporter can be termed transporter modifiers. Comprehensively, the biological transport modification could be conveniently clubbed into three classes:

1. Membrane Permeability Modification,
2. Enzyme Modification and
3. Transporter Modification.

All these modifications can be observed normally in diseased states proving as examples for further investigations in normal patients. Sometimes in diseased states the gastro intestinal membranes are stripped off layer by layer or totally sealed for any of the pathological reasons, thereby altering the bioavailability compared to a normal subject. A brief overview of these processes would help better understand these concepts of increasing drug absorption.

Membrane Permeability Modulation

Once dissolved, a drug encounters several barriers (such as mucus layer, the unstirred water layer, the epithelial cell layer and its underlying tissue layers) sequentially during transport from the intestinal lumen into the blood. It is generally believed that the permeation of epithelium lining the intestine is the rate-limiting step. There are two pathways a molecule can traverse across epithelial layer and reach systemic circulation,

1. the transcellular pathway which requires the drug to penetrate the intestinal cell membranes and
2. the paracellular pathway in which diffusion occurs through water filled pores of the tight junctions between the cells. In a transcellular pathway, both active and passive processes may be involved. Each of these processes is different.

Active mechanism of transport across the membranes involves the drug binding to a transporter, then gets deposited into the cytoplasm and further is transported to the other side of the membrane to reach systemic circulation. This may require energy that might come from various cellular and non-cellular sources. Fortunately or unfortunately, this transport mechanism is very much controlled with several inhibitors or activators and sometimes could be, as perceived without complete assessment, very toxic to the body. In a passive mechanism of transport the molecule partition into the membranes followed by diffusion through the cytoplasm and then comes out to the other side. Different cell membranes possess different lipid content and proteins. This ordered arrangement of different chemicals to form a perfect barrier helps in the homeostasis of a cell. Diffusion of molecules from simple lipid bilayer constitutes passive mechanism of transport. A molecule that is ionic in the intestinal fluids and has passive mechanism of transport across gastrointestinal tract membranes would never pass through the membrane. This is because of the very low permeability of ionic compounds into the lipid bilayers. In these conditions the bioavailability of this molecule would be very low. The solution that would help, is to modify the membrane properties transiently, during which the ionic compound reaches systemic circulation and then gets distributed in the body. Subsequently, the membrane can get corrected and normalization would proceed. This can increase the bioavailability for these kinds of molecules. These kinds of experiments could be conducted simply in a laboratory using liposomes. Liposomes can be simply defined as spherical lipid bilayers forming cellular like structures. When phospholipids are hydrated, they spontaneously form lipid sacs. Paracellular drug transport can be investigated using these liposomes. Already formed liposomal sacs could be incubated with drug solution and the encapsulated material is determined from time to time. After a series of calculations, the permeability of drugs can be very closely predicted with the help of the data generated. Since proteins are not present in the membranes, the permeability values of only the drugs or new chemical entities with passive mechanism of transport are determined using these, may be called artificial cellular structures. Both active and passive processes may contribute to the permeability of drugs transported by the transcellular pathway. Each and every process is entirely different and some times all of them may be active for some drugs. In these peculiar situations, transport mechanism determination is very problematic. For the dissection of each and every pathway, it can consume lot of time and effort. If the mechanism is collaborative, in every likely the other techniques of drug absorption would aid in the penetration enhancement. Transport investigations across isolated biological membranes would be an alternative to further dissect the mechanism of transport of a molecule or a series of molecules. Since these biological membranes contain transporter proteins simulating natural system, obviously they would give very real estimations of transport processes. Careful estimations are required. Either excess or lower estimations may some times not give proper *in vitro – in vivo* correlations. Otherwise, biological means of enhancent would be essential for the benefit of the society in general. Several examples of modulating transcellular pathways can be found in the literature. Some of the examples are discussed in the chapter on drug transport mechanisms.

The other mechanism of transport that can be discussed in this context is the paracellular pathway. This is the path of a molecule using the intercellular spaces. A molecule can utilize this pathway based on its molecular size. The greater the size the greater is the restriction of the transport of a molecule with these properties. The bioavailability of ionic drugs could be increased by transient increase in the pore size of the paracellular space. Several modulators of both the paracellular path and membrane modifiers were previously investigated with success. An example will be discussed henceforth. A very recent discovery in this area is Zot protein. Fasano et al. identified *Zonula occludens* toxin (Zot), a 45 kDa protein elaborated by *Vibrio cholerae*, which activates a protein kinase C (PKC)-dependent complex intracellular cascade of events that regulate tight junction competency in the small intestine. Zot exerts its action on tight junctions by mimicking Zonulin, a ubiquitous molecule that regulates tight junction permeability. Zot is capable of binding to the Zonulin receptor on the luminal surface of the intestine and reversibly opening the tight junctions between intestinal epithelial cells. Studies suggested that Zot perturbs tight junctions and allows for the transport of agents across the intestinal mucosa to achieve higher concentrations in the systemic circulation. Zot significantly enhanced the flux of paracellular marker compounds mannitol and inulin, and two compounds, DM5 and paclitaxel, in the CACO-2 cell culture system, an *in vitro* representation of gastrointestinal tract. This is one of the best example currently popular. Several other agents were previously investigated. For the most times, these agents fall in two classes:

1. calcium chelators and
2. surfactants. However, these agents suffer from several disadvantages. Calcium chelators induce global changes in the cells including disruption of actin filaments, disruption of adherent junctions and diminished cell adhesion. The proteolytic nature of surfactants may cause exfoliation of intestinal epithelium, irreversibly compromising its barrier functions. COX inhibitors such as indomethacin inhibit regulation of epithelial permeability by reducing PGE2. Inhibitors such as indomethacin were previously shown to increase transcellular permeability of several molecules. This NSAID induced disruption of small intestinal integrity is preventable by concomitant prostaglandin administration including several other agents.

Enzyme Modulation

Although traditionally liver was considered the main site of metabolism of drugs that limit drug availability to the tissue, the presence of several CYP3A enzymes in the intestinal tract is found to play an important role in limiting the bioavailability of some drugs. Even before the drug is transported from the intestines to the circulation, metabolism may occur. These cytochrome P4503A4 (CYP3A) enzymes are expressed at high levels in mature villus tip of the enterocytes. Because of their topographic location in small intestines and because these are the first cells that a drug is exposed in the intestines, the drug substrates for this enzyme would be degraded inside the intestines before getting transported across the membrane, thereby limiting its bioavailability. Thus, the bioavailability of drug substrates for these enzymes or the prodrugs that are cleaved with these enzymes could be increased by co-administration with the enzyme inhibitors or enzyme activators, respectively. Some inhibitors of these enzymes include ellipticine, sulfaphenazole, quinidine, disulfiram, cimetidine and ketaconozole, etc. Activators include clofibrate, clofibric acid, ciprofibrate and gemfibrogil, etc.

As mentioned in the above paragraph, the intestinal tissue consists of some metabolizing enzymes. These enzymes include UDP-glucuronosyltransferases (UGTs), sulfotransferases (PSTs), and glutathione *S*-transferases (GSTs) exhibit a decreasing gradient along the intestinal wall, from duodenum to ileum. In human beings, the human intestinal CYP3A4 shows a slightly lower level at the duodenum before levels rise again at the jejunum, then finally decreasing toward the ileum. Similar expression is found in several animal species including long and short one, from mammalian to reptiles. However, in real time only human metabolism data in both normal and diseased conditions would be applicable. In studies pertaining to the perfused, rat small intestine preparations, significant metabolism was observed for acetaminophen, enalapril, and morphine. These are very simple experiments that can be done in a laboratory to obtain metabolism related absorption data. A prodrug, (-)-aminocarbovir, is converted to (-)-carbovir, when given luminally, whereas metabolism was either absent or negligible when the drug dose was given into the reservoir for systemic delivery, suggesting that it is significantly metabolized in the gastrointestinal tract and is definitely the limiting factor in the drug absorption of this compound. Interestingly, intestinal CYP3A4 levels in humans correlated well with rates of midazolam 1'- and 4-hydroxylation but failed to show a relation with the erythromycin breath test that is ordinarily used to correlate with liver CYP3A4 levels. This completes the story of drug metabolism as required currently in this textbook.

Transporter Modulation

Utilization or modulation of carrier-mediated or secretory transport systems in the gastrointestinal tract to increase the bioavailability of drugs is currently of a great interest. As a consequence, the molecular and functional characterization of transport proteins is emerging rapidly and significant numbers of drugs are shown to be substrates or inhibitors. Several transporters that are expressed in the gastrointestinal tract and are involved in drug transport include peptide transporter, glucose transporter, amide transporter, oligo peptide transporter, nucleoside transporter and monocarboxylic acid transporter. Generally, these are the transporters that act as gates to push drugs from within the intestinal tract into the systemic circulation. Some times they are limiting gates for some of the drugs of the same nature, as related to its chemistry. The known specific transport systems for organic anions can recognize the wide range of acidic and hydrophobic organic compounds. The enterocyte peptide transporter PEPT1 mediates the absorption of peptide-like drugs including beta-lactam antibiotics as well as valacyclovir lacking peptide bond. Frequently, transporters play a direct role in drug absorption from the intestines. The bioavailability of some drugs may significantly depend on carrier-mediated system. For example, the hPepT1 transporter—a H^{+}-symporter—is thought to be responsible for carrier-mediated uptake of various peptoid-like drugs such as cephalosporins, ACE-inhibitors, and 5′-amino acid ester prodrugs of antiviral nucleosides, acyclovir and AZT. Acyclovir itself is poorly absorbed, but as the 5′-amino acid ester, it is transported by hPept1 yielding enhanced bioavailability. The median bioavailabilities of acyclovir after administration of acyclovir and valacyclovir, a substrate for hPepT1, were 22 and 70%, respectively, in human subjects. Further examples of actively transported compounds are pravastatin and salicylic acid, which are transported by MCT1, a monocarboxylic acid transporter. The uptake of nateglinide, a novel oral hypoglycemic agent, appears to be mediated by proton-dependent transport system(s) distinct from MCT1. The co-administration of the substrates for these transporters so as to increase or decrease the transport of the substrate drugs could either increase or decrease the systemic levels of drugs. This could gravely affect or alter the systemic bioavailability of drugs that are the substrates for these transporters.

Similar to uptake transporters, several efflux transporters or also called secretory transport exist on the gastrointestinal membranes. Instead of taking a drug from within the intestinal tract into the systemic circulation, these transporters push a drug from systemic circulation back into the gastrointestinal tract, thereby reducing the bioavailability. Examples of these transporters include Multi-drug resistance associated protein (MRP) subfamility and P-glycoprotein. ABCB1, a member of the ABC superfamily (P-glycoprotein, MDR1) is a prominent efflux pump, which limits the uptake of substrates such as digoxin and cyclosporin. Lowes et al., 2003, suggested that an additional secretory pathway for digoxin, sensitive to the MRP-selective inhibitor MK-571, is likely to secrete digoxin from intestinal CACO-2 epithelia, an in vitro intestinal tract model. Further members of the large ABC family comprised of 48 known genes, might also contribute to reduced drug bioavailability. Grepafloxacin is secreted by ABCC2 and ABCB1, and irinotecan—used in the treatment of advanced colorecteral cancer—by ABCB1 and canalicular multispecific organic anion transporter (cMOAT). These examples demonstrate the complexity of drug membrane transport. It is likely that each drug serves as a substrate for several transporters, and moreover, transporters, ion exchangers, and ion pumps interact with each other to establish the cell's transport capacity. Thus, the modification of the transport properties helps in the increase of bioavailability of a drug.

Conclusions

As mentioned in this entire section, there is both great interest and immediate need for improving the oral bioavailabilities of various poorly bioavailable drugs. Maximizing oral bioavailability is therapeutically important because the extent of bioavailability influences plasma concentrations as well as the therapeutic and toxic effects, resulting after oral drug administration. Poorly bioavailabile drugs are inefficient because, a major portion of drug never reaches the plasma or exerts its pharmacologic effect. Moreover, a compilation of published results on structurally diverse drugs showed that the extent of bioavailability mainly depends on drug structure. Therefore, low oral bioavailability leads to high variability and poor control of plasma concentrations and effects. Intersubject variability would be particularly of concern for a drug with a narrow safety margin or a steep dose vs effect profile. In this chapter, several techniques to increase the drug bioavailability after oral administration along with the reason for such a need are discussed.

Questions for Practice and Exercise

1. Why are the methods to improve drug absorption important? Describe briefly in two paragraphs with citing very specific examples.
2. Describe the following methods used to improve drug absorption:
    1. drug particle size reduction,
    2. solid dispersions,
    3. micronization,
    4. nanocrystal technology,
    5. nanosuspension technology,
    6. Cyclodextrin technology
    7. Liposomes
    8. SMEDDS and SEDDS
    9. Solid lipid nanoparticles
    10. salt formation,
    11. prodrugs,
    12. permeation enhancers,
    13. biological methods,
    14. membrane permeability modulation,
    15. enzyme modulation, and
    16. transporter modulation.

Bibliography

1. The Practice of Medicinal Chemistry, Second Edition, Edited by Camille Georges Wermuth, Elsevier Publications, 2003.
2. Foye`s Principles of Medicinal Chemistry, Fifth Edition, David A. Williams and Thomas L. Lemke, Lippincott Williams & Wilkins, 2002.
3. Rowland M, Tozer T, Clinical Pharmacokinetics: Concepts and Application. 3rd ed. Philadelphia: Lea and Febiger, (1994).
4. Physiological Pharmaceuticals: Barriers to Drug Absorption, Second Edition, Authored by Neena Washington, et al, CRC Publication, (2001).
5. 'Drug Absorption Enhancement: Concepts, Possibilities, Limitations and Trends (Drug Targeting and Delivery), First Edition, Edited by A. G. De Boer and A.G. De Boer, CRC Press, (1994).

References

Chen Y, Lu Y, Chen J, Lai J, Sun J, Hu F, Wu W. Enhanced bioavailability of the poorly water-soluble drug *fenofibrate* by using *liposomes* containing a bile salt. Int J Pharm. 376:153-160 (2009).

CHAPTER 8

SALT SELECTION AND CHARACTERIZATION

- **Introduction**
- **Background**
- **Theory**
- **Properties Affected After Salt Synthesis**
- **Techniques**
- **Factors Affecting Salt Selection**
- **Characterization**
    - Structural analysis
    - Physico-chemical properties
    - Physical properties
    - Impurities
    - Stability studies
- **Conclusions**

Introduction

In the recent years, one of the most commonly employed practices of improving the properties of drugs is salt selection. Use of hydrochloride salts of drugs to improve the properties of a compound has been in practice for over several years. By 1977, nearly 43% of the FDA commercially marketed salts were hydrochlorides. In addition, mesylate salts were also common to alter the properties of drugs. These salts are generally converted back to the active component either in the intestines or at the active site. Unfortunately, this technique was restricted to a very few compounds of interest. However, with the increase in the availability of number of molecules for pharmacological screening and because of high-throughput synthesis and screening techniques, libraries of highly potent molecules with poor pharmaceutical properties are reaching the hands of a formulation scientist. Several techniques as discussed in length in this entire book could be investigated to improve the pharmaceutical properties of drug substances. One such technique, currently in vogue among the pharmaceutical scientists, is salt selection. Several important salt formers that are currently employed include hydrochloric acid, citric acid, palmoic acid, procaine, benzathine, arginine etc. The prominence of hydrochloric acid is slowly diminishing because of the toxicity associated with the release of hydrogen chloride once the salt is cleaved into the base and the hydrochloric acid. In addition high-throughput synthesis of pharmaceutical salts is also in active state of research, thereby enhancing the importance of salt selection technique in modifying the properties of a new chemical entity.

According to Remenar et al., 2003, “due to its central placement in chemical development and pharmaceutical research, salt selection is becoming increasingly automated to meet the need for rapid identification of crystalline salt forms in early development”. Right from the beginning, the goal of a pharmaceutical scientist is to develop a very stable compound that can reach the market place. However, if a compound is realized to be physically or chemically unstable- catalyzed by any of the processes in the development after a certain stage, it is likely that the entire process should be repeated with a new stable version of the compound or the project entirely dropped out. In addition, the physical or chemical instability during the process development may also alter the physiological and pharmacological behavior of a drug substance. Thus, it becomes mandatory not to overlook these developmental processes. The reasons that can be furnished for salt selection process thus include:

More soluble and stable salt form of a basic or acidic drug can be obtained.

1. Conversion of a compound to its crystalline form with improved aqueous solubility, chemical and physical stability, and high bioavailability relative to the freebase or acid of the active compound can be obtained.

2. High-throughput synthesis techniques can be used to obtain several salt forms of a compound in the early developmental stages.
3. The large number of salt forms synthesized would allow early identification of crystalline forms with desired properties.

A brief overview of the background, the theory and the modern high-throughput screening and characterization techniques are essential to understand the importance of salt formation in the new drug discovery process. This review comprehensively covers various aspects of salt formation including the fundamental theory, synthesis techniques, factors affecting the salt formation, characterization techniques, and case studies along with the regulatory considerations.

Background

The assessment of new chemical entities for salt screening has taken considerable attention only lately. Many thousands of compounds manufactured over several years in several countries using various synthetic methods are stored as libraries of structurally related compounds. These compounds are generally dissolved in dimethylsulphoxide (DMSO) solution and screened in an enzyme- or receptor-based assay system. If the number of "positive hits" produced is large, further screening and selection usually refine the numbers until a manageable number of "leads" is available. Many of these leads will show only weak or moderate activity and further refinement and optimization is invariably necessary. It is however very difficult to trace these "mislead" compounds. Thus, optimization procedures usually involve numerous structural modifications, aided by computational techniques, until a small number (usually 1-5) of highly active "candidates" remain. These candidates are usually free bases, free acids, or neutral molecules rather than their salts. Also, because of the generally higher molecular weights of modern drug substances and the increased use of DMSO solutions in the screening processes, it is becoming apparent that there is a tendency towards ever more lipophilic candidates being presented. Frequently, when first proposed as potential development candidates, they are often amorphous or partially crystalline. At this stage, little effort has been made to investigate formal crystallization procedures. The need for soluble drug substances has been recognized for many years before the introduction and innovation of "combinatorial chemistry". Although DMSO is used in screening, it cannot be further used because of toxicity. The other technique that is relevant in this chapter is salt screening or could be called as salt formation.

The first step in the salt formation is the identification whether the free base, its acid salt or base salt is required for evaluation at least theoretically. If the evaluation is proper, then further step can be preceded. Otherwise, the project and the investigator could stop and make transitions. On the other hand, if the decision were hassle free, then it would be a different story. The next step is to determine if polymorphic or pseudopolymorphic or amorphous forms exist. The compounds are recrystallized in several solvents to obtain desirable physical form of the drug substance. If a desirable crystal form is obtained, then this crystalline product is recovered and examined using different techniques. In the case of mixture production, the number of these different forms is identified and also if any, the existence of hydrates or solvates is identified. Preliminary information on the inter-relationships between the different forms could be determined, even at this early stage. This ensures that the different physical forms of the salts are investigated very prior to further proceeding with the formulation development so that these transitions could not be seen during the next investigations. Then the routine tests including stability tests, analytical methods for activity, for degradation products and for chiral purity, electrophoresis, shelf-life determinations, physical properties like specific surface area, size, true density, bulk powder density, wettability, melting range, optical rotation, cosolvent solubilities, propellant solubility, intrinsic aqueous solubility and finally excipient compatibility are determined. As larger quantities of drug substance and samples are available the variation in each of the physical batch of the salt produced are studied. These properties include crystal size, shape, character, etc. along with the repetition of some of the previous tests. If everything is fine and ideal and the final salt form is selected, then the formulation development along with further clinical trials etc. is continued. Otherwise, salt formation for this molecule could be stopped. Prior to initiating the formulation development the other aspect to be considered is to modify the recrystallisation conditions to obtain greater batch-to-batch uniformity and ideality in the physical properties of the candidate of interest.

Theory

The attraction and dissociation forces between atoms lead to the formation of molecules and ions, whether organic or inorganic. For instance, inorganic salt such as NaCl (sodium chloride) is an association between sodium and chloride ions and exist as solid on storage. However, when placed in water it dissolves rapidly into sodium and chloride ions to form sodium chloride solution. The other water-soluble salts are NaCl, LiBr, KI, NH_4NO_3 and $NaNO_2$. On the other hand, inorganic salts such as $BaCl_2$, MgI_2, Na_2SO_4, Na_3PO_4 are poorly water soluble. Solute-solute interactions between the ions within these salts are stronger thereby making the compounds poorly water-soluble. On the other hand, organic compounds are formed because of very strong and often resonating association between carbon and hydrogen. These organic structures are either linear or cyclic. A great many of these are either weak acids or weak bases, and their solubility is largely dependent on the polarity of the chemical groups. Apart from the attractive and dissociation forces, factors such as the rate of diffusion of water into solids, the rate of diffusion of ions into the aqueous media, the temperature, the pH of the solution all influence the solubility of organic and inorganic compounds.

Inorganic chemists very well know the assay of individual ions for over hundred years. These techniques lead to the proposal of the basic theories of solubility. Practically, the solubility of a substance is determined by adding the excess of a compound into water and then allowed to equilibrate over a period. The insoluble portion, if any, is filtered and the soluble ions are assayed to determine the amount of soluble portion. Because of the development of assay procedures for inorganic ions, the solubility theories first reported were those related to inorganic substances. Some of the theories were later applied to solubility of organic compounds. These theories generally include dielectric constant, solvatochromic polarity parameters, pH, temperature, and diffusion coefficient as the factors that influence the solubility of organic or inorganic compounds. Several complex solubility theories were proposed later. These theories included several unfathomable parameters that influence the solubility of both organic and inorganic compounds. Because of their complex nature, these theories are not yet applicable to pharmaceuticals in general and drugs in common. May be they would barge into the solubility of pharmaceuticals after some time. Some of the current basic principles as applied to the solubility of drugs are discussed below.

Most of the drugs are either weak acids or weak bases. Their solubility in water is generally low. These could be made into salts by the reaction with corresponding base or acid, respectively. Generally, acidic or anionic drugs are relatively insoluble in water. These compounds can form salts with dilute sodium hydroxide, carbonates, and bicarbonates. Examples of such drugs include methesculetol, theophylline and ascorbic acid. On the other hand, basic drugs form salts with weak acids. Earlier examples studied include the alkaloids, sympathomimetic amines, antihistamines, local anesthetics etc. Atropine sulfate and tetracaine hydrochloride salts are formed by the reaction of these basic compounds with acids.

In the current scenario of the drug synthesis, large numbers of chemical entities are generally generated because of high throughput screening techniques. A database of chemicals is generally prepared when a discovery group synthesizes a series of molecules. The first information that is collected with regard to these molecules is the pKa value of the ionizable group and the logP value of the compound. At this stage based on the pK_a values of the ionizable groups, a list of potential salt forming agents (counter-ions) could be selected, for each candidate based on list available in the literature. Then subsequent studies are performed for further evaluations. Since most of the compounds available for salt screening are either weak acids or weak bases, the theories of solubility of weak acids and weak bases will be applied. These theories are discussed below.

Solubility of Weak Acids and Weak Bases

Most of the commonly occurring drugs or new chemical moieties at the end of the chemical synthesis are either weak acids or weak bases. Because solubility is important in pharmaceutical aspects to prepare a liquid formulation or evaluate the bioavailability of a compound after oral or intramuscular administration, one of the first physical properties determined is its aqueous solubility in a wide range of pH values. After determining, further formulation development is continued, for pharmacological, toxicological and preclinical investigations with new chemical moieties and for clinical and market formulation evaluations for generic compounds. Thus, solubility determination of these weak acids and weak bases is a very important aspect. Figure 8.1 shows a classical pH-solubility profile of a weakly acidic drug. Scientists in this area spent much of the time in their earlier investigations. Subsequently, examples of pharmaceutical compounds were investigated. This theory as developed will be illustrated for an example drug, flurbiprofen. Flurbiprofen is an antianalgesic anti-inflammatory compound. It has two distinct regions in its pH-solubility curve and

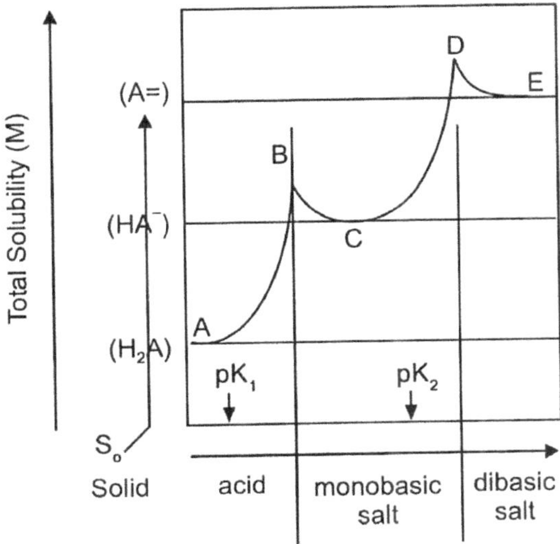

Figure 8.1 Classical solubility profile of a salt with two weakly acidic groups.

could be conveniently termed Bottom and Top. In Bottom (pH <7.3 in the figure), the excess solid phase in equilibrium with the saturated solution is the free acid. In top (pH > 7.3), the excess solid phase is the sodium salt. In Bottom, the total solubility is described by the following equation:

$$S = [HA] + [A^-]$$

$$S = S_o\,[1 + (k_a)/[H^+]]$$

Where, S is the total solubility at any given pH, S_o is the intrinsic solubility of the free acid, [HA] and $[A^-]$ represent concentrations of the undissociated and dissociated forms, respectively, in solution, and k_a is the acid dissociation constant defined as

$$K_a = \frac{(H^+)(A^-)}{(HA)}$$

The total solubility in bottom region is described by,

$$S = (1+[H^+]/[k_a]\ \sqrt{K_{sp}}$$

$$K_{sp} = [Na^+][A^-]$$

Where, K_{sp} is the solubility product of the salt

For a weakly acidic compound, the observation at $pH << pk_a$ (e.g., by 2 units), the solubility is practically independent of pH and remains at S_o. At $pH > pk_a$, the solubility increases exponentially with pH (i.e., log S increases linearly with pH). At a certain pH value, the log-linear relationship of solubility with pH abruptly ends, the solubility plot enters bottom region. The pH value where the two regions intersect is the pH of maximum solubility, referred to as pHmax. Thus, the two equations describe the entire pH-solubility profile of this mono-protic acid. In these situations, the consideration was that the activity coefficients are equal to unity in the above equilibria. Similarly this theory can be extrapolated to weakly basic drugs.

RBx 9841. HCl is a new chemical moiety currently in clinical investigation by Ranbaxy Research Laboratories for the treatment of overactive bladder. It is a novel M3 muscarinic receptor antagonist. It belongs to a class of phenyl acetamides. It is a basic compound, and a hydrochloride salt was thus synthesized to develop a safe and stable oral formulation. Apart from solid dosage forms like capsules and tablets, the aim for preclinical studies was to develop a liquid solution and a syrup formulation. This molecule is soluble in water and methanol. The solubility in water is pH independent over a range of 2.0 to 9.0. pk_a of this molecule as determined using potentiometric titration is 9.57. This pK_a suggests that the unionized form of this molecule would be present in the entire gastrointestinal tract. Thus, this molecule may not undergo pH dependent absorption from the gastrointestinal tract. At any given area of gastrointestinal tract, it is very likely that the molecule exists as a salt that has good oral bioavailability, as is indicated by its bioavailability profile. However, as per the current investigations, it is likely that in higher pH conditions such as those found in the intestinal tract during stress, the bioavailability may be increased and action may be elicited very quickly compared to that found in the normal conditions. The other explanation for its increased bioavailability, in stress conditions that may lead to decreased pH, is the common ion effect. The common-ion effect of HCl on the solubility of the salt at $pH<pH_{max}$ is significant. In the gastro intestinal tract, hydrochloride salts are particularly sensitive to the common chloride ion effect. Any minor differences in the solubility at different salt concentrations at $pH<pH_{max}$ are due to the effects of activity coefficients. This theory was further developed by several other scientists, as found in the literature and was thence termed pH_{max} theory. This theory was able to explain several other molecular behaviors. Similarly, several examples can be found in the literature. Some of the examples for the observation of such a phenomenon include terfenadine and papaverine. In close networks, these phenomena have been explained by several other theories. Since the protonated base can be considered as an acid corresponding to the free base, it is possible to characterize both, acids and bases with the same parameter, i.e. the acid ionization constant. The K_a or the pK_a, respectively, is the key parameter indicating the strength of an electrolyte. Thus, this is the first physical property determined by any chemist as the first step in new drug discovery process.

In Situ Salt Screening

In Situ Salt Screening is interrelated to salt synthesis. However, these kinds of salts are produced in the system rather than synthesized. The basic principles of utilization are the same as mentioned in the previous section. However, these salts are produced inside the intestinal tract so as to increase or decrease the bioavailability of a compound. It utilizes the changes in pH in the GIT to achieve this effect. Say for instance, RBx 9841.HCl is administered into stomach at very high doses. This definitely elicits action. However, upon co-administering with lime, its bioavailability is decreased. Basically, the precipitation of the base from the salt form is more likely the reason for decreased bioavailability in these conditions. On the other hand, the bioavailability of the same molecule would be more in higher acidic conditions, which could be seen with increased acidity with the time after administering lime along with this drug. This is one example of *in situ* salt formation. Similarly, salicylic acid administration along with lime would enhance its bioavailability after a certain time when it entirely exists as an acid rather than a salt, which may be seen in the later stages after co-administration with lime. This is another example of *in situ* salt formation.

Dissolution of Weak Acids and Weak Bases

To better understand the theory of absorption of drugs and the role of salt forms of drugs in increasing the bioavailability, comprehension of the theory of dissolution of weak acids and weak bases is essential.

Absorption from Solution

A drug given orally in solution is subjected to numerous GI secretions and, to be absorbed, must survive encounters with low pH and potentially degrading enzymes. Usually, even if a drug is stable in the enteric environment, little of it remains to pass into the large intestine. Drugs with low lipophilicity (ie, low membrane permeability), such as aminoglycosides, are absorbed slowly from solution in the stomach and small intestine; for such drugs, absorption in the large intestine is expected to be even slower because the surface area is smaller. Consequently, these drugs are not candidates for controlled release.

Absorption from Solid Forms

Most drugs are given orally as tablets or capsules primarily for convenience, economy, stability, and patient acceptance. These products must disintegrate and dissolve before absorption can occur. Disintegration greatly increases the drug's surface area in contact with GI fluids, thereby promoting drug dissolution and absorption. Disintegrants and other excipients (eg, diluents, lubricants, surfactants, binders, dispersants) are often added during manufacture to facilitate these processes. Surfactants increase the dissolution rate by increasing the wettability, solubility, and dispersibility of the drug. Disintegration of solid forms may be retarded by excessive pressure applied during the tableting procedure or by special coatings applied to protect the tablet from the digestive processes of the gut. Hydrophobic lubricants (eg, magnesium stearate) may bind to the active drug and reduce its bioavailability.

Prediction of Solubility

Solubility is understood as the concentration in a solution found in equilibrium with an excess of the solid solute at a given temperature. It is generally accepted that solubility in aqueous media is the most crucial physiochemical property of a drug substance. In order to get an estimate of the solubility of a non-electrolyte at a very early stage, many computational approaches have been made. Among them, a surprisingly simple and yet effective tool is available, the General solubility Equation (GSE) as developed and refined during the last two decades by Yalkowsky and his coworkers using a thermodynamically sound approach for establishing a semi-empirical correlation:

$$\text{Log } S = 0.5 - 0.01(M_p - 25) - \log K_{ow}$$

Where S is the molar solubility of the solute, K_{ow} the octanol/water partition coefficient, which can be calculated from the structural formula (ClogP), M_p is the melting point (in centigrade) as the only experimental data, representing the easiest accessible descriptor of the strength of a solids crystal lattice. Based on the assumption, that the non-ionized form of an electrolyte may be regarded as a non-electrolyte, an extension of the GSE has recently been proposed. By simply combining the above equation with the solubility-ionization relationships, it is possible to construct pH solubility profiles for acids, bases and zwitterions.

Dissolution Rate

Dissolution rate determines the availability of the drug for absorption. When slower than absorption, dissolution becomes the rate-limiting step. Overall, alteration of formulation is done to alter the dissolution rate. For example, reducing the particle size increases the drug's surface area, thus increasing the rate and extent of GI absorption of a drug whose absorption is normally limited by slow dissolution. Dissolution rate is affected by whether the drug is in salt, crystal, or hydrate form. The Na salts of weak acids (eg, barbiturates, salicylates) dissolve faster than their corresponding free acids regardless of the pH of the medium. Certain drugs are polymorphic, existing in amorphous or various crystalline forms. Chloramphenicol palmitate has two forms, but only one sufficiently dissolves and is absorbed to be clinically useful. A hydrate is formed when one or more water molecules combine with a drug molecule in crystal form. The solubility of such a solvate may markedly differ from the nonsolvated form; eg, anhydrous ampicillin has a greater rate of dissolution and absorption than its corresponding trihydrate.

Dissolution Theories: Older and Newer as Related to the Salt-formation

The term dissolution refers to the overall process by which a solid compound dissolves in a liquid medium, while dissolution rate is the kinetic descriptor giving the rate at which the dissolution takes place. The concept of solubility, on the other hand, implies that the process of dissolution has reached equilibrium, and the solution is saturated. Dissolution rate of solids is of paramount importance in the development of pharmaceutical products and quality control. Salt formation is one of the most commonly employed techniques to improve dissolution of weakly acidic or basic drugs. A number of theories of the dissolution of solids have been proposed. However, the simple diffusion model may be adequate to describe the dissolution behavior of most pharmaceutical solids in aqueous and non-aqueous media.

In this theory, it is proposed that around a solid particle, there always exists a layer or stagnant film of thickness 'h' during the process of dissolution. This is called a stationary layer. The concentration of the solute molecules exists as C_s to C from outside to inside. Mixing occurs outside this layer. This rate of mixing determines the thickness of the outer layer. The smaller the mixing, the thicker is the coat. Outside this layer the concentration is always C. This area can be termed the bulk phase. Several transitions of molecules other than the molecule of interest may effect the bulk phase and as such the transfer in the presence of these external agents can be either higher or lower according to the charge imparted by these agents. The other aspect is the particle size of the drug substance. The smaller the surface, the lesser is the diffusion. Accordingly,

$$DM/dt = DSC_s/h$$

Or simply,

$$J = DC_s/h$$

Where J is the flux of dissolution (this is in the sink conditions). When C is considerably less than the drugs solubility, C_s, the system is represented by sink conditions, and concentration C may be eliminated from Noyes-Whitney's equation to obtain the above equation. In the derivation of the above equation it is considered that h and S are constant, which is not the case as described previously. The same equation can be applied to the dissolution of pharmaceutical salts, either hydrophilic or hydrophobic with necessary modifications and alterations.

Eerikainene et al. (2005), observed a markedly slower release of sodium indomethacin trihydrate from granules when calcium hydrogen phosphate dihydrate was included in the formulation. The conclusion from this study was that the formation of calcium salt of indomethacin, is less water soluble than the sodium salt. This explanation is easy because of the low solubility of a drug. However, with water-soluble salts of drugs, the solubility is generally very high compared to the mother drug. In these situations, simple dissolution studies may not be helpful to predict and propose dissolution theories. In these situations, a non-disintegrating compact of the drug-salt is prepared and the release of the drug from this two-component system (drug and drug-salt that exists in the dissolution medium) is studied and the corresponding theories proposed.

In the simple case of a non-disintegrating compact composed of two components, a and b, the classical theory for the diffusion-controlled dissolution of two-component mixtures predicts, for non-interacting components, that the solubilities ($C_{S\,a}$, $C_{S\,b}$), diffusion coefficients (D_a, D_b), and the relative proportion (N_a, N_b) of the two components control dissolution in the steady state. According to this model, three different situations are possible at the solid-liquid interface during dissolution, depending on the relative amounts of the components present. At the critical mixture ratio, defined by:

$$N_a/N_b = D_aC_{sa}/D_bC_{sb}$$

both components coexist at all times at the solid-liquid interface and dissolution profiles of each component will be linear from the surface of the disc under sink conditions. At all other weight ratios, one or other component forms a porous layer at the interface, which represents an additional barrier retarding the dissolution of the receding phase. Thus, when $N_a/N_b > D_aC_{S\ a}/D_bC_{Sb}$, the dissolution rate of A (dW_a/dt) per unit surface area (G_a) will be given by the Nernst-Brunner equation:

$$G_a = dW_a/Sdt = D_aC_{sa}/h$$

where S is the surface area and *h* the diffusion layer thickness. The dissolution rate of *b* decreases with time to reach a limiting value defined by:

$$G_b = dW_b/Sdt = N_bG_a/N_a$$

In the case of mixtures of the two components, a and b, in ratios such that phase b dissolves fast enough to leave a layer of pure *a* behind, the time required to reach steady state, *t*, is given by the following equation:

$$T = K_1\{S_2\text{-}e(K_1/K_2\text{-}h^{)}/t[1\text{-}\exp^{(-K2tS2/K1}e)]\}$$

Where $K_1=A_{ah}/D_aC_{sa}$, $K_2=A_b/D_bC_{sb}$, S_2 is the coordinate value representing the a + b mixture-phase a boundary, A_a and Ab are the amounts per unit volume of a and b in the mixture, and T and e represent the tortuosity and porosity fo layer a, respectively.

When a large difference (i.e., orders of magnitude) exists between the component solubilities, deviations from this model may occur. Mixtures low in the more soluble component approximate to matrix-controlled dissolution. Carrier-controlled dissolution may occur in mixtures low in the less soluble component. The drug (less soluble) can be either molecularly dispersed in the soluble excipient or dispersed as fine particles. Dissolution of the excipient can cease to be hindered by a surface drug layer and the excipient can act as a carrier, bringing drug into the dissolution medium as it dissolves. This extension of carrier phase dissolution control to higher drug weight fractions than predicted by the two-component model is a consequence of the disparate solubilities of carrier and drug.

When the drug is considered to be molecularly dispersed in the carrier, drug release is dependent on the product of the carrier dissolution rate, G_b, and the ratio of amounts of drug and carrier present, A_a/A_b:

$$G_a = G_bA_a/A_b$$

Recently O'Connor and Corrigan (2002) developed a solubility theory called "Salt conversion model (SCM)", that can be conveniently applied for the dissolution of pharmaceutical salts. SCM theory was developed to predict dissolution of a salt of an ionizable drug and an ionizable excipient capable of forming a salt with the drug. Deviations from the model at high weight fractions of base and, in the case of the systems containing the more soluble drug, at low weight fractions of base were attributed to carrier-controlled dissolution. The current work with regard to the solubility of potential salts, which may form between the drug and ionizable excipients can be conveniently applied for any of dissolutions of pharmaceutical salts. Similarly there are several other theories to explain the dissolution behaviour of salt forms of drugs.

Properties Affected After Synthesis

Asalt is definitely different from the original drug. Salts surround the drug molecules forming clusters. The salts obtained after salt selection, screening and synthesis process are different from salts in the solution. The bond lasts for a long time. In the very beginning of the synthesis in every likely the cluster can have the same properties as that of the drug. However, with time when the bonds become solid, the properties keep changing till a final stable state is obtained. Study of these properties could result in the betterment of the formulation and the salt as such. Some of the salts slowly pick up one or two molecules of water and slowly form hydrates. Others may attach to several other similar clusters of molecules to form crystals. The crystals then have several water molecules to further lead to different polymorphic characters of the crystals. This depends on the environment in which the crystal is stored in.

Most of the times the two drug molecules are similar in nature. This leads to the formation of a uniform crystal. Otherwise, there is a possibility of contamination, if a salt is formed along with drug substance with the presence of an impurity. The best solution for this case is that the impurity has to be removed and the salt is formed at this stage. This would aid in the formation of appropriate crystal, which would be easy to characterize, and the formulation development would be very systematic. Otherwise, the resulting product may be very erratic. If the molecule of interest is potent, each and every issue is very critical. On the other hand, if the molecule is not protecting, there is enough leverage to be applied to make different attempts and transitions for productivity. In this case, if after several attempts, the result is not productive, the resulting salt can be conveniently discarded. However, the exercise is not futile because the lessons learnt in this respect are helpful to further proceed with the development of the salts of other drug candidates. This kind of investigation is also helpful in the high throughput screening techniques with several drug candidates screening together for salt synthesis at one time. Intelligent estimations and manipulations at this stage would further assist in the development of suitable salt forms of several drug candidates at one time point. In this situation, the investigation of the alterations of the properties of the resulting salts helps. Several properties are noticed to be altered during salt synthesis process. These include hygroscopicity, morphic state, crystallinty, melting point, chemical stability, corrosiveness etc. The change in these properties can be conveniently explained based on the above hypothesis.

Techniques

The first time a pharmaceutical scientist encounters salt formation technique in his mind is during the formulation development to be supplied for initial screening in animal models or cell culture studies. Most of the currently generated drugs are poorly soluble in water. For *in vitro* screening in cell culture models, a drug has to be solubilized in distilled water. Because of the poor solubility of these molecules, a solution of the compound in distilled water with the help of DMSO or other co-solvents is made and this is administered to test the *in vitro* efficacy. However, upon such administration, it is always likely that a compound could be insoluble during the *in vitro* cell culture screening, and thus the efficacy would be either an artifact or the compound could be thrown into the sink even though it has high activity. Under this circumstance, salt formation would be very helpful. The salts of the drugs thus formed would be soluble and thus could be used in cell culture screening. This is the first consideration. The second consideration is during formulation development. *In vivo* studies of promising molecules are typically conducted using suspension formulations of the free acid or base. Often, however, such dosing practices result in low or insufficient exposure due to poor oral absorption, making it difficult to evaluate these compounds. In such cases, extensive formulation work may be needed in order to achieve adequate exposure. One way of reducing this workload is to adopt high-throughput processes. One formulation technique that could be used by this process is salt-synthesis and screening. The synthesis of salts has been there for long time. However, adequate research is only achieved very recently. Very commonly a salt could be synthesized in a laboratory in a test tube. But high-through put could be achieved with the help of computers employing advanced software with all the techniques including statistical and very latest algorithms that could definitely increase the output of salt screening process in the current drug industrial setup. The techniques that can be routinely used in a laboratory set up are tabulated below.

Table 1

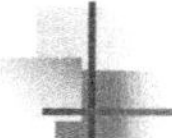

Synthesis Methods

- **Synthesis in test tubes**
- **High through put synthesis techniques**
  - **6-well plate**
  - **24-well plate**

High throughput synthesis process is currently used for salt-selection and screening. Several systems are commercially available for such a synthesis. Currently, all the processing steps such as salt formation, formulation optimization for simple formulations, solid-state characterization of the salt-formation are automated. In these automated systems, the hardware manipulates as little as 40 mcg of solid compound, or 2.5 μl of liquid, allowing hundreds of thousands of experiments to be rapidly performed using the amounts of compounds typically available during the early lead optimization. As per some of the manufacturers' suggestions, greater than 1500 experiments can be performed and analyzed with only 200 mg of the new chemical entity in less than a week and the screens could be performed in parallel. A simple laboratory experiment can also be designed. In this, the reaction can be performed in a 96-well plate. A simple protocol could be as below:

Table 2

Protocol for Salt Formation: A Microplate Technique

Preparation of an NCE solution in a suitable volatile solvent

↓

Addition of these solutions into a microplate well

↓

Addition of concentrations of each counter ion in equimolar proportion into each well

↓

Microscopic observation at regular intervals for the appearance of crystals

↓

Identify the crystal formation

↓

Initiate the large scale crystal formation

↓

Evaluation of crystals using dynamic vapor sorption analyser, Differential scanning calorimetry (DSC), thermogravimetric Analysis (TGA) or hot stage microscopy

↓

Definition of the salt and the stoichiometry with the use of HPLC, infrared and other spectroscopic techniques

Factors Affecting Salt Selection

Pharmaceutical salts are the other important forms of drugs. These salt forms have been investigated for over several years to increase the bioavailability of drugs across the biological membranes and to increase their stability, apart from offering several other advantages. Simply, a pharmaceutical salt can be defined as a salt form of a drug with improved properties. This drug can be either a small molecule or a macromolecule. The salt can be a small anion, a small cation or large molecule. Salts for erythromycin were synthesized and investigated for over several years to reduce the bitter taste and increase its bioavailability. Similarly, salt forms for several small molecules have been synthesized and investigated. The other class of salts called as **"Large molecule salt forms"** could be used for extended or targeted delivery. Generally, salt form is cleaved to form the active drug for its action to be elicited. Another class of salt forms is **"local delivery drug salts"**. Drugs for local delivery such as to the skin, the eyes, or the lungs predominantly belong to the class of local delivery drug salts.

Table 3

Factors Governing the Choice of the Salt Former

- Acidity or basicity of the ionisable group of the NCE
- Safety of the counter-ion used for conjugation
- Toxicological and pharmacological implications of the selected salt former
- Drug indications
- Route of administration
- Intended dosage form

Salt selection is a very important aspect of salt formation. Several factors affect salt selection. Some of the very important factors are presented in the Table 3. Not all the salts that are available in the market are helpful to cure the problem associated with a drug. Not all the conditions are helpful in the synthesis of a salt form of a drug. Not all the salts are selected for a particular utility of a drug. Not all the salts are accessible in the market all over the world for a particular selection. Not all the salts are used to prepare a particular formulation.

pK_a

The selection of acids or bases for salt formation is chiefly decided with regard to the physico-chemical properties. When a salt is formed, the acid transfers a proton to the conjugate base, which in turn must be selected to be ready for accepting the proton. This is generally the case if the pK_a of the acid is at least two units lower than the pK_a of the base. This corresponds to a situation where in water both components are ionized to a degree of at least 99%. Strong mineral acids such as HCl (pK_a=-6) or H_2SO_4 (pK_a=-3) could form solid salts with the anti-helminthic **flubendazole** having a pK_a value as low as 4.1, whereas with acetic acid or with benzoic acid (pK_a=4.2) an attempt to prepare a salt would not be successful with such a very weak base. For basic drugs, Gould (1986) has published detailed physicochemical relationships along a decision analysis procedure including useful tablets of salt-forming agents. Some of the very common salts used in salt selection are tabulated below.

Table 4

Classification of Common Pharmaceutical Salts: Anions

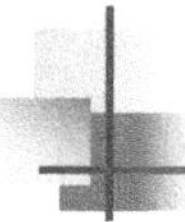

Class	Salts
Inorganic acids	Hydrochloride, hydrobromide, sulfate, nitrate, phosphate
Sulfonic acids	Mesylate, esylate, isothionate, tosylate, napsylate, besylate
Carboxylic acids	Acetate, propionate, maleate, benzoate, salicylate, fumarate
Anionic amino acids	Glutamate, aspartate
Hydroxyacids	Citrate, lactate, succinate, tartrate, glycollate
Fatty acids	Hexanoate, octanoate, decanoate, oleate, stearate
Insoluble salts	Pamoate (embonate), polystyrene sulfonate (resinate)

Table 5

Classification of Common Pharmaceutical Salts: Cations

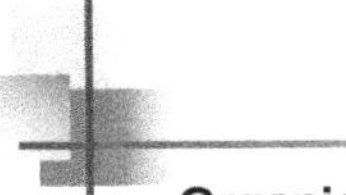

Organic amines	Triethylamine, ethanolamine, triethanolamine, meglumine, ethylenediamine, choline, procaine, benzathine.
Insoluble salts	Procaine, benzathine
Metallic	Sodium, potassium, calcium, magnesium, zinc
Cationic amino acids	Arginine, lysine and histadine

Resulting pH

The next parameter to be considered is the pH of the aqueous solution of a salt form of a drug. Using several equations, the final pH of the solution could be calculated without even measuring, with the aid of a device. The importance of pH is exemplified with the help of a weakly basic tranquillizer **chlordiazepoxide** (pK_a=4.6). The volumes of solutions in the gastro-intestinal tract, the pH values at different sites of the intestinal tract, the known solubility of the nonionized base in water, the solubility of the salt in water were either considered or determined and subsequently the resulting concentrations of this drug in the gastrointestinal tract estimated as follows: The calculated pH for a solution containing 50 mg/ml as a hydrochloride salt was 2.7. At this pH, as different equations predicted, the solubility of hydrochloride salt was 200 mg/ml. Taken together in tandem, with this solubility, it could be concluded that a hydrochloride salt for this molecule is the best option. If the absorption site for this molecule is the stomach where the pH is very low in the acidic range, history from earlier investigated salt studies repeats in such assessments for the bioavailability of a similar molecule, to be on the higher side for this molecule. In this situation an acetate salt of chlordiazepoxide would make little sense for three reasons:

1. the pK_a of acetic acid is just the same as that of the drug base;
2. an equimolar solution of base and acetic acid would have a calculated pH of 4.78, at which pH in 1ml a mere 4 mg of the base are soluble, a solubility value not really worthwhile for a salt;

3. if a solid acetate were feasible it would, on contact with water or humid air, release the volatile acetic acid, and the solid drug base would be left behind. Very unfortunately thus this salt is not suitable for chlordiazepoxide when hydrochloride salt is working fine. In this aspect, another basic example of phenazopyridine could further elucidate this effect.

The pH-solubility profile of **phenazopyridine** as determined by the addition of HCl or NaOH solutions to its aqueous suspension was identical to that of its hydrochloride salt except during phase transition from base to salt. With the addition of HCl to a suspension of the base, the pH dropped to a certain point and then remained constant until a supersaturated solution was formed. Only after a high supersaturation did precipitation of the hydrochloride salt occur. The solubility of the salt decreased at low pH due to a common ion effect. Unlike solubility profiles, the pH-intrinsic dissolution rate profiles of the base and its salt differed greatly. At low pH, the dissolution rate of the hydrochloride salt decreased with an increase in HCl concentration, whereas the dissolution rate of the base increased. The self-buffering action of the base and the increase in solubility, leading to a supersaturation of the diffusion layer was responsible for the increase in its dissolution rate with a lowering of the pH of the medium. Good conformity with the Noyes-Whitney equation was demonstrated when the solubility values under pH conditions such that the diffusion layer thickness approaches zero (Cs,h = 0) were used rather than solubilities under pH conditions of the bulk media (Cs). Supersaturation of the dissolution medium was observed during dissolution of the hydrochloride salt at pH 7.

The Common-ion Effect

While the preference for preparing hydrochloride and sodium salts is favored by the physiological abundance of Cl^- and Na^+ ions, these can also bring about negative effects. One of them is the suppression of solubility, which becomes particularly evident with hydrochlorides and sodium salts of moderate to low intrinsic solubility, as per several current references. This may be because of the presence of very similar smaller ions of the same kind, e.g. in physiological saline, in the stomach and in blood, causes a reduction of solubility by the law of mass action. Several examples can be mentioned: One of the famous and older examples is terfenadine hydrochloride. The 'common-ion effect' depresses the solubility of **terfenadine** hydrochloride in water (2 mg/ml at pH of approximately 5) down to a tenth when 0.05M NaCl is added. The solubility of diclofenac sodium in water is 21.3 mg/ml, but 6.7 mg/ml in physiological saline. Under the same conditions, the corresponding figures for **4-(5,6-dimethyl-2-benzofuranyl)-piperidine** hydrochloride, an experimental antidepressant, are 3.8 and 0.44 mg/ml, respectively. Solubility and dissolution rate of hydrochlorides administered orally may be further suppressed by the common-ion effect, since the chloride ion is present at concentrations between 100 and 140 mg/l in gastric fluid. There are examples of **pyrimidine derivatives** whose hydrochlorides are even less soluble than the free bases. Thus, these examples suggest that either historical salts with proven track record in terms of thorough research and scientific evaluations are to be considerd further or just to be on the safer side, avoiding toxic salt forms is an alternative. In this respect, high throughput screening techniques helps in salt synthesis and selection to expedite and aid in comprehensive investigations.

Market Requirements

This is a very peculiar issue as related to either prodrugs or salt forms. Prodrugs are generally synthesized for drugs that are already in the market and demonstrated some success. However, as per the regulatory considerations, several issues crop up with the prodrugs. On the other hand, salt selection is entirely different. Salts are currently synthesized right at the stage of the synthesis of drugs. Regulatory issues may not be significant until the salt itself is very toxic. However, these are definitely not like prodrugs. The toxicity is generally aroused in the very early stages during the selection as related to salt selection. In either case, market requirements some times become very important. For instance, ketotifen is an antihistamine drug used for ocular allergies. It is currently marketed as **ketotifen fumarate**. The reason for the selection of this salt form is that the drug is highly lipophilic and thus the business would be closed for ocular therapy several years ago when drug delivery systems were not discovered and the need was to develop a solution form. Ketotifen fumarate is a water-soluble salt and helped in the development of an ocular solution. However, the drawback with such a therapy is that repeated dosing of the solution form is required because of very poor bioavailability of drugs into the target tissues in the eye after topical administration. Several techniques are currently available to develop ocular drug to improve the residence time of this drug in the eye. Keeping silence in these situations and compromising on the solution form would be a non-issue when the competition is becoming stiff in the market place and mostly with the availability of other compounds, however potent this molecule is. Thus, the necessity for a very positive molecule currently is to simply develop a salt form. The best pick for a salt that could be of market use would be a bulk salt with sustained release properties and high lipophilicity. Thus, selection of a salt like pamoate, also called embonate, would be helpful. The characterization and other investigations and regulatory filings as per the current requirement would be easy with this salt rather than developing a prodrug. This is a very simple example of a salt form. Similarly several other examples can be furnished.

Patent Issues

Patent issues as related to either the salts used for infringing the original innovators drugs or their salt forms would be sometimes very tricky, time consuming and may cost a lot to the company. One recent example as related to the patent infringements of salt form will be briefed. This example is a very good learning experience for non-lawyers handling the salt forms of drugs in any stage of its development. Currently (as of 2004) a case is pending as related to Novarsc. Pfizer developed this compound. It is used in the treatment of hypertension, chronic stable angina or vasospastic angina. Novarsc has been evaluated for safety in more than 11,000 patients in U.S. and foreign clinical trials. In general, treatment with Novarsc was well-tolerated at doses up to 10 mg daily. Norvasci is **Amlodipine besylate**. It is a white crystalline powder with a molecular weight of 567.1. It is slightly soluble in water and sparingly soluble in ethanol. Tablets are formulated as white tablets equivalent to 2.5, 5 and 10 mg of amlodipine for oral administration. In addition to the active ingredient, amlodipine besylate, each tablet contains the following inactive ingredients: microcrystalline cellulose, dibasic calcium phosphate anhydrous, sodium starch glycolate, and magnesium stearate. Pfizer's original patent on Novarsc expired last year but was extended for several years because of the long delay at the FDA over the safety issue in allowing the drug to come to market. The issue in this case was whether the patent protected both the chemical structure of Novarsc and a host of sister compounds, or salts. Dr. Reddy's applied to the FDA for a so-called 505(b) (2) approval to market its version of the drug. However, later Pfizer realized that this product infringed its rights on Novarsc and filed a lawsuit. A federal appeals court has reversed the decision of the lower court and thus Dr. Reddy's Laboratories Ltd. was barred from selling its version of Pfizer's Inc. hypertension drug Novarsc. Novarsc had sales of over $4 billion in 2003. The lower court had ruled that Dr. Reddy's version of the drug violated Pfizer's patent that covered all aspects of the chemical amlodipine. Dr. Reddy's had hoped that the patent did not cover all molecules of the chemical, and at the same time it argued that it could use the research data that Pfizer used to get the FDA to approve Novarsc. Thus, this simple example illustrates how costly it could be in improper evaluations and judgements as related to patent infringement of new chemical drug substances.

Availability, Need and Requirement

Erythromycin is produced by a strain of *Saccaropolyspora erythraea* and belongs to the macrolide group of antibiotics. It is basic and readily forms salts and esters. Erythromycin ethylsuccinate is the 2'-ethylsuccinyl ester of erythromycin. It is essentially a tasteless form of the antibiotic suitable for oral administration, particularly in suspension dosage forms. The chemical name is erythromycin 2'-(ethylsuccinate). Sulfisoxazole acetyl or N'-acetyl sulfisoxazole is an ester of sulfisoxazole. Chemically, sulfisoxazole is N'-(3, 4- dimethyl-5-isoxazotyl) sulfanilamide. Erythromycin ethylsuccinate and sulfisoxazole acetyl, when reconstituted with water as directed on the label, the granules form a white, cherry flavored suspension that provides the equivalent of 200 mg erythromycin activity and the equivalent of 600 mg of sulfisoxazole activity per teaspoonful (5 ml).

Molecular Weight

The amount of the salt obtained at the end of salt synthesis would be a very important factor. Since new drug discovery is becoming very competitive and several leads and their salts are prepared at one time right from the initial stages of the project, the screening of these salts in cell culture studies, in animal models and their toxicological evaluations become very competitive. In this respect, the weight obtained from one of the high-througput techniques like that prepared out of a 96-well plate technique would become very important. If the molecular weight of the drug is very large and the molecular weight of a suitable salt at the end of screening is also very large, then the amount required for initial cell culture screenings and pharmacological evalutions would be very high. Thus, it is always a challenging environment even to develop new and convenient salts for several of the new molecules coming up in the market currently. In addition, the physical state at the end of the synthesis is also an important issue. The primary factor that should be considered is the crystallinity of the resulting salt form. Crystallinity in a salt affords a means of purification and removal of unwanted impurities. Lack of crystallinity (i.e., the salt is amorphous) normally would be expected to lead to severe problems and uncertainties, if the product intended to be developed in a solid, oral dosage form. The prospect of unexpected and uncontrolled crystallization at some stage with just one batch, creating a product recall, is something that the quality, regulatory, and marketing groups could not live with. Absence of crystallinity is often less of a problem if the dosage form intended is a liquid. A balance is always the requirement in terms of molecular weights of the initial and the end products. Examples: **Procaine Penicillin and Benzathine Penicillin.**

Convenience

Not all the drugs are administered by oral route. Not all the drugs are needed to be administered by oral route. Keeping in view the requirements, ease, convenience and the best possible route for a particular treatment, salts are for convenience sake synthesized and sold in a pharmacy. For example, sodium salts of **acetazolamide, aciclovir, aescin, diclofenac, furosemide, phenytoin** are administered by parenteral route, while the acid forms are administered by peroral route. **Diclofenac** is administered as a diethylamine gel by topical route.

Benproperine is only administered by oral route as embonate or a phosphate. **Bromperidol** is administered as base and lactate only by oral route. **Clomethiazole** is administered as edisilate salt in the form of syrup by oral route, while edisilate is administered as solution by parenteral route. **Theophylline** is administered by oral route while its sodium glycinate salt is administered by parenteral route. **Scopolamine** base is administered by topical route, its borate salt is administered as a solution into the eye, its bromide salt is administered by parenteral route. **Flupentixol** and **fluphenazine** decanoates are administered by parenteral route while hydrochloride salts are administered by oral route. **Meclozine** is administered as base in the form of a suppository while its hydrochloride salt is administered by peroral route. Finally, **phenytoin** is administered as a sodium salt by parenteral route while its acid form is administered by oral route.

Targeted Release

Drug targeting can be achieved by several means. This area of pharmaceutical research has been in vogue for several decades after the innovatory medicine of allopathy has been introduced successfully. Some of the targeted release systems are lipososomes, immunoconjugated nanoparticles, prodrugs etc. Size is the criteria with liposomes. After injecting intravenously, smaller liposomes are found to be lodged in the liver because of the size of the capillary bed in the liver. Similarly immunoconjugated nanoparticles could be targeted to a specific tissue that expresses the target protein at higher levels. Prodrugs are degraded into active drugs at the site of the presence of the enzyme thereby resulting in the targeted release of the drug. However, salts forms are very tricky. With the very commonly used salt forms of drugs, cleavage occurs generally in the intestines before the drug reaches systemic circulation, where it may be clouded with salts of interest before getting absorbed into the cells. Lipophilic drugs are easily taken up into the cells because of their hydrophobicity. However, binding with the systemic salts is very low and thus all the cells will take up this molecule. On the other hand, there are some specific tissues in the body and during certain stages of the human beings life cycle, the pH is different from the rest of the cells. This could be either because of the differential expression of enzymes controlling homeostasis of the surrounding environment or because of recycling of the transport protein during a certain period of 24 hours that may lead to alterations in the pH only at that particular time. In these situations, the best method is to conjugate a hydrophilic drug with a large hydrophobic salt that could be cleaved only during that time of night and only near certain cells and thus gets absorbed only into these cells, thereby leading to the targeted release. This phenomenon can be conveniently used to prepare salts for targeted release of drugs. A simple example along with the physiology at this stage will be illustrated.

Cholesterol gallstone disease (CGD) has a high prevalence in the United States, where 20 million patients are treated for this disease annually. The major events leading to the disease include supersaturation of bile with cholesterol, rapid precipitation of cholesterol crystals in the gallbladder, increased bile salt hydrophobicity and inflammation of the gallbladder. Of these events, precipitation of cholesterol crystals from supersaturated bile is a prerequisite for gallstone formation, and has been observed in 70% of patients with acute, formerly idiopathic, pancreatitis. In bile, cholesterol is solubilized in mixed micelles together with bile salts and phospholipids. Under supersaturated conditions, the sterol is solubilized by phospholipids into vesicles, called liquid crystals. As monohydrate crystals enucleate from these cholesterol-enriched vesicles, they aggregate, fuse and eventually precipitate into larger pathogenic crystals that lead to the disease. The treatment for this disease would be to target bile formation and stop at the gallbladder site. **Lithocholic acid and its derivatives** can be used in this condition. Several lithocholic acid analogs were synthesized and their role to treat the condition was examined in one study. Several studies indicated the interrelation ship between lithocholic acid and a protein called VDR. In the mechanism process one more protein called VDR may be involved. Thus, VDR agonists, as is lithocholic acid is, are helpful in this situation. Of the several salts developed LCA acetate was found to be more effective. LCA acetate is the most potent of these VDR agonists. It binds directly to VDR and activates the receptor with 30 times the potency of LCA and has no or minimal activity on FXR and PXR. **LCA acetate** effectively induced the expression of VDR target genes in intestinal cells. Unlike LCA, LCA acetate inhibited the proliferation of human monoblastic leukemia cells and induced their monocytic differentiation. The group that investigated this salt proposed a docking model for LCA acetate binding to VDR. The development of VDR agonists as salt forms derived from bile acids should be useful to elucidate ligand-selective VDR functions. Thus, it is very likely that the acetate salt form is more effective than its base in terms of targeting the drug to the active site. Similarly, several examples could be found in the literature.

Stability and Compatibility

Salt forms can have an effect on the chemical stability of the drug. If a potentially reactive salt-forming agent has been chosen unwittingly, the resulting salt may decompose under certain conditions. Such cases have been reported for fumarate and maleate salts. A pH-dependent adduct formation with maximum reactivity at pH = 5 took place with the dimaleate of the development compound **PGE-7762928** (two basic nitrogens; $pK_a1=4.3$; $pK_a2=10.6$). Further, with the selective serotonin reuptake inhibitor suproxetine maleate hemihydrate, the interaction of the primary amine groupd with the anion in aqueous solution (optimum pH range 5.5 – 8.5) resulted in adduct formation. Similarly several examples can be found in the literature. Similarly, Powell found a dramatic difference in stability between the phosphate and the sulfate salts of **codeine** in solution at room temperature (1986). Whereas the phosphate solution had a shelf-life of 1.1 years, the extrapolated shelf life of the sulfate was 44 years. The low stability of the former was ascribed to a catalytic effect of the phosphate anion on the degradation of codeine.

Characterization

After salt synthesis occurs, its characterization is important as is for any drug candidate. With salts, it becomes more important because of the aim of increase in the properties of drug candidate with salt synthesis. In this aspect various properties such as structural analysis, physico-chemical properties, physical properties, impurities and stability studies are investigated. Most of the important properties are very briefly discussed in this section as related to the pharmaceutical salts. One of the examples that was published recently as related to the physico-chemical properties is described in the table. Most of the techniques employed are the same as those used to characterize the drug substances.

Table 6

An Example: Comparison of Properties of RPR 127963 and its Salts

Test	Result for free base anhydrate (RPR 127963)	Result for mesylate salt (RPR 127963)	Result for sulfate salt (RPR 127963)
Solubility (mg/mL)			
Ethanol	190	0.6	0.2
Propylene glycol	35.4	0.7	1.7
PEG 400	188	0.2	0.2
Dimethylsulphoxide	>500	14	110
N-methylpyrrolidone	>400	4.4	8.5
Glycerol	42	n.d.	2.7
Intrinsic dissolution Rate, mg/min/cm^2	0.35	7.3	7.7
Powder flow	n.d.	Good, but becomes much worse with increasing humidity	Sticks slightly

Structural Analysis

Several of the very common methods of structural analysis for any characterization are listed in the table. These are the very routine techniques that are currently used for structural analysis of small as well as large molecules. These are not discussed here henceforth. However, the physical state i.e., solid-state characterization is a very important investigation as related to salt formation. As most pharmaceutical drugs are administered as solids, it is very important that solid-state characterization of salts is a very important aspect. Several kinds of physical structures associated with pharmaceutical salts as described in the section of "Factors Affecting Salt Selection" are possible. Of the several salts that are produced out of several thousands using the combination of drugs of similar nature targeting a particular diseases and high-throughput screening as is a possible method for new drug discovery, the final number of potent molecules along with the salts after the final step would be 5-6, that enters preclinical stages and further would be associated with the highest ball-park for future clinical investigations and worth investment by a company. In this regard, solid-state charaterization would also be in tandem with synthesis as a high-throughput screening method. Currently, microscopy can be conveniently used for preliminary screening of salt form synthesis in a high-through put set up. In this set up, the drug is added in either organic solvent or an aqueous solvent in the presence of various buffering agents. Different salt formers as per the requirement are added into these plates. The formation of the crystals can be monitored on a timely basis using microscopic evaluation. The final form of the salt form can be very appropriately picked up in this process. Some of the techniques described in the table can be used for solid-state characterization of pharmaceutical salts.

Table 7

Characterization: Structural Analysis

- Mass spectroscopy
- H NMR
- C NMR
- IR spectrum
- UV spectrum
- Florescence spectrum
- Elemental analysis

A satisfactory salt form of a drug molecule must be technically feasible and suitable for full-scale production and its solid-state properties maintained batch-wise as well as over time. Comparison of the solid-state properties of different salt forms of a drug molecule may be quite complicated, especially when the salt form(s) exist as different solid phases. Different solid phases may arise during crystallization and pharmaceutical processing and include polymorphs, amorphous forms and solvates (often termed pseudopolymorphs). Polymorphism is often defined as the ability of a substance to exist as two or more crystalline phases that have different arrangements and conformations of the molecules in the crystal lattice. Amorphous solids, unlike polymorphs, are not crystalline because the arrangement of the molecules is disordered. Solvates contain molecules of the solvent of crystallization in a definite crystal lattice. Solvates in which the solvent of crystallization is water are termed hydrates. Because moisture is the part of the atmosphere, hydrates of drugs may be formed rather easily, especially with salts, on account of the dipolar water molecules and constituent ions. Most of the details of the crystal structures are described in chapters 1 through 4 and can be conveniently applied to salt forms of drugs. In addition, the worthy discussion would be as related to the synthesis of pharmaceutical salts during various physical and chemical stresses used during the step of achieving a particular salt. It is necessary to know the thermodynamic relationships between drug substance and solvent (s), and the factors that govern the final crystallization process for the reproducible manufacture of the required solid phase of the drug. Because effects associated with temperature, pressure, humidity (water and moisture), solvents, and excipients are involved in processing solid forms of the active drug molecule, it is important to understand the detailed parameters relevant in the choice of its appropriate salt form (s).

Physico-chemical Properties

The fundamental physico-chemical properties are consequences of the underlying crystal structure of the salt obtained after synthesis. In constrast, the wear and tare on a particular salt form could reduce the crystalline nature and the particle size of a particular salt form. The ball-park in this regard is to judiciously conduct the experiment after carefully storing these salt-forms rather than performing the experiment indiscreetly. Melting points lower than 100°C can cause problems during mechanical handling and processing. In particular, melting or lumping can occur when comminution by milling is attempted. Some times corrosiveness of the resulting salt form could be very problematic.

Table 8

Characterization: Physicochemical properties

- Melting range
- pKa
- C log P/log P[a]
- Preliminary polymorphism study
- X-ray diffraction
- Aqueous solubility
- pH-solubility profile
- Cosolvent solubilities
- Propellant solubility

Salts of weak bases with strong acids need to be tested whether or not they are corrosive on tableting tools. Such profiles are studied in preformulation programs, but some of the properties must already be known before the decision for the final salt form is made. Several of these physico-chemical properties listed in the table are the first properties investigated for salt forms of drugs. Most of these properties are discussed in chapter 1 through 4.

Physical Properties

Physical properties are very essential investigations for any solid. It is very interesting if the physical properties are altered. Currently, several robotic methods with several new instruments are being used in the pharmaceutical industry to determine the physical properties. A clear description of these physical properties and their description can be refered from chapters 1 through 4. Unfortunately, comprehensive description is not the idea of this textbook, and thus even in these chapters only a very brief outline of these properties is presented. Interested readers and the investigators related could do more reference with relevant literature.

Table 9

Characterization: Physical Properties

- **Hygroscopicity**
- **Microscopy (SEM/optical)**
- **Particle size (Malvern)**
- **Size reduction (Sonication)**

Impurities

Stability can be some times a very important issue as related to salt synthesis. The related substances, the degradation products, and the chiral purity can be determined using any of the standard analytical tools. However, the real issue is the correction of the stability. The following steps can be conveniently used to achieve the desired stability of a particular salt form:

(a) Increase hydrophobicity of acid
(b) Use carboxylic rather than sulfonic or mineral acids
(c) Use acid of higher pKa to reduce pH of adsorbed water
(d) Decrease solubility
(e) Increase crystallinity

The following steps may be the consequences of a change:

1. Reduced hygroscopicity
2. Improved resistance to attach by environmental agents

Table 11

Characterization: Impurities

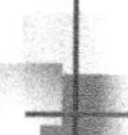
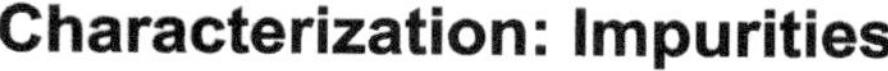

- Related substances
- Degradation products
- Chiral purity

Stability

A list of stability studies is presented in the table that can be investigated as a part of salt screening. The methods of dissolution of the salt along with the active acid or base can be investigated as a part of stability studies.

Table 12

Characterization: Stability studies

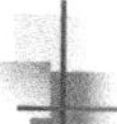

- Stability to hydrolysis (pH 2, 7, 10)
- Stability to oxidation (Peroxide/peracid)
- Stability to photolysis

Conclusions

Salt screening is a very wide area currently very routinely used in the pharmaceutical industry. Because of several new chemical moieties being generated very frequently every likely the productivity has to increase. Currently, several new innovations are being made in this area. It is very essential for a pharmaceutical scientist to keep in touch with these developments. This chapter presented a brief overview of the salt screening process in the pharmaceutical industry.

Questions for Practice and Exercise

1. Why salt selection is important? What are the reasons that could be furnished for salt selection (salt-screening) process?
2. Discuss the case study of RBx 9841. HCl as a pharmaceutical salt? Particularly specify the several inter-related factors.
3. Elaborate "*in situ* salt screening to increase drug absorption".
4. Why is the understanding of the concepts of dissolution of weak acids and weak bases important for investigations associated with salt synthesis techniques?
5. Explain drug absorption and the need for salt forming in the modification of drug absorption. How is the bioavailability affected with salt formation? Explain both solution and solid forms of salts.
6. Mention briefly the theories of dissolution and explain their application in the use of pharmaceutical salts.
7. Present a brief introductory note on the change in the properties of a drug that are affected after salt synthesis.
8. Describe the different techniques used in salt formation.
9. What are the different factors that affect salt formation? Briefly describe.

References

1. Remenar JF, Morissette SL, Peterson ML, Moulton B, MacPhee JM, Guzman HR, Almarsson O.Crystal engineering of novel cocrystals of a triazole drug with 1,4-dicarboxylic acids. J Am Chem Soc. 2003 Jul 16;125 (28):8456-7.
2. Eerikainene, Cavallari C, Albertini B, Rodriguez L, Rabasco AM, Fini A. Release of indomethacin from ultrasound dry granules containing lactose-based excipients. J Control Release. 2005 Jan 20; 102(1): 39-47.

3. O'Connor KM, Corrigan OI. Effect of a basic organic excipient on the dissolution of diclofenac salts. J Pharm Sci. 2002 Oct; 91(10): 2271-81.
4. Gould, P.Salt selection for basic drugs. Int. J. Pharm. 1986, 33, 201-217.
5. Powell MF. Enhanced stability of codeine sulfate: effect of pH, buffer, and temperature on the degradation of codeine in aqueous solution. J Pharm Sci. 1986 Sep; 75(9):901-3.

Bibliography

1. The Theory and Practice of Industrial Pharmacy, Third Edition, Edited by Leon Lachman, Herbert A. Lieberman, and Joseph L. Kanig, Lea & Febiger Publications, 1986.
2. Physical Characterization of Pharmaceutical Solids (Drugs and the Pharmaceutical Sciences: a Series of Textbooks and Monographs), First Edition, Edited by Harry G. Brittain, Marcel Dekker Inc., 1995.
3. New Drug Development: Regulatory Paradigms for Clinical Pharmacology and Biopharmaceutics (Drugs and the Pharmaceutical Sciences: a Series of Textbooks and Monographs), First Edition, Edited by Chandrahas G. Sahajwalla, Marcel Dekker Inc., 2004.
4. The Practice of Medicinal Chemistry, Second Edition, Edited by Camille Georges Wermuth, Elsevier Publications, 2003.
5. Foye`s Principles of Medicinal Chemistry, Fifth Edition, David A. Williams and Thomas L. Lemke, Lippincott Williams & Wilkins, 2002.
6. Physical Pharmacy: Physical Chemical Principles in the Pharmaceutical Sciences, Third Edition, Alfred Martin, James Swarbrick and Arthur Cammarata, Lea & Febiger Publications, 1983.
7. Pharmaceutical Dosage Forms and Drug Delivery Systems, Seventh Edition, Howard C. Ansel, Loyd V. Allen, Jr., and Nicholas G. Popovich, Lippincott Williams & Wilkins, 1999.
8. Pharmaceutical Salts: Properties, Selection, and Use, First Edition, Edited by P. Heinrich Stahl and Camille G. Wermuth, Wiley VCH, 2002.

CHAPTER 9

PRODRUGS: DESIGN, KINETIC STUDY AND SYNTHESIS

- Introduction
- Design
- Kinetic Studies and Characterization
- Biotransformation Pathway Identification
- Enzymatic Models
- Analytical Methods
- Pharmacokinetics
- Examples in Clinics
- Synthesis
- Safety and Regulatory Considerations
- Conclusions

Introduction

A prodrug is a drug conjugate with improved properties. A drug for a prodrug is mostly a small molecule, an intermediate size molecule, a peptide, a protein, a macromolecule or a polymer. Conjugation of these molecules with a desired side chain or a macromolecule can be conveniently synthesized with the help of several chemical, enzymological and biochemical techniques. Generally, a prodrug is cleaved to form the active drug for its action to be elicited.

Paracetamol was the first drug actively investigated for prodrug drug formation. Prodrugs for paracetamol were synthesized and investigated for over several years to reduce the hepatic toxicity and increase its bioavailability. Approximately 7.0% of all marketed medicines currently in the Germany can be included in the category of prodrugs. Blockbusters currently in the USA, European and Asian markets are omeprazole, simvastatin, lovastatin, enalapril, and aciclovir. The recent innovations in the prodrugs are for controlled and sustained release of active drugs either at the site of absorption or at the site of the target. About 49% of these prodrugs are activated by hydrolysis, and 23% are bioprecursors activated by biosynthetic reaction such as metabolism in the liver.

Prodrugs are conveniently classified into small molecule prodrugs, polymeric prodrugs and soft drugs. Prodrugs for small molecules are termed small molecule prodrugs. Most of the marketed prodrugs are small molecule prodrugs. A polymeric prodrug consists of a drug conjugated to a polymer. These prodrugs are generally used for extended or targeted delivery or for altering various properties of drug substances. Soft drugs are active analogues of existing drugs deactivated in a predictable and controllable way after achieving their therapeutic role. Drugs for local delivery such as to the skin, the eyes, or the lungs predominantly belong to the class of soft drugs. Several prodrugs, esp. small molecule prodrugs have been synthesized for various reasons and some of these are slowly being renegade because of the introduction of latest and more powerful prodrugs with the blockbusters always existing in the market. Two famous blockbusters in the pharmaceutical market and to the scientific community are prodrugs for propranolol and diethylstilbestrol. Shrewd selection of the molecules and proper design may result in better prodrug market. This review highlights the basics and advancements in the area of prodrugs.

Design

Albert A, a French scientist, first used the term prodrug in a paper published in Nature in 1958. Eversince, very active research has been undertaken in the area of prodrug development leading to ample lessons for a prodrug scientist. The area is very vast, that prodrugs have been developed for small molecules to macromolecules, from the modification of physico-chemical properties to controlled release systems. Sparingly soluble salts of penicillin, say for example, are the salts that have been used for over several years to promote higher blood levels and bring about better distribution. For instance, ampicillin was conjugated to form lipophilic pivampicillin to produce higher blood levels of the parent compound. New erythromycin prodrugs that are available are tasteless and stable in aqueous suspensions. The parent molecule is protected with chemical groupings that are eventually lost in the tissue, where the drugs then become effective antibacterial agents. Before further discussing the design of a prodrug comprehensively, the reasons to develop prodrugs are:

1. To improve the physico-chemical properties of a small molecule drug: These physico-chemical properties include the solubility and dissolution, organoleptic properties, pain at the site of administration and the chemical stability of the drug.
2. To enhance the bioavailability of a small molecular or a macromolecular drug: This can be achieved either by increasing the passive permeability of a drug candidate across biological membranes, by targeting a drug to the transporter with high velocity across biological membranes, by improving the resistance of a drug candidate to the metabolic enzymes, by targeting a drug to particular cells of an intestinal tract to increase the permeability or by targeting surface antigen to increase the permeability.
3. To control and sustain the release and action of a drug in the intestinal tract or at the target site.
4. To home a small molecule drug or a macromolecule. The home could be a target tissue such as lung, brain, liver, colon, cancer tissues, joints, bones, tumors or coud be a cell or group of cells

The design of prodrugs is based on the data obtained from the *in vitro-in vivo* hydrolysis, tissue uptake, pharmacokinetic-pharmacodynamic, pharmacological and cell culture studies. Based on the results, the structural moiety involved in the hydrolysis is determined and the need for prodrug synthesis is evaluated. Subsequently, this structure is further modified with different functional groups to prevent the hydrolysis in the presence of different enzymes that may be required for its activity. If the mechanism of action were hydrolysis, this would be a proper approach. On the other hand, if the requirement were not hydrolysis but a different one, then the specific reason would be identified and determined. However, in many cases it is an enzyme and it is generally a protein. The current trend in this area is to use structure-based drug design, especially as it is applied to the rational generation of new enzyme inhibitors and thus prodrugs. Established methods and approaches are being applied to an ever-increasing breadth of enzyme targets of varying structural determinants with good success.

Simple examples are presented regarding the computer aided drug design followed by its application in the design of prodrugs for various purposes.

In the last several years, many compounds with HIV-1 integrase inhibitory activity have been identified. However, due to their low potency or high toxicity, none have entered clinical trials. Unlike HIV-1 protease or HIV reverse transcriptase, no crystal structure of the enzyme-inhibitor complex has been published as of today, nor there is a crystal structure of the enzyme itself. This has hindered the structure-based design of HIV-1 integrase inhibitors. In the absence of a 3D structure of the enzyme, 3D database pharmacophore searching has provided researchers with the opportunity to identify new leads. 3D database pharmacophore searching is useful if inhibitors are known and adequate models and databases are available. A conformational search was performed on a tetrameric coumarin structure, with low micromolar activity, by varying the torsion angles. From the resulting low energy conformations, a 3-point pharmacophore model was developed by measuring the distance between atoms a to d. This is the general method of pharmacophore query using any of the databases. One of the databases, National Cancer Institute (NCI) 3D database, USA, containing 206,876 compounds was used. The search resulted in the identification of 340 compounds with a similar pharmacophoric pattern. Using criteria such as market availability, chemical diversity and *in vivo* availability for selection, 29 computer-identified compounds were subjected to an integrase inhibition assay. Compounds 2-5, where the highlighted atoms that matched the pharmacophore query, are the most potent of the ten compounds showing integrase inhibitory activity, with IC_{50} values of < 30 microM.

Crystallographic structural details of the mode of binding for many enzyme inhibitors have led to the development of numerous pharmacophore models. A graphical analysis of hydroxylated benzylideneanilines and benzylamines interacting with epidermal growth factor receptor-associated tyrosine kinase (PTK) has provided a minimal structural pharmacophore for two distinct ligand substrate binding sites within the PTK domain. It has been proposed that one binding site of PTK can accommodate a planar molecule with hydrogen bond donor groups approximately 10 Å apart. A second proposed binding site corresponds to the inhibitor lavendustin A in which there is a hydrogen bond donor between the two aromatic rings. Inhibitors of PTK, an enzyme involved in cell signaling mechanisms, could be potential therapeutic agents against numerous forms of malignancy. Furthermore, a new mode of binding of acetylcholine (ACh) to acetylcholinesterase (AChE) was discovered using full force field energetics that might lead to the development of improved Alzheimer's disease drugs. Detailed and accurate molecular representations of enzyme-inhibitor interactions are best determined by experimental methods such as X-ray crystallography. Data, however, is not always available to the medicinal chemist especially during the early stages of an enzyme-inhibitor design project. Computer-assisted protein homology modeling (or comparative protein modeling) is an approach that attempts to relate the amino acid sequence of a protein to its 3D structure. In this approach, homology of the primary protein structure is related to a protein structural family generating the 3D atomic coordinates for that protein based upon selected templates. This method was used to explore potential inhibitors of pyrophosphate-phosphofructokinase(PPi-PFK) from *Entamoeba histolytica* based on the crystal structure of ATP-PFK from *Bacillus stearothermophilus*.

Another example that can be cited in this case is the design of FK228 (Depsipeptide) as a natural prodrug for the inhibition of class I histone deacetylases (HDACs). FK228 (formerly named FR901228), also known as depsipeptide, is produced by *Chromobacterium violaceum* and shows potent *in vivo* antitumor activity against both human tumor xenografts and murine tumors. A Phase I study of FK228 in the Medicine Branch, National Cancer Institute showed that cutaneous T-cell lymphoma patients had a complete or partial response· Thus, FK228 is at least a novel and potentially effective agent for patients with T-cell lymphoma. This molecule strongly inhibits histone acetyltransferase enzymes (HDAC). However, FK228 has no apparent chemical structure that interacts with the HDAC active-site pocket. FK228 is a bicyclic depsipeptide that is structurally distinct from other HDAC inhibitors, such as TSA, TPX and butyrate. Reduction of an internal disulfide bond of FK 228 yields two free sulfhydryl groups (to form red FK), one of which is potentially accessible to catalytic residues in the active-site pocket. Inside the cell this occurs because of cellular reducing activity. Crystallographic studies using the HDAC-like protein-TSA complex have shown that TSA inserts its long aliphatic chain into the tube-like pocket and inhibits enzyme activity by interacting with the zinc and active-site residues through its hydroxamic acid at one end of the aliphatic chain. Because redFK has a 4-carbon-long chain between one of the sulfhydryl groups and the cyclic depsipeptide core, this sulfhydryl group is probably accessible to the residues in the active-site pocket. There is only one conserved cysteine residue (Cys-151 for HDAC1) in the pocket of all of the HDAC enzymes identified thus far. It therefore seemed possible that redFK interacts with the cysteine residue to form a covalent disulfide bond between redFK and the enzyme. To test this possibility, this group introduced a single amino acid exchange from Cys-151 to Ser in HDAC1 (C151S), and the drug sensitivity of this mutant enzyme was examined. The C151S mutant was still sensitive to redFK, although the IC_{50} was higher than that for wild-type enzyme. Further docking simulations using X-ray crystallographic data of the HDAC-like protein was performed. The position of the sulfur atom of redFK is 5.83 Å apart from the conserved cysteine residue (Cys-142) corresponding to Cys-151 in HDAC1. On the other hand, the sulfur atom is located at a position allowing interaction with the active center zinc via a water molecule. These results strongly suggest that redFK reversibly interacts with the zinc, thereby reversibly inhibiting the enzyme activity in a manner similar to TSA. Thus, it is likely that finding may explain why FK228 is more effective than other classical HDAC inhibitors such as TSA, TPX, and butyrate in *in vivo* models. On the other hand, if the binding were not proper this molecule would not be a proper fit and definitely would be out of the ballpark of the other inhibitors. Fortunately, these *in silico* methods are very helpful in reducing the time of discovery atleast several folds, for instance 10-fold, compared to using the normal older techniques of *in vitro* and simple *in vivo* investigations. The unique properties of FK228 thus obtained provide a new basis for further development of HDAC inhibitors as antitumor agents on these lines. Similar would be the design of any class of prodrugs for a suitable enzyme using computer-aided drug design. Further, referencing would give a comprehensive picture. The example currently presented is with regard to a very huge molecule and its prodrugs. Currently, all the molecules involved in this class of prodrugs may not occupy as such huge numbers because of their poor water solubility and still the infancy of this group of medicinal agents. However, further extractions and investigations in natural products would comprise many of such molecules for life threatening diseases such as AIDS and cancer; very likely the market for these large molecules may go up. Because of their general poor formulation properties prodrugs would be better alternatives for these classes of molecules and thus the example presented in this section is very suitable for the current to near future explorations in drug discovery. Extrapolations with regard to small molecule prodrugs could be made on the similar lines. However, a very simple description of the method of using computers in prodrug design was thus presented.

Kinetic Studies and Characterization

Kinetics of release and degradation of a prodrug is an important consideration in prodrug design. A simple understanding of mechanism of degradation and rate of degradation would help in better appreciation of this area. Kinetic studies and characterization helps in very stable and freelance kind of design of prodrugs, rather than spending lot of effort, abruptness and borrowing from precedence type of models, which, some times, may not only cost lot of money but also may eventually result in redoing everystep in the drug discovery right from the design to initial formulation steps to the regulatory filings. This is the very simple reason for systematic stability investigations that would help progress prodrugs with very low cost expenditure. Right from the introduction into the gastrointestinal tract and to the release of the drug at the site of action or its release during the sojourn, the reaction kinetics, the pharmacokinetics and pharmacodynamics are all important for its action and activity. Half-life of the prodrug per sé and it's solution or enzymatic degradation are the important factors in the evaluation of better pharmacological action of the prodrug compared to its parent drug.

Stability studies with prodrugs can be simply divided into degradation pathway identification, enzymatic studies and analytical methods useful in such investigations. Degradation pathway is the main initial investigation for prodrugs' design. Enzymatic studies and analytical methods help in identification of the degradation pathway and the rates of formation. Each of these sections will be elaborated:

Biotransformation Pathway Identification

The initial investigations and thoughts on the design of these experiments should constitute the aim and role of these prodrugs. Once the role of these prodrugs is identified, the project is initiated and the work started.

For instance, in one study, the aim was to develop prodrugs that are more lipophilic than their parent drugs in order to be able to cross cell membranes and to be absorbed from the gastrointestinal tract. For this purpose, the compounds should be stable in the strongly acidic medium of the stomach and stay intact before being absorbed and reaching the target cells. They are aimed to release the parent drug *in vivo*, preferably by an enzymatic mechanism. The surface receptors for extracellular nucleotides, both purine and pyrimidine, are called P2 receptors. P2 receptors are divided into two categories based on molecular structure and signal transduction mechanisms: P2Y (G-protein coupled receptors) and P2X (ligand-gated ion channels). These receptor subtypes are found in the central and peripheral nervous system, the cardiovascular system, the endocrine system, lungs, intestines, muscle, and the immune system. Antagonists of these subtypes may display antithrombotic properties and CNS effects. Because of their role in the CNS, these molecules are potential therapeutic agents to treat CNS ailments. The vast majority of P2 receptor antagonists known to date are also anionic molecules, e.g., suramin, Reactive Blue 2, PPADS, and derivatives thereof. All of these molecules share a common partial structure containing one or several phenylsulfonate moieties. Yan and Miller (2004) investigated the development of the prodrugs of a new class of P1 and P2 receptor antagonists. These belong to the class of aryl sulfonic acid groups. The negatively charged phosphate groups of P2 agonists and the negatively charged sulfonate groups of P2 antagonists are believed to bind to the positively charged amino acid residues which are typically found in the ligand binding pocket of P2 receptors. Thus, very likely these classes of molecules are likely agents to act as P1 and P2 receptor antagonists and are of potential use in the treatment of CNS diseases. Due to the low pKa value of free sulfonic acid groups (pKa < 1), sulfophenylxanthine derivatives and P2 antagonists with phenylsulfonate structure are depronated under physiological conditions. This means that they do not penetrate into the central nervous system (CNS) and thus are only peripherally active.

However, to be able to investigate CNS effects *in vivo*, e.g. a potential neuroprotective effect of P2 antagonists, penetration into the brain is essential. In addition, because of their polar character, sulfonates are not readily able to cross cell membranes and thus can hardly be absorbed from the gut if they are perorally used, if a systemic effect is desired. In addition, if a CNS effect is required, they should penetrate into the brain and release the drug at the site of action.

The salient features for the design of prodrugs include:

1. The prodrugs should be more lipophilic than their parent drugs in order to be able to cross cell membranes and to be absorbed from the gastrointestinal tract.
2. The compounds should be stable in the strongly acidic medium of the stomach.
3. They should stay intact before being absorbed and reaching the target cells.
4. They should release the parent active drug *in vivo*, preferably by an enzymatic mechanism.
5. The studies should clearly elucidate the conversion pathways from the prodrug to the active drug. Although this is sometimes very tedious, it would help in the clarity of further studies.
6. The studies should be able to determine the reaction rates of the kinetic reactions along with the identification of the path of the reaction. Reaction rate kinetics is helpful in identifying a prodrug that could cleave at the site of action, and possesses desired or increased half-life in the plasma. Usually a series of prodrugs is synthesized as a process of design of prodrugs.

Ester prodrugs of compounds bearing acidic groups are described in the coming discussion. Such prodrugs are well known for carboxylic and phosphoric acids, but not for sulfonic acids. Two kinds of sulfonic acid derivatives are conceivable as potential prodrugs: amides of sulfonic acids (sulfonamides) or sulfonic acid esters.

Sulfonamides are highly stable *in vivo* and therefore are unsuitable as sulfonate prodrugs. In constrast, sulfonic acid esters are relatively unstable since they may react with nucleophiles *in vitro* and *in vivo*. Reactive sulfonic acid esters are used in synthetic organic chemistry (e.g. mesylates and tosylates) and as anticancer agents (busulfane, treosulfane) due to their alkylating properties.

However, the stability of sulfonic acid esters greatly depends on the substitution pattern. Highly stable esters could be obtained, if suitable, electron-withdrawing, deactivating substituents are introduced. A series of prodrugs with several electron withdrawing and deactivating substituents were synthesized. Initial stability studies were performed with nitrophenyl esters of tosylate, namely o-, m-, and p-nitropheynyl tosylate as model compounds. The reaction kinetics was investigated. These studies were initiated because of non-availability of stability data regarding model compounds in the literature. Literature investigations could also help in this direction as memories of instructions for further synthesis as requested by the chemists involved in the research. One of the compounds of this series, m-nitrophenyl tosylate was quite stable over a large pH range, m-nitrophenyl esters of xanthine phenylsulfonic acids were selected as potential prodrugs for further synthesis, stability and receptor binding investigations. The most frequently used analytical method for stability is HPLC. However, because the synthesized xanthine sulfonic acid esters are very lipophilic, they are insoluble in most common HPLC solvents, such as methanol, acetonitrile, H_20, etc. Therefore, capillary electrophoresis with a diode array detector (DAD) was used for the analyses. Compared with HPLC, CE is advantageous in many regards including speed, versatility, low running costs, high separation efficiency, and the requirement of only very small sample volumes.

As a first step, the chemical stability was investigated. Expected hydrolysis products were determined with the help of CE/UV analyses. Chemical stability of the esters was calculated. The hydrolysis by hydroxide ions followed a first-order kinetics. Hydrolysis rates and half-lives of the esters were collected. Since their structures were similar, their half-lives were comparable and were very close to each other. Keeping this as a reason, only one compound was selected and investigated to perform further *in vitro* stability tests. Its biological stability was determined in fetal calf serum, simulated gastric acid, and rate liver homogenate. The stability test in simulated gastric acid was performed for 4h since drugs usually do not stay in the stomach any longer. The compound selected was quite stable in these conditions and thus was selected for further studies. In the next step, hydrolysis of this compound in fetal calf serum was determined as an indicator for the stability of the m-nitrophenyl sulfonate esters in blood serum. The hydrolysis of this compound was very slow with a half-life of 16h following a zero-order kinetic study. Finally, metabolism in liver enzymes was investigated. The hydrolysis followed first-order kinetic reaction. Although, the enzymes responsible for degradation were unknown, there was significant degradation of this compound into the parent compound in the presence of metabolic enzymes. Thus, the ester was very stable in simulated gastric acid as well as in serum. However, it was readily hydrolyzed by incubation with rat liver homogenate, indicating an enzymatic pathway of hydrolysis. The results from this study indicate that this prodrug after oral administration is quite stable in the intestines, followed by quick absorption into the blood, where it is quite stable in the plasma, followed by rapid enzymatic biotransformation in the liver. Thus, this prodrug can be conveniently administered for systemic treatments.

However, if the target were brain, as is the case with these latest classes of compounds, then a totally different variety of ballpark studies would be needed. Along with these studies, degradation in the brain homogenates would also be investigated. If the enzymes are purely available, then simple studies are adequate. However, if the enzymes are not purely available, then animals would be sacrificed followed by brain tissue homogenate preparation. Instead of only one prodrug that was used previously, several other prodrugs that are also quite stable in the liver homogenates will be selected for further studies. The biotransformation studies in the brain homogenates. The presumed end result is that the prodrug travels across the blood-brain barrier and gets degraded into the active drug in the brain homogenates. Prior to studying degradation in the brain homogenates, the transport and stability of the prodrugs across the blood brain barrier would be investigated. If the prodrug travels across the BBB perfectly and gets metabolized into the active drug at the site of action, then the prodrug approach for this molecule is fine. All the results as a whole are helpful in the characterization of the pathway for this prodrug. Subsequently, several other prodrugs can be synthesized on these lines. The reaction kinetics' determination would facilitate the development of very efficient prodrugs for this class of drugs. The final result and the solution of these studies is the identification of biotransformation pathway from intestines to the brain to its activity.

Enzymatic Models

Enzyme models, apart from various buffers are very essential in the investigations of pathway determinations of a prodrug. These enzyme models could include tissue lysates, cell cultures, tissue cultures, microbial cultures and pure enzymes. A brief description of each of these models will be henceforth presented in this section:

Tissue Lysates

Tissue lysates can be conveniently prepared in a laboratory. After collecting the animal tissues, in the presence of selected enzyme inhibitors or cold temperature, the tissue is be homogenized to obtain tissue lysates. The prodrugs are incubated in these homogenates and from time to time the homogenates are collected and assayed for the drug. Currently, many tissue homogenates are available in the market. Since, the marketed ones are validated and are generally homogenized, they are the most preferred ones. As an example, Zyagen sells ready-to-use rat and mouse tissue lysates. Zyagen provides researchers with access to high quality tissue lysates (total protein) for rat and mouse tissues that might be difficult to obtain because of the size, anatomical complexity, or high protease activity. Tissue lysates are derived from adult Sprague Dawley rats and Swiss Webster mice strains. Tissues are dissected and homogenized in RIPA lysis buffer supplemented with SDS and a cocktail of protease inhibitors to minimize proteolysis. The extracted protein is precisely quantified, and packed in 1.5-ml tubes at a concentration of 3 mg/ml. Protein is stable for one year if stored at -80°C. The quality of protein as indicated by the absence of smear (no degradation) and sharpness and resolution of protein bands is verified by denatured SDS-PAGE with Coomassie blue staining. The integrity of protein is tested by immunoblotting using specific beta-actin antibody. The extracted protein is ready for immediate use in Western blotting, immunoprecipitation, SDS-PAGE, isoelectric focusing gels, metabolism studies and SDS-capillary electrophoresis. Different tissue lysates that are currently marketed include whole brain, heart, colon, kidney, liver, lung, ovary, placenta, skeletal muscle, skin, small intestine, spleen, stomach, testis, thymus and uterus.

Cell Cultures

Cell cultures are the very common models of *in vitro* investigations of metabolism and degradation. These include cell suspensions, cell cultures and cellular fractions. In the present context only the hepato cultures will be discussed. However, as mentioned in the tissue culture sections, the appropriate tissue and cell culture can be obtained and used based on the requirement of the prodrug design. However, keeping in view the importance of liver, where the drugs under go major transformation, only hepatic cultures will be discussed. Cell suspensions, cell cultures and cellular fractions represent *in vitro* model systems characterized by preserved integrated cell metabolism. Compared to subcellular models, these systems have several advantages: Firstly, enzyme cofactors need not be added to an incubation system. Second, the risk of unstable enzymes' loss is minimized. Third, intracellular compartment integrity is maintained and metabolic reactions remain interconnected and occur naturally, which is difficult to obtain during experiments on sub-cellular levels.

Hepatocyte Suspensions

Isolated hepatocytes and hepatocyte suspensions are a successful example of a cellular model that is used routinely during the development of new drugs and in the investigation of metabolic or toxic effects of xenobiotics.

The following summarizes important points that should be considered when utilizing this model: Hepatocytes are usually obtained after a two-step collagenase action on the liver tissue. Collagenase disrupts intercellular contacts and communication systems. However, preservation of normal intercellular contacts is considered critical for preservation of some important features of differentiated cells. Remarkably the cells lose their polar character and change shape after collagenase digestion. Proteolysis also damages the enzyme and receptor apparatus of cells. It impairs their biophysical characteristics and transport capabilities as well. Nevertheless, the cells are capable of repairing membrane defects and may preserve the majority of their functions. Utilization of hepatocytes in suspension is limited by their survival period during which they can exhibit metabolic activity. This is why cell suspensions can be used only for a period of four to six hours.

If hepatocytes in suspensions survive only for hours and tissue slices last a few days, liver cell cultures can be maintained for weeks. Cell cultures are different from tissue slices in that they represent only chosen cell types, most typically only one type, whose isolation is technically difficult and time demanding. It is also necessary to prevent them from overgrowing other cell types and protect them against contamination and infection. Cell-to-cell interactions are very different in cell cultures. Confluent cell monolayers are typical by their abnormal cell surface-to-cell volume ratio or cell surface-to-protein content ratio. The cells have a much larger contact area with their surroundings than they have *in vivo* or in tissue homogenates.

Subcellular Fractions

Subcellular fractions involve membrane vesicles, microsomes, cytosol and isolated biochemical entities such as proteins etc. Preparation of such subcellular fractions is relatively simple and these can be stored in a frozen state for relatively long periods of time. It is, however, necessary to add proper co-substrates and co-enzymes to the incubation systems when sub-cellular fractions are used. Microsomes allow us to study both phase I reactions and phase II biotransformations. They can be used preferentially for screening and for preparatory purposes to obtain a required amount of material, e.g. for identification of metabolites. However, cytosolic enzymes, for example, cannot detect important transformations catalyzed, using this system. Thus, the results should be interpreted with caution.

Pure Enzymes

Pure enzymes can be isolated in a laboratory using a variety of techniques. However, these enzymes are also available in the market and could be conveniently used in metabolism studies. Several companies now sell the enzymes isolated from various tissues in a pure form.

Microbial Cultures

Metabolism was previously studied using liver homogenates or several of the techniques mentioned previously. However, the recent fashion in this area is to use microorganisms to investigate the metabolism of compounds. This is a very wide subject. However, keeping in view, its nature and importance, a very small description of the application of microbial cultures in the investigations of drug metabolism will be described henceforth. Envirogen's is one of the companies that sells microbial cultures to be used in several biocatalysis reactions. Extensive collection of degradative bacteria is a unique and valuable tool for biocatalysis as marketed by Envirogen. The production of enantio-pure epoxides using toluene-oxidizing bacteria was demonstrated. They also developed a collection of esterase producing bacteria that resolve racemic mixtures of aromatic esters that could create novel enzyme production and purification systems for producing commercial scale quantities of esterase enzymes. Another library of strains useful for selective oxidation of alkanes was also produced. In addition, these microbial systems offer several other advantages. The technology has become increasingly important in recent years, primarily because of the ability of biological systems to perform reactions in a stereo-specific and regio-specific manner.

Analytical Methods

Analytical methods useful in prodrug studies include UV-spectrophotometry, HPLC, HP-TLC, and capillary electrophoresis etc. These techniques are used in studying the biotransformation reactions, their kinetics and other miscellaneous investigations, as related to prodrug design and development. These techniques are very briefly described in this section.

UV-Spectrophotometry

Light from both sources enters the monochromator where it is dispersed by a concave holographic grating. Monochromatic light exits the monochromator and illuminates the sample. A single photodiode detector measures the amount of light that passes through the sample. When organic molecules in solution, or as a liquid, are exposed to light in the visible and ultraviolet region of the spectrum, they absorb light of particular wavelengths depending on the type of electronic transition that is associated with the absorption. Those parts of a molecule that can be directly associated with an absorption of ultraviolet or visible light, such as the carbonyl group, are called chromophores. Basically, each of a chromophore has specific absorption wavelength at which it absorbs the UV light. The spectrum associated with the entire molecule is termed as UV spectrum. This UV spectrum determines the nature of a drug substance. The extent of absorption depends on the concentration of the substance, including several other parameters, when the drug substance is in a solution form. This is the basic principle using which a spectrophotometer works. This instrument can be conveniently used in the prodrug design for the measurement and determination of spectrum associated with individual components.

High-Pressure Liquid Chromatography (HPLC)

A physical method of separation in which the components to be separated are distributed between two phases, one of which is stationary (stationary phase) while the other (the mobile phase) moves in a definite direction. This is the basic principle involved in chromatographic techniques.

Chromatography always involves use of two phases:

1. a "mobile" phase, which is usually the liquid, and
2. a "stationary phase", which is usually the solid support that the liquid mobile phase runs through. The stationary solid phase is usually held in a glass pipe, or column, and the liquid mobile phase passes through the stationary phase, often simply due to gravity pulling it.

Research with thin-layer and column chromatography showed that separations are much more effective when the stationary phase is a very thin layer on the surface of very small and very uniform spherical beads. Thus evolved high pressure liquid chromatography. However, resistance to flow of the mobile phase is very much higher, and in order to get a useful flow of a liquid mobile phase, e.g., 1 - 3 milliliters/minute, pressures of around 15 Mpa (about 2,000 psi) must be applied to the mobile phase. It is possible to apply such pressure from a cylinder of compressed gas, but most systems use a reciprocating piston pump or diaphragm pump with some means of damping the pressure fluctuations from the piston. The sample is usually dissolved in the mobile phase before injection. Columns are typically 4.6mm ID (6mm OD) stainless steel tubing 250mm long. A typical packing will have octadecylsilyl (C_{18}-Si-) (ODS) groups bonded to 5μm silica beads. The packing is held inside the column by “frits”, discs with pores about 0.5μm in diameter. Liquid chromatography with the stationary phase less polar than the mobile phase is called “reverse phase”, but is now the common situation. The mobile phase is very often not just water but a mixture of water with methanol (CH_3OH) or acetonitrile (CH_3CN). “Solvent programming”, a stepwise or continuous change (gradient elution) of the mobile phase composition, is used to speed up separations, like temperature programming in gas chromatography.

"Chiral"columns have been developed relatively recently to separate optical isomers. This separation is important because many pharmaceuticals are active in only one chiral form. For instance, natural Vitamin E is D-α-tocopherol, while half of synthetic Vitamin E is the less active L- isomer.

Different kinds of detectors are used in identifying the chemicals separated out in the detector cells as a process of separation. A refractive index (RI) detector responds to most components, but is not very sensitive. An ultraviolet (UV) detector is quite sensitive for molecules which absorb ultraviolet light, and a variable wavelength UV detector can be set to the absorption maximum for a particular molecule of interest, or to a short wavelength where most molecules absorb. A diode array detector (DAD) disperses the transmitted light into a spectrum, providing an absorption spectrum of each component that absorbs ultraviolet light. A fluorescence detector measures fluorescence emitted from components that have absorbed ultraviolet light. Amperometric systems measure electron flow that oxidizes or reduces certain components (sugars, for instance). Polarimetric detectors are generally not very sensitive. However, they detect components that are optically active. Mass spectrometric detectors are the recent additions. They are very sensitive and effective in identifying the metabolites.

High Pressure Thin Layer Chromatography (HPTLC)

Thin layer chromatography involves the use of a particulate sorbent on an inert sheet of glass, plastic, or metal. The solvent is allowed to travel up the plate with the sample spotted on the sorbent just above the solvent. Depending on the sorbent, the separation can be either partition or adsorption chromatography (cellulose, silica gel and alumina are commonly used). The major advantage of TLC is the disposable nature of the plates. Samples do not have to undergo extensive cleanups as they would for HPLC. The other major advantage is the ability to detect a wide range of compounds cheaply using very reactive reagents (iodine vapours, sulfuric acid) or indicators. Non-destructive detection (fluorescent indicators in the plates, examination under a UV lamp) also means that purified samples can be scraped off the plate and analyzed by other techniques. There are special plates for such preparative separations, and there are also high-performance plates that can approach HPLC resolution, also called high-pressure thin layer chromatography (HPTLC). The sorbent material (e.g. silica gel 60) has a finer particle size and a narrower particle size distribution (classification) than conventional TLC material. HPTLC layers are characterised by an improved surface homogeneity and are thinner. The advantages are: improved resolution, shorter analysis times, higher detection sensitivity, and in-situ quantitation. It is sufficient to apply nanoliter or nanogrammes of sample (Nano-TLC).

Capillary Electrophoresis (CE)

Capillary electrophoresis uses a small fused silica capillary that has been coated with a hydrophilic or hydrophobic phase to separate biomolecules, pharmaceuticals or small inorganic ions. A voltage is applied and the materials migrate and separate according to charge under the specific pH conditions, as happens in electrophoresis. The capillary can also be used for isoelectric focusing of proteins. The use of salt or vacuum mobilization is no longer required. The major advantages of CE are speed of method development and low operating costs. A low pH phosphate buffer is usually sufficient to analyse a wide range of basic drugs and peptides. For example, in one regulated forensic laboratory a pH 2.7 phosphate buffer was shown to be capable of screening 550 basic drugs. Acidic species can be analysed successfully at high pH. Borate, which has a natural pH of 9.4, is the standard buffer and has been used in the forensic lab to analyse 100 acidic drugs. The typical volume of aqueous buffer used per day is in the order of 10-100ml. This compares favourably with HPLC, where litres of waste organic solvent are produced per day.

Developed in the early 1990s, capillary electrophoresis (CE) is now an established technique. The use of CE is routine in many hospitals and clinics, particularly for analysing serum proteins and disease markers. This technique can be conveniently used in prodrug development. The technique has also dramatically increased throughput for DNA profiling in criminal investigations. CE data have been shown to be credible evidence in law courts, and forensic testing laboratories have published validated procedures. Pharmaceutical companies make extensive use of CE, in particular for chiral separations, and the technique is widely accepted by regulatory authorities such as the US Food and Drug Administration.

Pharmacokinetics

Pharmacokinetic comparison of a drug and its prodrug is one way of evaluating its efficacy. For a prediction, obviously the degradation kinetics of the prodrug in a suitable buffer and a specific tissue of interest, and taken together, the pharmacokinetics would indicate the efficacy of a prodrug. However, this is only helpful in comparing a series of prodrugs of a particular drug candidate. For somebody who is further interested in evaluating in depth, a clear elucidation of the biotransformation picture would be essential. Routine chemical analytical techniques such as UV, IR, NMR and mass spectroscopy are used in the characterization of prodrugs, whether macromolecular or small molecular. These techniques include UV, IR, NMR, and mass spectroscopy.

For the purpose of pharmacokinetic determinations and evaluations, the drug and the prodrug are administered generally by intravenous route and by oral routes with a very convenient dosage form. Very simple pharmacokinetic parameter comparisons would be enough for evaluating the efficacy of a prodrug over the original drug. The concentration of the active drug and its prodrugs in the plasma and in several tissues of interest viz., liver, toxicity eluciting tissue and the target tissue at specific points of time is determined. Prior to such investigations, a very proper method of identification of the compound in the plasma and the tissues of interest would be very essential. Since the structure of the drug and its prodrug would be very close to each other, very likely, a very sensitive and current method is needed to be used. Some of the techniques of separation are described in the previous section along with some of the detection techniques. However, very sophisticated analytical techniques of identification of the drug, its prodrug, and also its metabolites can be used as of today. Things become more complicated if the analysis is required in the plasma and tissues of interest. However, these are basic steps that can be preceded in prodrug efficacy determinations. The best way for pharmacokinetic comparisons is noncompartmental analyses of plasma-time curves after oral and intravenous administrations. Any available pharmacokinetic software packages such as WinNonlin, version 2.1 can be conveniently used for this purpose. The simple parameters that could be used include C_{max}, AUC, AUMC, half-life, releative bioavailability and MRT.

Clinical Examples

Enalapril

Enalapril is an ACE (Angiotensin converting enzyme) inhibitor. ACE is an important enzyme that forms Angiotensin II, which causes constriction of blood vessels thereby enhancing the blood pressure. Enalapril lowers the blood pressure by inhibiting the ACE enzyme and thereby relaxing the blood vessels. Relaxing the arteries not only lowers the blood pressure but also enhances the pumping efficiency of a failing heart and improves cardiac output in patients with heart conditions. Enalapril converts to an active metabolite enalaprilate in the liver. Enalaprilate itself is poorly absorbed when administered orally but may be given directly into the blood in aqueous solution. Enalapril is a lipid soluble and relatively inactive prodrug with good oral absorption (60% to 70%). The conventional pharmacokinetics suggest a rapid peak concentration at 1 hour and rapid clearance (undetectable by 4 hours) by de-esterification in the liver to a primary active diacid metabolite enalaprilate.

Propranolol

Propranolol, a beta-adrenergic blocking agent, is a widely accepted and clinically effective cardiovascular agent indicated in the treatment of angina pectoris, hypertension and cardiac arrhythmia. It has very low and variable bioavailability after oral absorption. The reasons are extensive presystemic metabolism including hepatic and the intestinal mucosal cell metabolism. In addition, it is a poorly soluble molecule. Other routes of delivery such as transdermal, rectal and nasal routes have been explored to enhance the delivery of propranolol. These routes by-pass the hepatic and intestinal metabolism and thus enhance the bioavailability. However, because of the ease of administration, oral route is the preferred route of administration. Thus, the other possibility is to develop the prodrugs of propranolol that avoid degradation in the liver and the intestines. One of the major metabolites of propranolol is glucoronide. The most suitable prodrugs would shield the glucoronide-binding site. O-Acylation is helpful in such a shield. Studies demonstrated that o-acylation is helpful in reducing the presystemic metabolism. In addition, since esterases are very common in human body, acylation would solve both reduced bioavailability and also would cleave the molecule in the systemic circulation and thus enhances the bioavailability. Garceau et al., 1978, synthesized a hemisuccinate ester of propranolol and tested its bioavailability in a beagle dog. It was found that the bioavailability after hemisuccinate ester administration was eight times higher than an equal dose of propranolol. The molecule also resulted in favourable pharmacokinetics suggesting that the prodrug approach was helpful in enhancing the bioavailabiliy of propranolol. Another group synthesized and tested ester prodrugs of propranolol and found that these molecules elevated the bioavailability by reducing the first-pass metabolism after oral administration. This was a very important case study and would be used as a lesson for over several years in the prodrug design. Unfortunately, none of these molecules are currently in the market. Hopefully, one of the prodrugs of propranolol would be in the clinic soon.

Viramidin

Modern design techniques were used in the design of a new prodrug viramidin, a prodrug of ribavarin. This molecule is currently being investigated for human use for the treatment of chronic hepatitis C. Ribavarin is a nucleoside analog with a broad spectrum of activity against a variety of RNA and DNA viral infections. At present, a combination of ribavirin and pegylated interferon-alpha is the standard for the treatment of chronic hepatitis C. One study reported that after 30 minutes of intramuscular injection of ribavarin in rats, the drug was well distributed in all the tissues, except in the brain. The liver had the highest concentration of ribavarin, which rapidly decreased with time. At 8 hours, the liver still retained the highest concentration of the drug, suggesting that the molecule has the best pharmacokinetic properties for liver targeting. However, ribavirin has dose limiting toxicity. Hemolytic anemia is the side effect. After ribavarin enters the circulation it accumulates in red blood cells and is metabolized into various phosphorylated derivatives. Because of the lack of phosphatase activity in erythrocytes, these phosphorylated metabolites are trapped intracellularly and accumulat over a period of time leading to hemolytic anemia. The adverse effect often necessitates dose reduction and discontinuation of therapy in a vast majority of patients. Therefore, currently new ribavirin derivatives with reduced toxic effects are being explored. One such derivative is 3-carboximidine derivative, viramidine. Whole body autoradiography in rats suggested that viramidine actively accumulates in the liver, its target tissue and its accumulation in RBCs is considerably reduced compared to that of ribavarin. In the system viramidine is converted back to ribavarin by the process of deamination.

An enzyme-activated prodrug approach was used in this prodrug design. Many purine nucleoside prodrugs used for the treatment of viral infections such as hepatitis and AIDS are deaminated and activated. The enzyme responsible for these conversions is adenosine deaminase (ADA). Atomic level investigations into this enzyme were performed using complexation with a transition state analog, 6-hydroxy-1,6-dihydropurine ribonucleoside (HDPR). Modeling the binding of ground state of adenosine by replacing with HDPR in the active state suggested that ADA initiates hydrolytic deamination with Asp295 acting as general base to assist the zinc-bound water molecule for a nucleophilic attack at the C6 position of adenosine. Non-specific hydrophobic interactions as well as specific interactions are used in the binding of the substrate to its site. One interaction is believed to be important for catalysis and two other interactions important for substrate recognition and binding affinity. Upon further analysis, it was concluded that ADA should be able to tolerate major structural alteration on the ribose unit but not on the purine. Thus, a sound prodrug should have the three specific hydrogen bonds for the purine and the two with 5'-hydroxy should be preserved. This is the case with all the antiviral nucleoside prodrugs. Of all the ADA-activated prodrugs, it was found that viramidine is the only one that misses the critical N3-Gly184 hydrogen bond and this was given the explanation for very high k_m value for viramidine. It was also concluded that since viramidine is an ADA-activated prodrug, it suggests that it is possible to design a prodrug by employing a non-cognate five-membered ring base in the place of purine, retaining most of the critical interactions. Thus, such a modeling made the design of prodrugs relatively easy and straightforward. The same principles can be applied to the design of other prodrugs. This is a classic example of prodrug design using latest *in silico* technologies introduced into the medicinal chemistry.

Types

As discussed in this entire chapter, a variety of prodrugs are investigated. For the convenience of the reader, a list of the prodrugs is given below. This list would help in the library investigations.

1. Carrier linked prodrugs
2. Bioprecursor prodrugs
3. Site-specific chemical delivery systems
4. Macromolecular prodrugs
5. Drug-antibody conjugates
6. Enzymatically activated oxidation reaction prodrugs
7. Enzymatically activated reduction reaction prodrugs
8. Enzymatically activated hydrolysis reaction prodrugs
9. Oxidation activated prodrugs
10. Reduction activated prodrugs
11. Hydrolysis activated prodrugs

Synthesis

Ever since the prodrug concept was introduced several synthetic methods have been employed. Basically, the reactions are similar to routine chemical reactions with enormous literature available with individual prodrugs. However, a very few classic examples of the synthesis are presented here for each class of molecule.

1. Soluble Prodrugs for Parenteral use

Soluble prodrugs are synthesized as a first step to develop a parenteral formulation for a poorly soluble drug and to develop a water-soluble oral formulation. For example, prodrugs of tocopherol are synthesized to reduce the oxidation potential of tocopherol and also to increase its water solubility. These are acetate and acid succinate esters. Several other groups are used in the synthesis of water-soluble prodrugs. The classic examples that were investigated for such water-soluble prodrugs include tocopherol, hydrocortisone, benzimidazole carbendazoles like mebendazole and albendazole, cephalosphorins, beta-lactam antibiotics, anticancer drugs like etoposide, antihypertensive drugs like prazosin, antiasthmatic drugs like BI-L-266 and antiepileptic drugs like fosphenytoin. The reaction is simple with the drug being mixed with the suitable linker and with suitable reaction conditions a prodrug is obtained.

2. Prodrugs to Improve Passive Oral Drug Delivery

The linkers that improve the passive oral drug delivery are generally esters connected to carboxylic acids group or amino-acid groups of water-soluble drugs. Sometimes, a double or a triple ester can also be used. These molecules upon crossing the intestinal membranes are distributed and then subsequently get converted to the original compound to elicit its action. The drug thence follows its course of pharmacokinetic-pharmacodynamic activity. A variety of enzymes responsible for the cleavage of the molecules are ubiquitous in the system. There are ample of reports published with respect to the linkers. Some of the linkers used for such a purpose are mentioned in the table below. The classic drugs that have been investigated to improve passive oral drug delivery include foscarnet, disodium chromglycate, angiotensin II receptor antagonists like losartan, angiotensin converting enzyme inhibitors such as enalapril, NSAIDS like diclofenac, phenytoin, nucleoside based antiviral drugs, beta blockers such as propranolol, and finally peptide drugs and peptidomimetics.

3. Prodrugs for Targeted Delivery

This topic includes a variety of agents targeting cells, microbes and tissues. However, only a few classic examples will be presented here. These include targeting viruses with site-selective activation, e.g., acyclovir; targeting the colon, e.g., glycosidic and glucurodinic prodrugs of agents such as dexamethasone, nalaxone and menthol for colon targeting (glycosidases and glucuronidases are abundantly present in colon), sulfasalazine for colon targeting (metabolism to the active drug by bacterial microfloral enzymes); targeting the liver (bile acid prodrugs of chlorambucil, thyroid hormone, HMG-COA inhibitors), lactosaminated albumin, lactosylated poly-L-lysine prodrugs of antiviral compounds (targeting parenchymal liver cells); amine containing drugs targeting the brain; targeting with antibodies (antibody drug conjugates and antibody-directed enzyme prodrug therapy (ADEPT)) for anticancer molecules to target tumour cells. Some of the techniques of the conjugation are well developed and these drug-macromolecule conjugate entities are known for a long time since 1958 when the first synthesis of drug-polymer conjugates appeared in literature. Most of the other synthesis techniques are very common reactions routinely used in the chemistry laboratories. These techniques are discussed and presented in length at several places for over several years and very well perceived, understood and investigated by pharmaceutical and chemical scientists.

4. Polymeric Prodrugs

Polymeric prodrugs have evolved into a very useful class of drug delivery agents. Numerous conjugates have been prepared for applications ranging from passive drug targeting to controlled release. Various chemical linkers such as esters, carbonates, carbamates, C=N linkage, and amides are used. Polymeric conjugates are grouped into two broad categories: "permanent conjugates" and 'prodrugs". In a permanent conjugate, the half-life of the cleavage of the linkage is greater than the half-life of the conjugate itself. On the other hand, the polymer conjugate is dissociated to the polymer and the conjugate with the linkage broken down in the system before the action of the drug is elicited and the drug thus follows its pharmacokinetic and pharmacodynamic pathways as known to every pharmaceutical scientist. This class of conjugates is termed as prodrugs, as the prodrugs, by definition, are cleaved into the active drug before it is activated. However, the other class also would belong to the class of conjugates and the use is the same as that of prodrugs and is thus discussed as a part of this section. Although a lot of research has been done in this area with several of the molecules in clinical trials, none of these conjugates is in the market at this time either because of the severe side effects or uselessness or toxicity associated with such a kind of delivery systems. However, they will be discussed because of their historical significance in the subject of prodrugs. These studies can be used to advantage to the scientists working in the area of prodrugs.

A. Synthesis of Ester Conjugates

The clearance of protein drugs by reticular endothelial drugs can be reduced considerable by using ester conjugates with macromolecules. For example, Interferon alpha 2B was conjugated with polyethyleneglycol to increase its plasma circulation time to 10-fold when compared to the native form, after intravenous administration. There is abundant literature available with regard to the synthesis of ester conjugates. Several drugs like doxorubicin, camptothecin, daunorubicin, podophyllotoxin were conjugated with polymers and proved to be effective in enhancing the physico-chemical and pharmacokinetic properties. Here, one of the synthesis reactions used to conjugate a small molecule and a polymer will be detailed. Schoenmakers et al., 2004 described the conjugation of a low soluble anticancer drug paclitaxel, which was coupled using a hydrolysable linker to a polyethylene glycol macromonomer via a conjugate addition reaction between a thiol and an acrylamide. In this synthesis reaction, the macromonomers were synthesized in three steps with an average yield of 70%. In the first step PEG-3400-diacrylamide was synthesized. A drug was then coupled to a linker, a protected mercaptoacid, to the hydroxyl moiety of the model drug. This allowed easy purification of the small molecule conjugate. In the final step, the linker-conjugated drug is further conjugated to the polymer via a conjugated addition reaction also known as Michael-type addition. This reaction did not required any coupling group and generated no residual groups that would be difficult to obtain a pure conjugate. According to the author, the synthetic methodology employed was relatively simple and applicable to any hydroxyl-containing group.

B. Synthesis of Carbonate Conjugates

To illustrate this reaction, the development of carbonate conjugates of camptothecin prodrugs as described by Groot et al., 2002 will be presented. The first prodrugs of camptothecin and 9-aminocamptothecin that are activated by the tumour-associated protease plasmin are reported. The tripartite prodrugs consist of a tripeptide sequence recognised by plasmin, which is linked to the 20-hydroxyl group of the camptothecins via a 1,6-elimination spacer. After selective *N*-protection of 9-aminocamptothecin with an Aloc group, the promoiety (tripeptide–spacer conjugate) was linked to camptothecin or 9-Aloc-9-aminocamptothecin via a 20-carbonate linkage by reacting parent drugs with the *p*-nitrophenyl carbonate activated promoiety in the presence of DMAP. Both prodrugs showed to be stable in buffer solution and both parent drugs were released upon incubation in the presence of plasmin. Furthermore, the prodrugs showed an average 10-fold decreased cytotoxicity with respect to their parent drugs upon incubation in seven human tumour cell lines.

C. Synthesis of carbamate conjugates

A recently published synthesis of PEG conjugates of alsterpaullone, a CDK inhibitor with carbamate as the linker are described by Greenwald et el., 2004 will be illustrated as an example for a carbamate conjugate synthesis. This group adopted two different methods of synthesis. In both methods the indole group of the drug was conjugated. In the first approach, the indole group was activated by reaction with p-nitrophenylchloroformate to produce a reactive carbamate. This was then condensed with a monoblock diamine to form a urea bond followed by deblocking and conjugation to PEG. In the second method, the carbamate was produced using the anion of the indole. Both the compounds were highly water soluble, stable in buffer and released the active drug *in vitro* and *in vivo*.

D. Synthesis of C=N linkages

C=N linked prodrugs are of varied types. However, in this context only hydrozones, that are more popular, are discussed. The popularity of hydrazone is that this bond is quite stable at physiological pH 7.4. However, when subjected to pH 5.0, it is cleaved to form the original molecule. The most popular examples are the prodrugs PEG-doxorubicin and PEG-paclitaxel. One of the synthesis methods for doxorubicin will be discussed, as reported by Rodrigues et al., (1999). In this paper, they synthesized doxorubicin maleimide conjugates containing an amide or acid-sensitive hydrozone linker coupled to different analogs of PEGs to obtain PEG conjugates which are purified by size-exclusion chromatography. The conjugates thus obtained showed no *in vitro* activity. However, the acid-sensitive PEG-doxorubicin conjugates retained their ability to bind to calf thymus as shown by fluorescence and visible spectroscopy studies.

E. Synthesis of Amide Prodrugs

Amide bonds are very stable to aqueous hydrolysis at physiological pH and to enzymatic hydrolysis by esterases. Thus, these prodrugs are the best prodrugs to form permanent drug-polymer conjugates. Hinds and Kim (2002) synthesized these types of conjugates of insulin. Electrophilically activated derivatives of low-molecular-weight monomethoxy poly(ethylene glycol) (mPEG) were chemically coupled to insulin via its amino groups at positions phenylalanine-B1 or lysine-B29, with an amide bond being formed between the polymer and protein. This site-specific conjugation retained the physico-chemical properties of insulin. On the other hand pegylation of insulin almost completely eliminated the resultant conjugates' immunogenecity, allergenecity, and antigenecity. The low-molecular-weight monomethoxypoly(ethylene glycol) was prepared by reacting insulin in a dimethylsulfoxide –triethylamine (DMSO-TEA) mixture. The mixtures of proteins thus obtained were purified to get a PEG-insulin conjugates. Insulin is a standard therapy for the treatment of diabetes. However, it is still marred with lot of formulation problems. One of the best ways discovered by scientists is a prodrug approach. The other approach is controlled release that is also achieved by prodrugs. However, several other methods of achieving controlled release are currently in the process of development and are being investigated.

Safety and Regulatory Considerations

Although most of the times prodrugs are similar to the original drugs in terms of safety, some times the safety of these prodrugs compared to the original drug may be totally different and the regulatory filings may be different compared to the filings of the original drugs. The following are some of the safety and regulatory issues to be kept in mind in the prodrug design and development in tandem:

1. The preclinical safety issues for a prodrug are similar to the safety of the active drug including the methodologies and conclusions.
2. When drugs, whose metabolism is P450IID6-dependent, are given to poor metabolizers, the serum levels achieved are higher, sometimes much higher, than the serum levels achieved when identical doses are given to extensive metabolizers. To obtain similar clinical benefit without toxicity, doses given to poor metabolizers may need to be greatly reduced. In the case of **prodrugs** whose actions are actually mediated by P450IID6-produced metabolites (for example, **codeine** and **hydrocodone**, whose analgesic and antitussive effects appear to be mediated by morphine and hydromorphone, respectively), it may not be possible to achieve the desired clinical benefits in poor metabolizers.
3. Although bioequivalence technically refers only to comparisons of two formulations administered at the same dose, the principles of bioequivalence can be used in other situations. These situations include modified release formulations, prodrugs and formulation with increased bioavailability. In these situations, the safety of a prodrug is established and it is equivalent to any other formulation. Thus, the same priniciples of bioequivalence holds true for a prodrug as is for a formulation.
4. During Phase-I clinical trials, it is desirable to rapidly and safely assess the effective dose in humans. PK-guided dose escalation is the normal routine. The PK studies are also used in the effective dose calculation with preclinical pharmacokinetic and pharmacodynamic studies. Clinical dose selection process for a prodrug may be the same in situations when AUC of an active metabolite is the same as that of AUC of the drug substance.
5. Safety assessment is an important aspect during dose escalations with prodrug. With respect to total drug exposure, represented by AUC (0-infinity), if high-dose prodrug is bioequivalent to high-dose active drug, then it is fine, if the safety of the prodrug is determined in this dose range in preclinical studies to be continued for phase I clinical trials.
6. Ribavirin, part of the current first-line combination therapy for the treatment of chronic hepatitis C, has side effects-in particular, hemolytic anemia-that is frequently dose limiting. Based on animal studies, viramidine, a prodrug of ribavirin, is converted to ribavirin in the liver. Viramidine dosing yielded 50% higher ribavirin levels in the monkey liver but only half in plasma and red blood cells compared to ribavirin dosing. At the same dose, it also had a safer profile than ribavirin in a 28-day toxicity study in monkeys. This would be a safer prodrug of ribavarin. This would be any other situation parallel to other prodrugs. Safety is the criteria.

Conclusions

Gene transcription is known to human race for several centuries. However, this concept is used in the treatment of human beings in modern times only. Adenoviral vectors were the first homing devices used to target the genes into human cells. However, their use has been marred by toxicity and lack of targeting. The very recent innovation in this area is to modify the properties of genes and increase their cellular delivery. The latest of such uses is the development of prodrugs for the genes. This chapter did not discuss any of these latest issues in drug discovery because of its still infancy nature and toxicity associated with gene delivery. However, a variety of concepts regarding prodrug design and development are presented in this chapter.

Questions for Practice and Exercise

1. Define
    1. Prodrug and
    2. Softdrug.

    Explain the differences between the two.
2. Why is the design of a prodrug essential for some classes of drugs?
3. Define the following:
    1. a biotransformation pathway,
    2. biotransformation pathway identification,
    3. design of a prodrug,
    4. route of administration, and
    5. pharmacokinetic parameters.
4. Explain rationally and systematically the design of a prodrug.
5. What are the different studies that are performed during a prodrug development?
6. Describe step-by-step how prodrugs are designed using computer-modeling techniques. Take one specific example from the literature.
7. A. Use the example of the development of prodrugs for HIV-1 integrase inhibitory activity from this textbook. B. Explain using the example of the design of FK228 (depsipeptide) as a natural prodrug for the inhibition of class I histone deacetylases (HDACs) using computer-aided investigations.
8. What are the salient features for the design of prodrugs? Mention briefly the various pharmacokinetic methods that are useful in the development of prodrugs?

9. A. What are the different cell culture methods used in the development of prodrugs? B. How are tissue lysates useful in the prodrug design? C. How are hepatocyte and cell culture suspensions useful in the prodrug design? D. How are subcellular fractions helpful in the design of prodrugs? E. How are pure enzymes useful in the design of prodrugs?
10. How are microbial cultures useful in the design of prodrugs?
11. Cite the following examples in clinics as prodrugs and explain in detail about these prodrugs
    1. Enalapril,
    2. Propranolol, and
    3. Viramidin.
12. List the different categories of prodrugs that would help in the library investigations.
13. Explain the synthesis of prodrugs useful for
    1. parenteral use,
    2. improving oral drug delivery, and
    3. for targeted delivery.
14. How are the various polymeric prodrugs synthesized? Explain in detail the
    1. synthesis of ester conjugates,
    2. synthesis of carbonate conjugates,
    3. synthesis of carbamate conjugates,
    4. synthesis of C=N linkages, and
    5. synthesis of amide prodrugs.
15. What are the safety and regulatory considerations that are considered in the development and use of prodrugs?
16. Describe briefly the following analytical methods
    1. UV-Spectrophotometry,
    2. High-Pressure Liquid Chromatography (HPLC),
    3. High-Pressure Thin Layer Chromatography (HPTLC),
    4. Capillary Electrophoresis.

References

1. Stella V. Pro-drugs: an overview and definition. In: Higuchi T, Stella V, eds. Prodrugs As Novel Drug Delivery Systems. ACS Symposium Series. Washington, DC: American Chemical Society; 1975:1-115.
2. Stella VJ, Charman WN, Naringrekar VH. Prodrugs. Do they have advantages in clinical practice? Drugs. 1985;29:455-473.
3. Albert A. Chemical aspects of selective toxicity. Nature. 1958;182:421-423.
4. Stella VJ, Himmelstein KJ. Prodrugs and site-specific drug delivery. J Med Chem. 1980;23:1275-1282.
5. Stella VJ, Himmelstein KJ. Critique of prodrugs and site specific delivery. In: Bundgaard H, ed. Optimization of Drug Delivery. Alfred Benzon Symposium 17. Copenhagen, Munksgaard; 1982:134-155.
6. Sinkula AA, Yalkowsky SH. Rationale for design of biologically reversible drug derivatives: prodrugs. J Pharm Sci. 1975;64:181-210.
7. Yan L, Muller CE. Preparation, properties, reactions, and adenosine receptor affinities of sulfophenylxanthine nitrophenyl esters: toward the development of sulfonic acid prodrugs with peroral bioavailability.J Med Chem. 2004 Feb 12;47(4):1031-43.
8. Garceau Y, Davis I, Hasegawa J. Plasma propranolol levels in beagle dogs after administration of propranolol hemisuccinate ester.J Pharm Sci. 1978 Oct;67(10):1360-3.
9. Wu JZ, Larson G, Walker H, Shim JH, Hong Z. Phosphorylation of ribavirin and viramidine by adenosine kinase and cytosolic 5'-nucleotidase II: Implications for ribavirin metabolism in erythrocytes.Antimicrob Agents Chemother. 2005
10. Wu JZ, Lin CC, Hong Z. Ribavirin, viramidine and adenosine-deaminase-catalysed drug activation: implication for nucleoside prodrug design. J Antimicrob Chemother. 2003 Oct;52(4):543-6.
11. Wu JZ, Larson G, Walker H, Shim JH, Hong Z. Phosphorylation of ribavirin and viramidine by adenosine kinase and cytosolic 5'-nucleotidase II: Implications for ribavirin metabolism in erythrocytes. Antimicrob Agents Chemother. 2005 Jun;49(6):2164-71.
12. Wu JZ, Walker H, Lau JY, Hong Z. Activation and deactivation of a broad-spectrum antiviral drug by a single enzyme: adenosine deaminase catalyzes two consecutive deamination reactions.Antimicrob Agents Chemother. 2003 Jan;47(1):426-31.

13. de Groot FM, Busscher GF, Aben RW, Scheeren HW. Novel 20-carbonate linked prodrugs of camptothecin and 9-aminocamptothecin designed for activation by tumour-associated plasmin. Bioorg Med Chem Lett. 2002 Sep 2;12(17):2371-6.

14. Greenwald RB, Zhao H, Xia J, Wu D, Nervi S, Stinson SF, Majerova E, Bramhall C, Zaharevitz DW. Poly(ethylene glycol) prodrugs of the CDK inhibitor, alsterpaullone (NSC 705701): synthesis and pharmacokinetic studies. Bioconjug Chem. 2004 Sep-Oct;15(5):1076-83.

15. Rodrigues PC, Beyer U, Schumacher P, Roth T, Fiebig HH, Unger C, Messori L, Orioli P, Paper DH, Mulhaupt R, Kratz F. Acid-sensitive polyethylene glycol conjugates of doxorubicin: preparation, in vitro efficacy and intracellular distribution. Bioorg Med Chem. 1999 Nov;7(11):2517-24.

16. Hinds KD, Kim SW. Effects of PEG conjugation on insulin properties. Adv Drug Deliv Rev. 2002 Jun 17;54(4):505-30. Review.

Bibliography

1. New Drug Development: Regulatory Paradigms for Clinical Pharmacology and Biopharmaceutics (Drugs and the Pharmaceutical Sciences: a Series of Textbooks and Monographs), First Edition, Edited by Chandrahas G. Sahajwalla, Marcel Dekker Inc., 2004.
2. The Practice of Medicinal Chemistry, Second Edition, Edited by Camille Georges Wermuth, Elsevier Publications, 2003.
3. Foye`s Principles of Medicinal Chemistry, Fifth Edition, David A. Williams and Thomas L. Lemke, Lippincott Williams & Wilkins, 2002.
4. Rowland M, Tozer T, Clinical Pharmacokinetics: Concepts and Application. 3rd ed. Philadelphia: Lea and Febiger, 1994.
5. Fundamentals of Clinical Trials, Third Edition, Authored by Lawrence M. Friedman, Curt D. Furberg, David L. DeMets, Springer Mathematics Series, 1998.
6. The Theory and Practice of Industrial Pharmacy, Third Edition, Edited by Leon Lachman, Herbert A. Lieberman, and Joseph L. Kanig, Lea & Febiger Publications, 1986.
7. Physical Pharmacy: Physical Chemical Principles in the Pharmaceutical Sciences, Third Edition, Alfred Martin, James Swarbrick and Arthur Cammarata, Lea & Febiger Publications, 1983.

8. Pharmaceutical Dosage Forms and Drug Delivery Systems, Seventh Edition, Howard C. Ansel, Loyd V. Allen, Jr., and Nicholas G. Popovich, Lippincott Williams & Wilkins, 1999.

9. Hydrolysis in Drug and Prodrug Metabolism: Chemistry, Biochemistry, and Enzymology, First Edition, by Bernard Testa, Joachim M. Mayer, Wiley-VCH, 2003.

10. Enzyme-Prodrug Strategies for Cancer Therapy, First Edition, Edited by Roger G. Melton and Richard J. Knox, Kluwer Academic Press, 1998.

11. D.Fleisher, B.H.Stewart and G.L.Amidon, *Design of prodrugs for improved gastrointestinal absorption by intestinal enzyme targeting*, in: Methods in Enzymology, Drug and Enzyme Targerting, 112, 360, 1985 K.S.Widder and R.Green (Eds.), Academic Press, N.Y.

12. Polymeric Drugs and Drug Delivery Systems, First Edition, Authored by Raphael M Ottenbrite and Sung Wan Kim, CRC Press, 2000.

13. Design of Prodrugs, First Edition, Authored by Bodor, N, Elsevier, Amsterdram, 1985.

14. Quantitative Chemical Analysis, Sixth Edition, Authored by Daniel C. Harris, W.H. Freeman, 2002.

15. Principles of Instrumental Analysis, Fifth Edition, Authored by Douglas A. Skoog, F. James Holler, Timothy A. Nieman, Brookes Cole, 1997.

CHAPTER 10

REGULATORY AFFAIRS

- **Introduction**
- **Forensic Pharmacy**
- **Minimum Requirements to Handle Drugs Intended to be Administered for Therapeutic Benefits**
- **Who is a Pharmacist? What are the Basic Needs for a Person to be a Pharmacist?**
- **History**
- **Acts and Guidelines**
    - The Drugs and Cosmetics Act, 1940 and Rules, 1945
    - Conduction of Clinical Trials
    - Guidelines to Good Manufacturing Practices (GMP)
    - Prevention of Cruelty to Animals Act, 1960
    - Intellectual Property Rights
    - Birth of Generics: The Hatch Waxman Act of 1984
- **Pharmacopoeia**
    - Introduction
    - British Pharmacopoeia
    - Indian Pharmacopoeia
    - United States Pharmacopoeia
- **Definitions**
- **Conclusions**

Introduction

According to several earlier investigations and observations over several years, around everyday consumption of medicines as related to their indications were called by someone passports to heavens, others nice therapies and some others essential needs. As a result, several drugs related committees were started and ultimately lead to the further growth of these oral drug regulatory departments. The eventuality resulted in specialized confinement of these dosage forms in the commercial market in the very earlier years of modern drug development, as ordered by the governments of several countries. This is especially true when the actual dosage of a drug in a formulation is 1 mg to 2 mg. The other needs for such a kind of regulatory departments could be illustrated by these particular examples. The quality of drugs and formulations imported into developing countries having a tropical climate may be adversely affected if their formulations and storage conditions are not optimized. In these situations, the very early stability testing in the countries of production or in the countries of selling prior to the formulation introduction into the local market is compulsory. However, without such proper investigations, if the product is in the market, and this instability phenomenon is noticed while it is in the market, then most likely this formulation could be withdrawn from the market. A regulatory agency authorizes or looks after such matters. The other example as mentioned below could better illustrate the need for drug regulatory departments.

The definition of a "new drug" along with the definition of several other pharmacy related vocabulary by USA regulatory agencies were modified several times. However, the major modification is related to the definition of a new drug. Probably the most significant and taller provisions of the 1962 Drug Amendments relate to "new drugs". The definition of a "new drug" was expanded beyond that of the original 1983 definition, for which lack of general recognition by qualified experts as to a drug safety for intended purpose was the sole criterion. Currently, the older complicated definitions are no more existing and in place more simple and well-defined definitions have been lately in use. All these uses are definitely based on these new definitions and all the older definitions are no more in vogue. Thus, accordingly any deviations from these rules could result in the arrest or revoking or shutting down of a drug or for instance any drug related formulation business. All the new businesses should definitely keep these in mind before the start of any activity or an occasion. For these reasons regulatory agencies were initiated. Thus, regulatory agencies play a major role in oral drug industry. Keeping in view lot of coverage of oral formulations in the pharmaceutical industry, this author perceived that this current textbook definitely should have a well-defined chapter for this topic. As a result, some of the related areas at the outset of today's oral pharmaceutical industry are discussed.

Forensic Pharmacy

The word 'forensic' is derived from the Latin term 'forencis' meaning forum which signifies a public place, market place or a place of assembly for judicial and other business. Thus a place where everybody is given an opportunity of debate may be called a forum. These are the basic working places in ancient civilizations. It is definitely the continuity, as may not be visualized to lay or unintelligent personalities, which still governs some of the basic governing bodies all over the world. As the human kind progressed it is the continuum in many factors which still could be visualized in the market places. Thus, forensic pharmacy is definitely not an old subject of interest for human kind. Eversince any kingdom or any empire has reached a zenith the people, their methods, and the culture was definitely adopted by the next set of people ruled under a different emperor, although a different one. Thus, what we perceive here at this time as a subject of forensic pharmacy is an old one. During this transition lot of things might have got changed or matured or culminated. However, the basics which remained the same are the fundamental keys for the progress of the current forensic pharmacy. It is always better as the civilization is progressing any science has also to progress. Old methods in the minds or acts of the community should be tailored according to the maturity. Money is always there with any rung of the society. However, development reflects the maturity of this rung. Thus, as could be visioned this science is very cheap at this time. Slowly modernization is entering into this field without lack of accelerated progress. As the progress into allopathy medicine continued, several laws and legislations were conveniently and clearly adopted which entered into the bigger circles of pharmacy community at this time. Several case studies and examples of set backs and draw backs further resulted in weeding out the older disadvantages associated with older laws and thus this field is always progressing although very slowly. According to NK Jain (2005), "development of laws in general and those related to drugs and pharmaceuticals in particular cannot be looked into in isolation. Development of forensic pharmacy runs parallel to the development of medicine. According to one medical historian, Henry Siegerist, every culture has developed a system of medicine and medical history is but one aspect of the history of culture. It must be a sound belief that the first doctor was the first man because he had to survive against so many odds like sickness and accident. Drugs and medicines developed out of necessity. Vedic medicine was still reining the control among the common man till the Arabic or Unani Tibb system was brought into India by Muslim rulers". Modern training in forensic pharmacy is very essential for every pharmacist to attain ideal heights in his professional progress. Tacitly these statements also hold true for the current medical fashion i.e., allopathy medicine or western medicine.

Minimum Requirements to Handle Drugs Intended to be administered for Therapeutic Benefits

It is not only the pharmacists who handle drugs intended for therapeutic benefit. It could be lab technicians, microbiologists, surgical technologists, etc. Thus, very proper minimum requirements to handle drugs intended to be administered for therapeutic benefits are essential. Any person who could be taken into a company or a research organization intended for routinely handling the drugs should definitely know these aspects. One technologist who may routinely handle drugs is a surgical technologist. Keeping in view the requirements to handle drugs for this person this section will be elaborated.

Surgical technologists, also knows as surgical or operating room technicians or scrubs, help during surgical operations under the direction of registered nurses, surgeons, and other surgical workers. Operating room teams, of which surgical technologists are part, typically comprise surgeons, nurses, and anesthesiologists. Prior to the surgery, technologists prep get the room ready by placing surgical tools and equipment and sterile dressings and liquids in their appropriate places. They ensure that all equipment is functioning properly, and prepare the patient for the operation by disinfecting the part of the body where the incision will be made and removing any hair that may be present there. They move the patient to the room, properly position them on the table, and use sterile "drapes" to cover them. Technologists are also responsible for checking the patient's vital signs and records, and helping doctors and nurses put on their gloves and gowns. During the operation, technologists hand tools and supplies to the doctors and surgeon assistants as they request them. They also count equipment, such as needles, sponges, and other instruments, to ensure that nothing is left inside the patient. They may be required to handle lights, suction equipment, and sterilizers. They also assist with specimens to be taken to the laboratory by collecting and caring for them. Following the surgery, technologists restock the room with supplies and may transport the patient back to their room to recover. Many a times they also handle drugs.

Handling of Drugs by a Surgical Technologist

A surgical technologist should know the basic principles of pharmacology. He should be able to identify basic drugs used by the surgical patient, their side effects & the common dosage. The technologist should have wide knowledge about proper response to drug reactions and demonstrate safe practice when using drugs on the sterile field. He/she should also be aware of the legal responsibilities of the surgical technologist in handling drugs and solutions. He should be able to develop both written and verbal communication skills, utilize critical and creative thinking skills, acquire organizational, leadership and administrative skills, as well as solve ethical dilemmas in real-world situations when dealing with drugs, especially new drug substances. Some of these issues could be applied for other professionals who are required to handle drugs. These issues are further discussed. Drugs could be classified into safe drugs and hazardous drugs, although all the drugs are generally considered as hazardous. These definitions vary depending on the safety and toxicity profiles of the compounds. However, keeping in view the perspective of the current topic, hazardous drugs will be cited in elaboration. Some of these drugs could be orphan drugs, whose mention could be very much necessary at this juncture as these drugs may be potentially dangerous and further there is a lack of enough statistical evidence of the safety and toxicity of such drugs in human beings.

Hazardous drugs are drugs that pose a potential health risk to health care workers who may be exposed during preparation or administration. Such drugs require special handling because of their inherent toxicities. While most drugs are hazardous because they are cytotoxic, drugs from other categories are potentially harmful (such as the antiviral agent gancyclovir). Currently, the term "hazardous" is preferred over "chemotherapy" or "antineoplastic" because is it is more inclusive of drugs that present a risk. The below table presents criteria for defining hazardous drugs.

Criteria for Defining Hazardous Drugs
Drugs that meet one or more of the following criteria should be handled as hazardous: • Carcinogenicity • Teratogenicity or developmental toxicity • Reproductive toxicity • Organ toxicity at low doses • Genotoxicity • Structure or toxicity similar to drugs classified as hazardous using the above criteria
From Preventing Occupational Exposures To Antineoplastic And Other Hazardous Drugs In Healthcare Settings.

A list of drugs that should be handled as hazardous can be found from respective regulatory authorities all over the world. In the United States of America (USA) Appendix A of the electronic document available from the Centers for Disease Prevention and Control (CDC) mentions this list. The Ames test measures genetic mutations in bacteria after exposure to compounds. Ninety percent of known carcinogens test positive on this test. The test is reliable during drug excretion in the urine, which is usually within 48 hours of exposure. It has neither high sensitivity nor specificity. Several other studies followed that demonstrated risks from occupational exposure to chemotherapy.

The Occupational Safety and Health Administration (OSHA), whose mission is to protect the health and safety of workers, became interested in the occupational risk of handling chemotherapy agents in the early 1980s in the USA. During a visit to a northern California hospital, California, USA, OSHA became aware of the facility's chemotherapy preparation practices. The subsequent investigation resulted in the facility being cited for failure to provide protection for the pharmacists. The safe handling program that was implemented was described in the American Journal of Hospital Pharmacy and became the basis for the first American Society of Hospital Pharmacists (ASHP) Technical Assistance Bulletin on Handling Cytotoxic Drugs. After several years of published data suggesting harm from occupational exposure to chemotherapy drugs, OSHA published guidelines for the safe handling of those agents. The guidelines described the equipment, garments, and work practices aimed at protecting pharmacists and nurses from exposure. While the guidelines are not considered as standards, enforceable by law, the guidelines are responsible for hospitals and other health care organizations' implementation of safe handling precautions. In the 1970s and 1980s it was common practice for nurses to perform drug preparation activities in medication rooms on nursing units. The main route of exposure to hazardous drugs (Below Table) was thought to be inhalation of drug aerosols generated during preparation. To reduce this risk, OSHA guidelines state that cytotoxic drug preparation must be performed in a biological safety cabinet (BSC) in a designated area, usually a pharmacy. A BSC has vertical airflow that moves away from the worker, as opposed to horizontal airflow that moves away from the product toward the worker. Vertical airflow protects the worker, while horizontal airflow is designed to protect the sterile product from contamination. Air leaving a BSC is filtered through a HEPA (high efficiency particulate air) filter.

Routes of Exposure to Hazardous D
• Inhalation of aerosolized drug • Dermal absorption • Ingestion • Injection

The OSHA guidelines suggest that drugs may leak during the manipulations required to reconstitute powders and the transfer of drug from one container to another. Since contamination has been found on the outside of biological safety cabinets and on floors around them, it is clear that such engineering controls do not always contain the hazard. Incorrect operator technique can interfere with airflow and allow the escape of drug aerosols. Accidental drug spills obviously contribute to surface contamination.

After several years of experience in this area, the following suggestions were made:

- Biological safety cabinets (BSCs) provide imperfect protection against hazardous drug exposure. Other types of ventilated cabinets may provide containment, but are not currently available in pharmacies
- Routine handling activities can result in contamination of the worker and work environment.
- There is frequent and persistent contamination of the environment where hazardous drugs are handled.
- Dermal absorption of hazardous drugs as a result of contact with contaminated surfaces is another potential route of exposure.
- Failure to use personal protective equipment can result in inadvertent contamination of clothing.
- Workers who are not directly involved in activities related to hazardous drug handling are at risk for exposure.
- Drug exposure can result in drug absorption that can be measured.

Magnitude of Exposure to Occupational Hazardous Drugs

While most hazardous drugs are used in the treatment of persons with cancer, they are also used for non-oncology indications, such as rheumatoid arthritis, lupus, nephritis, and multiple sclerosis. For example, methotrexate is used as a medical treatment for tubal ectopic pregnancy. The increasing use of such drugs outside the oncology arena increases the number of health care workers who may be potentially exposed. It is estimated that as many as 5.5 million health care workers have the opportunity for exposure to hazardous drugs in the workplace. Most patients are in a health care setting such as a hospital, clinic, or physician's office when receiving hazardous drugs, but some patients are treated in the home. By far, health care workers at greatest risk for exposure are pharmacists who prepare hazardous drugs, and nurses who may both mix and administer the drugs. However, all other individuals involved in both direct and indirect care of persons who receive such drugs should be considered potentially exposed.

"Procedures for proper handling and disposal of anticancer drugs as well as NCEs ***should be considered***. Several guidelines on this subject have been published. There is ***no general agreement*** that all of the procedures recommended in the guidelines are necessary or appropriate." Clearly, there is evidence to the contrary. The NIOSH Hazardous Drug Safe Handling Working Group proposed more than three years ago that appropriate language be substituted, but the FDA has not adopted the recommendation. The group was informed that the process of replacing the language in every applicable package insert would be monumental.

Personal Protective Equipment for Hazardo
• Gowns – disposable, made of fabric that has low-permeability to the agents in use, with closed-front and cuffs, intended for single use. • Gloves – powder-free, labeled and tested for use with chemotherapy drugs, made of latex, nitrile, or neoprene. • Face and eye protection when splashing is possible. • A NIOSH-approved respirator when there is a risk of inhaling drug aerosols (such as spill clean up).

Components of a Safe Handling Program

The development of a safe handling program requires multidisciplinary planning in the pharmaceutical industry setup from the input from administration, medicine, nursing, pharmacy, risk management, safety, and environmental services staff. Such interdisciplinary groups should review national guidelines regularly and develop policies and procedures based on the guidelines. The purpose of the *Alert* is to inform health care workers of the continuing risk of exposure and to outline the responsibility of employers and health care workers related to safe handling. The employer responsibilities include:

1. Developing policies and procedures for the safe storage, transport, administration, and disposal of hazardous agents.
2. Identifying those hazardous drugs used in the facility and determining methods for updating the list.
3. Making guidance documents such as Material Safety Data Sheets (MSDS) available to health care workers who handle hazardous drugs.
4. Requiring that all employees who handle hazardous drugs wear personal protective equipment (PPE) designated for the purpose (Table).
5. Requiring a BSC for the preparation of hazardous drugs.
6. Prohibiting eating, drinking, etc. in areas where hazardous drugs are handled.
7. Providing mandatory training for all employees based on their hazardous drug handling tasks.
8. Developing a hazardous-drug spill management policy and procedure.
9. Setting forth a plan for medical surveillance of personnel handling hazardous drugs.

10. Addressing in a policy workers' hazardous drug handling during pregnancy. The Oncology Nursing Society recommends that employers provide alternate duty to employees who request other assignments due to pregnancy, the desire to conceive, or breast-feeding.
11. Monitoring compliance with safe-handling policies and procedures.

The Health Care Worker Responsibilities Include

- Participating in training before handling hazardous drugs and updating knowledge based on new information.
- Referring to guidance documents as necessary for information regarding hazardous drugs.
- Utilizing BSCs in drug preparation.
- Consistently using recommended gloves, gowns, and face and respiratory protection.
- Washing hands after drug handling activities and removal of PPE.
- Disposing of materials contaminated with hazardous drugs separately from other waste in designated containers.
- Cleaning up hazardous drug spills immediately according to recommended procedures.
- Following institutional procedures for reporting and following up on accidental exposure to hazardous drugs.

Who is a Pharmacist? What are the Basic Needs for a Person to be a Pharmacist?

A pharmacist is a person who routinely handles drugs, compounds them and delivers them to the patient based on the requirement or as per the suggestions of a physician. Thus, he has to know about drugs, their chemistry, pharmacology, physiology of the patient, aeitiology of the diseases, formulation development aspects, drug interactions, pharmacokinetics, jurisprudence, etc. and a practicising pharmacist should be able to give such information orally provided a patient, a higher authority or a doctor requests for as the need is. Thus, he has to know about these facts on the tip of the mouth. So, a pharmacist requires a thorough and memorable knowledge of the information about the drugs which he dispenses. In addition a pharmacist is definitely different from a compounder or a dispenser which are used in the old days. However, this field is now a days very sophisticated and accordingly a pharmacist is trained. Currently, several questionnaires, question banks, etc. are available in the market which are routinely memorized by a pharmacist for his day to day activities. This is apart from several other books routinely referred by this person which includes USP, IP, BP, JP, etc. which are subsequently discussed. In addition, several countries have their own methods of allowing a trained person in pharmacy to practice pharmacy. Although in India this is not rigorous as of today, a day would come when the practice would be very much similar to that found in the modern western countries.

History

History comes to the pen of a poet, an author or an historian. This is what the saying is. This could be the saying that holds true with the development of any civilization, science or technology. However, there is a lot of background which cannot be ignored. As per the religion, science is a bane and is a curse also. Thus, human progress has to be carefully made. This is especially true with scientific or technological progress. Rules have been made eversince such acceleration of the human development has been discovered and made. History of regulatory departments of some countries is presented here.

USA, Europe and Japan

The U S. Food and Drug Administration (USFDA) is a scientific, regulatory, and public health agency that looks after accounting for 25 cents of every dollar spent by consumers. Its perview include most food products (other than meat and poultry), human and animal drugs, therapeutic agents of biological origin, medical devices, radiation-emitting products for consumer, medical, and occupational use, cosmetics, and animal feed. USFDA was started in 1862 with a single chemist in the US Department of Agriculture. It now has a staff of approximately 9,100 employees and a budget of $1.294 billion in 2001, comprising chemists, pharmacologists, physicians, microbiologists, veterinarians, pharmacists, lawyers, and many others. About one-third of the agency's employees are in the offices other than those located in Washington, D. C. area, staffing over 150 field offices and laboratories, including five regional offices and 20 district offices. Currently scientists at FDA evaluate applications for new human drugs and biologics, complex medical devices, food and color additives, infant formulas, and animal drugs. Also, the FDA monitors the manufacture, import, transport, storage, and sale of about $1 trillion worth of products annually at a cost to taxpayers of about $3 per a persone living in the USA. Investigators and inspectors regularly visit several facilitie (as of today more than 16,000 facilities a year), and arrange with state governments to help increase the number of facilities checked.

Beginning as the Division of Chemistry and then (after July 1901) the Bureau of Chemistry, the modern era of the FDA dates to 1906 with the passage of the Federal Food and Drugs Act; this added regulatory functions to the agency's scientific mission. The Bureau of Chemistry's name changed to the Food, Drug, and Insecticide Administration in July 1927, when the non-regulatory research functions of the bureau were transferred elsewhere in the department. In July 1930 the name was shortened to the present version. FDA remained under the Department of Agriculture until June 1940, when the agency was moved to the new Federal Security Agency. In April 1953 the agency again was transferred, to the Department of Health, Education, and Welfare (HEW). Fifteen years later FDA became part of the Public Health Service within HEW, and in May 1980 the education function was removed from HEW to create the Department of Health and Human Services, FDA's current home. To understand the development of this agency is to understand the laws it regulates, how the FDA has administered these laws, how the courts have interpreted the legislation, and how major events have driven all three.

FDA included several duties on its list after the election of Franklin Roosevelt and the death of embodiment of the 1906 act in 1930. The duties included legally mandated quality and identity standards for foods, prohibition of false therapeutic claims for drugs, coverage of cosmetics and medical devices, clarification of the FDA's right to conduct factory inspections, and control of product advertising, among other items. The FDA itself exemplified the state of affairs in the marketplace by assembling a collection of products that illustrated shortcomings in the 1906 law. It included Banbar, a worthless "cure" for diabetes that the old law protected; Lash-Lure, an eyelash dye that blinded many women; numerous examples of foods deceptively packaged or labeled; Radithor, a radium-containing tonic that sentenced users to a slow and painful death; and the Wilhide Exhaler, which falsely promised to cure tuberculosis and other pulmonary diseases. A reporter dubbed this exhibit "The American Chamber of Horrors," a title not far from the truth since all the products exhibited were legal under the existing law.

Languishing in Congress for five years, the bill that would replace the 1906 was ultimately enhanced and passed in the wake of a therapeutic disaster in 1937. A Tennessee drug company marketed a form of the new sulfa wonder drug that would appeal to pediatric patients, Elixir Sulfanilamide. However, the solvent in this untested product was a highly toxic chemical analogue of antifreeze; over 100 people died, many of who were children. The public outcry not only reshaped the drug provisions of the new law to prevent such an event from happening again, it propelled the bill itself through Congress. This was neither the first nor the last time Congress presented a public health bill to a president only after a therapeutic disaster. FDR signed the Food, Drug, and Cosmetic Act on 25 June 1938.

The new law brought cosmetics and medical devices under control, and it required that drugs be labeled with adequate directions for safe use. Moreover, it mandated pre-market approval of all new drugs, such that a manufacturer would have to prove to FDA that a drug were safe before it could be sold. It irrefutably prohibited false therapeutic claims for drugs, although a separate law granted the Federal Trade Commission jurisdiction over drug advertising. The act also corrected abuses in food packaging and quality, and it mandated legally enforceable food standards. Tolerances for certain poisonous substances were addressed. The law formally authorized factory inspections, and it added injunctions to the enforcement tools at the agency's disposal.

In the late 1960s and 1970s the FDA lost some of its responsibilities but acquired many more. Shortly after the FDA became a part of the Public Health Service, the Department of Health, Education, and Welfare transferred several functions administered by other PHS agencies to the FDA, including regulation of food on planes and other interstate travel carriers, control over unnecessary radiation from consumer and professional electronic products, and pre-market licensing authority for therapeutic agents of biological origin. The latter originated under the predecessor of the National Institutes of Health in the Biologics Control Act of 1902, which followed the deaths of thirteen children from a tetanus-tainted batch of diphtheria antitoxin in St. Louis, and nine pediatric fatalities from similar circumstances in Camden, New Jersey. (At right, a scientist in FDA's Center for Biologics and Research is conducting research on the organism that causes the childhood disease pertussis.) Congress had authorized the FDA to regulate consumer products such as potential poisons, hazardous toys, and flammable fabrics in a number of laws dating back to 1927, but this function was transferred to the Consumer Product Safety Commission in 1973.

Changes in the work of the FDA have come rapidly in the past 20 years, shaped at least in part by political pressure, consumer activism, and industry involvement. Patient advocacy groups influenced a law to stimulate industry interest in developing so-called orphan drugs for rare diseases, and they played a role in the agency's development of accelerated techniques for drug approval, beginning with drugs for AIDS. Congress passed a law that simultaneously extended patent terms to account for time consumed by the drug approval market acceptance and facilitated the market acceptance of generic human and animal drugs to offer a lower-cost alternative to brand name pharmaceuticals. Also, Congress instituted procedures for industry to reimburse the FDA for review of drugs and biologics to speed the agency's evaluations.

The other country, which has significant history, related to drug regulatory authority is Germany. Since World War II, the United States and Germany have experienced a similar growth in government bureaucracies. New and expanded agencies faced similar pressures to draw upon scientific and medical expertise when making decisions. Regulatory agencies overseeing the pharmaceutical industry in the two countries developed and maintained their authority in similar ways by demanding premarket testing and formal application for market approval.

New drugs achieve marketable status only if the manufacturer complies with government guidelines for testing and provides authorities with evidence of their safety and efficacy. In both countries, drug companies must pay for clinical trials, oversee the clinics that test drugs, and then submit formal results to the government. Likewise, regulatory agencies in both countries assess "user fees" to companies that want to expedite the review process.

Therapeutic cultures are active in three primary arenas: legislative/regulatory mandates, scientific testing in clinical trials, and oversight of adverse drug reactions. Because of their different therapeutic cultures, the distribution of authority among the quartet of actors in medical policy has shifted frequently in the United States, but remained comparatively stable in Germany. In one key feature of medical policy, American regulators delineated a strict boundary between premarket testing and market approval, whereas their German counterparts adopted a more flexible approach that blurred the line between pre- and postmarket oversight. More recently, differences between their therapeutic cultures promoted the emergence of disease-based interest groups targeting regulatory policy in the United States, while few such organizations sought to change regulatory approaches in Germany. Despite claims that U.S. tort law impedes innovation and is extremely costly to manufacturers, liability is not uniform across product categories. Contraceptives, vaccines, and drugs taken during pregnancy are especially subject to liability claims in the United States. Thus three products, the Dalkon Shield contraceptive, Bendectin (a treatment for pregnancy-related nausea), and silicon breast implants have composed the majority of liability litigation in the health care sector during the past three decades.

A dominant technological product, such as a blockbuster drug that outsells its competitors, is not always chosen for its technical superiority alone. Instead, a variety of social factors and informal judgments help determine technological "winners." Similarly, proving drug safety and efficacy involves a body of informal practices and testing methods, no matter how hard regulators and practitioners seek to follow a standardized testing regime. Clinical trials are loci for social, ethical, and even moral debates about appropriate therapies, just as they serve to reinforce social roles for patients and physicians. As a result, the testing methods and results are often very controversial. The therapeutic cultures of the

United States and Germany form the backbone of this study, and the rest of the chapters are organized around sites where they are active: legal and regulatory structures, experimental methods and testing approaches, and surveillance and postmarket controls. Each of these areas is presented chronologically; thereby offering three different passes through the same historical period. The conclusion explores how findings from each of these arenas relate to contemporary plans for international regulatory harmonization, and speaks to the future of relations among the state, physicians, industry, and patients. German drug laws, in contrast, were linked to broader concerns in the health care system regarding the distribution of authority across the network of physicians, industry, and the state. Since physicians had more control over constructions of "the patient," few groups articulated political demands for either greater regulatory protections or speedier drug approvals. Case studies of Terramycin, thalidomide, and propranolol reveal that clinical trials served different functions in the therapeutic cultures of the United States and Germany. The FDA enforced the use of quantitative testing methods and imposed methods for statistical evaluation of test results between 1950 and 1980. Formal testing procedures were a means to demonstrate objectivity and helped shield the agency from criticism and public controversy. In Germany, on the other hand, trials were integral to defining physicians' authority in relation to the state and key to establishing new professional norms for medical care after World War II. Clinical trials carried out in the period between 1950 and the mid-1970s were generally integrated into overall patient care in Germany, rather than forming distinctive testing sites as in the United States.

Japan is one of the leading countries in terms of pharmaceuticals and it is worth mentioning about its history of drug regulatory affairs. Interestingly, in Japan, the Ministry of Health, Labour, and Welfare (MHLV) was established by the merger of the Ministry of Health and Welfare and the Ministry of Labour on January 6, 2001, according to the government program for reorganizing government ministries. This MHLV department established in 1938 is the in charge of the improvement and promotion of social welfare, social security and public health. The role of MHLV is the same as the role of the newly established department. Systematic government regulations requiring all medicinal products to be registered for sale started in the 1950s. This includes the experiments right from the inception of the market acceptance protocols. Most of these pharmaceutical regulations subsequently followed US FDA principles as mentioned before. However, “Pharmaceuticals and Medical Devices Evaluation Center” department established on July 1st 1997 to built up the government's evaluation capacity for securing safety and preventing harmful side effects of pharmaceuticals has been playing a major role in the market acceptance of a new drug and formulation. This center evaluates quality, efficacy and safety of each prescription drugs and medical devices as well as proprietary drugs, quasi-drugs and cosmetics that are purchased directly by the general public. The evaluation process is, taking a newly developed drug as an example, as follows: on accepting the market acceptance process to the Minister for Health, Labour and Welfare from a pharmaceutical company, the center leaves the data reliability survey to the external institution. The consideration is conducted from the scientific point of view by an evaluation team consisting of several officials whose backgrounds are pharmaceutical science, medicine, dentistry, veterinary, bio-statistics and otherwise, to make an evaluation report on the drug. The report is submitted to the Pharmaceutical Affairs and Food Sanitation Council (PAFSC) that is a consultative body of the Minister. Based on the agencies recommendations, the concerned ministry finalizes the decision of accepting and importing the formulation or the drug, accordingly within the scheduled time or the acceptance may be made earlier on special occasions as scheduled as mentioned before with the american situation.

India

In India testing of pharmaceuticals and their formulations including toxicity studies and pharmacological outcomes was not observed in the beginning of the current century. However, with the First World War some companies were started and then began the process of drug regulation and market acceptance. These laws were based on some of the earlier laws that were introduced by British rule in India. Two of the laws, The Poisons Act and the Dangerous Drugs Act were passed in 1919 and 1930, respectively. The Opium Act was adopted as early as 1878. Indian Government in 1931 for the cause of rapid expansion of the pharmaceutical production and drug market has set up a committee called Drugs Enquiry Committee under the Chairmanship Lt. Col. R. N. Chopra. This committee's role was to initiate and proceed with sifting enquiries into the whole matter of drug production, distribution and sale by inviting opinions and meeting concerned people. After several enquiries and examinations of the data, accordingly, the Chopra Committee submitted a voluminous report to the government suggesting creation of drug control machinery at the center with branches in all provinces. In addition, this committee was instrumental in the establishment of a well-equipped central drug laboratory with competent staff and experts in various branches for data standardization work by making proper huge recommendations. Accordingly, investments and divestments in the establishment of smaller and newer laboratories with special focuses on provinces were suggested. In this regard, the committee was asked to list the names and addresses of the licensed pharmacists with the permission of central pharmacy council and the provincial pharmacy councils. The outbreak of the Second World War in 1939 delayed the introduction of legislation on the lines suggested by the Chopra Committee that the Indian government contemplated and considered as urgent. This was the time of swadeshi movements and the rejection and acceptance of foreign goods and imports. This also included pharmaceuticals. With time the scenario changed. The Drugs Act was passed in 1940 partly implementing the Chopra recommendations. With the achievement of independence in 1947 and subsequently, the rest of the required laws were placed on the Statute Book as a Good Samaritan perspective.

In 1985, the Narcotic Drugs and Psychotropic Substances Act was enacted repealing the Dangerous Drugs Act 1930 and the Opium Act of 1878. At present the following Acts and Rules made there under that govern the manufacture, sale, import, export and clinical research of drugs and cosmetics in India.

- The Drugs and Cosmetics Act, 1940
- The Pharmacy Act, 1948
- The Drugs and Magic Remedies (Objectionable Advertisement) Act, 1954
- The Narcotic Drugs and Psychotropic Substances Act, 1985
- The Medicinal and Toilet Preparations (Excise Duties) Act, 1956
- The Drugs (Prices Control) Order 1995 (under the Essential Commodities Act)

Some other laws

There are some other laws that have a bearing on pharmaceutical manufacture, distribution and sale in India. The important ones being:

1. The Industries (Development and Regulation) Act, 1951
2. The Trade and Merchandise Marks Act, 1958
3. The Indian Patent and Design Act, 1970
4. Factories act

Thorough understanding of these laws before filing for a market acceptance process of a new drug or a formulation would be essential as detailed in subsequent sections. In addition, the comprehension of these laws would help in betterment of India at this time, as of 2004. Some of the above concerns with latest opinions, subjects and discussions, further elaborations with regard to the current perview are discussed in this section in general and most of the laws are published in the government gazettes.

Acts and Guidelines

Several acts and guidelines are currently in place to deal with the regulatory affairs associated with the development and utility of new drug substances. Some of the very important ones as relevant to India are described below.

The Drugs and Cosmetics Act, 1940 and Rules, 1945

The Drugs and Cosmetics Bill was passed by the Central Legislative Assembly and it received the assent of the Governor General on 10th April, 1940 and thus became the Drugs and Cosmetic Act, 1940. This act seeks to:

(i) Regulate import of drugs and cosmetics into the country in order to prevent entry of substandard or harmful drugs and cosmetics.

(ii) Exercise control over the manufacture of drugs and cosmetics in the country so that no substandard or spurious drugs or cosmetics are produced.

(iii) Provide for the regulation of sale and distribution of drugs and cosmetics whereby only qualified and trained persons could undertake their handling, compounding and distribution.

(iv) Regulate the manufacture and sale of Ayurvedic, Sidda and Unani drugs, wherever applicable.

The act also provides for the constitution of two "Boards" namely the Drugs Technical Advisory Board and the Ayurvedic and Unani Drugs Technical Advisory Board to advise the Central and State Governments on technical matters arising out of the administration of this Act and to carry out the other functions assigned to it by this Act. It also provides for the establishment of two Drugs Consultative Committees, one for allopathic and the other for the Ayurvedic, Siddha, and Unani drugs to advise the various Governments and Boards on matters tending to secure uniformity throughout the country in the administration of the Act. There are two Schedules to the Drugs and Cosmetics Act and thirty Schedules to the Rules. However, keeping in view the limitations of this textbook and the orientations, only Schedule Y will be henceforth discussed. This schedule deals with the requirements and guidelines on the conduction of clinical trials.

1. Conduction of the Clinical Trials

(a) Nature of trials: The clinical trials required to be carried out in the country before a new drug is approved for marketing depend on the status of the drug in other countries. If the drug is already approved/marketed, Phase III trials are usually required otherwise trials are generally allowed to be initiated at one phase earlier to the phase of the trials of the other countries.

Phase I and III trials are necessary if the new drug substance is discovered in India but Phase I trials may be omitted if the new drug substance is discovered in other countries and the Phase I data is already available.

(b) Permission for trials: Permission to initiate clinical trials with a new drug may be obtained by applying in Form 12 for a test license (TL) to import or manufacture the drug. Such permission is given in stages. The application shall be accompanied by:

   (i) Data appropriate for various phases of clinical trials.
   (ii) Protocol for proposed trials.
   (iii) Case report forms to be used.
   (iv) Names of investigators and Institutions.

   Permission to carry out clinical trials with a new drug is issued along with a TL in Form II. For new drugs having potential for use in children, permission for clinical trials in the paediatric age group is normally given after Phase III trials in adults are completed. However, if the drug is of value primarily in a disease of children, early trials in the paediatric age group may be allowed.

(c) Responsibility of Sponsor/Investigator: Sponsors are required to submit to the licensing authority an annual status report on each clinical trial. In case a trial is terminated, reason for this should be stated. Any unusual, unexpected or serious adverse drug reaction (ADR) detected during a trial should be promptly communicated by the sponsor to the licensing authority and other investigators. In all trials an informal, written, voluntary consent must be obtained from each voluntee/patient in the prescribed Forms.

Data required to be submitted with the application for permission to market new drug

For filling the application for permission to market a new drug substance the data under the following heading is required:

(i) Clinical and Pharmaceutical Information
(ii) Animal Toxicology
   (a) Acute Toxicology
   (b) Long Term Toxicology
   (c) Reproduction Studies: Fertility Studies, Teratogenicity Studies, Prenatal Studies
   (d) Local Toxicology
   (e) Mutagenicity and Carcinogenicity

(iii) Animal Pharmacology
(iv) Human/Clinical Pharmacology (Phase I)
(v) Exploratory Trials (Phase II)
(vi) Confirmatory Trials (Phase III)
(vii) Special Studies e.g., bioavailability and dissolution studies, etc.

Phase I Trials

The objective is to determine the maximum tolerated dose in humans; pharmacodynamic effects; adverse effects, if any, with their nature and intensity; and pharmacokinetic behaviour of the drug as far as possible. These studies are carried out in healthy and adult males, using clinical, physiological and biochemical observations.

Phase II Trials

In Phase II trial, a limited number of patients are studied carefully to determine possible therapetic uses, effective dose range and further evaluation of safety and pharmacokinetics. Normally 10-12 patients should be studied at each dose level. These studies are usually limited to 3-4 centres and carried out by clinicians in the concerned therapeutic area and having adequate facilities to perform the necessary investigations for efficacy and safety.

Phase III Trials

The purpose of these trials is to obtain sufficient evidence about the efficacy and safety of the drug in a larger number of patients, generally in comparison with a standard drug and a placebo suspension as appropriate. If the drug is already approved/marketed in other countries, Phase III data should generally be obtained on at least 100 patients distributed over 3-4 centres primarily to confirm the efficacy and safety of the drug in Indian Patients when used as recommended in the product monograph for the claims made.

If the drug is a new drug substance discovered in India, and not marketed in any other country, Phase III data should be obtained on at least 500 patients distributed ove 10-15 centres. In addition, data on adverse drug reactions observed during clinical use of the drug should be collected in 1000-2000 patients. The selection of clinicians for such monitoring and supply of drug to them will need approval of the licensing authority. The reports of the complete clinical trials shall be submitted by the applicant duly signed by the investigator withing a stipulated period of time. It is important to state if any restrictions have been placed on the use of the drug in any other country e.g. dosage limits, exclusion of certain age groups, warnings about adverse drug reaction, etc.

Likewise if the drug has been withdrawn from any country, such information should also be furnished. Marketing information in the form of product monograph should comprise the full prescribing information necessary to enable a physician to use the drug properly. It should include description, actions, indications, dosage precautions, drug interactions, warning and adverse reactions.

Guidelines to Good Manufacturing Practices

Maintaining the quality of drugs is basically the responsibility of manufacturer and the Good Manufacturing Practices (GMP) guidelines are a means to assure this very quality. A draft of GMP regulations was prepared in 1975 which could be finalized and implemented in 1988, in the form of amended Schedule M. Schedule M is revised for dosage forms. The revised Schedule M also requires documentation at every stage of production, validation for processes and equipment; efficient Standard Operating Procedures (SOP) during different stages of manufacture and quality control operations; training of technical personnel involved in the manufacture and testing. There are different sections in the Schedule M of the Drugs and Cosmetics Act, 1940 and Rules, 1945. A list of these Schedules is mentioned henceforth. Some of the sections are discussed in different chapters of the textbook. The Government of India, Department of Health and Sciences could furnish further details. Part I of Schedule M deals with Good Manufacturing Practices relating to Factory premises and materials while Part II deals with the Plant and Equipment for manufacture of drugs.

Part I – Good Manufacturing Practices for Premises and Materials

1. General requirements
    - (i) Location and surroundings
    - (ii) Buildings and premises
    - (iii) Water system
    - (iv) Disposal of waste
2. Warehousing area
3. Production area
4. Ancillary areas
5. Quality control area
6. Personnel
7. Health, clothing and sanitation of workers
8. Manufacturing operations and controls
9. Sanitation in the manufacturing premises

10. Raw materials
11. Equipment
12. Documentation and records
13. Labels and other printed materials
14. Quality assurance
15. Self inspection and quality audit
16. Quality control system
17. Specifications
    1. For Raw materials and Packaging materials
    2. For Product Containers and Closures
    3. For in-process and bulk products
    4. For finished products
    5. For preparation of containers and closures
18. Master formula records
19. Packaging records
20. Batch packaging records
21. Batch process records
22. Standard operating procedures (sops) and records, regarding
    (i) Receipt of Materials
    (ii) Sampling
    (iii) Batch Numbering
    (iv) Testing
    (v) Records of analysis
23. Reference samples
24. Reprocessing and recoveries
25. Distribution records
26. Validation and process validation
27. Product recalls
28. Complaints and adverse reactions

29. Site master file
    - (i) General information
    - (ii) Personnel
    - (iii) Premises
    - (iv) Equipment
    - (v) Sanitation
    - (vi) Documentation
    - (vii) Production
    - (viii) Quality control
    - (ix) Loan licence manufacture and licensee
    - (x) Distribution, complaints and product recall
    - (xi) Self-inspection
    - (xii) Export of drugs

Part II-Requirements of Plant and Equipment

Part II of Schedule M recommends the requirements of plant and equipment for the manufacture of drugs under the following sections:

- (i) External preparations
- (ii) Oral liquid preparations
- (iii) Tablets
- (iv) Powders
- (v) Capsules
- (vi) Surgical Dressings
- (vii) Ophthalmic preparations
- (viii) Pessaries and Suppositories
- (ix) Inhalers and Vitrallae
- (x) Repacking of Drugs and Pharmaceuticals
- (xi) Parenteral preparations

For most of the sections an area of minimum 30 sq. meters has been recommended for the basic installation along with an ancilliary area of 10 sq.meters. For certain products like tablets, a minimum area of 60 sq. meters and for parenterals, a minimum area of 150 sq. meters has been recommended. Detailed requirement with respect to the machinery required for each section has been provided. Areas for formulations meant for external use and areas for formulations meant for internal use shall be separately provided to avoid mix-up even though they are from the same category of formulations. Separate equipment and manufacturing and packaging areas shall be provided for penicillin and non-penicillin products.

Prevention of Cruelty to Animals Act, 1960

The use of animals has been long in pharmaceutical field. Dogs, cats, rats, mice, and other species that are found very commonly are routinely used in the studies of the investigations with oral drug delivery industry. In this regard, the first animals to be used for such investigations are dogs. The reason for their use is their common availability on the whole of the globe. Especially ancient man living near the coastal areas thought that these species have developed their own instincts to survive in the disease conditions. With the modern therapy the initial testing was done by dissolving the drug in water and administer into the test animals. In this regard also dogs are very convenient. The new drug could be just dissolved in water or solubilized in solvents like DMSO or dispersed in food and then administered very conveniently into dogs. However, with the increased sophistication the research is needs to be expedited. On the other hand, dogs are not convenient to handle and currently with regulations in place, only a particular kind of species of dogs that may be very costly are to be used in such investigations. Subsequently, several other species were introduced in pharmaceutical investigations.

Use of animals in experiments for establishing the therapeutic efficacy and safety of drugs is generally unavoidable but causing them unnecessary pain or suffering is both unethical and inhuman. The Act of prevention of cruelty to animals act, 1960 laid specific rules to treat the animals used in the pharmaceutical industry for drug and formulation testing. This Act provides rules for preventing unnecessary pain and cruelty to animals. In the Act, Animals have been defined to include all species of animals (except man) as well as all species of birds. The term cruelty has not been precisely defined but it roughly means inflicting unnecessary pair or suffering to animals. The objective of this law is "The Prevention of Cruelty to Animals Act was enacted in 1960 to prevent the infliction of unnecessary pair or suffering on animals as well as to prevent cruelty to animals. The Act extends to the whole of India except the State of Jammu and Kashmir". The Act provides for the constitution of committee to look after the various aspects of experimentations on animals and to supervise and control their use for experimentation thereby saving them from any avoidable pain or injury.

This committee consists of the following members:

(i) Two members each of the Indian Council of Medical Research, Indian Council of Agricultural Research, and Council of Scientific and Industrial Research nominated by the Central Government.

(ii) Two members representing Universities granting medical and veterinary degrees nominated by the Central Government.

(iii) One member each of the Lok Sabha and the Rajya Sabha to be elected by the Houses, respectively.

(iv) Five persons actively involved in the promotion of animal welfare nominated by the Central Government.

The committee is required to take all proper measures to make sure that animals used for scientific experiments are not subjected to unnecessary pair or suffering before, during or after the experiments. The committee is authorized to make the rules which provide for the following matters:

(i) If the experiments are performed in an Institution, the head of the Institution shall be responsible for making sure compliance with the provisions of the Act and where the experiments are carried out by individuals, they shall be qualified and be responsible for avoidance for cruelty to the animals.

(ii) The experiments should as far as possible be performed while the animals are under the influence of an anaesthetic and if the animals are thereby injured during the course of experimentation that their recovery would involve serious suffering, they should be destroyed while still insensible.

(iii) Where small animals such as rats, frogs, rabbits, etc. could be used for an experiment, the use of large animals should be avoided.

(iv) If it is possible to substitute the use of animals by devices such as models, films, charts, books etc., such substitution should be made.

(v) Experiments on animals should not be performed just for the sake of acquiring manual skill.

(vi) Animals intended to be used for experiments should be properly looked after before and after the experiments and records of experiments performed should be maintained.

Intellectual Property Rights

Intellectual property is the property associated with the innovations specific to a particular location, region or a person. Thus, sometimes it is the property of a locality of people or group of people or a particular person. These intellectual properties could be again divided into patents, trademarks, copyrights and trade secrets. A **Patent** differentiates a society from the individual inventor. This could be a contract between the society as a whole and an individual inventor. This social contract gives the inventor the exclusive rights to prevent others from making, using, and selling a patented invention for a fixed period of time in return for the inventors disclosing the details of the invention of the public. Thus, patent systems do not allow the disclosure of information to the public by rewarding an inventor for his or her works. The use of patents have been tentatively discovered in middle ages in England and subsequently several countries adopted the concept of patents. Currently and during the course of the sojourn, several modifications and amendments were always in place as per the convenience and social needs. **Trademarks** and service marks are primarily intended to indicate the source of goods and services and to distinguish the trademarked goods and services from others. They also symbolized the quality of the goods or services with which they are used. A **Copyright** is an exclusive right to reproduce an original work of authorship fixed in any tangible medium of expression, to prepare derivatice works based upon the original work, and to perform or display the work in the case of musical, dramatic, choreographic, and sculptural works. A **Trade Secret** is information that is secret or not generally known in the relevant industry and that gives its owner an advantage over competitors. Most of these are very much relevant to oral pharmaceutical systems and are discussed very briefly in this section for the benefit of the reader of this textbook. Currently, intellectual properties for individual countries fall under each country's intellectual property laws. However, as a global way several organizations and laws like world trade organization, Trade Related Aspects of Intellectural Property Rights, Patents Law etc. are used in the discussions associated with the intellectual properties. Some of these issues as related are very briefly and comprehensively discussed henceforth.

India as a founder member of WTO is obliged to introduce TRIPs compliant (Trade Related Aspects of Intellectual Property Rights) IPR regime in January 2005. The Government has already passed the Patents (Second Amendment) Act and the Patents (Amendment) Bill 2003 has been placed before Parliament and it is referred to the Select Committee. There are several positive features in the Patents Act such as 20-year patent life, etc. However, some deficiencies like broadening the scope of Compulsory Licensing and lack of clarity on Data Exclusivity and Importation as a Working of Patent are worrisome factors. OPPI is working actively with the Government to correct these deficiencies and to ensure TRIPs compliant regime in India. Recently, two Exclusive Marketing Rights (EMRs) in pharmaceuticals have been granted by the Government, one for anti-cancer drug, GLIVEC (Imatinib Mesylate) of Novartis India and other for NADOXIN (Nadifloxacin), an antibiotic of Wockhardt Ltd.

Compulsory Licensing

While OPPI honours use of Compulsory Licensing for national emergencies, it has grave concern due to widening the scope of Compulsory Licensing provisions. While the health concerns of the Government are appreciated, raising the commercial threshold of Compulsory Licensing by giving sweeping CL provisions across the board is not justifiable.

Exclusive Marketing Rights (EMR)

The Patents (First) Amendment Act, 1999 provided mailbox applications and Exclusive Marketing Rights (EMR) in line with Articles 70.8 and 70.9 of TRIPs with retrospective effect from January 1, 1995. However, several EMR applications are pending for approval due to ambiguities in the law.

Bolar Provision

The Bolar exemption strikes a careful balance between promoting invention and ensuring that consumers have timely access to cheaper generics, after the expiry of the patent. OPPI wants Government to explicitly state that Bolar provisions shall be used only for R&D and not for manufacturing and stockpiling.

Data Exclusivity

The discovery, development and bringing to market a new drug requires the originator to conduct extensive chemical, pharmacological and clinical research and testing and generate data for submission to the Drug Regulatory Authority for marketing approval of the new drug. This activity takes 8 – 10 years of painstaking efforts. The data generated in such work is proprietary to the originator and needs to be protected. OPPI has requested the Government to amend the Schedule 'Y' of the Drugs & Cosmetics Act to include provision for Data Exclusivity for a period of 6 years from the date of marketing approval.

Misconceptions and Facts

Several myths have been propounded by the anti-Patent lobby. Most of these are based on conjecture and are unsupportable on facts. The two most frequently employed are "High Prices" and "Impact on Local Industry". Both of these are addressed below:

Myth of 'High Priced Medicines after Change in Patent Laws'

A myth is propagated that after introduction of Patent Act, in compliance with TRIPs provisions, the prices of medicines will accelerate and medicines will become unaffordable for people. This fear is due to a lack of understanding of how the transition to a Patent Regime works and how pharmaceutical prices are determined. Patents can never be awarded retrospectively. Patents can only apply to new discoveries. The transition provisions of TRIP's ensure that patents in India will only be granted for totally new discoveries, post 1st January 1995. Since patents of over 95% of the drugs available in India and on WHO List of Essential Drugs have expired, these drugs will continue t be available at current prices. Also, National Pharmaceutical Pricing Authority (NPPA) have a power to control the prices of Drugs if found excessive.

It should be noted that it takes anywhere between 10-15 years for a new drug to be granted registration by Drug Authorities of any country after which marketing permission is given. This registration period comes out of the overall patent life of the medicines, which is now almost universally 20 years from the date of application. A discoverer thus enjoys at best only 5-10 years of Exclusive Marketing for recovering the cost of research. The number of new drugs registered worldwide each year is between 25-35.

What this essentially means is

(a) Within the transition period (1995-2004) allowed for India, not more than a handful of new drugs will actually qualify for any form of exclusivity.

(b) Even after India commences granting patents, by the time patented products become a significant proportion of those already available locally; it will be another 10-15 years i.e. 2015-2020.

(c) It is not correct to believe that Multinational Corporations (MNCs) have only one price for a product every where in the world and as such the price charged in India will be exorbitant. There are several examples to show that even when the product is unique, it is introduced in India at a price significantly lower than in Western countries. Most international manufacturers will base their pricing strategy for countries, like India, on "affordability criteria".

There is empirical evidence (Study by the National Economic Research Associates –NERA, Washington – January 1998 and Study by Dr. Heinz Redwood entitled 'New Horizons in India' - 1994) to show that prices do not rise after IPR.

A study of prices in 6 therapeutic categories (anti-ulcerants, anti-depressants, calcium antagonists, non-narcotic analgesics, broad-spectrum penicillins and ACE inhibitors) in 9 countries: (South Korea, Mexico, Hungary, Taiwan, Brazil, Argentina, Egypt, Jordan and Turkey) demonstrates that strengthening IPR does not have a measurable impact on real or nominal prices of existing drugs.Globally, only 15 to 20 new drugs enter market every year and only a few of them are commercial successes. At the same time, each year patents expire for earlier products. On an average there will not be more than 15 to 20 patented products in any market. Newer products, being more effective, ultimately lead to lower per day cost of therapy to the patient. Beyond all these, in India drug prices are administered by Government.

Myth of 'Damage to Local Industry'

As has been stated earlier, the effective period of exclusivity enjoyed by a patent holder is, at best, 5-10 years. Once patent life ends, other manufacturers are free to market 'generic versions' of the same products. Worldwide, generic markets are growing at a rate faster than that of patented products. There will therefore always be a large generic market in India and this will continue to be dominated by Indian companies. In conclusion, India should adopt a strong world class patent law without further delay for the following reasons:

1. Development of Science and Technology

In the research world today, where collaboration and alliances are the order of the day, ability to network within the world community of scientists will be strengthened only if we have strong IPR.

2. Attracting Foreign Investments in Technology and Research

World class and TRIPs compliant law will bring to India the benefits of investments, funding of R&D and technological development. Funding of R&D is a major hurdle today. India can attract funds from abroad if it gives the right signals. Out of total Foreign Direct Investment (FDI) Approvals during the period August 1991 to December 1998, the Pharmaceutical Industry accounted for a meagre 0.44% of the total.

3. Reverse Brain Drain

IPR will provide challenging opportunities to retain scientific talent in India and attract our scientists and researchers from abroad back into the national mainstream.

4. Creation of Wealth

The wealth of nations is created by Intellectual Property. Recognition of IPR will change our scientific culture from 'copying' to 'creativity'. For all this to happen, India should have a Patent Law, which is clear and unambiguous and comparable to the best statutes available to IPR. A well-drafted legislation will minimize litigation and disputes.

Birth of Generics: The Hatch Waxman Act of 1984

US congress passed the Hatch Waxman Act in the year 1984 for the benefits of the consumers in an attempt to stop the dominance and monopoly of the innovator and to encourage the use of cheaper and equally effective drugs as the innovator. This has promoted the generic drugs and encouraged the generic manufacturers to bring cheaper versions of the brand name drugs without compromising the quality of the product.

The act which gave rise to the generic drug industry was passed as amendments of the Federal Food, Drug, and Cosmetic Act (FFD & C). The main objectives of the act were to:

1. **Offset the drug approval delay**: Early before the passage of this act, the innovators used to encounter a delay in approval of their New Drug Applications (NDA) for brand name product which eventually affected their brand entry in the market and financial losses.
2. **Bring healthy competition and to avoid price rise**: Early before its passage there was no scope of the generics to enter the market until the patent term of the innovator has expired as no provisions of challenging the validity of the innovator patent was there. Also there were not many benefits expected by the generic in investing capital to relaunch another version of already existing brand of the drug after its patent expiry. This product monopoly kept competition away and the drug prices high as per the innovators will.
3. **Make life easier for the generic**: Generic manufacturers used to face a lot of difficulties in doing all the pre-clinical and clinical studies as done by the brand name manufacturers to get their generic approved. The act was passed keeping one eye on the interests of both the brand name and the

generic drug manufacturers providing almost equal benefits to both. The benefits received by the brand name manufacturers are:

1. Regulatory delays in brand approval were deciphered.
2. The market exclusivity and the 'effective patent life' (the time left when the drug comes into the market after drug development and FDA approval) was extended from 8.5 years (1980) to 13 years (late 1980s) and now it's nearly 16-17 years.

The benefits received by the generic manufacturers are:

1. The generic could challenge the validity of the patent issued to the innovator,
2. The act provided with the stipulation to file an abbreviated new drug application (ANDA) and to leave out the expensive pre-clinical and clinical trials as done by the innovator and provided with the provision of relying on the safety and efficacy data of the innovator drug and to perform a much cheaper substitutable study called 'bioequivalence' to establish equivalence with the innovator.
3. As per the act, once approved the generic gets an exclusivity period of six months to rule the market along with the innovator during which no other generic can be given approval.

The FDA publishes the information on every approved drug product in the "Approved Drug Products with Therapeutic Equivalence Evaluations" which we also know by the name of "Orange Book". It lists the NDA's and ANDA's along with the expiry dates of patents and generic exclusivities. It is a ready reference of brand name drug products for the generic companies who usually use this information to identify the reference for developing their generic versions. The Orange book also contains certain therapeutic equivalence codes. An A- prefixing product is considered to be substitutable and B- prefixing is a safe and effective product for use but is regarded inequivalent and non-substitutable with the brand namedrug product

ANDA certifications

While filing an ANDA, the generic manufacturer is required to file one of the following four possible certifications on the subject of the reference brand name patent listed in the Orange Book.

1. **Para I certification**: There is no patent for the drug listed in the orange book
2. **Para II certification**: Patent is listed but has expired
3. **Para III certification**: Patent is listed, is valid but the generic wants approval to market the drug once the pertinent patent expires

4. **Para IV certification**: The generic manufacturer either challenges the validity of the brand name listed patent asserting it to be invalid or fake, or it affirms not to cross the fringe of the brand name patent claims.

   Para IV certification is the most critical of all and gives rise to almost all the anti-competitive practices associated with the Hatch Waxman amendments of the FFD and C act.

Approval process

Many of the points for the requirement for generic and brand name drug approval are the same. The generic must have the same active ingredient, same route of administration, same dosage form, with same strength and condition of use. Chemistry (components and composition), Manufacturing, and Controls (specifications and tests, packaging and stability) are rigorously reviewed by both the new drug reviewers and the generic drug reviewers. Labeling is also reviewed and has to be identical in most aspects (generic may delete portions of labeling protected by patent or exclusivity, bottle size need not be the same). The same FDA field inspectors inspect the manufacturing facilities for generics and for the innovator products. These facilities must be up to date with respect to good manufacturing practices or GMPs and must have documentation that they are able to manufacture the products for which they have applications. The differences in the applications, as previously stated, are the clinical studies and animal studies required for the new drug application and the bioavailability studies that have to be conducted to define the drug's interactions and adverse events. A surrogate for these studies is the bioequivalence study that has to be submitted for the ANDA. Showing in the bioequivalence study that the active ingredient is absorbed at the same rate and extent as the reference product allows the generic to rely on the findings of safety and efficacy of that product.

Pharmacopoeias

Pharmacopoeias are basically official compendias. Once a product reaches a market place and is very routinely used for treatment, then this product is evaluated at several stages as is the case for day-to-day commodity`s quality control. For a drug, all the dosage forms available for this particular drug, the assay methods, quality control specifications, are all compiled at one place as an easy reference to industries, drugs inspectors, quality control departments, drug regulatory authorities and pharmacies. These compendia are termed pharmacopoeia. The information related to each of the drug is termed a monograph. Several countries have their pharmacopoeia at this time. Some of the very important pharmacopoeias as relevant to Indian Pharmaceutical Industry are henceforth discussed here.

Indian Pharmacopoeia

The origin of Indian Pharmacopoeias goes back to the publication of the Bengal Pharmacopoeia and General Conspectus of Medicinal Plants 1844, generally known as the Bengal Pharmacopoeia. The pharmacopoeia was prepared by William Brooke O'Shaughnessy and published by order of the Government. Its main focus was on indigenous drugs though it included some products imported from Europe. The first Pharmacopoeia of India was published in 1868. It was prepared under the authority of the Secretary of State for India in Council by an Indian Pharmacopoeia Committee constituted in 1865. Edward John Waring edited this pharmacopoeia. The Pharmacopoeia contained the drugs official in the British Pharmacopoeia 1867 and also some selected indigenous drugs. Moodeen Sheriff prepared Supplement to the Pharmacopoeia of India 1868 that was published in 1869. Subsequently, several editions of pharmacopoeia were released and were in practice for over several years.

Three amendment lists were issued in respect of certain monographs included in the Indian Pharmacopoeia 1996. One meeting of the IP Committee was held to approve the amendment lists and to review the progress in publication of a Veterinary Supplement to the IP 1996 containing 55 monographs of veterinary biologicals and 113 monographs of non-biologicals that are under process. Although a Pharmacopoeia was in place for drugs in India, a permanent building and a permanent council are not in place yet. In this regard, there was a very recent convention and decision committee set up by Union Minister for Health, 2002. The proposal to set up a permanent Indian Pharmacopoeia Commission (IPC), cleared by the Union Minister for Health last year, will be operationalised by the year-end. Announcing this at the the Pharmaceutical Analysts Convention 2003 organised by the Indian Drug Manufacturers Association and European Pharmacopoeia Commission, Mr Nitya Anand, Chairman, IP Committee, said the IPC would be set up at Ghaziabad in Uttar Pradesh. While infrastructure details are being worked out, the IPC would use the state-of-the-art laboratory at Ghaziabad for developing standards. Currently, the committee is looking at building a more structured system wherein the Commission does not have to refer to (different) groups to get even small issues sorted out. The IPC will be more autonomous. While the decision to set up the Commission and related infrastructure was agreed in principle, now the decision to actually set it up has been taken.

British Pharmacopoeia

The BP is the authoritative collection of standards for United Kingdom medicinal substances and an essential reference point for everyone involved in their research, development and manufacture. Complete with formulated preparations and Veterinary substances, British Pharmacopoeia 2004 assures complete compliance within the United Kingdom and Europe. As of today, BP is supplied in three formats; a boxed five volume set for quick reference, a CD-ROM for quick and easy searches and a comprehensive, searchable website, updated daily and accessible anywhere in the world by the utility of passwords. In addition, all European Pharmacopoeia material up to and including Supplement 4.8 is integrated into the text of BP 2004.

United States Pharmacopoeia

According to the United States Pharmacopoeia committee, a United States Pharmacopoeia helps to make sure that consumers receive quality medicines by establishing state-of-the-art standards that pharmaceutical manufacturers must meet. As the world's most highly recognized and technologically advanced pharmacopeia, USP provides standards for more than 3,800 medicines, dietary supplements, and other health care products.

Definitions

Definitions to the words like drug, animal feed, etc. should be known to all the personal working in the oral drug industry. Some of these definitions are mentioned below.

Drug

According to the Drugs and Cosmetic Act, 1940, Ayurvedic, Sidda or Unani drugs includes all the medicines intended for internal or external use for or in the diagnosis, treatment, mitigation or prevention of disease or disorder in human beings or animal manufactured exclusively in accordance with the formulae described in the authoritative books of Ayurvedic, Sidda and Unani-Tibb system of medicines specified in the First Schedule.

Animal Feed

The term “animal feed” means an article which is intended for use for animals other than man and which is intended for use as a substantial source of nutrients in the diet of the animal, and is not limited to a mixture intended to be the sole ration of the animal.

Label and Labeling

The term “label” means a display of written, printed, or graphic manner upon the immediate container of any article; any a requirement made by or under authority of this Act that any word, statement, or other information appearing on the label shall not be considered to be complied with unless such word, statement, or other information also appear (s) on the outside container or wrapper, if any there be, of the retail package of such article, or is easily legible through the outside container or wrapper. The term "labeling" means all labels and other written, printed, or graphic matter upon any article or any of its containers or wrappers, or labels accompanying such article.

Recalls

A recall is a term used to withdraw a product from the market for either its inefficacy, partly efficacious, toxic effects with new drugs, toxic effects with certain batches of a drug after this has been already released into the market. As concerned with the terminal definition of withdrawl of a batch, the better term that is used is "stock recovery". Removal of a product that is still entirely under the direct control of the manufacturer, even though it may have been shipped interstate to one or more branch warehouses, also is not classified as a recall, provided no stock has been distributed to the trade. These removals are termed "stock recoveries" as mentioned before and do not appear on the public recall list. Usually, however, checks are made on the adequacy of these retrievals to cover ultimate disposition of the merchandise. The FDA classifies all recalls into one of three categories. Category I recall represents an emergency situation in which the drug poses a hazard that is immediate, long-range, and life-threatening. The second type of recall is Category II, a priority situation in which the consequences of the offending drug remaining on the market may be immediate, long-range, or potentiall life-threatening. The final recall classification is Category III. This is a routine situation in which the threat of life is remote or non-existent. Adulterated or misbranded products come under this category. Example. Labeling violations not involving a health hazard. Such recalls are required only to the wholesale level, and press releases are usually not issued.

New Drug Application (NDA)

A new drug application consists of details including the research, clinical results and the mathematics written in a very systematic manner to be sent to the concerned office for the approval of this drug and its formulations. This application generally includes

1. detailed reports of the preclinical (animal studies);
2. reports of all clinical (human) studies;
3. information on the composition and manufacture of the drug and on the controls and facilities used in its manufacture; and
4. samples of the drug and its labeling.

Abbreviated New Drug Applications (ANDA)

These are the short forms of the long forms of drug applications. These are very compiled by the pharmaceutical industries. In these situations, all the necessary information regarding the new drug application is not needed. Information submitted in an abbreviated NDA may be limited to a table of contents, label and labeling copy, a statement as to the prescription or OTC nature of the drug, and the components of the new drug. If the finding that the drug requires only an abbreviated new drug application also specifies that there must be included adequate data to asure the biological activity of the drug, and for preparations claiming sustained action, such data should show that the drug is available at a rate of release that will be safe and effective.

Conclusions

The laws and regulations governing the pharmaceutical industry are basically to protect the consuming public by attempting to provide drugs of consistent quality, purity, and efficacy. In this regard, several laws and amendments as related to and encompassing various aspects of the manufacture, clinical approval and marketing of oral pharmaceuticals are very routinely published. This chapter itself consists of information regarding the arena of the oral pharmaceutical industry. In addition, the final point at this juncture would be that several bodies and charters are involved in this area. Thus, judicious study of the laws, the practices and the associated amendments before any proper judgement regarding these poisonous chemicals to be drugs of human benefit is drawn, is very essential. This chapter definitely presents a very brief outlay of drug regulatory affairs in oral industry in India at this time.

Questions for Practice and Exercise

1. Briefly introduce oral drug regulatory departments and guidelines.
2. Write a note on forensic pharmacy.
3. What are the minimum requirements to handle drugs intended to be administered for therapeutic benefits?
4. Discuss the criteria for defining the hazardous drugs.
5. How could the list of the hazardous drugs help a person handling new drug substances?
6. Define a new drug.
7. Write a note on OSHA and its role in the new drug discovery process.
8. Elaborate the different functions of OSHA.

9. How is the safety to the human beings to hazardous drugs ensured? Explain in detail.
10. Write a note on NIOSH.
11. Write a note on the historical development of various oral drug industry regulatory authorities in A. USA, B. Europe, C. Japan, and D. India.
12. Write a note on
    1. the drugs and cosmetics act, 1940 and rules, 1945,
    2. conduction of clinical trials,
    3. guidelines to good manufacturing practices (GMP),
    4. prevention of cruelty to animals, and
    5. intellectual property rights.
13. Write a note on Pharmacoepia.
14. Mention about
    1. British Pharmacoepia,
    2. Indian Pharmacoepia and
    3. United States Pharmacoepia.
15. Define
    1. drug,
    2. animal feed,
    3. label and labeling,
    4. recalls,
    5. new drug application (NDA), and
    6. abbreviated new drug applications (ANDA).

Bibliography

1. Scheinberg, IH and Walshe, JM (eds). 1985 Orphan Diseases and Orphan Drugs. Manchester University Press, London.
2. Nunn, JF. (1996). Ancient Egypt Medicine. University of Oklahoma Press, Norman, Oklahoma.
3. Dispensing Pharmacy, RM. Mehta, Vallabh Prakashan Publishers.
4. History of Pharmacy in India, Harkishen Singh, Vallabh Prakashan Publishers. Vol-1. Pharmacopoeias and Formularies, Vol-2. Pharmaceutical Education, and Vol-3. Pharmacy Practice.

5. A Textbook of Forensic Pharmacy, NK Jain, Vallabh Prakashan Publishers.
6. Drug Store and Business Management, RM Mehta, Vallabh Prakashan Publishers.
7. Pharmaceutical Jurisprudence and Ethics (Forensic Pharmacy), Dr. S.P. Agarwal and Rajesh Khanna, Birla Publishers.
8. Question bank for pharmacy, gate and other competitive exams, Dr. D.R. Krishna, Jupiter Printers and Publishers.
9. New Drug Development: Regulatory Paradigms for Clinical Pharmacology and Biopharmaceutics (Drugs and the Pharmaceutical Sciences: a Series of Textbooks and Monographs), First Edition, Edited by Chandrahas G. Sahajwalla, Marcel Dekker Inc., 2004.
10. Sigerist, H. 1951. History of Medicine, vol. 1, Primitive and archaic medicine, Oxford University Press, New York.
11. Burger, A. (1990) Comprehensive Medicinal Chemistry, Pergamon Press, Oxford.
12. Griffin, JP (1995). Famous names in toxicology. Mithridates VI of Pontus, the first experimental toxicologist. Adverse Drug React. Toxicol. Rev. 14: 1-6.
13. History of the Pharmacopeia of the United States. In: United States Pharmacopeia, 23rd rev. Rockville, MD: United States Pharmacopeial Convention, Inc., 1995.
14. The United States Pharmacopeia, 23rd rev. Rockville, MD: United States Pharmacopeial Convention, Inc., 1995.
15. Mathiew M. New Drug Development: A Regulatory Overview. 3rd ed. Cambridge, MA: PAREXEL International Corporation, 1994.
16. Smith CG. The Process of New Drug Discovery and Development. Boca Raton, FL: CRC Press, 1992.
17. 60 FR 11263-11268. International conference on harmonization; guideline on the assessment of systemic exposure in toxicity studies, 1995.
18. Spilker B. Guide to Clinical Trials. New York: Raven Press, 1991.
19. Drug Safety Evaluation, First Edition, Authored by Shayne Cox Gad, Wiley-Interscience, 2002.
20. Safety Pharmacology in Pharmaceutical Development and Approval, First Edition, Authored by Shayne C. Gad, CRC Press, 2003.
21. 2004/2005 OSHA Handbook, First Edition, Authored by OSHA Inspectors, Pennsylvania Chamber of Business and Industry, 2004.

22. Introduction to Patent Law (Introduction to the Law), First Edition, Authored by Janice M. Mueller, Aspen Publishers, 2003.
23. 2005 Physicians' Desk Reference, 59th Edition, Authored by Medical Economics, Physicians; Thomson HeathCare, 2004.
24. Harrison's Principles of Internal Medicine 16th Edition – Authored by Dennis L. Kasper, et al., McGrawHill Professional, 2004.
25. Indian Pharmacopoeia 1996, Controller of Publications, 1996.
26. Japanese Pharmacopoeia 2002, by Japanese Pharmacopoeia Commistion, Stationery Office Books, 2002.
27. British Pharmacopoeia 2004 by British Pharmacopoeia Commission, Stationery Office Books, 2004.
28. US FDA Generic Approval Process, Ind J Pharm Edu and Res 43(3):232-240 (2009).

CHAPTER 11

ORAL FORMULATIONS

- **Introduction**
- **Conventional Formulations**
  - Liquids
  - Powders and Granules
  - Solids
  - Quality Control
- **Novel Drug Delivery Systems**
  - Solid Dosage Forms
  - Innovative Drug Delivery Systems
- **Trouble Shooting Oral Product Manufacture**
  - DLVO Theory
  - Powder Flow
  - Drug-Excipient Interaction
- **Stability Testing**
- **Pharmaceutical Plant Design**
- **Good Manufacturing Practices**
- **Concusions**
- **References**
- **Bibliography**

Introduction

From time immemorial oral route was commonly used in the administration of therapeutic agents. Both plant and inorganic drugs were routinely administered by oral route in the form of powders, solutions, suspensions, etc. However, with the discovery of benzene structure by Kekule, the era of synthetic chemistry began. Several new chemicals were synthesized or isolated from plant products as pure compounds. These compounds were more effective than the existing therapies. In the beginning, these were administered as powders, solutions, suspensions and pellets. With the advent of new technologies, tablets and capsules came into vogue. These dosage forms offered more advantages compared to already available modes of administration. The technology of tablets and capsules is currently in a very advanced stage. Several millions of tablets and capsules are manufactured in a short span of time. These dosage forms are capable of incorporating miniscule doses of very potent drugs.

Novel Drug Delivery Systems for oral route aids in site-specific release, sustained release and bioavailability enhancement of a drug. Delivery systems like liposomes, microspheres, nanospheres, prodrugs etc., incorporating molecules with low bioavailability, high potency or macromolecules are currently being investigated. Although conventional systems such as tablets, capsules, and liquids are in advanced stages, in some circumstances, they are not helpful. This is especially true with molecules such as peptides, proteins, antisense oligonucleotides and genes. Permeability of these molecules across gastrointestinal tract membranes, apart from high enzymatic degradation, is generally low. These molecules could be incorporated into particulate systems with high permeability through the biological membranes. The other situation is the enhancement of bioavailability. Sustained release tablets, suspensions, liquids to enhance the residence time thereby enhancing the bioavailability were developed. In addition, fancy systems such as gastric floatation systems, high-density systems, mucoadhesive systems, magnetic systems, unfoldable, extendable or swellable systems, superporous hydrogel systems have been researched to localize or increase the retention time of the drug in the gastro-intestinal tract. The other practical area is the development of prodrugs. Lately, it has been identified that several transporters exist for substrates like amino acids in gastro-intestinal tract membranes. Several classes of drugs or drug-amino acid conjugates or prodrugs could be developed that could use this target transporter to reach the systemic circulation at an enhanced rate, thereby enhancing the bioavailability of the therapeutic agent. This chapter deals with some of these oral systems.

Conventional Formulations

Liquids

The potent nature and low dosage of most of the very poorly soluble and low dose drugs obviates the need of conventional dosage forms in their original form. Thus, thorough investigations into these conventional dosage forms from a different angle would be needed. Different liquid dosage forms currently in the market include solutions, elixirs, emulsions, suspensions and syrups. All these formulations along with other fluid kind of formulations could be clubbed together to form conventional liquid dosage forms. In special cases like very poorly insoluble drugs, this very conventional dosage form clubs could be discarded and novel dosage forms for these kinds of molecules could be investigated. However, keeping in view the bottom line use of these dosage forms and their ease of manufacture, they are discussed in length with specific examples and that is because of the very important relevance here. In this regard, besides providing the mechanism for the safe and convenient delivery of accurate dosage, liquid dosage forms are needed for additional reasons that include:

(a) providing liquid preparations of substances that are either insoluble or unstable in the desired vehicle (e.g., suspensions)
(b) providing clear liquid dosage forms of substances (e.g., syrups, solutions)
(c) providing rate-controlled drug action (e.g. suspensions)

Solutions

In physico-chemical terms, solutions could be prepared from any combination of solid, liquid, and gas, the three states of matter. The very commonly used soda drink consists of carbondioxide in water. The very commonly used coconut water consists of several water-soluble components and ions. The very commonly used camphor water consists of camphor dissolved in water. In very old days these were very commonly used in the pharmacies for several reasons. However, the present context is in terms of the preparation of solutions for toxicological, preclinical and clinical and market formulations. When an NCE is first synthesized, the physico-chemical parameters that are investigated include pH solubility and stability and solubility in various solvents. If this NCE is water-soluble then a solution formulation is preceded for further toxicological evaluations. If the NCE is poorly soluble in water, cosolvents could be used to increase the solubility of poorly soluble compounds, resulting into a solution formulation. Cosolvents such as ethanol, propylene glycol, and glycerol are very commonly used. By different mechanisms these promote the solubility of NCEs. Sometimes, if it becomes imperative, 100% ethanol, propylene glycol, and glycerol are used as solvents for preparing toxicological and preclinical supplies.

Otherwise, a better alternate formulation is recommended and the process proceeded. Examples of marketed solutions include theophylline oral solution and ergocalciferol solution.

The other aspect in this regard is the salt formation. A drug possessing acidic or basic group when conjugated with the corresponding base or acid could be made into a solution dosage form. Once a compound is synthesized as a series of compounds and a decision has been made that these compounds are most likely to possess activity, manufacture of the activity testing, toxicological and preclinical supplies is the next step. Most of the toxicity supplies do generally use one of the highest possible doses. These solutions often times are toxic to the animal models. Desperate manufacture of formulations is the priority. A company does not want to loose a very promising and potential compound at this stage. If things went wrong here, the pharmaceutical company as well as human kind could have lost a very potential molecule to be used further. In this context if the compound is not water soluble or likely to possess some flawed properties like sticky nature etc. the best alternative a chemist precedes is to synthesize its water-soluble salts. These drug-salts are used to prepare the preclinical and toxicological supplies. If everything is fine, the same salt could be used to prepare clinical supplies and market formulation for this drug. Examples of such formulations include Nortriptylline HCl Oral solution, Fluoxetine HCl oral solution, Diphenoxylate HCl and Atrophine Sulfate Oral solution, Loperimide hydrochloride oral solution. In big pharmaceutical companies, the toxicological and preclinical supplies are needed everyday. That is the reason why salt screening is the best alternative at this stage. Currently, high through put screening is one of the best alternatives. During olden days, because it would require long and tedious process of preparing salts, the very common hydrochloride salt was used routinely. However, this salt cannot go into market most of the times with NCEs because of the likely toxic effects. In addition, the modern high-throughput screening is able to synthesize several salts of one NCE at one time, thus salt-screening currently is very actively and conveniently used in this stage of drug discovery. Although some times salt screening may not be helpful (when the compound does not has an acidic or basic group) it is always a very good beginning option and a learning exercise for a formulation scientist, in the development of solution formulations.

Suspensions

Suspensions are basically solid drugs dispersed and suspended in a liquid medium. There are several reasons for preparing suspensions. For one thing, certain drugs are chemically unstable when in solution but stable when suspended. For many patients, the liquid form is preferred over the solid form of the same drug because of the ease of swallowing and flexibility in the administration. Suspensions could be liquids or dry powders. Dry powder suspensions are powder mixtures containing the drug and suitable suspending and dispersing agents, which upon dilution and agitation with a specified quantify of vehicle (generally purified water) results in the formation of a suspension suitable for administration. Drugs that are unstable if maintained for extended periods of time in the presence of an aqueous vehicle (for example, many antibiotic drugs) are most frequently supplied as dry powder mixtures for reconstitution at the time of dispensing.

A pharmacist before manufacturing or supplying a suspension should know very well the characteristics of a continuous phase and the dispersed phase. Occassionally, the dispersed phase is in tandem with the continuous phase and on these occasions drugs are wetted in the continuous phase. However, in most of the situations, the dispersed phase is not easily wetted with the continuous phase. On these occasions wetting agents are generally used in the formulation of suspensions. Examples of wetting agents include alcohol, glycerin, and other hygroscopic liquids. They function by displacing the air in the crevices of the particles, dispersing the particles, and subsequently allowing the penetration of dispersion medium into the powder. Apart from the wetting agent, a suspension generally has a viscosity promoter and a suspending agent along with preservatives and other excipients. In a laboratory scale, a mortor or a homogenizer are used in the preparation of a suspension. The drug is first wetted if required. The dispersion media is prepared using suspending agents such as HPMC, tragacanth, acacia and methylcellulose. The drug is slowly added into the mortor containing the dispersion media and triturated to obtain a suspension. If a homogenizer is used, the entire content is added together and then the suspension is prepared by homogenization. However, larger mixers are used in large-scale manufacture. Some examples of mixers are presented later in this chapter.

Nanosuspensions: Special Case

Currently, large numbers of new drug candidates emerging from drug discovery programmes are water insoluble. These are therefore poorly bioavailable and resulting in abandoned development efforts. These compounds could be called "brick dust" candidates. The current focus is to rescue these candidates by formulating them into crystalline nanosuspensions. Apart from improving the solubility, these nanosuspensions improve the pharmacokinetic properties. Insolubility issues of the older compounds resulted in a model change in NCE investigations and thus offering novel solutions for innovative drugs of the current and the future. Nanosuspension formulation technology has evolved to meet the needs of drug screening programs that stress a perfect fit of current and future compounds into hydrophobic receptor pockets. Nanosuspension technology is ideally suited for drugs with a high crystal energy, which renders them insoluble in lipid as well as aqueous vehicles. The following advantages are offered by nanosuspension technology:

1. The solid state of the nanosuspension confers high weight per volume loading, which is ideal for depot delivery in which administration volume is constrained and high drug levels must be administered.
2. The reduced particle size entails high surface area, thereby increasing the dissolution rate to overcome solubility limited bioavailability.
3. Surfactants, utilizing electrostatic and steric stabilization mechanisms, coat the nanoparticles, thereby preventing their agglomeration and ensuring pharmaceutical stability.
4. Methods of manufacture involve crystallization, building nanocrystals up from the supersaturated solution state, as well as making larger particles smaller by homogenization or milling.
5. Pharmacokinetic profiles for injectables vary from rapidly soluble in the blood, to slowly dissolving, after which macrophage uptake and subsequent release greatly prolong drug delivery, while minimizing peak height. For several drug classes, this leads to improved safety, which permits higher dosing and improved efficacy.
6. Regional delivery confers increased efficacy to local target organs, while minimizing systemic toxicity, and has been demonstrated for the central nervous system, lungs and topically.
7. Numerous solubility-related issues in oral administration of drugs can be resolved, and include increased rate and extent of absorption, reduced variability of absorption, faster onset of action, higher peak drug level, improved dose proportionality and reduced fed/fasted effects.

Emulsions

Mankind knows emulsions for several centuries. Milk is a natural emulsion. It incorporates several water-soluble and oil soluble vitamins along with several other nutritional supplements. An emulsion is a heterogenous system consisting of oil droplets dispersed in an aqueous media and stabilized using a surfactant, or vice-versa. The best and the very oldest example of a therapeutic emulsion is garlic milk. British herbalist Grieve 16 suggested using garlic milk as dewormer. This is manufactured by boiling garlic bulbs mashed in cow or buffalo milk. Oil-soluble ingradients move into the lipid. Water-soluble ingradients move into the aqueous phase. The potency of garlic (Allium sativum) has been acknowledged for > 5000 years. It is used in India every day as a component of food from time immemorial. Garlic is helpful in several disease states. Garlic acquired a reputation in the folklore of many cultures over the centuries as a formidable prophylactic and therapeutic medicinal agent. Some of the diseases that garlic is useful do not have any proper current treatment in allopathic medicine. As such several labs around the world recently undertook several investigations on garlic. The chemistry of garlic is quite complex and likely developed as self-protective mechanisms and other insults. Several sulfur containing constituents such as allicin, typical volatile components such as diallyl sulfide (DAS), diallyl disulfide (DADS), and several water-soluble components such as S-allyl cysteine (SAC), sallylmercaptocysteine (SAMC) and aged garlic extract (AGE) exist in garlic. For oral delivery of such a kind of formulation that consist a mixture of components, as mentioned before, an emulsion is a best choice because during the processing and preparation of garlic milk the water soluble components reach water phase and the oil soluble components reach oil phase of the milk. This is one example. Similar is the principle of any drug containing emulsion. After an emulsion is prepared using any of the techniques, the water-soluble drugs reach the aqueous phase and the water insoluble drugs reach the lipid phase. Water-soluble drugs those are unstable in the intestinal tract such as peptides and hydrophobic drugs with low oral bioavailability such as class II drugs could be conveniently incorporated into an emulsion with added advantages.

Peptide drugs are currently in fashion in pharmaceutical research. However, the main problem with peptide drugs is their instability in the gastro-intestinal tract. A solution form of peptides further aggravates the situation. Alternate formulations to incorporate peptide drugs that include nanoparticles, microparticles and liposomes are complex in terms of theory and manufacture. The best and simple alternative in this situation is an emulsion. The peptides get incorporated into the aqueous phase of the emulsion. Once the liquid is administered by oral route, the emulsion gets dispersed. If it is an o/w emulsion, then the emulsion is stable in aqueous environment. Thus, the drugs remains in the aqueous phase and slowly gets dispersed to reach the intestinal mucosa where it reaches the systemic circulation after getting absorbed from the intestinal mucosa. The other advantage is that this formulation could also incorporate some water-soluble enzyme inhibitors in the aqueous phase that could further protect the peptide from degradation. The second situation may arise because of the dissolution problems associated with poorly soluble components. A suspension formulation is the general formulation that is adopted as the first step for oral delivery. However, in the case of poorly soluble drugs, which are limited by dissolution, the oral bioavailability is generally poor. On the other hand, when an emulsion is released into the lumen of the gut it disperses to form a fine emulsion. The drug remains as a solution in the gut, avoiding the dissolution step that frequently limits the rate of absorption of hydrophobic drugs from the crystalline state.

Emulsions are the most common forms of liquid oral dosage forms. These are prepared by shearing oil and water phase in the presence of an emulsifier as mentioned before. This shearing could be achieved using a mortor or a homogenizer kind of equipment. In smaller scales, a homogenizer is a very convenient method of preparing an emulsion. Shearing due to a homogenizer is higher compared to a mortar and pestle. Thus, a homogenizer forms a uniform emulsion at appropriate shear compared to a mortar-pestle technique. In any emulsion preparation, the main problem associated is creaming and cacking. Creaming occurs because of the separation of lipid phase together by coalescence of droplets into thick layer. Breaking occurs because of total loss of thermodynamic stability of individual oil and aqueous phase resulting in total physical separation of the individual phases. This generally occurs because of the inactivity of the surfactant at the interface. Use of high shearing equipment in both laboratory scale and large-scale manufacture helps in the development of a very elegant emulsion formulation.

Syrups

Syrups could be defined as solutions high in sucrose, but containing little or no alcohol (ethanol). Thus, syrup formulations consist of drugs incorporated into viscous sugar based liquid solution. Advantages of syrups include:

1. flavoured (helps compliance);
2. viscous (good for retention);
3. prevent breakdown (stabilize).

Syrups were very common formulations in earlier days when the drugs were not in large number. It is very convenient to formulate syrups. It promotes the viscosity to the formulation, some times as such increases the solubility of drugs, and helps in taste masking. Different cosolvent systems could be incorporated to enhance the solubility of a poorly soluble compound. Syrup based formulations existed in several ancient medicines. However, with the increase in the number of NCEs available particularly poorly water-soluble NCEs and the availability of other dosage form with advances in suspension, tablet, capsule, nanoparticle, macroparticle technologies, the prominence of syrups decreased. However, in special conditions like padeatric or geriatric formulations, syrups are the first choice. These dosage forms are particulary helpful for the formulation of bitter or highly potent drugs. Taste masking is obviously important with bitter drugs, especially for kids and with hightly potent drugs, dose adjustment is an important criterion. Dose adjustment and swallowing is very easy with a syrup formulation. Several drugs have been incorporated into syrups. Examples include acetaminophen, erythromycin, clarithromycin and azithromycin. It is also likely that when these drug substances are incorporated into water, their bitterness may further increase. The best suitable formulation in these situations is a syrup formulation. Currently, the trend is towards the development of sustained release syrup formulations. Unfortunately or fortunately, as such only a few drugs have been investigated for such a kind of formulations. Published and in-house data suggests that low permeability excipients such as sorbitol (or mannitol), in amounts used in typical syrup formulations, can significantly reduce bioavailability of drugs that also exhibit low intestinal permeability. In these situations, artificial sweeteners help in the formulation development. Examples of commercially available syrups include Ampicillin Dry Syrup, Amoxycillin Dry Syrup, Antacid Syrup, B Complex Syrup, Chloramphenicol palmitate syrup, Meperidine HCl syrup, Dicyclomine HCl syrup, Oxybutynin Chloride syrup, Chlorpromazine syrup, Dimenhydrinate syrup, Prochlorperazine Edisylate syrup, Promethazine HCl syrup, Sodium valproate syrup, Chlorpheneramine Maleate syrup, Cyproheptadine HCl syrup, Hydroxyzine HCl syrup, Lithium citrate syrup, Amantadine syrup, Albuterol sulfate syrup, metaproterenol sulfate syrup, lactulose syrup, Pyridostigmine Bromide Syrup, Pseudoephedrine Hydrochloride Syrup, Ipecac Syrup, Guaifenesin Syrup, Metoclopramide Syrup, Aminocaproic Acid Syrup, and Cloxacillin syrup.

Syrups are most frequently prepared by one of four general methods, depending on the physical and chemical characteristis of the ingradients. These methods are

1. solution of the ingradients with the aid of heat,
2. solution of the ingradients by agitation without the use of heat, or the simple admixture of liquid components,
3. addition of sucrose to a prepared medicated liquid or to a flovored liquid, and
4. by percolation of either the source of the medicating substance or of the sucrose. However, for the official syrups there is no officially designated method for preparation. These methods are described here briefly.

Heating method is used when the ingradients in syrup are stable to the heat. These ingradients could be either stable drugs or drugs that are non-volatile. In this method sugar is generally added to the purified water, and heat is applied until solution is affected. Other heat stable compounds are added to the hot syrup, the mixture allowed cooling, and its volume adjusted to the proper level by the addition of purified water. As syrup is decomposed by heat, they cannot be sterilized by autoclaving. On the other hand, boiled water is generally used in the preparation followed by the addition of preservatives. The addition of preservatives offers microbial stability to syrup and increases the shelf-life. In any case, heat labile drugs are not incorporated into syrups using this method.

Inversion of sugar is major problem associated with normal syrups prepared by the method of heating and dissolving. This may result in eventual crystallization of the sugar in the preparation upon storage, which is not desirable. This may also impart bitterness beating the need for a syrup dosage form for bitter drugs. The other situation is where the drugs are not stable to the heat. In these situations, sucrose and other formulating agents may be dissolved in purified water by placing the ingredients in a vessel of greater capacity than the volume of syrup to be prepared, thus permiting thorough agitation of the mixtures. This technique could be called as **"Solution by Agitation without the aid of heat"**. This process is more time-consuming than that utilizing the aid of heat. In addition, sugar doesnot crystallize on the wall of the container permitting proper dosing and offering required viscosity to the preparation. This is a very common observation in the preparation of syrups using this method. When water-soluble ingradients are added to thick syrup, they do not easily mix and form uniform syrup immediately. Such kinds of situations take long time before a formulation of a drug using this trick is employed in the syrup manufacture.

The third technique of preparing syrup involves the "**addition of sucrose syrup to a medicated liquid or to a flavored liquid**". In plant or animal products occasionally the drug substance is contained in a liquid mixture. This could be called medicated liquid or a flavored liquid. In these situations, the placebo syrup is manufactured. Eventually, this syrup is added to medicated liquid or a flavored liquid and mixed to form a dosage form. Such formulations were common places in an apothecary or a pharmacy shop in ancient times. The source of the drug or the medicine is obtained separately before the final formulation is taken care. Controlled situation is needed for these kinds of preparations. Again crystallization to the walls would be a major issue. As long as the crystallization is considered and avoided the method is very fine. The present generation of very poorly soluble drugs could be conveniently incorporated into syrup forms using these dosage forms. Currently, these would be helpful for long-term preformulation and clinical testing of syrup dosage forms of new chemical entities. The other advantage would be to solubilize a drug into a cosolvent system and then add this to the syrup formulation. As an example, a leading pharmaceutical company in India (Ranbaxy Research Laboratories, Gurgaon, Haryana, India) is in the process of developing a dosage form for oral and IV pharmacokinetic studies in the preformulation stages. This molecule is a water insoluble analog of an already existing salt form of a drug. This new molecule was dissolved in DMSO and its activity tested in cell culture and animal models. The molecule demonstrated equal potency as that of the original proven molecule. That was the reason of pursuing this molecule for further studies. Interestingly this NCE could be used to treat anti-inflammatory diseases in young children. The next step would be to test the molecule in padieatric conditions. Since it is water insoluble, for investigating its pharmacokinetics, the best approach for both oral and IV studies is using cosolvent systems. After several trials, the drug was solubilized in a mixture of water: PEG 300: tween 80 and ethanol. Several trials were needed because of its poor solubility in water. It was highly soluble in ethanol. However, there is a limitation of the amount of ethanol in an oral dosage form. Exceeding more than 10% ethanol in a formulation resulted in dizziness in rats. Thus, it is necessary to avoid such high levels of ethanol. After adding very little amounts of tween 80 in the formulation it was found that the drug was solubilized in this cosolvent system. This cosolvent mixture could be conveniently incorporated into syrup to form a padietric formulation.

The fourth method could be conveniently called "**Percolation of either the source of the medicating substance or of the sucrose**". This is very similar to the third method. However, generally in limited amounts and preparations such as Ipecac syrup are manufactured using this technique. In the percolation method, either sucrose may be percolated to prepare the syrup, or the source of the medicinal components may be percolated to form an extract to which sucrose or syrup may be added. The second method definitely has two different steps, one, the preparation of the extraction of the drug and then the preparation of the syrup. This is like the preparation of vegetable pickles. Two parts,

1. one of the vegetables and
2. the second of the oils. Both components are mixed and allowed several days before the ripening of the pickle. The extract is like vegetables and the syrup is like the second oily portion. The osmotic pressure imparted by the oil prevents microbial growth in a pickle. Similar is the principle in preservative-free syrups as mentioned henceforth.

Generally, a 60% to 80% of sucrose is incorporated into syrups at the end of the manufacture. However, sucrose is a very good medium for the growth of microorganisms. The aqueous sugar medium of dilute sucrose solutions is an efficient nutrient medium for the growth of microorganisms. On the other hand, concentrated sugar solutions are resistant to microbial growth due to the unavailability of water to support microbial growth. Syrup has a specific gravity of about 1.313, which means that each 100 ml of syrup weighs 131.3 g. Because 85 g of sucrose are present, the difference between 85 g and 131.1 g or 46.3 g or ml of purified water are used to dissolve the 85 g of sucrose. The solubility of sucrose in water is 1 g in 0.5 ml of water; therefore, to dissolve 85 g of sucrose, about 42.5 ml of water would be required. Thus, only a very slight excess of water (about 3.8 ml per 100 ml of syrup) is employed in the preparation of syrup. Although not enough to be particularly amenable to the growth of microorganisms, the slight excess of water permits the syrup to remain physically stable under conditions of varying temperatures. If the syrup were completely saturated with sucrose, under cool storage conditions some sucrose might crystallize from solution and, by acting as nuclei, initiate a type of chain reaction that would result in the separation of an amount of sucrose disproportionate to its solubility at the storage temperature. The syrup would then be very much unsaturated and probably suitable for microbial growth. As formulated this way, the official syrup is both stable and resistant to crystallization as well as to microbial growth. This is similar to the preparation of a pickle. This method does avoid the use of a preservative in a syrup formulation. By proper use of sugar amounts the perculation method could be conveniently used in the preparation of preservative-free syrups. The other methods could also be conveniently used in such final formulation results.

Manufacture of Liquid Orals

Since liquid orals are one of the very early dosage forms attempted or developed in the arena of allopathy medicines, their manufacture has become common places. The concepts of manufacture of these dosage forms (especially solutions) either for age-old drugs, recent (10 to 20 year old) drugs or very new chemical drug substances (very young or in the investigational arenas) are the same. Since these dosage forms (solution dosage forms) are very docile a practically intelligent formulator would first attempt to develop this liquid oral however complex this molecule is. For recent drugs however tough they are the market requirements some times aim for liquid orals in the solution form for improved properties. It is better to work on these because the pharmacologist, the formulation, the clinical scientist and the marketing personal are very well aware of the therapeutic end points with these molecules then spending a lot of time on new drug substances. For new drug substances with very tough properties, suspension, emulsion or nanoparticle formulation would be better ideas. Although all these formulations come under liquid orals as manufacture is concerned solution dosage forms are preferable. Not always very docile molecules come into the hands of a formulation. The manufacture of these dosage forms as principle wise or practice wise is well investigated and studied and practised.

Laboratory Scale

The processing and preparation of liquid orals in the laboratory scale could be discussed as a whole in one section. The physics and chemistry of the manufacture of these liquid dosage forms is almost the same. That is the reason it is convenient to discuss these formulations clubbed together. Liquid orals are prepared in the laboratory using mortor pestle, sonicator, lab-scale homogenizer, grinder, vortex, ultrasonicator, emulsifier, centrifuge and mixer techniques. In a small-scale manufacture of liquids, large-scale used equipment such as big homogenizer, grinders, and ultrasonicators are generally not used because of several disadvantages. The main reason is improper mixing. Due to the laminar flow regime in a small-scale, mixing becomes difficult if not impossible. That is one main reason why a mortor and pestle are the best to manufacture an emulsion or a suspension in a laboratory scale. Recent innovations in this area suggest new principles in mixing for small-scale manufacture of liquids. A novel microdevice for passively mixing liquid samples based on surface tension and a geometrical mixing chamber was recently developed. In another investigation, a micromixer recently developed used a constantly changing time dependent flow pattern inside a two sample liquid plug is created as the plug simply passes through the planar mixer chamber. This device requires no actuation during mixing and is fabricated using a single etching process. The effective mixing of two coloured liquid samples is demonstrated with very positive results. Several other physical forms of micromixers are currently being developed. A different group analysed mixing in an active chaotic advection micromixer. The micromixer consists of a main rectangular channel and three cross-stream secondary channels that provide ability for time-dependent actuation of the flow stream in the direction orthogonal to the main stream. Three-dimensional motion in the mixer was investigated. Numerical simulations and modelling of the flow were studied. It was shown that for some values of parameters a simple model could be derived that clearly represented the natural of the flow. Particle image velocimetry measurements of the flow are compared with numerical simulations and analytical models. A measure for mixing and the mixing variance coefficient (MVC) were determined. Mixing was substantially improved with multiple side channels with oscillatory flows, whose frequencies increased downstream. The optimization of MVC results for single side-channel mixing indicated the dependence of MVC on frequency was not monotone. There was a local minimum. Residence time distributions derived from the analytical model demonstrated Lagrangian velocity profile flattened over the steady flow. Taylor-dispersion effects were still present for the micromixer configuration in this current study. These new set-ups are currently investigated for laboratory scale manufacture of suspensions.

Large-Scale

Oral liquid pharmaceuticals encountered in a pilot plant or a manufacturing set up is either solutions, suspensions, or emulsions. All other liquid dosage forms could be conveniently grouped into the three above groups. Once an NCE reaches the formulation division from a chemistry group, the first thing is to select a suitable oral formulation. Generally, in a preclinical set up the formulation first selected is a liquid. Formulation laboratory after several permutations and combinations develop a suitable liquid formulation for preclinical studies. If it is decided by the project team that this would be a market feasible formulation, then its scale-up will be considered. Scale-up of these dosage forms presents a different set of processing concerns that must be considered. Although a formulation is optimized and validated in laboratory scale, it is not that easy to take this formulation to large-scale manufacture. For instance, a molecule that is formulated as a suspension in the lab-scale using either a mortor-pestle technique or a homogenizer technique may elicit very good physical and chemical stability properties in the lab, however the preparation process may be very difficult in manufacturing scale. There may be crystallization issues similar to those found in the syrups at the end of manufacture or there may be clogging, lump formation etc in large-scale manufacture which may not be observed in small laboratory scale manufacture. These issues are to be very carefully considered during the large-scale manufacture. It is not that these issues are not observed in small-scale manufacture. However, in such manufacture they are not observed and these problems are manifested in large-scale manufacture. In addition, mixing is the chemical process that is used in the small-scale or large-scale manufacture of these liquid formulations. If the mixing is inappropriate, there is always a chance of phase separation. That is the reason why validation is essential for the manufacture of these kinds of formulations right from the beginning. Since the processes and manufacturing involved with all the liquid formulations is the same, their method of manufacturing is simply and carefully described together in this section.

Equipment such as vertical screws, V-blender, single planetary mixer, plough shear, planetary mixer, kneader mixer, battery mixer, double cone mixer and double planetary mixer are the very common equipment used in the manufacture of liquid dosage forms. The pictures of some of the equipment used are presented. When an emulsion is prepared in a small-scale this problem may not be elicited. However, on large-scale manufacture this is definitely a big issue. In these preparation methods, lot of care has to be taken. Most of the times during such a manufacture, large volume mixing tanks are used to form the emulsion through the action of a highspeed impeller. As desired, the product may be rendered finer by passage through a colloidal mill, in which the particles are sheared between the small gap separating a high-speed rotor and the stator, or by passage through a large homogenizer, in which the liquid is forced under great pressure through a small valve opening. Industrial homogenizers have the capacity to handle as much as 100,000 liters of product. This is the maximum volume limit for industrial homogenizers that are applied in the manufacture of the groups of liquid oral dosage forms, amenably. This is very commonly used equipment for manufacture of liquid orals. The manufacture of emulsions is an illustration of the manufacture of a liquid oral. The principle is the same for the manufacture of any liquid oral, whether it is a suspension, syrup, an emulsion, or a solution. Few of the common priniciples and the very recent investigations that are involved in the manufacture of these liquid orals in small and large-scale manufacture is mentioned henceforth.

Simple solutions are the most straight forward to scale-up. Generally, tanks are used in such dosage form preparations. Size and suitable mixing capability is the key in the manufacture. Many equipment possess heating/cooling capabilities to effect rapid dissolution of components of the system. Adequate transfer systems and filtration equipment are required, but they must be monitored to assure that they can clarify the product without selectively removing active or adjuvant ingredients. Liquid pharmaceutical processing tanks, kettles, pipes, mills, filter housing are frequently made out of hard ware. This makes things complicated because of the corrosive actions that are to be taken into continous monitoring. The larger the size of the tank the greater would be the need for maintenance. The other way of reducing such a reaction is to use glass or Teflon coating on the surface of the tanks. Cracking, breaking, flaking and peeling would be the common problems associated with these kind of tanks. In the scale-up of a suspension and an emulsion, more parameters and phenomenon are to be kept in the mind. In a laboratory scale, the addition of the suspending agent and the dispersion should be kept in mind and should be added very carefully. The type of mixers, pumps, and mills, and the horsepower of the motors, should be carefully selected based on the scale-up performance. The equipment is selected according to the size of the batch and the maximum viscosity of the product during the manufacture process. Once scale-up is achieved, the manufacturing would be a key issue. The reproducibility of the process is a very important. Batch-to-Batch variations have to be carefully kept in control. Any deviations would be a disaster to the entire batch. Thus, validation of the manufacture process is a main issue. Several factors have to be kept in the mind for such considerations.

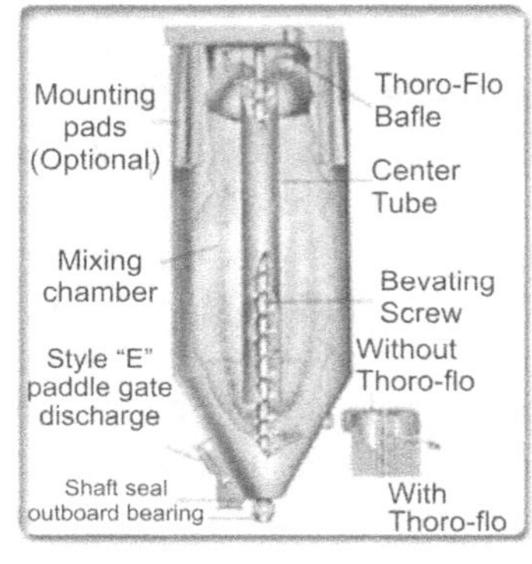

Vertical Screws

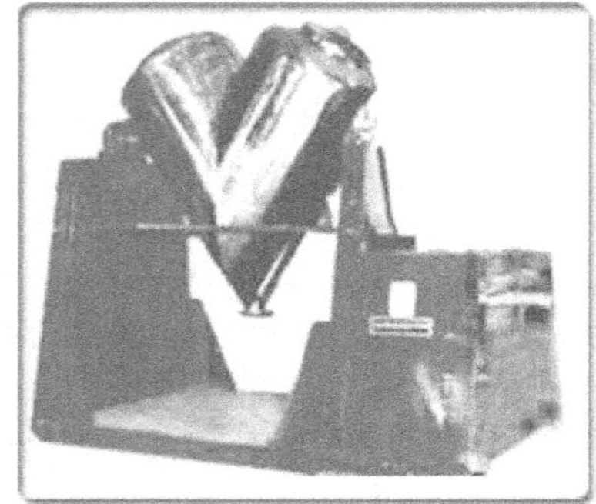

V-Blender

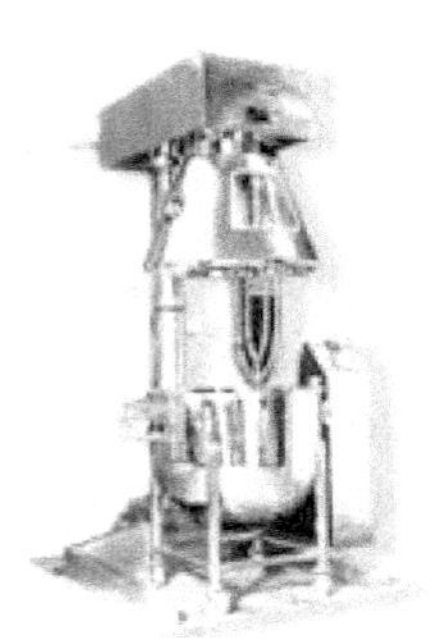

Single Planetary Mixer

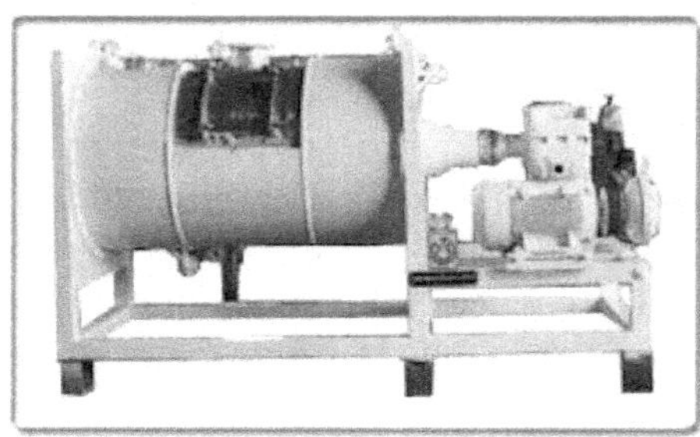

Plough Shear

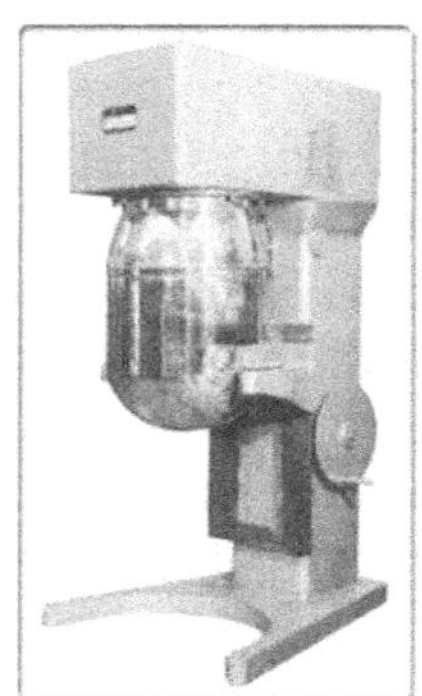

Planetary Mixer

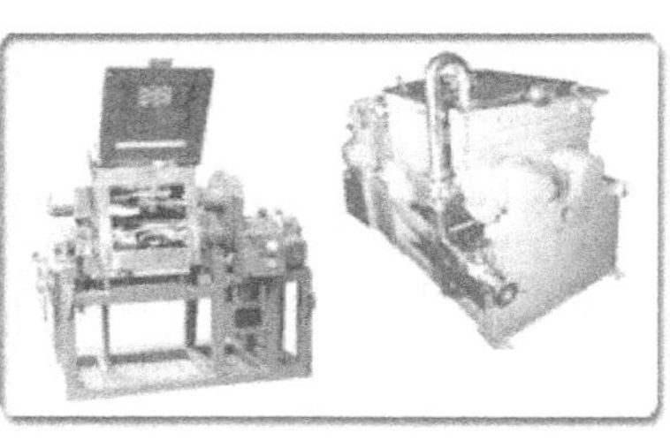

Kneader Mixer

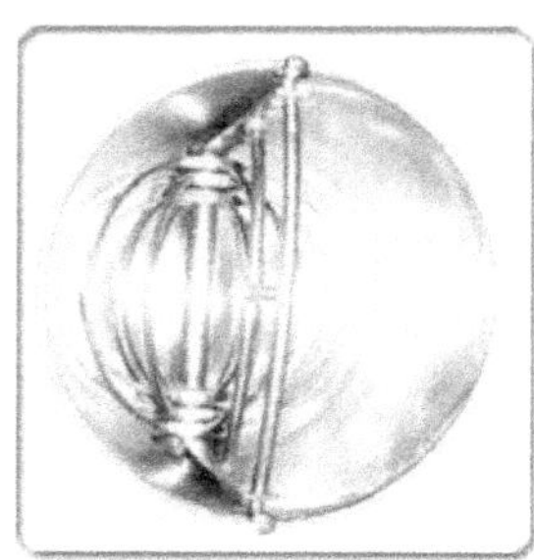

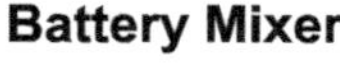

Battery Mixer

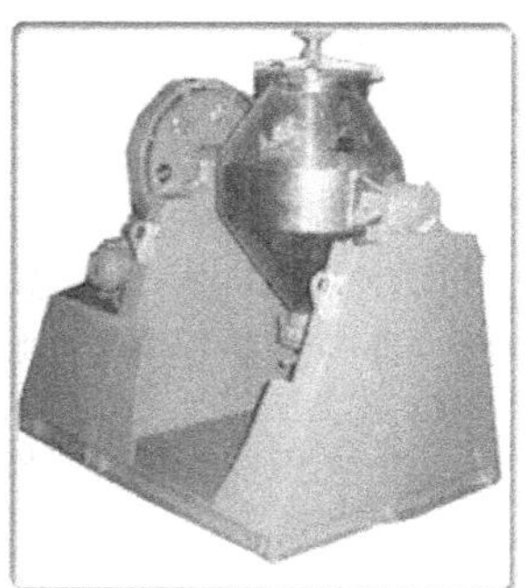

Double Cone Mixer

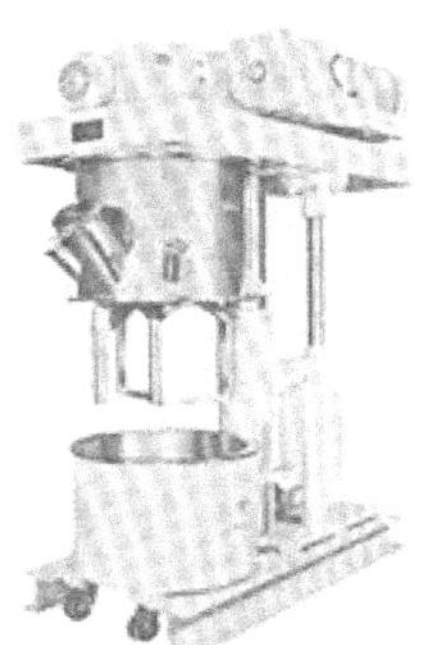

Double Planetary Mixer

Powders and Granules

As of today these are the very interesting and age-old dosage forms as solids are concerned. With the advancement of tablets these dosage forms prominence diminished although some times very commonly used. However, these dosage forms could be used to develop formulations very quickly for very early new drug substances for very new drug investigations. These are definitely respectable dosage forms for the new drug substances for the new drug investigations.

Overview

In very ancient times, powders were very common places in the apothecaries for oral administration of medicines. Drugs were mixed with orally compatible solid substances, mixed thoroughly and then given orally. However, as the time passed by it was realized that the dose with the powders is not properly delivered. In these situations, if a very potent drug is incorporated into a powder, it would have been further deliterious. Powder dosage form delivery was thus an art. A skillful pharmacist would be required for proper delivery of powder dosage form to a patient. However, the technology has slowly transformed.

A common statement that could have appeared in the literature before the sophistication of capsule and tablet dosage form would clearly emphasize the transition between a powder dosage form to a solid dosage form as relevant to market formulation and the then current scenerio would be as follow. Customer demand should focus in varying proportions on the mixture quality and the market appeal of the final product form. Patients are no longer passive; increasingly, manufacturers are required to present the product in forms that are well accepted by patients. The customer-led development of powder inhalants and skin penetrants suggests that the slow succession of dosage forms from 'shake the bottle' prescriptions through to rolled pills, capsules and the all- dominating tablet might not yet be finished and might even gather further momentum in the future. The market for powder-based products is large and is growing. Products such as foodstuffs, cosmetics, ceramics, detergents, powdered metals, plastics and abrasives share many of the processing challenges faced by the pharmaceutical industry and can frequently provide alternative process outcomes. From that stage, currently very few medicated powder formulations are available in the market. Over recent decades, all these other industries have undergone a rapid transition from a processing art to a processing science. The art of manufacturing requires the acquisition of manufacturing skills based on experience generated over a long period of time and requires a stable, consistent market for its products. Intense competition in these industries has led to the manufacturing process becoming customer-led rather than technology-led and has instigated the requirement that the process should be flexible to meet changing customer demands.

Now it is the age of tablets and capsules and other oral sustained release dosage forms. Although currently, the powdered dosage forms are not in vogue, definitely they are used in the manufacture of other dosage forms like granules, capsules and tablets. However, since these dosage forms mainly consist of powder and mixing is a physical process in the preparation of powders, definitely a brief description of powders is very essential. Alongside, the most common modification of powders is granules. Rather than a powder directly incorporated into a capsule or a tablet, the powders are blended into granules. Granules enhance the fluidity of the powder form and regulate the delivery of appropriate amounts of drugs, thereby enhancing the homogeneity of these dosage forms. Sometimes granules are also administered orally. In this context, some theory would be good for the description of physical nature involved in powders, granules, capsules and tablets.

Manufacturing

Mixing is a central operation associated with powder and granule manufacture. This process has to be customer sensitive. A generic mixer selection can be made based on an information input of the mixture formulation, the product quality requirements and the process limitations imposed by the nature of the product. The procedure will highlight any selection compromises that are needed to resolve conflicting requirements from the three data inputs.

Mixing as a Unit Chemical Engineering Process

Although the weight proportions of a formulation are usually fixed, there is considerable freedom at the formulation stage to vary the morphology of the ingredients and hence their flow characteristics. For mixing to occur, individual particles must be given the opportunity to relocate themselves repeatedly within the bulk of the mixture. To generate such movement the particles can be tumbled, kneaded, fluidized, sheared, scooped or impacted within a mixer with a variable level and type of energy input. Whatever the imposed mixing mechanism, the ability of individual particles to move independently within the bulk powder is evidently an important characteristic and leads to a broad division of powder-mixing processes into 'free-flowing' and 'cohesive' (non-free-flowing) mixtures. The free-flowing powder moves smoothly with well-defined planes of movements whereas the cohesive powder exhibits 'stick-slip' motion with irregular surface characteristics. Particle size is probably the dominant influence on the type of flow regime. The gravitational force associated with a large particle is much larger than any restraining interparticulate force with the result that individual particles retain their freedom of movement. As the particle size decreases, various interparticulate forces can potentially dominate and the particles attempt to retain a structured arrangement. The actual transition size will be a function of the nature of the interparticulate forces and other particle characteristics, but in general terms it can be stated that particles of nominal diameter greater than 50 μm tend to be free-flowing whereas particles of nominal diameter less than 50 μm tend to be cohesive.

From both marketing and processing perspective, free-flowing powders have many desirable features, but the disadvantage of these mixtures is that they can be subjected to segregation or 'unmixing' on a severe scale. The same freedom that allows a particle to move smoothly and independently of its neighbours enables it to preferentially move in a particular direction. Even if a mass of free-flowing powder is 'satisfactorily' mixed, great care has to be taken in subsequently handling the mixture. Storage and handling processes can destroy the mixture quality that has been so carefully created and only when the mixture has been 'frozen' at its final point of usage can the mixture be regarded as safe.

For the free-flowing mixture, the art of the process engineer is often to restrict the freedom of movement of individual particles; however, for the cohesive mixture the problem is reversed. The cohesive system has a natural structure that must be repeatedly broken down in order to give individual particles within that structure an opportunity to relocate themselves. Problems of mixture quality can arise in processes that demand a finely textured product. It is commonly found that although the scale of segregation of cohesive mixtures is small, the intensity of segregation can be high. This is caused by small agglomerates of individual mixture ingredients retaining their structure throughout the mixing process. The strength of these agglomerates and the ability of different mixers to break them down to the scale of the individual particle is a central study of cohesive mixtures.

A subject of considerable industrial interest is the achievement of an ordered structural arrangement of particles, which could improve the typically limiting random particle arrangement. If the shape and surface characteristics of the constituent particles can be manipulated so that the particles prefer to adhere to a dissimilar particle, an orderliness is introduced into the mixture that gives a better mixture quality than that for random mixing. Particularly attractive is the so-called 'coating process' wherein fine minor component mixture constituents adhere preferentially onto a relatively coarse carrier particle. Such a mixture carries the double advantage of having free-flow characteristics for handling whereas still retaining a high mixture quality.

A poor mixture will have a large scale of segregation and a high intensity of segregation whereas a good mixture will have a small scale of segregation and a low intensity of segregation. Mixtures with identical scales of segregation will differ in quality if the amount of dilution of the segregated patches is different, as will mixtures of constant dilution but varying scale of segregation. The role of a mixer is to reduce the scale of segregation and to lower the intensity of segregation. Although these two definitions are helpful in describing the role of the mixer, they give no indication of the 'end point' in the mixing process. To what extent should the scale and intensity of segregation be reduced within the mixer? What is the end point of the mixing operation for a particular process?

As the scale and intensity of segregation are reduced, the mixture passes through a critical mixing state during which it changes from an 'unsatisfactory' to a 'satisfactory' mixture for a particular process. The identification of this critical quality or scale of scrutiny is perhaps the most important step in the performance analysis of a mixture. Any mixture will be unsatisfactory if scrutinized closely enough because the scale of scrutiny will then approach the scale of individual elements. Thus, in the case of the dispersion of a pigment in plastic, the **scale of scrutiny** on the plastic surface will normally be a small area incapable of resolution by the human eye. Microscopic examination of the plastic places higher demands on the mixture because the area examined, and hence the scale of scrutiny, is reduced. The smaller the scale of scrutiny demanded by a product application, the greater the difficulty the mixer will have in achieving a satisfactory mixture. For meaningful results a mixture should be sampled at a size equal to or less than the scale of scrutiny required by the mixture application. The control of the mixture quality is then based on a statistical assessment of a selection of such samples. The variance of a component in several samples is a measure of the consistency or quality of the product. The smaller the variance, the better is the mixture. Such a measure gives a graded assessment of mixture quality, which enables process trends to be followed and problems to be predicted and avoided. The sample variance value alone gives no absolute assessment of mixture quality; this value has to be related to the limiting mixture variance values of complete segregation and of randomized mixing. The variance of the randomized mixture is the more helpful datum of comparison because it usually represents the attainable mixture quality in an industrial process and represents a random positioning of the components within the mixture with no segregation or preferential positioning. The limiting random variance can be calculated for most industrial mixtures.

Traceability is rapidly becoming a requirement for all the process industries. For the pharmaceutical industry it is an essential requirement and usually precludes the 'open-ended' continuous mixing route. If **batch integrity** is to be maintained from the loading of the mixture ingredients through mixing to the final packaging of the product then intermediate storage and handling should be minimized and all process equipment should be capable of easy flushing and cleaning. A mixing vessel that can be transported between the loading, mixing and packaging operations would have many advantages. Further, easy access for sampling is desirable.

There are a very large number of mixers and mixer manufacturers and the temptation to choose 'the same as last time' can be strong. The **mixer selection** problem can be simplified considerably by grouping most mixers under the broad descriptive headings of convective, tumbler, impaction and high shear. These categories will be reviewed giving generic descriptions and their relative merits under the three information input headings.

Convective mixers relocate groups of related particles within a static shell by means of a rotating impeller. The shell can be a trough, a double trough, a vertical cone or a cylindrical hopper; the impeller can be a blade, a ribbon, an Archimedian screw, a Z-blade or a paddle. Rotational speeds are typically five to 30 revolutions per minute. They are probably the most frequently used group of industrial powder mixers. Examples of convective mixers include Hosokawa Nauta mixer and a Ribbon Blender.

The greatest advantage of convective mixers is their ability to handle a wide range of process materials from free-flowing powders to pastes and doughs. In the powder sector, the mixing mechanism of pushing and relocating groups of particles minimizes the opportunity for segregation and optimizes the mixture quality. Cohesive powders mix well but risk searching out unswept corners of the mixer to lodge as dead spots. Because of the static shell, the mixers are accessible for sequential ingredient additions, for heat transfer and for the addition of liquid sprays. The disadvantages of this generic group of mixers are that they risk contamination with their moving parts, are difficult to access for cleaning and sampling, and have to be carefully integrated with the overall process.

Simple mixer shell shapes are rotated horizontally on bearings and mixing occurs by the powder within the mixer tumbling and cascading on the free surface. A variety of simple shapes such as cubes, double cones and V-shapes are used with rotational speeds of typically five to 30 revolutions per minute. Tumbler mixers can handle free-flowing and cohesive powders but not pastes or doughs, and quality is a problem. Free-flowing powders can segregate relatively dramatically on the tumbling surface and the emptying process frequently reinforces this segregation. Weakly structured powders will be broken down within the mixer but small agglomerates or aggregates of an ingredient might remain intact. The degree of fill of the mixer can also affect mixture quality leading to inflexibility in the batch size. Although quality will always remain a problem, the tumbler mixer has significant process advantages. The simple shape enables the mixer to be manufactured in a wide variety of non-contaminating materials, gives good access for both cleaning and sampling, and has no internal bearings contacting the product. Interaction with the mixing process for heat transfer, liquid addition or the stage-wise addition of ingredients is difficult.

Impaction mixers represent a significant increase in energy input into a mixture because the blade rotates at speeds within the range of 2000 to 3000 revolutions per minute within a static vessel, similar to a kitchen food processor. Frequently, an impaction element is introduced along the axis of rotation of a tumbler mixer to present the possibility of an alternative mixing mechanism. The impaction mixer finds an important process niche as a combined mixer-granulator when the high tip speed of the blades can repeatedly break granules as they form and reform. The simple cylindrical or spherical shape of this class of mixer carries the advantages of ease of cleaning and of manufacture in a variety of materials and material finishes. For dry mixtures, the hold-up of fine material on the unswept walls of the vessel creates dead spots, and for a free-flowing powder the emptying of the mixer is vulnerable to physical or chemical segregation. There is good evidence that impactor blades are effective at breaking up aggregates of powder only down to a limiting size, and below that it is possible to have a small scale of segregation but with a high intensity of segregation. In some cases, though, this will limit the application of the impactor mixer.

High-shear mixers are industrial developments of the alchemist's mortar and pestle and the miller's millstone for the grinding of grain. Powder is 'pinched' between a moving and a static surface as in a Comil or between two moving surfaces as in a pair of pressurized rolls. The speed of rotation is low but the powder is subjected to a very high shear that will break down most aggregates. It is commonly preceded by a convective or tumbler mixer to give a general bulk quality before the conditioning of the mixture on a microscale in the high-shear mixer. In some cases the pressure exerted on the powder in the pinch zone is sufficient to consolidate it into a flake form. High-shear mixers tend to have a limited throughput rate and are reserved for those mixtures requiring homogeneity on a microscale.

Granulation

The moist agglomeration process, i.e. the wet massing, screening, and subsequent drying is often a critical unit operation. This unit process is termed as granulation. Granulation is performed to enhance the flowability of a powder. Drugs are incorporated into a mixture of diluent, disintegrant, color and other excipients as powders and then a granulating agent as solution or as a powder is added to the powder mixture and the granules of these powders are prepared by various methods. These methods include wet-granulation and dry-granulation. In a wet-granulation process liquid granulating agent is added, the wet dough is dried and then granules are manufactured out of it. In a dry-granulation method, the granules are manufactured by compressing a solid pellet of the equipment and further crushing it into pieces. The correct amount of granulating liquid and the correct monitoring and detection of the granulation kinetics are important issues. The method to monitor the kinetics needs to be robust and should be applicable for any batch size. In this context, the theory of scale-up and the monitoring of the moist agglomeration process are reviewed.

It has to be kept in mind that the production of granules in the pharmaceutical industry is still based on a batch concept. This concept offers many advantages with respect to quality assurance as a batch can be accepted or rejected. From experience, it is well known, however, that the scale-up of the batch size may lead to problems. This fact is due to the variety of the equipment involved and to the fact that there is a lack of well-known 'scale-up invariant' parameters. A survey of the granulation end-point detection procedure shows that the majority of the equipment manufacturers offer mixer/kneaders for the moist agglomeration process instrumented with a power consumption device. In this review, this and other approaches are discussed and emphasis is placed on how to best use the power consumption method.

For wet granulation in high-shear mixers, specific methods based on the liquid saturation and the consistency of the wet mass is described. Both parameters can be used to quantify the deformability of the wet granules, and relate well with the particle size of the end granules. In practice, the power consumption of the high-shear mixer is used for the monitoring of the wet granulation process, whilst for scale-up, it is helpful to use the underlying relationship between power consumption and saturation level or wet mass consistency. In fluid bed granulation the granulation process is different and the moisture content in the bed is the key parameter to control. This can be monitored directly by near infrared probes or indirectly with temperature probes. As a large number of inter-related variables can be adjusted to modify the process, computerized techniques have become popular for fluid-bed process control – fuzzy logic, neural networks, and models based on experimental design techniques are several examples. In addition, engineering techniques based on particle size population balance modelling are under development for both fluid bed and high-shear granulation.

Solids

Solids are currently very neat dosage forms in the pharmaceutical field. This field is very advanced with lot of personal trained on these lines atleast in India. As related to powders and pellets, the mixing unit process mentioned previously definitely explains the basic principles of tablet formulation and manufacture. Tablets were initially manufactured as triturates. Subsequently this science advanced to a very diverse group of solid dosage form that is now very prominent in the market. Although drug delivery units are currently vogue solid dosage forms still occupy the style of the pharmaceutical market.

Tablets

Tablets could be defined as solid dosage forms incorporating an active chemical agent to be intended for oral administration. Generally, a tablet is made up of a disintegrant, a diluent, a binder, a lubricant and a colorant, along with the active drug substance. Advantages of tablets include:

1. ease of administration;
2. a variety of doses could be incorporated;
3. ease and automation of manufacture;
4. patient compliant formulation unit;
5. millions of tablets could be manufactured within a short span; and
6. a variety of modifications that could enhance drug therapy are possible.

Prior to the introduction of tablets into the market liquid orals were common places. However, the disadvantages of these dosage forms include the change in the character of drugs upon storage and during manufacture. On the other hand, solid dosage forms slowly entered the formulation field. The first of these kinds of solid dosage forms are triturates. Triturates are molded tablets. However, with advanced technological introductions, tablets and capsules became prominent solid dosage forms. Tablets are available in different sizes, weights, hardnesses, thickness, disintegration and dissolution characteristics. At one time several drugs could be incorporated into a tablet to form a multi-drug tablet. As mentioned before, tablet forms of systems existed for long time before tablets became the whole and sole of drug delivery in the form of triturates. These triturates are hand made solid dosage forms. Tablets soon kicked triturates and other formulations in the market and started to rule the market. However, with the introduction of recent developments such as new delivery systems including nanoparticles, microparticles, implants etc. it is likely that the prominence of tablets in the market may falter in coming decades or centuries. These dosage forms are particularly helpful for the formulation of bitter and potent drugs. Taste masking is obviously important with bitter drugs, especially for kids and with highly potent drugs, dosage adjustment is an important criterion. Several drugs have been incorporated into tablets. Examples include aspirin, paracetamol, ephedrine, and digoxin. It is likely that these dosage forms could be incorporated into water, their stability may further go down. The best suitable formulation in these situations is a tablet formulation. Currently, the trend is towards the development of sustained release tablet dosage forms. Unfortunately or fortunately, as such lot of drugs have been incorporated for such a kind of formulations. Published and in-house data suggests that several excipients incorporated into tablets could significantly reduce bioavailability of drugs that also exhibit low intestinal permeability. In these situations, several permeability enhancers or salt forms of drugs could be incorporated as tablets. Examples of

Official tablets include acetaminophen, acyclovir, allopurinol, amitriptylline HCl, carbamazepine, ciprofloxacin, digoxin, enalapril, furosemide, griseofulvin, haloperidol, ibuprofen, loratadine, lovostatin, meperidine HCl, nitroglycerin, penicillin V, propanolol, verapamil HCl and Warfarin Sodium.

Currently, for oral administration, in the market, different kinds of tablets are available. These include compressed tablets, multiple compressed tablets, sugar-coated tablets, gelatin coated tablets, enteric-coated tablets, buccal or sublingual tablets, effervescent tablets, molded tablets, hypodermic tablets, dispensing tablets, instant disintegrating/dissolving tablets extended release tablets and vaginal tablets. The most commonly found tablets are compressed tablets. The manufacture and formulation ingredients are changed slightly to obtain the other kinds of tablets with a variety of uses. A brief definition of these special tablets followed by the description of the manufacture procedure of tablets as a whole will be described. The very common compressed tablet has the following ingradients: diluents or fillers; binders or adhesives; disintegrants or disintegrating agents; antiadherents, glidants, lubricants or lubricating agents or miscellaneous excipients. *Multiple compressed tablets* are prepared by subjecting the fill material to more than a single compression. The result is a multiple-layered or a tablet-within-a-tablet, the inner tablet being the core and the outer portion being the shell. *Compressed tablets* may be coated with a colored or an uncolored sugar layer. The coating is water-soluble and is quickly dissolved after swallowing. *Film-coated tablets* are compressed tablets coated with a thin layer of a polymer capable of forming a skin-like film over the tablet. The film is usually colored and has the advantage over sugar-coatings in that it is more durable, less bulky, and less time-consuming to apply. The new types of coated tablets are gelatin tablets. Unfortunately, their description is not that much and very latest literature could indicate their role. However, these tablets offer more advantage than the other kinds of coated tablets. *Enteric-coated tablets* pass through the stomach unchanged and then release the drug in the intestines. *Buccal or sublingual tablets* are flat, oval tablets are administered into the buccal pouch or beneath the tongue where the drug is released and is absorbed through the oral mucosa. *Chewable tablets* have a smooth, rapid disintegration when chewed or allowed to dissolve in the mouth, have a creamy base usually of specially flavored and colored mannitol. *Effervescent tablets* are prepared by compressing granular effervescent salts that release gas when in contact with water. Molded tablets are soft tablets designed for rapid dissolution. *Hypodermic tablets* are the tablets administered under the skin. *Dispensing tablets* are prepared by a pharmacist and incorporate large amounts of potent drugs. These tablets had the dangerous potential of being inadvertently dispensed as such to patients. *Instant-release tablets* disintegrate and dissolve in the mouth within one minute and are prescribed for pediatric and geriatric patients who have difficulty in swallowing tablets. *Extended release tablets* or some times called controlled release tablets are designed to release their medication in a predetermined manner over extended period of time. *Vaginal tablets* are uncoated and bullet- or ovoid-shaped tablets that are inserted into the vagina for localized effects.

Tablets are most frequently prepared by one of four general methods, depending on the stability and physico-chemical characters of a drug substance and the excipients. These methods are

1. wet granulation,
2. dry granulation,
3. slugging and
4. direct compression.

Single station tableting machine was commonly used in earlier days. However, the time taken for tablet compression is very high. This technique could be used for small-scale tablet manufacture and for laboratory investigations. Based on the number of stations, tablet machines could be classified into single station or multi-station. Based on the speed of tableting, they could be classified into slow speed, intermediate speed and high-speed. High-speed machines could manufacture several thousands of tablets in a very short span. On the other hand, several other intermediate speed-tableting machines also are available and these machines and methodologies are discussed in the chapter on pharmaceutical technology. Not all the time the same technique of tablet manufacture could be applied. The earlier drugs were highly compressible or docile to the manufacture. However, some of the recent drugs coming up because of high-through put techniques are not compressible and thus very special techniques or excipients are to be used in their manufacture. A brief overview of these techniques will be discussed henceforth.

Wet granulation is a widely employed method for production of compressed tablets. The steps in this process include:

1. weighing and blending of the ingredients,
2. preparing a damp mass,
3. screening the damp mass into granules,
4. drying the granules,
5. sizing the granules by dry screening,
6. adding lubricant and blending, and
7. Compression. Specified quantities of active ingradient, diluent or filler, and disintegrating agent are mixed by mechanical powder blender or mixer until uniform. Among the fillers used are lactose, microcrystalline cellulose, starch, powdered sucrose, and calcium phosphate. The choice of the filler

usually is based on the experience of the manufacturer with the material, its relative cost, and its compatibility with the other formulation ingradients. Disintegrating agents include crosscarmellose, corn and potato starches, sodium starch glycolate, sodium carboxymethylcellulose, polyvinyl polypyrolidone (PVP), crospovidone, cation-exchange resins, alginic acid, and other material that sell or expand on exposure to moisture and affect the rupture or breakup of the tablet in the gastrointestinal tract. Binders include acacia, cellulose derivatives, gelatin, glucose, polyvinylpyrrolidone, starch paste, sorbitol and tragacanth. As a first step the ingradient along with the drug are selected and the binder solution is added and mixed to form thick dough. This wet mass is passed through screen and the resulting granules are dried to obtain dried granules. These granules are then passed through the sieves to obtain granules of desired size. Then lubricant is added to improve the flowability of these granules. These granules are then compressed to obtain tablets.

In dry granulation method, entire mixture is added, blended very fine followed by compaction to obtain solid pellets. These pellets are generally bigger than the routine tablets. However, a disintegrant is missing. Once the tablets are manufactured, they are compressed to obtain small granules that are then passed through sieves to get dry granules of desired sizes. Subsequently, they are lubricated by the addition of a lubricant and then the other excipients that are missing are added and then compressed to obtain tablets. Generally, drugs that are not stable to moisture are incorporated using this technique. The third technique of preparing tablets is **slugging**. In a slugging process, after weighing and mixing the ingredients, the powder mixture is "slugged" or compressed into large flat tablets or pellets of about 1 inch in diameter. The slugs then are broken up by hand or by a mill and passed through a screen of desired mesh for sizing. Lubricant is added in the usual manner, and tablets are prepared by compression. Aspirin, which is hydrolyzed on exposure to moisture, may be prepared into tablets after slugging. Sometimes, slugs are prepared using roller compaction. Roller compactors are used to increase the density of a powder pressing it between high-pressure rollers at 1 ton to 6 tons of pressure. The densified material then is broken up, sized, and lubricated, and the tablets are prepared by compression. The roller compaction method is often preferred over slugging. Binding agents used in roller compaction formulations include methylcellulose or hydroxymethylcellulose (6 to 12%) and can produce good tablet hardness and friability.

The first tablets that were produced by **direct compression** were granular chemical like potassium chloride. These compounds possessed free flowing and cohesive properties that enables them to be compressed directly in a tablet machine without the need of wet or dry granulation. Thus, in a direct compression process, the active drug along with several excipients is mixed uniformly and this mixture is compressed to form tablets. The chemicals that are selected in a direct compression process are directly compressed. Drugs may not have direct compressible properties. However, it is wise to procure directly compressible active ingradients. Examples of directly compressible excipients include: filler, eg. spray-dried lactose, microcrystals of alpha-monohydrate lactose, sucrose-invert sugar-corn starch mixtures, microcrystalline cellulose, crystalline maltose, and dicalcium phosphate; disintegrating agents, eg. direct-compression starch, sodium carboxymethyl starch, cross-linked carboxymethyl cellulose fibers, and cross-linked carboxymethylcellulose fibers, and cross-linkded polyvinyl-pyrrolidone; lubricants, eg. magnesium stearate and talc; and glidants, eg. fumed silicon dioxide. Direct compression has tremendously improved the tablet production output. Several new excipients were synthesized to possess direct compressible properties. In addition, several NCEs that are synthesized at the present time are directly compressible.

Capsules

Capsules are gelatin shells incorporating drugs as powders or granules. Unfortunately, some drugs are generally not soluble in the gastrointestinal tract and may likely precipitate. In addition, several drugs that are incorporated as enteric coated tablets; several drugs that are designed to pass through the stomach for drug release and absorption in the intestine; several drugs that are designed for extended-release dosage forms, designed to provide prolonged release dosage forms; and several drugs that are incorporated as sublingual or buccal tablets, formulated to dissolve under the tongue or in the oral cavity to reach the systemic circulation could be conveniently incorporated as capsule dosage forms. These are thus several reasons for preparing capsules. For one thing, certain drugs that are to be administered extemporaneously, capsules are the best alternatives over tablets. The powder blend could be incorporated into the capsules and then administered. This could be quick and dirty and could be used in a dispensing pharmacy. Generally, hard gelatin capsules are used for this purpose. These capsules have been used in a dispensing pharmacy for over several years. On the other hand, some times liquid drugs or drugs formulated as liquids could be incorporated into a soft gelatin capsule and then administered orally. Thus, there are two kinds of capsules, one soft gelatin capsules and the second hard gelatin capsules. Basically, the ending of such formulations as evident was due to the sophistication of tablet formulations and introduction of several new kind of dosage forms including pellets, nanoparticles, microparticles, implants, sustained release liquids, gargles and beads. However, still capsules consume a significant market in pharmaceutical arena. Tablets are the priority. Compression technique has been well developed and evolved at the current settings. At the end, the goal is to better delivery of drugs orally.

A pharmacist before manufacturing or supplying capsules should know very well the characteristics of gelatin shells that are used in the preparation of a capsule. Hard gelatin capsule shells are used to manufacture most of the commercially available medicated capsules. They are also commonly employed in clinical drug trials, to compare the effects of an investigational drug to another drug product or placebo. The community pharmacist in the extemporaneous compounding of prescriptions also uses hard gelatin capsules. The empty capsules shells are made from a mixture of gelatin, sugar and water. As such, they are clear, colorless, and essentially tasteless. Gelatin is obtained by the partial hydrolysis of collagen obtained from the skin, white connective tissue, and bones of animals. In commerce, it is available in the form of a fine powder, a coarse powder, shreds, flakes, or sheets. Hard gelatin capsules are made out of this material. Hard gelatin capsules shells are manufactured in two sections, the capsule body and a shorter cap. The two parts overlap when joined, with the cap fittingl snugly over the open end of the capsule body. The shells are produced industrially by the mechanical dipping of pins or pegs of the desired shape and diameter into a temperature-controlled reservoir of melted gelatin mixture. Slowly after a series of steps including submerging, coating and drying, gelatin shells are prepared. After drying these are obtained as hard shells. Finally, the top portion and the bottom portion are attached to obtain an empty capsule shell. Empty gelatin capsules are manufactured in various sizes, varying in length, in diameter, and capacity. The size selected for use is determined by the amount of fill material to be encapsulated. Several series of mathematical calculations of dosings are done to fill the capsules. Soft gelatin capsules are made of gelatin to which glycerin or a polyhydric alcohol such as sorbitol has been added to render the gelatin elastic or plastic-like. Soft gelatin capsules, which contain more moisture than hard capsules, may have a preservative added as methylparaben or propyl paraben to retard microbial growth. Soft gelatin capsules may be manufactured to be oblong, oval or round. The manufacture of the batch is very tricky. Once a batch is lost, then there is definitely a loss of the drug, gelatin capsules and everything. This is because of the one step process involved in the manufacture of soft gelatin capsules.

Examples of official capsules include amoxicillin, ampicillin, cephalexin, diphenhydramine HCl, doxycycline Hyclate, erythromycin estolate, fluoxitine HCl, flurazepam HCl, gemfibrozil, griseofulvin, indomethacin, levodopa, loperaminde HCl, oxazepam, propoxyphene HCl, tetracycline HCl. Examples of some marketed soft gelatin capsules include acetazolamide, cyclosporine, digoxin, ethchlorvynol, ethosuximide and ranitidine HCl. Although tablets are in very advanced stages, capsules in some cases are still valid. The properties of drugs that are to be incorporated into hard gelatin capsules are entirely different from the properties of drugs to be incorporated into a tablet. Some of these properties include:

1. The flow properties should be average to moderately good.
2. Except for high-dose drug formulations, where a maximum of powder is forced into the capsule shells, there is no need for high compressibility and compactability of the formulations.
3. The majority of capsule formulations currently on the market does not include a disintegrant at all, or the formulations include materials such as starch, which, due to capillary activity ("wicking"), draw larger amounts of water into the powder plug helping in the dispersion and dissolution of the drug in the gastro-intestinal medium.

On the other hand, soft gelatin capsules are preferred for the following reasons:

1. Soft gelatin capsules are dosage forms suitable for administration of sensitive drugs posing technological problems.
2. They mask an unpleasant taste or smell of the drug and the colour combinations increase the safety of therapy by excluding interchangings.
3. Their manufacture is undemanding; it depends on the quality of gelatin and the gelatin mass for the shell of the capsules, on the properties of the fill, on mutual interactions between the fill and the shell, and on a special know-how, which is an unconditional precondition of successful manufacture of these dosage forms.
4. The oral delivery of hydrophobic drugs present a major challenge because of their low aqueous solubility. These drugs could be suspended, or emulsified and then put in soft gelatin capsules and administered orally. One such example is the incorporation of SEDDS. Self-emulsifying drug delivery systems (SEDDS) are isotropic mixtures of oils, surfactants, solvents and co-solvents/surfactants and are used for the design of formulations in order to improve the oral absorption of highly lipophilic drugs. These systems could be conveniently incorporated in soft gelatin capsules.
5. Several other uses of soft gelatin capsules currently investigated include sustained release of hydrophobic drugs and sustained release of peptide, protein and genetic drugs.

Pellets

Pellets are either non-pareil beads or tablet like solid dosage forms manufactured using a variety of novel techniques. Non-pareil beads are intended to be incorporated into capsules. The technique of preparing non-pareil beads is termed spheronization or also pelletization. The advantages of spheronization (pelletization) for the pharma industry include,

1. Facilitation of development of controlled and sustained release formulations.
2. Helpful in mixing otherwise incompatible formulations.
3. Enables uniform coating and accurate free flow filling into capsules.
4. Offers dust free packaging thereby reducing the risk due to toxic, environmental and explosive hazards.
5. Eliminates dust within the agro-chemical, pigment, and catalyst industries, thereby reducing risk due to toxic, environmental, and explosive hazards.
6. Reduces product settlement in transport.

The second forms of pellets are solids that are intended for oral administration. These are different from tablets. These pellets were in existence as sustained release systems for over several years. The common route of administration of these pellets is either subcutaneous or subdermal. These pellets could be defined as sterile, small, usually cylindrical-shaped solid objects prepared by compression and intended to be implanted subcutaneously or administered orally providing continuous release of medication. Very small pellets could be manufactured by some of the currently available technologies. Several polymers could be incorporated to form pellets. As a whole these pellets could be for many purposes. Oral administration of these pellets is however new. Especially for drugs like proteins, genes, peptides these pellets would be of help after oral administration. The other benefit of a pellet is repeated dose of the drugs could be conveniently incorporated into these pellets. Some times proper wax coating helps in protecting the drug in the gastrointestinal tract. They may help in releasing the drug at specified site of intestinal tract. Thus, this kind of pellet is an important oral dosage form, because of its numerous technological and pharmacotherapeutic advantages. The process of manufacture of pellets influences a number of formulation parameters. At one time the power of this technogy was tremendous for sustained release subcutaneous delivery. However, currently the orientation has changed its due course with new ideas introduced that include sustained release as well as oral release of drugs.

Triturates

In ancient times, tablets were administered as triturates. These are also called molded tablets. However, the commercial preparation of tablets by molding has been replaced by the tablet compression process. Still, these tablet triturates are in vogue in pharmacies for several reasons. These are intended to dissolve rapidly in the oral cavity. They do not contain disintegrants, lubricants, or coatings to slow their rate of dissolution. The base for molded tablets is generally a mixture of finely powdered lactose with or without a portion of powdered sucrose (5-20%). The addition of sucrose results in less-brittle tablets. In preparing the fill, the drug is mixed uniformly with the base, by geometric dilution when potent drugs are used. The powder mixture is wetted with a 50% mixture of water and alcohol sufficient only to dampen the powder so that is may be compacted. The solvent action of water on a portion of the lactose/sucrose base effects the binding of the powder mixture upon drying. The alcohol portion hastens the drying process. The mold that is used in the preparation of triturates is made of hard rubber, hard plastic, or die portion, and the lower part containing squat, and flat punches. This is a way of manufacturing triturates in olden days. However, currently several modifications in triturates as per the needs has evolved with the introduction of several new manufacturing techniques.

Recently triturate technology in modified version has presented viable dosage alternatives for patients who may have difficulty swallowing tablets or liquids. Traditional tablets and capsules administered with an 8-oz. glass of water may be inconvenient or impractical for some patients. For example, a very elderly patient may not be able to swallow a daily dose of antidepressant. An eight-year-old with allergies could use a more convenient dosage form than an antihistamine syrup. A schizophrenic patient in the institutional setting can hide a conventional tablet under his or her tongue to avoid their daily dose of an atypical antipsychotic. A middle-aged woman undergoing radiation therapy for breast cancer may be too nauseous to swallow her H2-blocker. Fast-dissolving/disintegrating tablets (FDDTs) or also called triturates are a perfect fit for all of these patients. These triturates disintegrate and dissolve rapidly in the saliva without the need for water. Some triturates are designed to dissolve in saliva remarkably fast, within a few seconds, and are true fast-dissolving tablets. Others contain agents to enhance the rate of triturate disintegration in the oral cavity, and are more appropriately termed fast-disintegrating tablets, as they may take up to a minute to completely disintegrate.

The target populations for these triturates are pediatric, geriatric, and bedridden or developmentally disabled patients. Patients with persistent nausea, who are traveling, or who have little or no access to water are also good candidates for triturates. With fast-dissolving/disintegrating dosage forms increasingly available, it will be likely that prescribers will recommend such products for their noncompliant patients. The ease of administration for these triturates, along with its pleasant taste, may encourage a patient to adhere to a daily medication regimen. Although a FDDT may not solve all compliance issues, it may be enough of an advance to be of therapeutic significance. The major advantage of this formulation is that it combines the advantages of both liquid and conventional tablet formulations, while also offering advantages over both traditional dosage forms. It provides the convenience of a tablet formulation, while also allowing the ease of swallowing provided by a liquid formulation. These formulations allow the luxury of much more accurate dosing than the primary alternative, oral liquids.

Manufacture of Solids

The manufacture of solid dosage forms is detailed in several textbooks and in a chapter in this book titled "Pharmaceutical technology" and thus is not discussed here in depth. However, an overview of tablet manufacture will be discussed henceforth.

A tablet press is used in the manufacture of a tablet. Currently several kinds of tablets presses are available in the market. These tablet presses are used for uniaxial pressing of powdered materials into shaped tablets or compacts. Tableting presses usually operate at high speeds. Parts can often be pressed and sintered to dimensional tolerance levels that do not require additional machining. For demanding applications, cold pressed and sintered parts may require subsequent coining/repressing, infiltration, hot pressing or forging to reach the required density and strength. Tableting presses are designed in two configurations: multi-station tableting press and single station presses. Single station presses consist of a single tool set (die and punch set) in a die table. Single action opposed ram presses use a die with both upper and lower punches. Anvil type presses have only a die and single lower punch. Single station compacting presses are available in several types basic types such as cam, toggle / knuckle and eccentric / crank presses with varying capabilities such as single action, double action, floating die, movable platen, opposed ram, screw, impact, hot pressing, coining or sizing. Multi-station tableting presses, also referred to as rotary presses, use a punch and die system with multiple stations or punches for compacting materials into tablets, or metal powders into simple flat or multilevel shaped parts like gears, cams, or fittings. Rotary types have a series of stations or tool sets (dies and punches) arranged in a ring in a rotary turret. As the turret rotates, a series of cams and presses rolls control filling, pressing and ejection. Pharmaceutical tablet and high volume metal part production facilities often use high-speed automatic rotary presses.

Currently, the trend in tablet technology is high speed tableting. Several contract manufacturers are helping out pharmaceutical companies in this high-speed tableting. The onset of high-speed tabletting posed a difficult problem in that the cohesive blend was required to flow consistently and at speed into the die of the tabletting plate. Granulating the cohesive mixture in a high-speed impaction mixer and granulator and then feeding a dried and free-flowing granular mixture to the tabletting machine satisfied the contradiction in flow requirements. The pre-mix followed by the granulation is optimal because the chemical uniformity of the product is achieved at the pre-mix stage, and at the tabletting stage any segregation associated with the free-flowing granules is physical rather than chemical.

The pre-mix stage is usually carried out in a tumbler mixer possibly with the aid of an impactor or intensifier bar. With a cohesive powder charge a tumbler mixer will not segregate the mixture and is capable of breaking up and mixing loosely structured systems. The use of an impactor along the axis of rotation will break up stronger structures but experience in the ceramic and cosmetic industries suggested that impaction will not be as effective as high shear in breaking down the microstructure of a mixture. Nonetheless, an effective and high-throughput process can be built about a combination of tumbler and high-impaction mixers. However, the sequencing of a tumbler mixer with a high-speed mixer granulator has lost the effective shearing action of the mortar and pestle, and if strongly structured aggregates are to be broken down in order to optimize the microstructure of the powder then a high-shear mixer needs to be introduced into the sequence.

The familiarity and availability of tumbler and high-impaction mixers within the industry can lead to quality-control problems when their clear roles in the high-speed tabletting process are forgotten. If the direct compression route to tabletting is attempted by omitting the granulation step then the flow characteristic of the bulk mixture has to be intermediate between cohesion and free flow in order to suppress segregation within the tumbler mixer whilst maintaining flow on the tabletting plate. The risk of segregation within the tumbler mixer is ever present in this delicate flow balance. If the alternative of using the high-speed impactor as a dry mixer is used, there are the combined risks of hold-up of powder on the unswept walls and segregation occurring on discharging the mixer. A new quality-assurance danger arises, as process segregation is possible. The tacit assumption that if a mixture is 'well mixed' within the mixer then the mixture quality can only be improved by subsequent handling is incorrect and the equilibrium nature of a mixture of a segregating powder can cause quality degradation downstream of the mixer. The possible use of a convective mixer and the careful sequencing and design of the downstream process are further very important steps in the mixing process. All of the above considerations if kept in mind, the tablet manufacturing becomes effective.

Tablet coating

Tablet coating is an integral part of tablet technology. A tablet is coated for several reasons including to: protect the medicinal agent from the environment; taste masking; provide special drug release properties; and to provide aesthetics or distinction to the product. The general methods of coating are sugar-coating tablets, film-coating tablets; enteric coating; fluid-bed or air suspension coating and compression coating. The first tablet coating developed was sugar coating. The process could be divided into the following steps:

1. waterproofing and sealing,
2. subcoating,
3. smoothing and final rounding,
4. finishing and coloring (if desired), and polishing.

Lot of time and money has been spent on sugar coating technology development and now this technology is very robust. Basically, the tablets are compressed. These are then added to the coating pan. Generally, these pans operate at 40° angle to contain the tablets whole allowing the operator visual and manual access. Several coating solutions such as subcoating, smoothing and final rounding coat, finishing and coloring coats are prepared in a syrup base with the appropriate ingradients. The coating is accomplished accordingly to enhance the coat and the size of the tablets including the coat. The first coating is waterproofing and sealing coat. Since the syrup is an aqueous coat and the coating process involves heat, definitely in every likely the tablet has to be protected from moisture to avoid drug degradation and the physical intactness of the tablet. This solution is alcohol based and the coat is done on the tablet with occasional warm blowing to prevent the tablets sticking together. Subsequently 3 to 5 subcoats of sugar-based syrup are applied. The purpose of this step is to give the tablets a round shape. The next step is smoothing and final rounding. This has 5 to 10 additional coating of thick syrup. Finally, finishing and coloring is achieved on the tablet.

In a film coating procedure, instead of sugar coat a flimsy coat is layed on the tablet. This technique was developed as an alterative to the sugar coating. Although sugar coating provides sustained release of the drug from a tablet, in every likely it almost doubles the size of a tablet and also very tedius and requires tremendous skill, as perfect control of each and every step is required.

Otherwise, the tablet batch is totally lost. To avoid these drawbacks, film coating was developed. In a film coating process, instead of using syrup based coating material, a film former solution is prepared and is coated over the tablet. Different ingradients of the film former solution include a film former, an alloying substance, a plasticizer, a surfactant, opaquants and colorants, sweeteners, flavors and aromas, glossant and volatile solvents. Tablets are film coated by the application or spraying of the film-coating solution on the tablets in ordinary coating pans. The volatility of the solvent enables the film to adhere quickly to the surface of the tablets. The film form solution coule be either aqueous or non-aqueous. Several problems are associated with tablet coating that is not discussed here. Interested reader should definitely consult further to become a skill master in coating technology. In enteric coating technique, a coat that dissolves based on the pH of the environment. Some enteric coatings are designed to dissolve at pH 4.8 and greater. Non-pareils could be coated with these kind of coatings and filled in a capsule for sustained and intestine targeted release. Very special equipment called fluid-bed or air suspension coating has been developed to automatize the entire process of coating. This is basically a spray coating of powders, granules, beads, pellets or tablets held in suspsion by a column of air. This is termed fluidized bed. Coating and drying of this fluidized bed are accomplished in this system by a variety of gadgets connected to the coating equipment. Compression coating is another kind of coating accomplished by the method of compression. A tablet is compressed first followed by the compression of the coat around this tablet. This needs very special equipment.

Color uniformity during coating is a very important consideration. Evaluation of tablet mixing within side vented coating equipment suggested the development of uniform color during coating. Baffle systems contained in a coating machine would help in unicorm coating. In one study, a colorimetric method was used to evaluate the time for uniform coating for different mixing baffle systems at different scales of equipment. The influence of tablet size was also determined. The inclusion of rabbit ear baffles in the small-scale equipment reduced the time to achieve color uniformity by 20 minutes. The design of baffle influenced the time for uniform color with a mixing efficiency rank order of tubular > ploughshare > rabbit ear. Upon scale-up, the efficiency of mixing seen at development scale remained equivalent in terms of the influence of baffle design. The study into the influence of tablet size revealed the importance that the total batch surface area has on the time taken to achieve color uniformity, with 7-mm diameter tablets having a higher surface area for an equivalent volume of product and taking 15 to 20 minutes longer to achieve color uniformity than 16-mm diameter tablets. These are some of the important considerations in a tablet coating procedure.

Quality Control of Conventional Dosage Forms

As such quality control is a very important aspect in pharmaceutical industries, however, for conventional dosage forms, the methods are well established with perfect validations and controls in place. Some times simple statistical methods are in place for such methodologies. The professional, social and legal responsibilities that rest with pharmaceutical manufacturers for the assurance of product quality are tremendous. Although, these methods for conventional dosage forms are very cheap, they still are routinely used in the companies. It takes several book volumes to just discuss the quality control of conventional dosage forms. Unfortunately, this is beyond of the scope of this text-book and thus a very brief outline of the quality control of conventional dosage forms clubbed together will be discussed.

The pharmaceutical manufacturer assumes the major responsibility for the quality of his products. Everything involved in the manufacture should be in tight control. These include:

1. Control of the sources of product quality variabilities including materials, methods, machines and men;
2. Ensurance of the correct and most appropriate manufacturing practices;
3. Assurance of the fact the testing results are in compliance with the standards or specifications and
4. Assurance of product stability and performance of other activities related to product quality through a well-organized total quality assurance. The ballpark and the bottom line is that the end result is totally compliant and patient and society safe. If things do not go properly at the end and after the product is launched, the recall of the product from the market is definite. Thus, care has to be taken before such things might have occurred. Prevention is better than cure is the bottom line.

Novel Drug Delivery Systems

Solid Dosage Forms

Rationale

Oral route is the most common route of administration of drugs because of the several advantages this route offers. The advantages include the ease of administration, least aseptic constraints and the ease of the manufacture of the dosage forms. Immediate release systems are the centerpieces among the oral dosage forms. Ideal character of a drug for these systems includes rapid dissolution, rapid absorption, low half-life and low metabolism in the gastrointestinal tract. However, for some drugs and under certain disease conditions, prolonged release of drugs would be needed. The characteristics features of these drugs include very short half-life and very low solubility in the gastro-intestinal tract. Exception to this rule, are the drugs that are inherently long-lasting. These drugs generally have prolonged half-life. These require only once-a-day oral dosing to sustain and equate drug blood levels and the desired therapeutic effect. These drugs are formulated in the conventional manner in immediate-release dosage forms. The other advantage of sustained release dosage forms is the improved patient compliance because of the reduced number of doses to be administered for the same amount of the drug. Basically, it could be said that the design of modified or sustained release dosage form is usually intended to optimize a therapeutic regimen by providing slow and continuous delivery of drug over the entire dosing interval whilst also providing greater patient compliance and convenience.

In addition, sustained release dosage forms help in reducing the toxicity associated with peaks and troughs noticed with conventional dosage form. Pharmacokinetically, when conventional dosage forms of drugs with low half-life are administered, the plasma profile demonstrates peaks and valleys associated with each administration. However, when doses are not administered on schedule, the resulting peaks and valley reflect less than optimum drug therapy. For example, if doses are administered too frequently, minimum toxic concentrations (MTC) of drug may be reached with toxic side effects resulting. If doses are missed, periods of sub-therapeutic drug blood levels or those below the minimum effective concentration may result, with no patient benefit. Extended-release tablets and capsules are commonly taken only once or twice daily compared with counterpart conventional forms that may need to be taken three to four times daily to achieve the same therapeutic level.

Design of a Sustained Release System

Practically two different approaches are generally used by pharmaceutical scientists in the design of a sustained release dosage form. The first approach is based on the modification of the physical and chemical properties of the drug and the second approach is based on the modification of the drug release rate characteristics of the dosage form that affect the bioavailability. Physicochemical properties of the drug substance could be modified by complex formation, drug-adsorbate preparation, or prodrug synthesis. Of these, prodrug synthesis is widely attempted and investigated. The other two techniques are not popular. In addition, the drug should possess appropriate functional group for such modifications. The second approach is the development of a sustained release system. This is popular because of the inherent advantage. The advantage being that the design is independent of the dosage form. The final formulation form could be a liquid suspension, a capsule or a tablet.

Several important factors should be considered in the design of a sustained release dosage forms. Not all the drugs are ideal. Drugs with longer biologic half-lives (e.g., digoxin –34 hours) are inherently long-acting and thus are definitely not suitable candidates. Until and unless there is a need for sustained released systems for these candidates, sustained release systems are not developed. For instance, single doses for such drugs often results in high peak concentrations and leads to toxicity. In these situations, a sustained release system reduces these side effects by prolonging the release of the drug. The other kinds of molecules are the drugs with narrow drug absorption zone. In these situations, because of the narrow requirement of absorption, a sustained release system may not be suitable. The important consideration of drug selection for sustained release dosage forms is its pharmacokinetics. Generally, multi-dose pharmacokinetics data is required prior to the design of a sustained release dosage form. A case study of a design of a sustained release dosage form will be presented henceforth.

Timmer and Sitsen (2003) investigated the pharmacokinetics of gepirone immediate release capsules and gepirone extended release tablets in healthy volunteers. Gepirone is a 5-HT agonist of azapirone class that has been studied for major depression. This molecule has a half-life of 3 hours and good oral bioavailability and undergoes extensive first-pass metabolism. Because of its rapid absorption and short half-life, gepirone must be administered atleast twice daily. The single dose administration has high peak concentrations and marked peak-to-trough fluctuations in plasma concentrations. Thus, the development of sustained released dosage forms was the obvious need. Selection of the proper dose and dosage interval is essential to obtain the desired therapeutic range. Elimination of drug level oscillations could be achieved through constant-rate intravenous infusion. However, it is not advisable in all the situations. Thus, the main objective of a sustained release dosage form is to provide a similar blood level pattern for upto 12 hours after oral administration of the drug. To design a best-sustained release dosage form, one must have thorough idea of the pharmacokinetic behaviour of the drug. In this case, gepirone was the drug of interest. This way of investigation would avoid repetitions and redundancies in the design of a sustained release dosage forms. Two 5-mg capsules of gepirone were administered by oral route to produce a controlled system. All dose were administered with water. Blood was collected and assayed for the plasma concentrations. The data thus obtained was evaluated by non-compartmental methods. The highest observed plasma concentration during a dosing interval and the corresponding sampling time were defined as C_{max} and T_{max}, respectively. The AUC and the area under first moment of the concentration versus time curve were calculated with trapezoidal rule. The absorption kinetics were determined using Wagner-Nelson method. Based on this data, extended release tablets were developed. Upon administration, these systems were able to obtain desired pharmacokinetics of a sustained release system. Similarly, suitable sustained release systems could be developed for any drug.

Mathematics of the Drug Release

The study of the drug release from a sustained dosage form is an important step in its design. A careful selection of polymers for sustained dosage form depending on the physico-chemical properties of a drug and the sustained release requirements is the first step. Looking at this feasibility, a dosage form is devised. The next step is to investigate the drug release mechanisms and sustained release affect of this dosage form. Based on these results, the alterations in the device are considered in its further design. Thus, release of the drug is a very important factor. During the release of drug from sustained release dosage form lot of factors are to be considered. Providing slow and continuous release of the drug over prolonged period of time during the requirement of the drug in the system is the main aim of oral controlled and sustained release systems. As mentioned before, different controlled and sustained release systems are available in the market. These include granules, capsules and tablets. Because of the low cost, the most commonly used sustained release systems are of matrix devices. Several equations have been proposed to describe the release profiles over a period of time. Fan and Singh et al., 1989 described some of these equations in detail. Siegel RA "modeling of drug release from porous polymers" in "Controlled Release of Drugs" (1989) is another classical kind of treatise on controlled release. Most of the proposed equations are based on diffusion kinetics that are reviewed in detail by Crank J. in book "The mathematics of diffusion". After ***in silico*** methods were introduced, the data was entered into the computers and new theories proposed, investigated and applied, respectively. In recent times, the temperature effects were also investigated according to various scientists and investigations. Higuchi equation and power law, the most commonly used equations to investigate drug release will be discussed henceforth.

Higuchi's Equation

Various pharmaceutical scientists have mathematically derived the release of the drug from these systems over several years. However, the famous equation that still explains the release of drugs from these delivery systems is Higuchi's equation. According to this equation, the release of a solid drug from a granular matrix involves the simultaneous penetration of the surrounding liquid, dissolution of the drug, and leaching out of the drug interstitial channels or pores. During its derivation a granule is defined as a porous rather than a homogenous matrix. The volume and length of the opening in the matrix are accounted, where

$$Q = \left\{ \frac{D\varepsilon}{\tau} (2A - \varepsilon C_s) C_s t \right\}^{1/2}$$

where ε is the porosity of the matrix and τ is the tortuosity of the capillary system, both being dimensionless quantities. Porosity is the fraction of matrix that exists as pores or channels in which the surrounding liquid could penetrate. Tortuosity is the increase in the path length due to branching and bending of the pores. The greater the tortuosity the greater is the path a molecule has to travel to be diffused into the surrounding media.

Higuchi demonstrated that during the initial release phase from a spherical system-until approximately 50% of the drug content in the vehicle has been released-the square root of time behavior is dominating, and then it depends on the design of the sustained release system. Taken together, a better model of release as predicted with each type of the sustained release systems, their geometrical factors, the porosity factors, the manufacture methods all play an important role. Thus, a scientist working in the area of the sustained release must judiciously use the release data and modern techniques in furthering their development. The practical benefit of these methods is to cut the number of experiments and use the lessons learnt over the past 40 years after Higuchi proposed his release equation, when optimizing the release kinetics of new controlled release dosage forms.

The final form of a sustained release matrix system may be a film, pipe, granule, a sphere or, more simply a cylinder. These forms are assumed because of the shape of the die or the method of manufacture, or the type of the sustained system. The sustained system may finally end up with a granular type device or a homogenous type device. The release of the drug from these systems follows a different pattern depending on the extent of release. Simple planar–system square-root-of-time law to estimate diffusion coefficients from a spherical systems provided that only the first part of the release process (before 50% is released) is used in the analysis. With homogenous systems, the porosity of the material is 1 and thus Higuchi equation for homogenous systems becomes,

$$Q = \left\{ \frac{D}{\tau} (2A - C_s) C_s t \right\}^{1/2}$$

Power Law

The other law that is routinely used for various purposes commonly used is the power law. This equation could be applied to release from any kind of delivery system. According to this law,

$$M_{t}) / (M_{\infty}) = Kt^{n}$$

Here (M_t) and (M_∞) are the absolute cumulative amounts of the drug released at time t and time infinity, respectively. K is the constant incorporating structural and geometrical characteristics of a sustained release device; n is the release exponent, indicative of the mechanism of drug release. When $n = 0.5$, the power law becomes equivalent to Higuchi's equation. This is derived for a short-term approximation of a solution for Ficks second law of diffusion for thin films. Peppas and co-workers used this equation and described its limitations (1985). Fickian diffusion and a case-II transport are represented in this equation. When $n=1$, the drug release rate is independent of time. This situation corresponds to zero-order drug release. Hence forth, this equation could be used for any situation with known polymer characteristics and the conditions of drug release. For instance, for slabs the release is a zero-order release because of the case-II transport seen with a slab. In this situation, the relaxation of the polymer occurs because of the imbibing of water. This is the rate controlling steps. Water acts as plasticizer to the polymer and reduces its glass transition temperature. Once the polymer is plasticized, the chains are relaxed and the polymer is transformed from plastic to rubbery state. This results in increased mobility of the macromolecules and thus volume expansion. This equation is mostly used for swellable matrices. The release mechanism in these conditions basically is influenced by polymeric water uptake, gel layer formation and polymer chain relaxation. The above equation helps in identifying the mechanism of release. A purely relaxation controlled drug release where $n=1$ is referred to as case II transport. Intermediate values indicate an anomalous behavior (non-fickian kinetic corresponding to coupled diffusion/polymer relaxation). Occasionally, values of $n > 1$ are observed, and in this case the release is termed as super case II kinetics.

Tablets

The extended drug action with oral dosage forms is achieved by affecting the rate at which the drug is released from the dosage forms and/or by slowing the transit time of the dosage form through the gastrointestinal tract. The rate of release from these systems is obtained by 1. modifying drug dissolution by controlling access of biological fluids to the drug through the use of barrier coatings; 2. Controlling drug diffusion rates from dosage forms; 3. Chemically reacting or interacting between the drug substance or its pharmaceutical barrier and site-specific biologic fluids.

Different types of sustained release tablets could include:

1. Delayed-Release Tablets
2. Extended-Release Coated Particle/Bead
3. Extended-Release Inert Matrix
4. Extended-Release Hydrophilic/Eroding Matrix
5. Extended-Release Microencapsulated
6. Extended-Release Osmotic

Delayed-release tablets

These are tablets coated with different polymers like cellulose acetate phathalate, carnauba wax, eudragit S and cellulose polymers intended for sustained release. In these systems a tablet containing the drug is punched. A coat of the polymer is built on the tablet. After the tablet enters the stomach, the polymer slowly dissolves or disintegrates thereby resulting in prolonged release of the drug. Depending on the type of the polymer the release profile is obtained. If the coat is made out of insoluble polymer, the drug is leached out of the tablet and a ghost tablet will result which is excreted. Generally, depending on the use of soluble or insoluble excipients, the final form of the tablet may be smaller or remains the same at the time of excretion, respectively.

Extended-release coated particle/bead

These are drug pellets coated with polymers compressed into tablets. These polymers include cellulose esters or polyvinyl acetate-crotonic acid copolymer or hydroxypropylmethylcellulose, etc. As mentioned before the final end products may be excreted as ghost capsules or the tablets totally dissolved. The advantage in this situation is desired release of the drug could be obtained; dose-dumping could be prevented; different combination of the drugs could be incorporated; depending on the thickness of the polymer coat of the beads timed-released tablets could be formed; placebo-beads could be incorporated in the group of the beads with different thickness to obtain repeat action tablets etc.

Extended release inert matrix

These tablets could be either drug impregnated in an inert, porous, plastic matrix or extended-release tablets with a core tablet of a non-erodible wax matrix coated with cellulose polymers. Drug leaches out as it passes slowly through the gastrointestinal tract. Extended matrix is excreted in stool.

Extended-release hydrophilic/eroding matrix

A hydrophilic matrix that swells and slowly erodes provides extended-release in these tablets. ex. sustained-release hydrophilic matrix system, based on the polymer hydroxypropyl methyl cellulose (HPMC).

Extended-release microencapsulated

These tablets are immediately dispersing drug microencapsulated with ethylcellulose and hydroxypropyl cellulose.

Extended-release osmotic

Controlled release “Gastrointestinal Therapeutic System” Osmotic system is the best example. Ingradients include polyethylene oxide, hydroxypropyl cellulose, and cellulose acetate. A controlled-onset extended release osmotic system.

Capsules

Different types of sustained release capsules includes:

1. Delayed-release capsules
2. Extended-release coated particle/beads

Delayed-release capsules

In these systems, the drug is distributed onto the beads, pellets, granules or other particulate systems. Using conventional pan-coating or air-suspension coating techniques, a solution of the drug substance is placed onto small inert nonpareil seeds or beads made of sugar and starch or onto microcrystalline cellulose spheres. The nonpareil seeds are most often in the 425 to 850 micrometer range whereas the microcrystalline cellulose spheres are available ranging from 170 to 600 micrometer. The microcrystalline spheres are considered more durable during production than sugar-based cores. Different coating could be achieved on these beads. These could be either aqueous or non-aqueous. Aqueous-based coating systems eliminate the hazards and environment concerns associated with organic solvent-based systems. These are capsules with non-pariel beads containing drug coated with different polymers like cellulose acetate phathalate, carnauba wax, eudragit S and cellulose polymers intended for sustained release. The variation in the thickness of the coats and in the type of coating material used affects the rate at which the body fluids are capable of penetrating the coating to dissolve the drug. Naturally, the thicker the coat, the more resistant to penetration and the more delayed will be the drug release and dissolution. Typically the coated beads are about 1 mm in diameter. They are combined to have three or four release groups among the more than 100 beads contained in the dosing unit. They are combined to have three or four release groups among the more than 100 beads contained in the dosing unit. This provides the different desired sustained or extended release rates and the targeting of the coated beads to the desired segments of the gastrointestinal tract.

Extended-release coated particle/bead

These are drug pellets coated with polymers and filled into capsules. The polymers include cellulose esters or polyvinyl acetate-crotonic acid copolymer or hydroxypropylmethylcellulose, etc. As mentioned before the final end products may be excreted as ghost capsules or the capsule totally dissolved.

Manufacture

Taken together, the manufacturing procedures for sustained release systems could be classified into granulation-layer containing therapeutics and compression processes. However, judicious selection of the choice of the ingradients, the manufacturing procedure, the dimensions of the solid dosage form and other formulation variables should be carefully considered to obtain a perfect zero-order release (desired release from a sustained release dosage form) with desired characteristics or specified drug release as demonstrated several times previously. These methods are described below.

Granulation-layer containing therapeutics

These could also be called encapsulated slow release granules. These were the first significant marketed sustained release beads. The first beads were non-pareil seeds (20/25-mesh sugar-starch granules) coated with an adhesive followed by powdered drug, and the pellets dried. This step repeated until the desired amount of the drug is coated. Several layers of barriers such as hydrogenated castor oil are coated as desired. However, this technology is modified and advanced rather than staying at individual coatings on nonpareil beads. The size of these beads as mentioned before could be altered by judicious selection of various formulation as well as manufacturing parameters. These beads could be filled into capsules or punched to form a capsule or a tablet as final products, respectively. According to Abdul and Poddar (2004), the following factors are to be considered while making granulation of active substances: granulation liquid percentage, massing step time, outlet target temperature during the drying step and milling screen apertures and the interaction between the amount of granulation fluid and the outlet temperature. The final product responses are classified into

(i) granulation physical characteristics (e.g. flowability, bulk density and particle size distribution);

(ii) extensometric responses (cohesion index, lubrication index, ejection strength, plasticity and elasticity);

(iii) tablet characteristics (thickness, weight variation, hardness and friability);

(iv) analytical results (content uniformity and dissolution profile).

Compression processes

These methods encompass simple tablet compression or moulded techniques. Granules of the drug with sustained release material are prepared as mentioned previous and then compressed into tablets or the drug mixed with sustained release excipients to obtain the tablet of desired shapes and sizes. The advantage of such a technique is that millions of tablets are manufactured because of the advanced stage in which this technology exists. However, to obtain a desired release profile, some times these tablets are moulded accordingly and coated with several layers of polymers. In those situations, the technology is slightly complicated. However, the manufacturing process parameters could be common for both the technologies. These parameters include turntable speed, compression force, hardness of compressed tablet, adhesion strength, polymer concentration in core and filler concentration in core.

Innovative Systems

Gastric retentive drug delivery systems

One of the reasons for the failure of oral controlled release systems is the transit time. For some drugs there is a very limited area available for absorption either because of the localized transport systems available for this drug in the gastro-intestinal tract or rapid transit of this drug in the intestines. On both these occasions, increased residence time of the drug in the intestines increases the bioavailability. Several attempts to extend the release time were researched. The most commonly attempted systems are:

1. intragastric floating systems,
2. high-density systems,
3. mucoadhesive systems,
4. magnetic systems,
5. unfoldable, swellable, extendable systems,
6. superporous hydrogen systems.

One of these systems is illustrated here. Steingoetter et al., (2003) developed a tablet dosage form labeled with superparamagnetic iron oxide (Fe_3O_4). Fe_3O_4, which is paramagnetic, induces a strong local reduction of the T2 relaxation time, causing a signal void in the resulting magnetic resonance images. Consequently, the intragastic position of an ingested labeled tablet could be traced by susceptibility artifact created in the image. Magnetic resonance image is used in this technique. The tablet consisted of Fe_3O_4 crystallites (1%), citric acid monohydrate (2.5%), sodium bicarbonate (2.5%), polyvinylpyrrolidone (1%), metolose (82%), magnesium stearate (1%) and lactose (10%). The crystallites were thoroughly mixed with the tablet compounds before drying of the tablet powder and final tablet formulation. Tablets were formed with a hydraulic press of appropriate size and compression force of 3 kN for 5 seconds. The tablet weighed 400 mg. In healthy human volunteers, 15 minutes after a meal the floating tablet was ingested together with 50 ml of water. Resonance measurements were taken at regular intervals to obtain images covering the entire gastric region (volume scan). The volunteers were not allowed to drink or eat during the four-hour scan period. The administered tablet demonstrated persistant-floating performance in all the volunteers independent of meal consumption. The design of this study is very interesting because of the evaluation technique for floatability of the dosage form. In routine studies, pharmacokinetics is investigated to evaluate the floatability of the dosage form. However, it is not amenable to dissect the differences between the efficacies of individual delivery systems. However, this study is neat because of the non-invasiveness of the technique used to evaluate the floatability of the delivery system.

Particulate systems

Particulate systems include liposomes, nanoparticles and microparticles. These are either biodegradable or non-biodegradable material made particles encapsulating or embedding either hydrophobic and hydrophilic drugs or macromolecules like proteins, peptides or genes. The advantage with these systems is the enhancement of oral bioavailability of molecules either by enhancing the dissolution of poorly soluble molecules or by protecting the molecules from gastro-intestinal degradation or by enhancing the penetration of the molecules through the biological membranes. Several publications consisting of vaccines, peptides and proteins encapsulated in liposomes, microparticles and nanoparticles either to enhance the activity or to increase the absorption of molecules is published over the past decade. In recent times, the interest has shifted to enhancing the oral bioavailability of the poorly soluble molecules by enhancing their dissolution in the intestinal fluids. Additionally, several studies done at tissue and cellular levels demonstrated that latex, polystyrene and DL-PLG copolymer particles with a size range of 50 nm to 20 □m are absorbed mainly through payers patches found in small intestine with little translocation occurring through non-lymphoid gut tissues. However, particulate technologies for oral delivery of drugs and macromolecules are still in the stage of investigation or in pre-clinical evaluations.

Liposomes are phospholipid bilayers encapsulating drugs either in the bilayers or in the aqueous internal compartments. These resemble biological cells because of their inherent phospholipid composition common to biological membranes. They enhance the solubility of molecules or increase the penetration across biological membranes because of the mechanism of transcytosis. Liposomes are manufactured either by dry film hydration, sonication or extrusion techniques. In all these situation phospholipids such as distearyl phosphotidyl choline, dimyrystyl phosphotidyl choline is formed into thin monolayers. These monolayers are subsequently hydrated to form vesicles or bag like structures in which the drug could be incorporated or embedded. Nano- and micro-particulate systems are particulates of the size ranges of nanometers and micrometers made of different material either degradable or biodegradable to be used for sustained release, enhancement of membrane permeation etc. as mentioned before. Either vaccines or protein drugs are embedded in these systems. These were one of the first sustained release delivery systems successfully attempted. Several modifications were then made onto these systems to obtain the desired assistance for the drug or vaccine of interest. Currently, polylacticacidglycolic acid copolymers are actively investigated.

Prodrugs

As mentioned before oral route is the most preferred route of administration of drugs. The optimal physico-chemical properties of synthetic molecules to allow high transcellular absorption following oral administration is well established and include a limit on molecular size, hydrogen bonding potential and adequate lipophilicity. For many drug targets, synthetic strategies are deviced to obtain balanced physicochemical properties required for high transcellular absorption and the structure-activity relationship for the drug target. There are drug targets with the SAR requires properties at odds with good membrane permeability. These include a requirement for significant polarity and groups that exhibit high hydrogen bonding potential such as carboxylic acids and alcohols. In these situations, prodrug strategies have been employed. The rationale behind the prodrug strategy is to introduce lipophilicity and mask hydrogen bonding groups of an active component by the addition of another moiety, most commonly an ester. An ideal ester should exhibit the following properties:

1. weak (or no) activity against any pharmacological target,
2. Chemical stability across a pH range,
3. High aqueous solubility,
4. Good transcellular absorption,
5. Resistance to hydrolysis during absorption phase,
6. Rapid and quantitative breakdown to yield high circulatory concentrations of the active component post absorption.

Some of the prodrugs currently marketed include omeprazole, simvastatin, lovastatin, enalapril and aciclovir.

Trouble Shooting Oral Product Manufacture

Development of oral formulations although is very common place in pharmaceutical industry, the trick of manufacturing elegant and stable formulations lies on some fundamental principles. In case of liquid oral formulations, whether solutions, emulsions and suspensions, although found to be simple, some principles that are used in their formulation is complicated. Especially, the formulation of emulsions and suspensions is a tricky thing. Understanding the principles of stability of colloids is essential. In this regard, knowing DLVO theory is essential. In case of solid dosage forms, whether powders, triturates, tablets or capsules, the knowledge of powder flow is essential. The principles of the manufacture of specialized products such as liposomes and nanoparticles are still a secret to most of the pharmaceutical industries. In this chapter, some essential concepts of the formulation of liquid orals such as emulsions and suspension along with the principles of powder flow will be discussed. Another area that should be known is the drug-excipient interaction. Although the formulation may be elegant, the stability may be compromised because of drug-excipient interactions. This aspect is also discussed in this section.

DLVO Theory

DLVO theory explains the formulation and stability of suspensions and emulsions. The charge on the surface of the drug particles/oil globules explains the type of association they hold in the stable state as a formulation. DLVO theory as applicable for suspensions is explained in this section. For emulsions it is self-explanatory. The charge on the surface of the drug particles explain the type of association they hold in the stable state as a formulation. The drug can be either suspended as floccules or segregated drug particles. The later types of suspensions are called deflocculated suspensions. The phenomenon and this behaviour are explained using DLVO theory. Most surfaces acquire a surface electric charge when they come in contact with aqueous surface. A solid charged surface when in contact with an aqueous medium possesses positive and negative ions. The counter ions are attracted towards the surface co-ions that ions of like charge are repelled away from the surface. This results in the formation of an electrical double layer, made up of the charged particles. The charges influence the distribution of ions resulting in the formation of an electrical double layer, made up of the charged surface and a neutralizing excess of counter-ions over co-ions distributed in a diffuse manner in the aqueous medium resulting into electric potentials. Zeta potential, φ_z, is a measurable indication of the potential existing at the surface of a particle. Its magnitude may be measured using microelectrophoresis or any other of the electrokinetic phenomena. The two parts of the double layer are separated by a plane, the stern plane. The stern plane occurs at a hydrated ion radius from the particle surface. The ions or molecules to be strongly adsorbed at the surface-termed specific adsorption rather than by electrostatic attraction. The specifically adsorbed ion or molecule may be uncharged e.g., with non-ionic surfactant. Surfactants specifically adsorb by the hydrophobic effect and impart effect on the stern potential.

According to DLVO (Derjaguin Landau Verwey and Overbeek) theory, in a dispersed system the interactions involved between particles are electrical repulsion and Van der Walls attraction. The total potential energy of interaction is addition of these parameters. The attraction predominates at small distance between the particles and hence the potential energy curve shows very deep primary minimum (Figure 1). As the distance between the particles get larger, the repulsive forces predominate and result in the formation of positive potential energy. Another minimum in the potential energy is achieved when the interparticle distances are further increased (Figure 2). In this case, the fall-off in repulsive energy with distance is more rapid than that of attractive energy. If potential energy at the positive side is large as compared to thermal energy of the particles the system would be stable. Otherwise the interacting particles will reach the energy depth of the primary minimum and lead to irreversible aggregation. If the secondary minimum is smaller than thermal energy the particles will not aggregate but will always repel one another leading to the formation of a deflocculated system. But if it is significantly larger than thermal energy, a loose aggregate will form with the ease of redispersibility by shaking i.e., flocculation occurs. The charge between the particles can be modified using selected large molecules or surfactants. Thus, the particles can be suspended using stearic stabilization or charge stabilization (Figure 3)

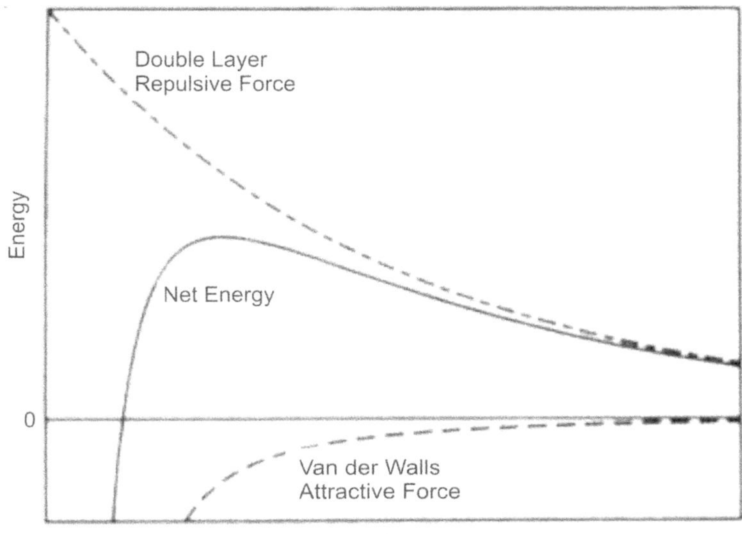

Figure 11.1 Schematic diagram of the variation of free energy with particle separation according to DLVO theory. The net energy is given by the sum of the double layer repulsion and the van der Waals attractive forces that the particles experience as they approach one another.

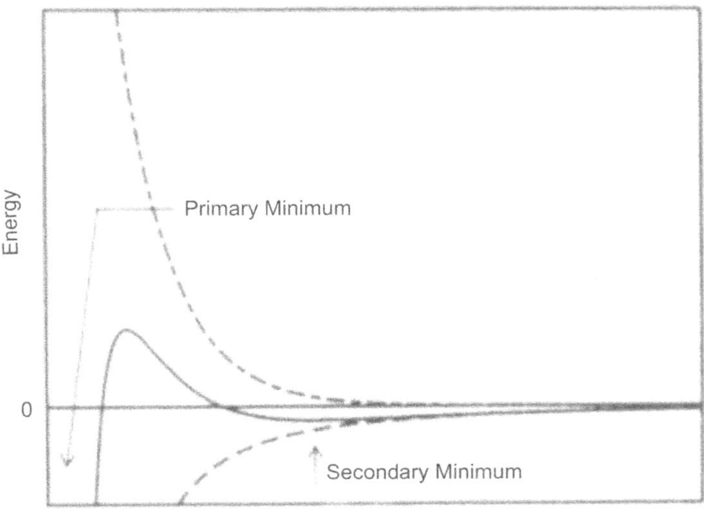

Figure 11.2 Schematic diagram of the variation of free energy with particle separation at higher salt concentrations showing the possibility of a secondary minimum.

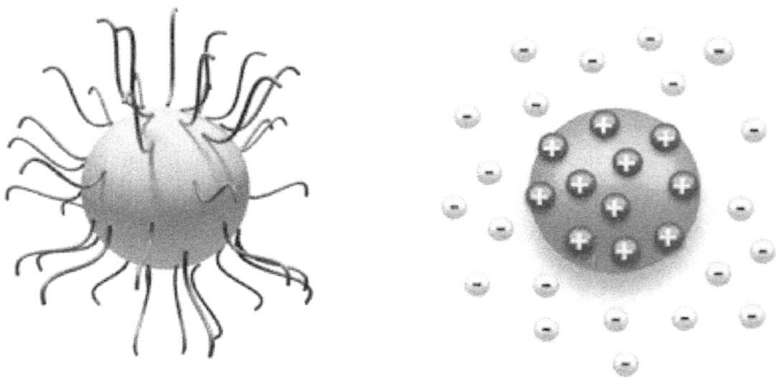

Figure 11.3 Types of colloidal stabilization.

In a deflocculated system containing a distribution of particle sizes, the larger particles naturally settle faster than the smaller particles. The very small particles remain suspended for a considerable length of time, with the result that no distinct boundary is formed between the supernatant and the sediment. Even when a sediment becomes discernible, the supernatant remains cloudy. When the same system is flocculated, two effects are immediately apparent. First, the flocs tend to fall together, so a distinct boundary between the sediment and the supernatant is readily observed; second the supernatant is clear, showing that the very fine particles have been incorporated into the flocs. The initial rate of settling in flocculated systems is determined by the size of the flocs and the porosity of the aggregated mass. Under these circumstances it is perhaps better to use the term subsidence, rather than sedimentation.

The other important issue is the settling of the dispersed material in the suspension. Those skilled in the art will recognize the fact that particle size of a specific particulate solid should be varied with the density of the particulate solid following the guidelines of Stokes' Law. Stoke's law relates the diameter of the particles, the density of the particle and the medium to the sedimentation rate:

$$dS/dt = d^2\,(\rho_p - \rho_M)g/18\eta$$

where dS/dt is the sedimentation rate,

d is the diameter of the particles,

ρ_p is the density of the particles,

ρ_M is the density of the medium,

g is the gravitational constant,

η is the viscosity of the medium.

Stokes equation was derived for an ideal situation with perfectly spherical particles in a very dilute suspension. It assumes the spherical particles settle without causing turbulence, without particle-to-particle collision and without chemical or physical attraction or affinity for the dispersion medium. Obviously, the typical pharmaceutical suspension contains particles which are irregularly shaped with a range of sizes, settling results in both turbulence and collision, and there is a reasonable affinity between the particles and suspension medium. However, the basic concepts of the equation offer an indication of the important variables for suspension of the particle and clues to formulation adjustments to decrease the rate of particle sedimentation. Thus, the influence of size, the viscosity of the medium and the density of the particle and the medium can be explained using the Stoke's equation.

The application of DLVO theory in the development of suspensions is described henceforth. The simple suspension involves the development of a uniform dispersion of deflocculated particles. After the size of the drug particles is reduced to the required, the dispersion in the aqueous medium is achieved. This is most often achieved with the help of surface-active agents. If wetting is needed, it is achieved appropriately as mentioned previously. After achieving a deflocculated suspension which most often results with the previous step, the formulation can be further tailored as per the requirement. Structured vehicles can be employed. Structured vehicles are generally aqueous solutions of polymeric materials, such as the hydrocolloids, that are usually negatively charged in aqueous solution. Typical examples are methylcellulose, carboxymethylcellulose, bentonite, and carbomer. The concentration employed will depend on the consistency desired for the suspension that, in turn, will relate to the size and density of the suspended particles. They function as viscosity-imparting suspending agents and, as such, reduce the rate of sedimentation of dispersed particles. Rheology of the suspensions is also an important issue to be considered. This is dealt in detail in standard textbooks.

Another interesting approach of developing suspensions is called controlled flocculation. When using the controlled flocculation approach, the formulator takes the deflocculated, wetted dispersion of particles and attempts to bring about flocculation by addition of a flocculating agent; most commonly, these are electrolytes, polymers or surfactants. The aim is to control flocculation by adding that amount of flocculating agent that results in the maximum sedimentation volume. Most of the times, a deflocculated suspension is an ideal and preferable suspension. However, often a drug is formulated as a flocculated suspension. The problems that arise when a drug is dispersed in a liquid include sedimentation, caking (leading to difficulty in resuspension), flocculation and particle growth (through dissolution and recrystallization). In practice the problems associated with aggregation are generally avoided. In many cases, lyophilization is practiced, so as to ensure redispersibility upon addition of water or other medium. There is also a problem of adhesion of drug to the walls of the container. This is especially true with low dose drugs. Although deflocculated suspension is most often preferred, some times flocculated suspensions are also considered. There are various states of flocculated and deflocculation. Unfortunately, the flocculated suspensions clear rapidly and the preparation often appears unsightly. The viscosity of the final formulation often depends on the floccules. In flocculated suspension, formed flocs will cause an increase in sedimentation rate due to increase in size of sedimenting particles. Hence, flocculated suspensions sediment more rapidly. Here, the sedimentation depends not only on the size of the flocs but also on the porosity of flocs. In flocculated suspensions the loose structure of the rapidly sedimenting flocs tends to preserve in the sediment which contain an appreciable amount of entrapped liquid. The volume of final sediment is thus relatively large and is easily redispersed by agitation. Use of flocculating agents result in the formation of flocs and thence flocculated suspensions. Controlled flocculation has also been used in the design of ophthalmic suspensions intended for the back of the eye. These formulations demonstrated additional benefits when compared to the existing formulations of the same drugs.

The sedimentation and the flocculation can be expressed quantitatively and can be further used in the formulation development. The first parameter is sedimentation volume and the second parameter is degree of flocculation. The sedimentation volume, F, is the ration of the equilibrium volume of the sediment, Vu, to the total volume of the suspension, Vo. Thus,

$$F = Vu/Vo$$

As the volume of suspension that appears occupied by the sediment increases, the value of F, which normally ranges from nearly 0 to 1, increases. In the systems, where F = 0.75 for example, 75% of the total volume in the container is apparently occupied by the loose, porous flocs forming the sediment. When F = 1, no sediment is apparent even though the system is flocculated. This is the ideal suspension for, under these conditions, no sedimentation will occur. Caking also will be absent. Furthermore, the suspension is esthetically pleasing, there being no visible, clear supernatant.

Flocculation is measured by a better parameter called as degree of flocculation, β, which relates the sedimentation volume of the flocculated suspension, F, to the sedimentation volume of the suspension when deflocculated, F_∞. It is expressed as

$$B = F/F_\infty$$

The degree of flocculation is therefore an expression of the increased sediment volume resulting from flocculation. If, for example, β has a value of 5.0, this means that the volume of sediment in the flocculated system is five times that in the deflocculated state. If a second flocculated formulation results in a value for β of say 6.5, this latter suspension obviously is preferred, if the aim is to produce as flocculated as possible. As the degree of flocculation in the system decreases, β approaches unity, the theoretical minimum value.

Powder Flow

Several pharmaceutical processes, including blending, transfer, storage, feeding, compaction and fluidization, involve powder handling. Although discussed for powders, the principles are the same for the flow of bulk solids-fine and coarse-such as dust, granulations and granules either as single substances or as multicomponent blends. The flow of powder during manufacturing dictates the quality of the product in terms of its weight and content uniformity. Flow also affects manufacturing efficiency, because it can determine whether bins can be used or hand scooping will be required, to what extent product (if any) is scrapped at the beginning or end of the run, and the allowable production rate of products (e.g., blend times and compression speeds). During formulation development, the flow of a blend may affect excipient selection and may dictate whether direct compression is used or some form of granulation is required. A full understanding of powder-flow behaviour is essential when addressing segregation problems. In extreme cases, the success or failure of a product is hinged on its flow behaviour during manufacturing. Given the importance of powder flow, the pharmaceutical industry still relies surprisingly heavily on flow properties that are poorly understood and applied.

A simple definition of powder flowability is the ability of powders to flow. By this definition, flowability is sometimes thought of as a one-dimensional characteristic of a powder, whereby powders can be ranked on a sliding scale from free flowing to non flowing. Unfortunately, this simplistic view lacks the science and understanding sufficient to address common problems encountered by the formulator and the equipment designer. Those who work with powder, whether in the lab or in production, quickly recognized that powder flow is complex. Flow behaviour is multidimensional and does in fact depend on many powder characteristics. For this reason no one test could ever quantify flowability. To address this multivariable problem, some suggest that all possible test values be considered; other porpose that these values be factored into a single flowability index. A more accurate definition of powder flowability is the ability of powder to flow in a desired manner in a specific piece of equipment. With this definition, the term free flowing, so commonly used, becomes meaningless unless the specific equipment handling the equipment is specified. The specific bulk characteristics and properties of a powder can affect flow and that can in principle be measured are known as flow properties. Examples of flow properties include density (compressibility), cohesive strength, and wall friction. These flow properties refer to the behavior of the bulk material and arise from the collective forces acting on individual particles (e.g., vander waals, electrostatic, surface tension, interlocking, friction.

The terms powder flow and powder flow properties should not be used synonymously. Powder flow is an observation and should refer to a description of how materials will flow (or did flow) in a given piece of equipment. Powder flow properties should refer to test results of the powder. Thus, when discussing or reporting flowabiltiy, one must include powder flow properties and handling equipment. Flowability is a factor for several processes in the pharmaceutical industry. These include:

1. Powder transfer
2. Powder storage
3. Separation of small quantity of powder from bulk
4. Blending
5. Compaction processes
6. Fluidization
7. Purely comparative, physical test methods to compare two powders.

For each of these applications, various types of handling equipment can be used. The flow behaviour of the same powder between applications may be quite different. For example, a powder that flows well through a bin may flow poorly at tablet press. In working with the technology available to industry today, each of the previously listed processes requires appropriate flow property tests to characterize and predict the actual flow behaviour within the equipment. Some of these tests are hence forth discussed.

Cohesive strength

By measuring the required shear force for various vertical loads, one can develop an relationship describing the cohesive strength of the powder as a function of the consolidating pressure. This relationship, known as a flow function, can be analyzed to determine the minimum outlet diameters for bins, press hoppers, blender outlets, etc. to prevent arching and ratholing. Other testing methodsuse the same principles of consolidation and shearing to determine the cohesive strength of the bulk powder. Annular (ring) shear testers product a rotational, rather a lateral, displacement between cell halves containing materials. Because of the unlimited travel that can be achieved with this type of test cell, the loading and shearing operations are more readily adopted to automation. Successful use of this test method to demonstrate differences in cohesive strength relating to handling characteristics has been discussed in industry.

Internal friction

Internal friction values are important when characterizing the flow properties of a powder. Such friction is caused by solid particles flowing against each other and is expressed as an angle of internal friction. This angle can be measured using cohesive strength tests mentioned previously.

Wall friction

Used in a continuum model, wall friction (particles sliding along a surface) is expressed as the wall friction angle or coefficient of sliding friction. The friction coefficient can be measured by sliding a sample of powder in a test cell across a stationary wall surface using a shear tester.

Bulk density

The bulk density of a given powder is not a single or dual value; rather it varies as a function of the applied consolidating pressure. Various methods can be used in industry to measure bulk density. These methods incorporate various-sized containers that are measured for volume after being loosely filled with a known mass of material and then measured again after vibration or tapping. USP24/NF 19 describes one frequently used approach for measuring the bulk (loose) and tapped density.

Permeability

The expansion of voids during flow can create air pressure gradients within the powder bed, resulting in flow-rate limitations when fine powders are handled. The permeability of powder controls the discharge rate that can be achieved. Permeability is measured as a function of bulk density. The method typically used involves measuring the flow rate of air at a specific pressure drop through a sample of known density and height. Once this relationship is determined, it can be used to calculate critical powder discharge rates tha will be achieved for steady-flow conditions through various orifice sizes.

Traditional Flow Property Tests

The most efficient means of measuring the effectivenss of a glidant in a powder blend is to compress the blend and determine weight variation. But this is an empirical model. Instead of theoretical models or detailed, complete, proven, empirical models to predict flow through a press feed frame, the industry relies on surrogate tests as indicators. Traditional tests are angle of repose, Carr indices,

Hausner ratio (the ratio of tapped to lose bulk density), minimum orifice diameter, and flow rate through a funnel. Shear cel and avalanche tests also are used, though less often. None of these small-scale tests simulate the state of aeration of powder before the feed frame nor th effects of the feed frame itself, both of which have a significant effect on the arching tendency and maximum flow rate of the powder. Most important none of these tests give a physical parameter directly linked to the flow at the press. Instead, it is hoped that flow-test result trends will correlate to tablet weight relative standard deviation (RSD), as may have been the case with a prior product or application. Arguably, tests for minimum orifice diameter and flow rate through a funnel seem more applicable for predicting th emaxium rate of compression because these measurements most closely simulate the need to fill a small die as fast as possible. However, rarely have published papers cited a strong correlation between any of these flow properties and weight variations during the creation of a dose.

Flow Properties as Comparitive Physical Test Methods

In many instances QC checks must be performed on powders to determine if certain attributes of the powder fall within a predefined range. These attributes include chemical composition, particle size, color, moisture and more often flow properties. QC checks can be made by a supplier before shipping raw materials, or by technicials for process control. The applicability of the flow property test highly depends on what the user is trying to capture. QC checks include angle of repose compressibility, Carr indices, the Johnson indicizer, flow funnels, minimum orifice diameter, dynamic angle of repose, or the Jenike & Johnson QC tester. Any flow property test could in principle be used as a QC test, and often the fastest, most convenient test is selected. This choice is acceptable, provided the user is aware of the test limitations. The different tests to measure the powder flow are clearly described in Remington.

Drug-Excipient Interactions

Although considered pharmacologically inert, excipients can initiate, propogate or participate inchemical or physical interactions with drug compounds, which may compromise the effectiveness of a medication. Excipients may also contain impurities or form degradation products that in turn cause decomposition of drug substances. Excipients are included in dosage forms to aid manufacture, administration or absorption. Other reasons for inclusion concern product differentiation, appearance enhancement or retention of quality. They rarely, if ever, possess pharmacological activity and are accordinly loosely categorized as inert. However, excipients can initiate, propogate or participate in chemical or physical interactions with an active, possibly leading to compromised quality or performance of the medication. Chemical interaction can lead to degradation of the active ingredient, thereby reducing the amount available for therapeutic effect; reaction products may compromise safety or tolerance. Physical interactions can affect rate of dissolution, uniformity of dose or ease of administration. Understanding the chemical and physical nature of excipients, the impurities or residues associated with them and how they may interact with other materials, or with each other fore warns the pharmaceutical technologist of possibilities for undesirable developments.

Excipients may have functional groups that interact directly with active pharmaceutical ingradients. Alternatively, they may contain impurities or residues or form degradation products that in turn cause decomposition of the drug substance. Excipients can be a source of microbial contamination. They can also cause unwanted effects such as irritation of skin or mucosal surfaces, sensitization reactions or adversely affect appearance or organoleptic properties. Excipients (like drug substances) are not exquisitively pure. In common with virtually all materials of mineral, synthetic, semi-synthetic or natural origin, manufacture involves using starting materials, reagents and solvents. Residues invariably remain after isolation. Low levels of residue can have a greater impact than might be expected, however, particularly where the ratio of excipient to drug is high, or where the residue has low molecular weight or acts as a catalyst. This is particularly true where an interaction product may pose safety questions and needs to be qualified by toxicology studies. Such complications often arise after mainstream safety studies have commenced, and can result in delayed or complicated programmes. Further, interaction between impurities/residues found in excipients and drug substances is another common source of incompatibilities. Peroxide impurities in povidone (binder) and crospovidone (disintegrant) have been identified as a source of degradation of an oestrogen receptor modulator, raloxifene. Table below illustrates how reactive chemical entities are commonplace in widely used excipients.

Excipient	Residue
Povidone, crospovidone, polysorbates	Peroxides
Magnesium stearate, fixed oils, lipids	Antioxidants
Lactose	Aldehydes, reducing sugards
Benzyl alcohol	Benzaldehyde
Polyethylene glycol	Aldehydes, peroxides, organic acids
Microcrystalline cellulose	Lignin, hemicullоses, water
Starch	Formaldehyde
Talc	Heavy metals
Dibasic calcium phosphate dehydrate	Alkaline residues
Stearate lubricants	Alkaline residues
Hydroxypropylmethyl/ethyl celluloses	Glyxol

Chemical interactions can result in the degradation of a medicament and thus reduce the fraction available for absorption. Different modes of drug decomposition exist. These are hydrolysis, oxidation, isomerization, photolyzation, polymerization. The modes of degradation of medicinal agents are tabulated below:

Hydrolysis	Oxidation	Isomerization	Photolysis	Polymerization
Methyl dopa	Calcitonin	Tetracycline	Riboflavin	Ceftazidime
Procaine	Ascorbic acid	Vitamin A	Folic acid	Ampicillin
Penicillin	Isoprenaline	Adrenaline	Nifedipine	

Direct interaction between actives and excipients is also a possibility. Excipients may b inorganic or organic in composition, synthetic or semi-synthetic or derived from biological or natural sources. Many possess functional groups that can interact with other materials. It may be possible on occasion to exploit such attributes to stability unstable materials, but more usually interactions lead to loss of quality. Different direct interactions include charge interactions, hydrogen-donating interactions, reactions with lactose, reactions with silicon dioxide.

Another type of interactions which commonly affect the quality of formulations is physical interactions. Some excipients are capable of adsorbing active ingradients to their surfaces and this has been used to enhance the surface area of drugs and optimize dissolution rate. Howeer, if forces of attraction are high, desorption may be retarded and absorption compromised. In a similar context, adsorption of a novel k-opoid agonist by microcrystalline cellulose led to incomplete drug release from capsules. Adsorption of finely divided excipients on to active ingradients can also occur and if such excipients are hydrophobic, dissolution rate and bioavailability may be retarded. Adsorption may also initiate chemical breakdown. Colloidal silica was shown to catalyze nitrazepam degradation in tablet dosage forms, possibly by adsorptive interactions altering the electron density in the vicinity of the labile azo group and thus facilitating attack by hydrolyysing entities. Although it is prudent to be aware of functional groups associated with drugs and excipients when considering possibilities for interaction, it must be stated that reaction on paper may not always occur in practice particularly in solid state. Many heterocyclic drugs contain amino groups. In accordance with the considerations above, lactose should be avoided as a formulation aid, but it is widely and successfully used in tablet and capsule dosage forms. Solution chemistry does not always translate to reactions in the solid state, particular in terms of rate of reaction, which may be the all-important consideration in a dosage form. Stereochemistry, local environment, degree of crystallinity or indeed drug-excipient ratio can mean that some potential interactions are more a problem in concept than reality.

Techniques to Measure Drug-Excipient Interactions

Several techniques are used to determine drug-excipient interactions. Currently, it is a common practice in pharmaceutical industry to first determine if an excipient is compatible and then use only those excipients that are compatible for drug. The assimilation of real-time stability and compatibility data is time-consuming and therefore it is desirable to obtain fast and reliable information about the possible interactions employing a suitable method. There is no universally accepted protocol for testing drug-excipient compatibility to date. Isothermal stress testing and thermal analysis of pharmaceutical substances are methods commonly used for this purpose. Differential scanning calorimetry (DSC) has been widely used as a rapid thermal method for assessing incompatibility between formulation components, since this method is fast, versatile and requires only milligrams of sample. Although a valuable technique, interpretation of DSC data can often be misleading. In most of the cases, interactions observed at accelerated temperatures may not occur at normal storage conditions. Also,m a solid-solid interaction does not necessarily indicate incompatibility, but might be beneficial in some cases. When two substances are mixed, the purity of each is reduced in the mixtures and DSC might not be able to discern a solid-solid interaction that is weak or non-existent. In isothermal stress testing, the binary mixtures of the drug and excipients in the presence or absence of moisture are exposed to high temperatures and drug content determined by a suitable analystical technique (mostly by HPLC). Other techniques such as differential thermal analysis (DTA) were previously used to study drug-excipient interaction. Other non-thermal methods that have been used to assess the drug/excpient interactions include infrared spectroscopy (IR), dissolution studies and X-ray diffraction.

Stability Testing

Stability testing is an important component of pharmaceutical product development. Once the formulation is developed, the stability of the drug in this formulation should be tested. The formulation can be any type of formulation. It could be final market formulation, or clinical trial formulation or toxicity supply formulation. Whenever there is any new formulation or change in an existing formula, the stability testing should be performed. The specifications may be different for different types of formulations. Different regulatory authorities have their own guidelines regarding stability testing. Different types of testing exist. Since most formulations are stored at room temperature over a period of time, the stability test should be conducted similar to their storage conditions. However, it may take long periods of time before a conclusion is drawn regarding the stability of a formulation. As a reason based on physical chemistry and chemical kinetic principles, accelerated stability testing has been developed. It should be known what happens to a drug when stored, and why we should we do stability testing for the formulations. Readers can refer other books for a knowledge on the fundamental principles of stability testing.

The purpose of stability testing is to provide evidence on how the quality of a drug substance or drug product varies with time under the influence of a variety of environmental factors such as temperature, humidity, and light, and to establish a re-test period for the drug substance or a shelf life for the drug product and recommended storage conditions. The choice of test conditions defined in this guideline is based on an analysis of the effects of climatic conditions in the three regions of the EC, Japan and the United States. The mean kinetic temperature in any part of the world can be derived from climatic data, and the world can be divided into four climatic zones, I-IV. Each of these climatic zones have their own guidelines.

One methodology to perform stability testing is illustrated below. As an example, a specific guidelines given by a regulatory authority (Nepal regulatory authority) are presented.

1. Accelerated stability testing on two batches should be conducted, one of which must be either commercial batch or a pilot-scale batch. A pilot batch should not be smaller than one eighth of the commercial batch. If accelerated stability testing was carried out on one laboratory batch, which was produced by similar manufacturing process and has the same composition of active ingredient/s and excipient/s as for the commercial batch, accelerated stability test on single commercial or pilot-scale batch should be acceptable. Accelerated stability testing should be done on 0, 3 and 6 months.
2. Initially real time stability testing should be conducted on two batches for the expected shelflife of the product, one of which should be commercial batch. One batch can be a pilot scale batch. Continuing real time stability study should be carried out on subsequent batches, as per the schedule and standard operating procedure approved by quality assurance department of the industry, taking into consideration any changes like equipment, process and source of raw material etc. Real time stability testing should be done on 0, 3, 6, 9 and 12 months on first year, every six-month on second year and once every year afterwards.
3. Stability testing should be conducted on the dosage form packaged in the container closure system proposed for marketing (including, as appropriate, any secondary packaging and container label).

4. Stability studies should include testing of those attributes of the pharmaceutical product that are susceptible to change during storage and are likely to influence quality, safety, and efficacy. The testing should cover, as appropriate, the physical, chemical, biological and microbiological attributes, preservative content (e.g. antioxidant, antimicrobial preservative). Analytical procedures should be fully validated and stability indicating.
5. One initial batch of the pharmaceutical product should be tested for antimicrobial preservative effectiveness (in addition to preservative content) at the proposed shelf-life for verification purposes.
6. If significant change occurs between three and six months' testing at the accelerated storage condition, the proposed shelf-life should be based on the real-time data available from the long- term storage condition.

   In general, "significant change" for a pharmaceutical product is defined as:

   (a) A 5% change in assay from its initial value, or failure to meet the acceptance criteria for potency when using biological or immunological procedures.

   (b) Any degradation product exceeding its acceptance criterion.

   (c) Failure to meet the acceptance criteria for appearance and physical attributes (e.g. colour, phase separation, re-suspendibility, caking, hardness). However, some changes in physical attributes (e.g. softening of suppositories, melting of creams, partial loss of adhesion for transdermal products) may be expected under accelerated conditions.

   (d) Failure to meet the acceptance criterion for pH (for liquid preparation).

   (e) Failure to meet the acceptance criteria for dissolution for 12 dosage units (tablet and capsule).
7. Stability studies for products stored in impermeable containers can be conducted under any controlled or ambient humidity condition.
8. If no significant change occurs during six-month's accelerated and real time stability testing, the product will be allowed to place in the market with a provisional shelf-life of up to twenty-four months. However, real time stability testing should be continued up to the proposed shelf-life. The manufacturer should have a system of recall in place so that the sale any batch which does not remain within the limit of approved product specification be stopped within twenty-four hours.

Expiry Date

The date given on the individual container (usually on the label) of a product up to and including which the product is expected to remain within specifications, if stored correctly. It is established for each batch by adding the shelf-life to the date of manufacture.

Once the pharmaceutical product has been registered, additional stability studies are required whenever variations that may affect the stability of the active pharmaceutical substance or pharmaceutical product are made, such as major variations like the following:

(a) Change in the manufacturing process.

(b) Change in the composition of the pharmaceutical product.

(c) Change of the immediate packaging.

9. The ongoing stability programme should be described in a written protocol, and results formalized as a report.
10. Condition of Climatic zone IV A will be applicable for Nepal, though the WHO document mentions Climatic Zone II. Condition for real time stability testing: 30°C ± 2°C/65% RH ± 5% RH; condition for accelerated stability testing: 40°C ± 2°C/75% RH ± 5% RH.

Parameters for stability testing

The following list of parameters for each dosage form is presented as a guide for the types of tests to be included in a stability study. In general, - appearance, - assay and - degradation products should be evaluated for all dosage forms, as well as preservative and antioxidant content if applicable. The microbial quality of multiple-dose sterile and non-sterile dosage forms should be controlled. Challenge tests should be carried out at least at the beginning and at the end of the shelf-life.The list of tests presented for each dosage form is not intended to be exhaustive, nor is it expected that every listed test be included in the design of a stability protocol for a particular pharmaceutical product (for example, a test for odour should be performed only when necessary and with consideration for the analyst's safety).

1. Tablets

   Dissolution (or disintegration, if justified), water content and hardness/ friability. For coated and coloure tablets aditional tests may require for texture and colour stability.

2. Capsules

   Hard gelatin capsules: brittleness, dissolution (or disintegration, if justified), water content, and level of microbial contamination.

3. Emulsions

   Phase separation, pH, viscosity, level of microbibial contamination, and mean size and distribution of dispersed globules.

4. Oral solutions and suspensions

   Formation of precipitate, clarity for solutions, pH, viscosity, extractables, level of microbial contamination. Additionally for suspensions, redispersibility, rheological properties, mean size and distribution of particles should be considered. Also, polymorphic conversion may be examined, if applicable.

5. Powders and granules for oral solution or suspension

   Water content, and reconstitution time. Reconstituted products (solutions and suspensions) should be evaluated as described in "Oral solutions and suspensions" above, after preparation according to the recommended labelling, through the maximum intended use period.

Minimum requirement for applying for the marketing approval of the product of one regulatory agency (to provide a sample)

1. Accelerated stability test result for at least one commercial batch, or pilot-scale batch intended to be placed in the market and produced using the same equipment and process approved for commercial batch. Accelerated stability testing should be done on 0, 3 and 6 months.
2. Real time stability study reports for 0, 3 and 6 month for the same batch for which accelerated stability testing is carried out.
3. Real time and acclerated stability test report should be self-explanatory and conclusion should be mentioned on the report.
4. Report of analysis from National Medicines Laboratory for the same batch for which accelerated stability report is being submitted.

State of Art stability Testing Conditions as per the ICH Guidelines

Different storage conditions are prescribed according to ICH guidelines. These include:

- 25°C/60% RH
- 30°C/65% RH
- 40°C/75% RH
- 25°C/40% RH
- 40°C/25% RH
- 25°C

- 60°C
- Refrigerator, 5°C
- Freezer, -20°C
- Freezer, -30°C
- Ultimate freezer, -70°C
- Photostability chamber – supports ICH
- photostability option II

Current Methodology in Stability Testing

Stability testing can be generally performed in the company itself in stability chambers. As there is a need for stability testing on various occasions, it is better to perform stability testing in the same company where the product is being developed. However, stability testing is also performed as an outsourcing job. This is specially advantageous as the company do not need to have a special stability testing department in the company. Further, as there are different types of products that need stability data, the huge burden of this exercise can be simply avoided using outsourcing companies.

Outsourcing testing facilities provide full stability testing and support services for all types of drug products, ranging from API, small molecules to biopharmaceutical drug products and drug-coated medical devices. The different services that they provide include:

- Stability protocol generation
- Stability testing
- Sample storage
- Stability data trending analysis
- Stability report generation
- Statistical analysis for shelf life confirmation

The different studies associated with stability testing that they can perform include:

- Preclinical stability
- Clinical stability
- Stability indicating method development
- Release testing
- Method transfer and analyst qualification
- Assay and impurities of various formulation

Accelerated Stability Testing

Studies designed to increase the rate of chemical degradation or physical change of a drug substance or drug product by using exaggerated storage conditions as part of the formal stability studies. Data from these studies, in addition to long term stability studies, can be used to assess longer term chemical effects at non-accelerated conditions and to evaluate the effect of short term excursions outside the label storage conditions such as might occur during shipping. Results from accelerated testing studies are not always predictive of physical changes.

Pharmaceutical Plant Design and Manufacture

Planning for new manufacturing capacity in the pharmaceutical industry is notoriously difficult. New potential blockbuster compounds are discovered that are predicted to have a big future yet can fail at the last hurdle. Thus, after considerable investment of both time and money in developing and testing many new chemical entities and medicinal products, some will reach the stage where there is a requirement for the manufacture of the product on a large scale. Older products coming 'off patent' may unexpectedly get a new lease of life meaning that existing production capacity has to be increased. Consequently many production facilities are built as multi-product or general purpose manufacturing units to cater for the wide variety of compounds, processing characteristics and volumes required. Now a days generic products are becoming popular both in Western countries as well as Eastern countries. Countries like India and China are popularly known for their generic product portfolio. Pharmaceutical manufacturing whether for new drugs or for generic products require considerable capital expenditure and are likey to be used for many years. It is necessary therefore to think very carefully about where the facility is located as well how it is constructed. One important consideration is whether the company should develop a new site or refurbish an existing one. In case of countries like India where generic products are the heart of pharma industry, in every likely the same principles hold true as is the case for product development of new drugs. Once the plant is developed, say for example, for liquid orals, for tablets, for capsules, for sustained release oral dosage forms for one particular drug, the same plant can be used for several drugs after carefully cleaning and washing the existing instruments. However, the plant has to be separate for these individual dosage forms. Upgrading or redesigning an existing site may often be a more cost-effective option but may not be always feasible. For example, there may be insufficient space to expand an existing site or it may be out dated and not suitable for upgrading. The company may also introduce a product type where there is no existing plant or the existing site may not be a suitable location.

Further, the location should be based on labour costs and availability, energy and construction costs,l environment legislation, likely opposition from local residents and local employment legislation (particularly for foreign companies). The chosen location must also have an acceptable local infrastructure including suitable road and air links, services such as electricity and water and availability of suitably qualified work force.

Different Types of Pharmaceutical Formulation Products

Before proceeding further, it is important that readers get an idea about different types of pharmaceutical formulation products. There are basically two types of products. The first is the formulation for the innovator drugs. Innovator has exclusivity period of ten years as per the current standards. Once this period is over, any company that is capable of producing and selling an equivalent product can do so. These types of products are called generic products.

A **generic drug** (generic drugs, short: generics) is a drug defined as "a drug product that is comparable to brand/reference listed drug product in dosage form, strength, route of administration, quality and performance characteristics, and intended use. It has also been defined as a term referring to any drug marketed under its chemical name without advertising.

Although they may not be associated with a particular company, generic drugs are subject to the regulations of the governments of countries where they are dispensed. Generic drugs are labelled with the name of the manufacturer and the adopted name (nonproprietary name) of the drug.

A generic drug must contain the same active ingredients as the original formulation. According to the U.S. Food and Drug Administration (FDA), generic drugs are identical or within an acceptable bioequivalent range to the brand-name counterpart with respect to pharmacokinetic and pharmacodynamic properties. By extension, therefore, generics are considered (by the FDA) identical in dose, strength, route of administration, safety, efficacy, and intended use. The FDA's use of the word "identical" is very much a legal interpretation, and is not literal. In most cases, generic products are available once the patent protections afforded to the original developer have expired. When generic products become available, the market competition often leads to substantially lower prices for both the original brand name product and the generic forms. The time it takes a generic drug to appear on the market varies. In the US, drug patents give 20 years of protection, but they are applied for before clinical trials begin, so the "effective" life of a drug patent tends to be between seven and 12 years. Prescriptions may be issued for drugs specifying only the chemical name, rather than a manufacturer's name; such a prescription can be filled with a drug of any brand meeting the specification. For example, a prescription for lansoprazole can be filled with generic lansoprazole, Prevacid, Helicid, Zoton, Inhibitol, or Monzlitum.

Site Master Planning

Despite the high-tech image of pharmaceutical facilities, many of today's manufacturing plants are over 20 years old and have developed in an unstructured manner. Support services often will have been provided individually on a project-by-project basis where with hindsight a more holistic approach would have been more cost-effective. Time pressures on new projects may have resulted in new facilities being located in the most convenient position rather than the best location for the overall site development.

Consequently many companies have identified the need for a more structured planning approach to their future site developments, involving:

- rationalisation of existing site facilities
- reduction in operating costs in support services
- surveying and census of newly acquired facilities
- upgrading for GMP, EHS or to incorporate new technologies
- improvements in flows and departmental relationships

Each pharmaceutical company understands its own business better than any other organisation and in this respect the site master plan is best undertaken by the company's own resource. However an external services provider can often add value by:

- bringing an independent and objective approach
- providing census techniques, questionnaires and workshops
- providing industry benchmarking
- offering specialist knowledge in key technology areas
- providing resources to enable the study

Pharmaceutical Plant Layout

Once the product is identified, it is set to manufacture. Before going further about the concepts of the manufacture, it is essential to know about plant layout. There are several possibilities for plant lay out. Depending on the convenience a specific layout can be designed. An example of plant layout is presented here for the convenience of the reader. There should be different areas to do different operations. It is shown in the figure below. Further, if there is a consideration for a big pharmaceutical company there could be various buildings including research center where products are developed, quality control area, and production area. The products that are developed in a small scale are generally developed in a research center. The scale up of these batches will be initiated and finally production batches are developed. This whole exercise is termed as technology transfer.

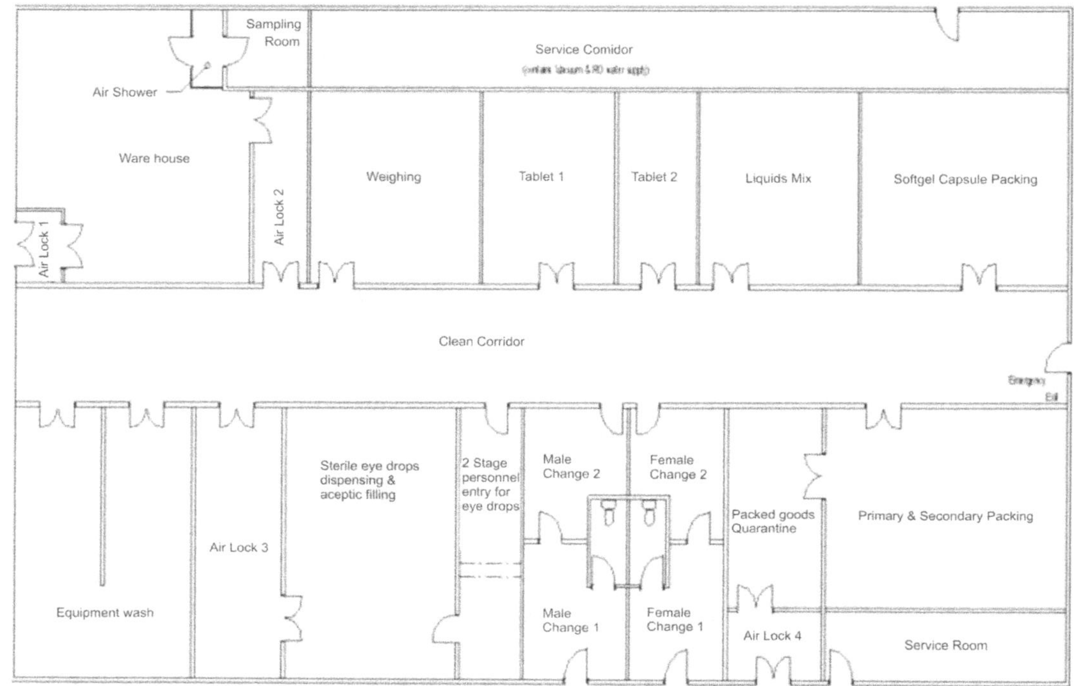

Typical Plant Layout.

Process Design

Once a formulation for a new candidate active compound has been identified or a generic product has been identified, a pharmaceutical company sets out to develop the manufacturing process. Almost without exception this results in the generation of a batch process though it is well understood that continuous processes are more efficient and cost only a fraction of the equivalent batch process. Good Manufacturing Practices (GMPs) have to be followed. Especially, guidelines for specific markets are given (More information is provided in chapter on GMPs). Speed-to-market and concerns over validation of the process have meant that a pharmaceutical company's approach to process development is conservative. Process Validation is important at this stage. More discussion on process validation is provided in the chapter entitled Process Validation. From a process engineer's point of view, it seems that the end result of a huge amount of engineering effort simply produces a scaled-up version of the laboratory plant. Pharmaceutical manufacturing processes are typically developed by a team of chemists, each of whom are individually responsible for small parts of the overall process and typically use simple laboratory glassware and equipment. Recently, however, operators are questioning why they constrain the kinetics, thermodynamics and fluid mechanics of pharmaceutical processes to the limited confines of a stirred tank. This is where the experienced process contractor, if involved early enough, can add value to the process development process. Analysed in a methodical manner, the specific characteristics of each process become evident and alternative processing methods then identified. One of the best methods available has been developed by Britest Ltd., a not-for-profit company founded in 1998, whose members include AstraZeneca, GlaxoSmithKline and Foster Wheeler. Britest's objective is to deliver major competitive benefits o chemical and pharmaceutical companies by designing the best processes and manufacturing strategy for each member, using a set of proprietary tools, known as the Britest tools. Utilising Britest methodology encourages the user to develop a greater understanding of the process as a whole, resulting in radically different options being considered. The Britest tools are a time-effective way of starting the development process and determining all the potential (and unfeasible) process options.

Metallurgy in Pharmaceutical Manufacturing

Metals are used in pharmaceutical manufacturing at various levels. All the utensils and manufacturing vessels are generally made up of metals. They are intended to be used for several years. Thus, proper case has to be taken. Also the life of the equipment should be as much as possible. Also, the metals should not contaminate the products. Further, now a day it is also important to consider the metallurgy of the entire building. Climate sensitive pharmaceutical manufacturing facility should be considered. Anyone involved in the design or construction of a climate-sensitive pharmaceutical manufacturing facility should consider the inherent benefits of exterior wall systems featuring insulated metal panels. With their exceptional thermal performance, these panels offer the highest insulating value per inch of any wall-insulating product on the market, resulting in significantly lower energy and operating costs.These wall systems also provide uniform insulating performance because the shape and thickness of the insulating material is maintained between two metal skins. In addition, tongue and groove installation ensures that the entire wall area is covered with insulation. Thus, these types of developing in the pharmaceutical manufacturing facility are important.

Good Manufacturing Practices

"**Good manufacturing practice**" or "**GMP**" are practices and the systems required to be adapted in pharmaceutical manufacturing, quality control, quality system covering the manufacture and testing of pharmaceuticals or drugs including active pharmaceutical ingredients and their formulations. These practices have tremendous impact on the quality of a product. Several countries have their own guidelines. Recently, these guidelines have been harmonized to meet international standards. Manufacturers are bound to legally follow these rules. Basic concepts of all of these guidelines remain more or less similar to the ultimate goals of safeguarding the health of the patient as well as producing good quality medicine. It is very interesting that the rules are very strict in some countries. For instance, in the U.S. a drug may be deemed adulterated if it passes all of the specifications tests but is found to be manufactured in a condition which violates current good manufacturing guidelines. Therefore, complying with GMP is a mandatory aspect in pharmaceutical manufacturing. The basic principles of GMPs are:

1. Manufacturing processes are clearly defined and controlled. All critical processes are validated to ensure consistency and compliance with specifications.
2. Manufacturing processes are controlled, and any changes to the process are evaluated. Changes that have an impact on the quality of the drug are validated as necessary.
3. Instructions and procedures are written in clear and unambiguous language. (Good Documentation Practices)
4. Operators are trained to carry out and document procedures.
5. Records are made, manually or by instruments, during manufacture that demonstrate that all the steps required by the defined procedures and instructions were in fact taken and that the quantity and quality of the drug was as expected. Deviations are investigated and documented.
6. Records of manufacture (including distribution) that enable the complete history of a batch to be traced are retained in a comprehensible and accessible form.
7. The distribution of the drugs minimizes any risk to their quality.
8. A system is available for recalling any batch of drug from sale or supply.
9. Complaints about marketed drugs are examined, the causes of quality defects are investigated, and appropriate measures are taken with respect to the defective drugs and to prevent recurrence.

GMP guidelines are not prescriptive instructions on how to manufacture products. They are a series of general principles that must be observed during manufacturing. When a company is setting up its quality program and manufacturing process, there may be many ways it can fulfill GMP requirements. It is the company's responsibility to determine the most effective and efficient quality process. Some of the principles related to GMP are presented in this chapter.

Different Types of Guidelines

There are several guidelines given by several organizations or regulatory bodies. Although these seem to be same, there is a variation among them. Also, these guidelines are amended from time to time.

GMPs are enforced in the United States by the US FDA, under Section 501(B) of the 1938 Food, Drug, and Cosmetic Act (21USC351). The regulations use the phrase "current good manufacturing practices" (cGMP) to describe these guidelines. Courts may theoretically hold that a drug product is adulterated even if there is no specific regulatory requirement that was violated as long as the process was not performed according to industry standards. The World Health Organization (WHO) has its own version of GMP guidelines. These are followed mostly by developing countries. European union also has its own guidelines. Similar GMPs are used in other countries, with Australia, Canada, Japan, Singapore and others having highly developed/sophisticated GMP requirements. In the United Kingdom, the Medicines Act (1968) covers most aspects of GMP in what is commonly referred to as "The Orange Guide", which is named so because of the color of its cover; it is officially known as Rules and Guidance for Pharmaceutical Manufacturers and Distributors. ICH (International Conference on Harmonization) guidelines have been released since 1999. All those countries signatories to ICH follow these guidelines. Guidelines exist both for manufacturing and testing of active raw material.

Enforcement

In European Union, GMP inspections are performed by National Regulatory Agencies (e.g., GMP inspections are performed in the United Kingdom by the Medicines and Healthcare products Regulatory Agency (MHRA)). The pharmaceutical companies in Republic of Korea (South Korea) are legislated by by the Korea Food & Drug Administration (KFDA). In Australia by the Therapeutical Goods Administration (TGA); in South Africa by the Medicines Control Council (MCC); in Brazil by the Agência Nacional de Vigilância Sanitária (National Health Surveillance Agency Brazil) (ANVISA); in Iran, in India GMP inspections are carried out by state FDA and these FDA report to Central Drugs

Standard Control Organization and Pakistan by the Ministry of Health;, Nigeri has NAFDAC and by similar national organisations worldwide. Each of the inspectorates carry out routine GMP inspections to ensure that drug products are produced safely and correctly; additionally, many countries perform pre-approval inspections (PAI) for GMP compliance prior to the approval of a new drug for marketing. Regulatory agencies (including the FDA in the U.S. and regulatory agencies in many European nations) are authorized to conduct unannounced inspections, though some are scheduled. FDA routine domestic inspections are usually unannounced, but must be conducted according to 704(A) of the FD&C Act (21USC374), which requires that they are performed at a "reasonable time". Courts have held that any time the firm is open for business is a reasonable time for an inspection.

Quality Management and Role of the Manufacturer

The manufacturer must assume responsibility for the quality of the pharmaceutical products to ensure that they are fit for their intended use, comply with the requirements of the marketing authorization and do not place patients at risk due to inadequate safety, quality or efficacy. The attainment of this quality objective is the responsibility of senior management and requires the participation and commitment of staff in many different departments and at all levels within the company, the company's suppliers, and the distributors. To achieve the quality objective reliably there must be a comprehensively designed and correctly implemented system of quality assurance incorporating GMP and quality control. It should be fully documented and its effectiveness monitored. All parts of the quality assurance system should be adequately staffed with competent personnel, and should have suitable and sufficient premises, equipment, and facilities.

General GMP Guidelines

Good manufacturing practice is that part of quality assurance which ensures that products are consistently produced and controlled to the quality standards appropriate to their intended use and as required by the marketing authorization. GMP are aimed primarily at diminishing the risks inherent in any pharmaceutical production. Such risks are essentially of two types: cross-contamination (in particular of unexpected contaminants) and mix-ups (confusion) caused by, for example, false labels being put on containers. Under GMP:

1. all manufacturing processes are clearly defined, systematically reviewed in the light of experience, and shown to be capable of consistently manufacturing pharmaceutical products of the required quality that comply with their specifications;
2. qualification and validation are performed;

3. all necessary resources are provided, including:
    (i) appropriately qualified and trained personnel;
    (ii) adequate premises and space;
    (iii) suitable equipment and services;
    (iv) appropriate materials, containers and labels;
    (v) approved procedures and instructions;
    (vi) suitable storage and transport;
    (vii) adequate personnel, laboratories and equipment for inprocess
    (viii) controls;
4. instructions and procedures are written in clear and unambiguous language, specifically applicable to the facilities provided;
5. operators are trained to carry out procedures correctly;
6. records are made (manually and/or by recording instruments) during manufacture to show that all the steps required by the defined procedures and instructions have in fact been taken and that the quantity and quality of the product are as expected; any significant deviations are fully recorded and investigated;
7. records covering manufacture and distribution, which enable the complete history of a batch to be traced, are retained in a comprehensible and accessible form;
8. the proper storage and distribution of the products minimizes any risk to their quality;
9. a system is available to recall any batch of product from sale or supply;
10. complaints about marketed products are examined, the causes of quality defects investigated, and appropriate measures taken in respect of the defective products to prevent recurrence.

Thus, the essential features of GMPS includes the guidelines for the following listed below. Guidelines are not provided for all the essential features here and could be obtained from WHO documents. The listed features are:

1. Sanitation and hygiene
2. Qualification and validation
3. Complaints
4. Product recalls
5. Contract production and analysis
6. Self-inspection and quality audits

7. Personnel
8. Training
9. Personal hygiene
10. Premises
11. Equipment
12. Materials
13. Documentation
14. Good practices in production
15. Good practices in quality control

The WHO guidelines for one essential feature of GMP will be illustrated below by taking Good Practices in Production as the Example

Good Practices in Production

1. *Principle*. Production operations must follow clearly defined procedures in accordance with manufacturing and marketing authorizations, with the objective of obtaining products of the requisite quality.
2. All handling of materials and products, such as receipt and cleaning, quarantine, sampling, storage, labelling, dispensing, processing, packaging and distribution should be done in accordance with written procedures or instructions and, where necessary, recorded.
3. Any deviation from instructions or procedures should be avoided as far as possible. If deviations occur, they should be done in accordance with an approved procedure. The authorization of the deviation should be approved in writing by a designated person, with the involvement of the quality control department, when appropriate.
4. Checks on yields and reconciliation of quantities should be carried out as necessary to ensure that there are no discrepancies outside acceptable limits.
5. Operations on different products should not be carried out simultaneously or consecutively in the same room or area unless there is no risk of mix-up or cross-contamination.
6. At all times during processing, all materials, bulk containers, major items of equipment, and where appropriate, the rooms and packaging lines being used should be labelled or otherwise identified with an indication of the product or material being processed, its strength (where applicable) and the

batch number. Where applicable, this indication should also mention the stage of production. In some cases it may be useful to record also the name of the previous product that has been processed.

7. Access to production premises should be restricted to authorized personnel.
8. Normally, non-medicinal products should not be produced in areas or with equipment destined for the production of pharmaceutical products.
9. In-process controls are usually performed within the production area. The performance of such in-process controls should not have any negative effect on the quality of the product or another product (e.g. cross-contamination or mix-up).
10. When dry materials and products are used in production, special precautions should be taken to prevent the generation and dissemination of dust. Provision should be made for proper air control (e.g. supply and extraction of air of suitable quality).
11. Contamination of a starting material or of a product by another material or product must be avoided. This risk of accidental crosscontamination arises from the uncontrolled release of dust, gases, particles, vapours, sprays or organisms from materials and products in process, from residues on equipment, from intruding insects, and from operators' clothing, skin, etc. The significance of this risk varies with the type of contaminant and of the product being contaminated. Among the most hazardous contaminants are highly sensitizing materials, biological preparations such as living organisms, certain hormones, cytotoxic substances, and other highly active materials. Products in which contamination is likely to be most significant are those administered by injection or applied to open wounds and those given in large doses and/or over a long time.
12. Cross-contamination should be avoided by taking appropriate technical or organizational measures, for example:
    - (i) carrying out production in dedicated and self-contained areas (which may be required for products such as penicillins, live vaccines, live bacterial preparations and certain other biologicals);
    - (ii) conducting campaign production (separation in time) followed by appropriate cleaning in accordance with a validated cleaning procedure;
    - (iii) providing appropriately designed airlocks, pressure differentials, and air supply and extraction systems;

(iv) minimizing the risk of contamination caused by recirculation or re-entry of untreated or insufficiently treated air;

(v) wearing protective clothing where products or materials are handled;

(vi) using cleaning and decontamination procedures of known effectiveness;

(vii) using a "closed system" in production;

(viii) testing for residues;

(ix) using cleanliness status labels on equipment.

13. Measures to prevent cross-contamination and their effectiveness should be checked periodically according to standard operating procedures.
14. Production areas where susceptible products are processed should undergo periodic environmental monitoring (e.g. for microbiological monitoring and particulate matter where appropriate).
15. Before any processing operation is started, steps should be taken to ensure that the work area and equipment are clean and free from any starting materials, products, product residues, labels or documents not required for the current operation.
16. Any necessary in-process controls and environmental controls should be carried out and recorded.
17. Means should be instituted of indicating failures of equipment or of services (e.g. water, gas) to equipment. Defective equipment should be withdrawn from use until the defect has been rectified. After use, production equipment should be cleaned without delay according to detailed written procedures and stored under clean and dry conditions in a separate area or in a manner that will prevent contamination.
18. Time limits for storage of eqiupment after cleaning and before use should be stated and based on data.
19. Containers for filling should be cleaned before filling. Attention should be given to avoiding and removing any contaminants such as glass fragments and metal particles.
20. Any significant deviation from the expected yield should be recorded and investigated.
21. Checks should be carried out to ensure that pipelines and other pieces of equipment used for the transportation of products from one area to another are connected in a correct manner.

22. Pipes used for conveying distilled or deionized water and, where appropriate, other water pipes should be sanitized and stored according to written procedures that detail the action limits for microbiological contamination and the measures to be taken.
23. Measuring, weighing, recording, and control equipment and instruments should be serviced and calibrated at prespecified intervals and records maintained. To ensure satisfactory functioning, instruments should be checked daily or prior to use for performing analytical tests. The date of calibration and servicing and the date when recalibration is due should be clearly indicated, preferably on a label attached to the instrument.
24. Repair and maintenance operations should not present any hazard to the quality of the products.
25. When the programme for packaging operations is being set up, particular attention should be given to minimizing the risk of crosscontamination, mix-ups or substitutions. Different products should not be packaged in close proximity unless there is physical segregation or an alternative system that will provide equal assurance.
26. Before packaging operations are begun, steps should be taken to ensure that the work area, packaging lines, printing machines and other equipment are clean and free from any products, materials or documents used previously and which are not required for the current operation. The line clearance should be performed according to an appropriate procedure and checklist, and recorded.
27. The name and batch number of the product being handled should be displayed at each packaging station or line.
28. Normally, filling and sealing should be followed as quickly as possible by labelling. If labelling is delayed, appropriate procedures should be applied to ensure that no mix-ups or mislabelling can occur.
29. The correct performance of any printing (e.g. of code numbers or expiry dates) done separately or in the course of the packaging should be checked and recorded. Attention should be paid to printing by hand, which should be rechecked at regular intervals.
30. Special care should be taken when cut labels are used and when overprinting is carried out off-line, and in hand-packaging operations. Roll-feed labels are normally preferable to cut labels in helping to avoid mix-ups. On-line verification of all labels by automated electronic means can be helpful in preventing mix-ups, but checks should be made to ensure that

any electronic code readers, label counters, or similar devices are operating correctly. When labels are attached manually, in-process control checks should be performed more frequently.

31. Printed and embossed information on packaging materials should be distinct and resistant to fading or erasing.
32. Regular on-line control of the product during packaging should include at least checks on:
    (a) the general appearance of the packages;
    (b) whether the packages are complete;
    (c) whether the correct products and packaging materials are used;
    (d) whether any overprinting is correct;
    (e) the correct functioning of line monitors.

    Samples taken away from the packaging line should not be returned.
33. Products that have been involved in an unusual event during packaging should be reintroduced into the process only after special inspection, investigation and approval by authorized personnel. A detailed record should be kept of this operation.
34. Any significant or unusual discrepancy observed during reconciliation of the amount of bulk product and printed packaging materials and the number of units produced should be investigated, satisfactorily accounted for, and recorded before release.
35. Upon completion of a packaging operation, any unused batchcoded packaging materials should be destroyed and the destruction recorded. A documented procedure requiring checks to be performed before returning unused materials should be followed if uncoded printed materials are returned to stock.

Conclusions

As if any development the role of innovation and reproducing are very important, the same was the role of the progressive development of conventional dosage forms in the development of the current formulation technology. From simple liquids and powders, the conventional dosage forms have developed into very advanced solid dosage forms. These advances could be clearly visioned from the market survey`s or the market outlook's. Some of the principles of these conventional oral dosage forms are discussed in this chapter. Other principles could be clearly visioned from the literature.

Novel drug delivery systems are the means of enhancing the therapeutic benefit of a drug. The efficacy of the medicament can have an immense effect by the method by which it is delivered. For some drugs optimum concentration range within which maximum benefit is obtained and minimum toxicity is produced is desirable. On the other hand, there are drugs which need to be effective for slowly developing diseases. These drugs are targeted by every day administration of drugs. If the halflife of the agents is very low, it could be trouble some to take 3 pills 3 times a day. In these situations, developing a novel drug delivery system which could deliver the drug appropriately by the way of taking only one pill per day is of immense benefit. Further, there are diseases that need the drugs to be delivered exactly at the site of the disease. From this, new ideas on controlling the pharmacokinetics, pharmacodynamics, non-specific toxicity, immunogenicity, biorecognition, and efficacy of drugs were generated. These new strategies, often called drug delivery systems (DDS), are based on interdisciplinary approaches that combine polymer science, pharmaceutics, bioconjugate chemistry, and molecular biology.

Once a formulation is developed in a laboratory, technology transfer is initiated. Technology transfer mainly deals with scale up of pilot batches to production batches. Production has to be performed in GMP compliant environment if a license to sell the product in the market. Depending on the market, the GMP guidelines vary. However, GMP guidelines are generally the same for all the agencies. However, changes do exist. As a result specific GMP has to be passed to get approval in that part of the world. In this chapter some general guidelines given by experts from WHO and are called WHO Expert Committee on Specifications for Pharmaceutical Products. These guidelines are generally being followed in developing countries like India.

This section covered the essential features used in the development and manufacture of oral formulations.

Questions for Practice and Exercise

1. What are the general disadvantages associated with some salts used for salt screening? Explain the disadvantages associated with hydrochloric acid salts? Infact this salt is very often found in the market, on contrary. Explain in terms of solution dosage forms.
2. What are the different techniques to improve the solubility of drugs?
3. Describe suspensions as liquid orals. What are nanosuspensions?
4. What are dry powdered suspensions?

5. Elaborate nanosuspensions. Explain its formulation and manufacture with suitable examples.
6. Describe emulsions as liquid orals.
7. Write in detail as it is from this chapter on "Syrups".
8. Mention, "manufacture of liquid orals?
9. Explain how powders transformed to granules and then to tablets.
10. Explain "mixing' as a unit chemical engineering process.
11. List and describe briefly all the mixers used in the manufacture of pharmaceutical solids used for oral administration.
12. Briefly describe granulation.
13. Write a brief note on granulation.
14. Describe (a) tablets, (b) capsules, (c) pellets, and (d) triturates.
15. Write a note on the manufacture of solid dosage forms and the quality control methods employed for these dosage forms (focus on tablet technology). Mention about latest trends in the tablet manufacture and tablet coating process.
16. Write a note on oral sustained release dosage forms.
17. Write about non-pareil beads and its applications to develop oral sustained release dosage forms.
18. Compare and differentiate the three sustained release dosage forms: matrix devices, reservoir devices and osmotic pumps.
19. Write about innovative drug delivery systems for oral administration.
20. Write a note on DLVO theory.
21. How are flocculated and deflocculated suspensions prepared?
22. Write about powder flow and powder flow properties.
23. What are the different tests used to measure the powder flow?
24. Write about drug-excipient interaction.
25. Write about stability studies of pharmaceutical products.
26. Write about plant design for a pharmaceutical plant.

References

1. Timmer CJ, Sitsen JM. Pharmacokinetic evaluation of gepirone immediate-release capsules and gepirone extended-release tablets in healthy volunteeers. J Pharm Sci. 2003 Sep;92(9):1773-8.
2. Fan LT, Singh SK. Introduction. In: Fan LT, Singh SK, eds. Controlled Release-A Quantitative Treatment. Berlin, Germany: Spinger-Verlag; 1989:4-5.
3. Fan LT, Singh SK. Diffusion-controlled release. In: Fan LT, Singh SK, eds. Controlled Release-A Quantitative Treatment. Berlin, Germany: Springer-Verlag; 1989:61-79.
4. Fan LT, Singh SK. Introduction. In: Fan LT, Singh SK, eds. Controlled Release-A Quantitative Treatment. Berlin, Germany: Springer-Verlag;1989:3.
5. Siegel R.A., "Modeling of Drug Release from Porous Polymers", in Controlled Release of Drugs: Polymers and Aggregate Systems (Rosoff M., ed.) VCH Publishers, Inc., New York, pp. 1-52 (1989).
6. Siegel R.A., Kost J. and Langer R. "Mechanistic Studies of Macromolecular Drug Release from Macroporous Polymers. I. Experiments and Preliminary Theory Concerning Completeness of Drug Release", *J. Controlled Release* 8, 223-236 (1989).
7. Peppas NA Analysis of Fickian and non-Fickian drug release from polymers. Pharm Acta Helv. 1985;60(4):110-1.
8. Abdul S, Poddar SS. A flexible technology for modified release of drugs: multi layered tablets. J Control Release. 2004 Jul 7;97(3):393-405.
9. Steingoetter A, Weishaupt D, Kunz P, Mader K, Lengsfeld H, Thumshirn M, Boesiger P, Fried M, Schwizer W. agnetic resonance imaging for the in vivo evaluation of gastric-retentive tablets. harm Res. 2003 Dec;20(12):2001-7.
10. Shah SP, Misra A. Liposomal amphotericin B dry powder inhaler: effect of fines on in vitro performance.Pharmazie. 2004 Oct;59(10):812-3.
11. Howard KA, Li XW, Somavarapu S, Singh J, Green N, Atuah KN, Ozsoy Y, Seymour LW, Alpar HO. Formulation of a microparticle carrier for oral polyplex-based DNA vaccines.Biochim Biophys Acta. 2004 Sep 24;1674(2):149-57.

12. Solaro R, Chiellini F, Signori F, Fiumi C, Bizzarri R, Chiellini E. Nanoparticle systems for the targeted release of active principles of proteic nature. J Mater Sci Mater Med. 2003 Aug;14(8):705-11.
13. Prescott JK, Barnum RA. On powder flowability. Pharmaceutical Technology, October 2000.
14. Crowley P, Martinin LG. Drug-Excipient Interactions.

Bibliography

1. The Theory and Practice of Industrial Pharmacy, Third Edition, Edited by Leon Lachman, Herbert A. Lieberman, and Joseph L. Kanig, Lea & Febiger Publications, 1986.
2. Physical Characterization of Pharmaceutical Solids (Drugs and the Pharmaceutical Sciences: a Series of Textbooks and Monographs), First Edition, Edited by Harry G. Brittain, Marcel Dekker Inc., 1995.
3. New Drug Development: Regulatory Paradigms for Clinical Pharmacology and Biopharmaceutics (Drugs and the Pharmaceutical Sciences: a Series of Textbooks and Monographs), First Edition, Edited by Chandrahas G. Sahajwalla, Marcel Dekker Inc., 2004.
4. The Practice of Medicinal Chemistry, Second Edition, Edited by Camille Georges Wermuth, Elsevier Publications, 2003.
5. Foye`s Principles of Medicinal Chemistry, Fifth Edition, David A. Williams and Thomas L. Lemke, Lippincott Williams & Wilkins, 2002.
6. Physical Pharmacy: Physical Chemical Principles in the Pharmaceutical Sciences, Third Edition, Alfred Martin, James Swarbrick and Arthur Cammarata, Lea & Febiger Publications, 1983.
7. Generic Drug Product Development: Solid Oral Dosage Forms (Drugs and the Pharmaceutical Sciences: a Series of Textbooks and Monographs), First Edition, Edited by Leon Shargel and Isadore Kanfer, Marcel Dekker, Inc. 2005.
8. Pharmaceutical Principles of Solid Dosage Forms, First Edition, by J.T. Carstensen, Technomic Publishing Company, 1993.
9. Drug Targeting and Delivery: Concepts in Dosage Form Design (Ellis Horwood Series in Pharmacological Sciences), First Edition, Edited by H.E. Junginger, Ellis Horwood Limited, 1992.

10. Pharmaceutical Dosage Forms and Drug Delivery Systems, Seventh Edition, Howard C. Ansel, Loyd V. Allen, Jr., and Nicholas G. Popovich, Lippincott Williams & Wilkins, 1999.

11. Pharmaceutical Salts: Properties, Selection, and Use, First Edition, Edited by P. Heinrich Stahl and Camille G. Wermuth, Wiley VCH, 2002.

12. Handbook of Dissolution Testing, Second Edition, by William A. Hanson, Aster Publication Corporation, 1991.

13. Pharmaceutical Dissolution Testing (Drugs and the Pharmaceutical Sciences: a Series of Textbooks and Monographs), First Edition, by Umesh V. Banakar, Marcel Dekker Publications, 1991.

14. WHO EXPERT COMMITTEE ON SPECIFICATIONS FOR PHARMACEUTICAL PREPARATIONS. WHO Technical report series 908.

CHAPTER 12

PHARMACOKINETICS

- **Introduction**
- **Fundamentals**
    - Biopharmaceutics
    - Pharmacokinetics
    - Mathematical Model
    - Pharmacokinetic Modelling
        - Empirical Modelling
        - Physiological Based Pharmacokinetic Modelling
        - Application of Various Modelling Techniques
- **Widely Used Models in Clinical Trials**
    - One Compartment Open Model
    - Multicompartment Models
    - Non-compartment models
- **Allometric scaling**
- **Software programs to calculate pharmacokinetic parameters**
    - WinNonlin
    - NonMem
- **New Drug Reporting and Approval: A Pharmacokinetic Perspective**
- **Clinical Trials**
- **Conclusions**

Introduction

Pharmacokinetics is the mathematical study of the movement of a molecule in the body after any route of administration.. Pharmacists, formulation scientists, physicians, clinical pharmacokineticists and medicinal chemists should be able to understand the basic principles of pharmacokinetics for their day-to-day practice. Essentially pharmacokinetics consists of study of the movement of molecules in the body after different routes of administration and subsequently applying these principles in preclinical and clinical investigations of a new chemical entity and in clinics for better patient treatment. It has been recently reported that the clinical development of 40% of drug candidates was discontinued due to unacceptable pharmacokinetic properties. Thus, pharmacokinetic investigations of early drug candidates are very crucial. A new chemical entity after its pharmacological activity is established is generally administered by oral route to determine its pharmacokinetic properties. The plasma samples are collected at regular intervals, the drug amounts determined and the data is further investigated to determine whether the molecule has promising pharmacokinetic properties or not. This review briefly outlines the principles of pharmacokinetics as applied to oral drug delivery and new drug discovery.

Fundamentals

In preclinical and clinical investigations, the pharmacokinetic parameters of a drug are derived from plasma-time profile after oral or intravenous administration of the drug. A drug administered as i.v. bolus elicits the profile shown in Figure 1. The concentration drops exponentially with time. However, this profile has several components that are not deciphered in the graph. Actually, there is an increase in the plasma drug levels because of the injection and immediate absorption into the system followed by sustained levels because of distribution and then declining levels due to elimination. However, these individual phases will not demonstrate in a plasma-time profile, because of simultaneous absorption, distribution and elimination in such a profile. These individual components are determined by mathematical derivations. Whatever the drug is, the physiological situation is, with appropriate design and kinetic analysis of the data, the appropriate pharmacokinetic parameters could be obtained. Some aspects of these experiments and the pharmacokinetic modeling are discussed here in brief.

Biopharmaceutics

To elicit therapeutic response, drugs should be present at the site of the need. Most of the times these cites will be receptors. Drugs have to be administered via some route so that they reach these cites. The very common route of administration of drugs is the oral route. Upon oral administration, drugs reach systemic circulation after passing through the gastrointestinal tract. Once in the systemic circulation, the drugs reach the site of action after passing through the blood vessels or the tissues. If the receptor or the site of action is in the blood the drug do not need to be transported out of the blood vessels. On the other hand, drugs can be directly administered into the systemic circulation with added advantages. However, such administrations are invasive. Similarly, drugs can be administered by a variety of routes so as to gain access to the site of the need. In the case, where the drugs also have to cross membranes, various properties of the drug and the tissue/membrane characteristics also influence the drug reaching the site of the need. Also, the vehicle/formulation by which the drug is administered also has a significant influence. The study of the formulation parameters, the route of administration, the drug characteristics, the tissue/membrane characteristics that influence the drug reach to the target site from the site of administration is called biopharmaceutics. Both the pharmacist and the pharmaceutical scientist must understand biopharmaceutics to comprehend the proper use and development of pharmaceuticals. Thus, biopharmaceutics involves factors that influence

1. the stability of the drug within the drug product,
2. the release of the drug from the drug product,
3. the rate of dissolution/release of the drug at the absorption site, and
4. the systemic absorption of the drug,
5. drug distribution to the site of need from the systemic circulation.

Drug distribution from the systemic circulation to the site of need/action is earlier not considered in biopharmaceutics. Now, it is different. The therapeutic response of a drug is normally dependent on an adequate concentration of the drug being achieved and then maintained at the site or sites of action of the drug. In the case of systemically acting drugs it is generally accepted for clinical purposes that a dynamic equilibrium exists between the concentration of the drug in blood and concentration of the drug at the site of action. It means that a linear relationship exists between the drug level in blood and drug concentration at the site of action. Therefore, drug concentration at the site of action can be predicted from blood concentration of drug. The is because the concentration of drug in plasma water (i.e. protein free plasma) is a more accurate index of drug concentration at the site of action than is concentration in whole plasma since a drug may often bind in a reversible manner to plasma protein. Only drug that in unbound (which is free and dissolved in plasma water) can pass out of the plasma through capillary endothelium and reach other body fluids and tissues and finally to its site of action. Thus, drug distribution is not considered as rate limiting membrane for drugs to reach target receptor from the blood. The effect of a drug probably depends on its concentration in the tissue in which it acts. Antibacterial activity may well relate closely to concentrations in plasma, because diffusion occurs fairly rapidly between plasma and extracellular fluids and infecting bacteria are on the whole extracellular. But the effectiveness of drugs acting on specific organs, for example cardiac glycosides, is likely to relate to the concentration in that organ, or some part of it, rather than to the concentration in plasma. It would therefore be useful to predict the concentration of a drug in different organs at various times after giving single or repeated doses. Although such predictions are based on another sister branch of biopharmaceutics, called pharmacokinetics, with the advent of novel delivery technologies and biotechnology based drugs, the whole definition of biopharmaceutics is changing. With the advent of biotechnology based drugs and drug delivery systems at nanolevel, drug distribution is also important rate limiting step for the drugs to reach the target receptor from the systemic circulation. Thus, although drug distribution is generally not studied as the class of biopharmaceutics, but with the advent of drug targeting it could be considered in biopharmaceutics under special circumstances.

Thus, **Biopharmaceutics** is a field of science that studies and develops methods to optimize the efficacy and safety of medicines. General aims can be e.g. to develop new routes of administration, increase the duration of drug activity or to improve drug targeting by the use of pharmaceutical nanotechnology. Biopharmaceutical knowledge is important in the field of research and industry, especially in clinical pharmacokinetics and pre-clinical studies, but biopharmaceutical expertise is also useful in local pharmacies to ensure effective and safe patient counseling.

The study of biopharmaceutics involves both in vitro and in vivo experimentation. *In-vitro* methods are procedures employing test apparatus and equipment without involving laboratory animals or humans. *In-vivo* methods are more complex studies involving human subjects or laboratory animals. These methods must be able to assess the impact of the physical and chemical properties of the drug, drug stability, and large-scale production of the drug and drug product on the biologic performance of the drug

Pharmacokinetics

Pharmacokinetics (PK) is the study of the fate of a drug in the body. It aims at quantitatively describing the processes that influence absorption, distribution, metabolism, and elimination (ADME) of a drug in the body. To analyze the PK profile of a drug, experimentally collected data, e.g., time series measurements of drug concentration in plasma or blood, is evaluated by means of mathematical modeling.The term *pharmacokinetics* was first introduced by F. H. Dost in 1953 in his text, *Der Bliitspiegel-Kinetic der Konzentrationsablaiife in der Frieslauffliissigkeit*. However, some of the subject matter was published before the word was coined. It is also of interest that the first English language review of the subject matter, published in 1961, was entitled the *Kinetics of Drug Absorption, Distribution, Metabolism and Excretion* and did not include the word *pharmacokinetics*. Pharmacokinetics has been defined in a number of ways. Literally, the word means the application of kinetics to *pharmakon,* the Greek word for drugs and poisons. *Kinetics* is that branch of knowledge which involves the change of one or more variables as a function of time. The purpose of pharmacokinetics is to study the time course of drug and metabolite concentrations or amounts in biological fluids, tissues and excreta, and also of pharmacological response, and to construct suitable models to interpret such data. In pharmacokinetics, the data are analyzed using a mathematical representation of a part or the whole of an organism. Broadly then, the purposes of pharmacokinetics are to reduce data to a number of meaningful parameter values, and to use the reduced data to predict either the results of future experiments or the results of a host of studies which would be too costly and time-consuming to complete. A similar definition has been given by other authors as follows: 'Pharmacokinetics is concerned with the study and characterization of the time course of drug absorption, distribution, metabolism and excretion, and with the relationship of these processes to the intensity and time course of therapeutic and adverse effects of drugs. It involves the application of mathematical and biochemical techniques in a physiological and pharmacologic context. To determine drug levels in biological fluids such as plasma, several biochemical and assay technique are possible. However, most of the time drug levels in the tissues should be assessed or determined. In this regard, assessing drug levels in the tissues become important. Reliable predictions would add to the understanding of pharmacological responses, and also would allow more accurate therapeutic use. Thus, the study of pharmacokinetics involves both experimental and theoretical approaches. The experimental aspect of pharmacokinetics involves the development of biologic sampling techniques, analytical methods for the measurement of drugs and metabolites, and procedures that facilitate data collection and manipulation. The theoretical aspect of pharmacokinetics involves the development of pharmacokinetic models that predict drug disposition after drug administration. To develop such models or (can also be called predictions), rates of transfer between plasma and tissues or components of tissues must be estimated. The whole body can be regarded as a very complex system of many compartments, and some sort of simplified model is essential. The application of statistics is an integral part of pharmacokinetic studies. Statistical methods are used for pharmacokinetic parameter estimation and data interpretation ultimately for the purpose of designing and predicting optimal dosing regimens for individuals or groups of patients. Statistical methods are applied to pharmacokinetic models to determine data error and structural model deviations. Mathematics and computer techniques form the theoretical basis of many pharmacokinetic methods. Classical pharmacokinetics is a study of theoretical models focusing mostly on model development and parameterization. Teorell was first to study compartment modeling. In Teorell's classical papers, only four compartments (site of administration, blood, tissues, excreta) were used, and complete equations using first order kinetics were shown to describe blood concentrations quite well.Extension of Teorell's equations to allow for tissues with several different rates of uptake leads to appallingly heavy algebra. This is regarding compartmental technique of assessing concentrations of drugs in various tissues. There are other methods of predicting drug levels in various tissues. These are basically classified into empirical or classical models and physiology-based pharmacokinetic models. Before pharmacokinetic modeling techniques are introduced, a general introduction of modeling is essential.

Mathematical Model

A *model* is a hypothesis using mathematical terms to describe quantitative relationships concisely. The predictive capability of a model lies in the proper selection and development of mathematical function(s) that parameterize the essential factors governing the kinetic process. The key parameters in a process are commonly estimated by fitting the model to the experimental data, known as *variables*. A *pharmacokinetic parameter* is a constant for the drug that is estimated from the experimental data. For example, estimated pharmacokinetic parameters such as k depend on the method of tissue sampling, the timing of the sample, drug analysis, and the predictive model selected.

A pharmacokinetic function relates an *independent variable* to a *dependent variable*, often through the use of parameters. For example, a pharmacokinetic model may predict the drug concentration in the liver 1 hour after an oral administration of a 20-mg dose. The independent variable is time and the dependent variable is the drug concentration in the liver. Based on a set of time-versus-drug concentration data, a model equation is derived to predict the liver drug concentration with respect to time. In this case, the drug concentration depends on the time after the administration of the dose, where the time: concentration relationship is defined by a pharmacokinetic parameter, *k*, the elimination rate constant.

Pharmacokinetic Modelling

Pharmacokinetic models are used to:

1. Predict plasma, tissue, and urine drug levels with any dosage regimen
2. Calculate the optimum dosage regimen for each patient individually
3. Estimate the possible accumulation of drugs and/or metabolites
4. Correlate drug concentrations with pharmacologic or toxicologic activity
5. Evaluate differences in the rate or extent of availability between formulations (bioequivalence)
6. Describe how changes in physiology or disease affect the absorption, distribution, or elimination of the drug
7. Explain drug interactions

If a simple model does not fit all the experimental observations accurately, a new, more elaborate model may be proposed and subsequently tested. Since limited data are generally available in most clinical situations, pharmacokinetic data should be interpreted along with clinical observations rather than replacing sound judgment by the clinician. Development of pharmacometric statistical models may help to improve prediction of drug levels among patients in the population. However, it will be some time before these methods become generally accepted.

Because a model is based on a hypothesis and simplifying assumptions, a certain degree of caution is necessary when relying totally on the pharmacokinetic model to predict drug action. For some drugs, plasma drug concentrations are not useful in predicting drug activity. For other drugs, an individual's genetic differences, disease state, and the compensatory response of the body may modify the response of a drug.

Empirical Modelling

The classical, i.e.,empirical, modeling approaches are classified into non-compartmental and compartmental methods. *Empirical models* are practical but not very useful in explaining the mechanism of the actual process by which the drug is absorbed, distributed, and eliminated in the body.

Non-compartmental technique

The non-compartmental technique relies on fitting a sum of exponentials function to the experimental data. Based on the estimated parameters, typical PK characteristics are determined to characterize the drug, e.g., area under the concentration time curve (AUC), elimination half-life (t1/2), total plasma clearance, etc..

Compartmental Technique

In compartmental technique, the body is typically divided into one, two, or three compartments that represent distributional spaces with identical kinetics. Within each compartment, drug distribution is assumed to occur instantaneously and homogeneously. The barriers between compartments represent rate-limited disposition processes, e.g., due to slow perfusion by the blood flow, limited permeability through membranes, active transporters, metabolic conversion, protein binding, distribution into tissue constituents, etc. The compartments are interconnected by first-order rate constants, while input rate constants may follow zero-order kinetics. Elimination is typically assumed to occur from the central compartment based on either a linear or a saturable Michaelis-Menten process. Compartmental PK analysis is based on dividing the organism into spaces with identical kinetics (compartments). Both, the model structure and the model parameters, are derived from the experimental data. The typical model finding procedure includes the development and parameter estimation of competing models. Model discrimination is based on a statistical criterion to select the model that best fits the experimental data. The compartmental PK models can then be used to describe and predict the concentration-time profile of the drug in plasma or blood.

The simplest compartment model depicts the body as a single compartment assuming homogenous distribution into accessible body spaces. More complex, often mechanism-based models (particularly models accounting for absorption from the gastrointestinal tract) exist.. Two- or three-compartment models are used to describe the PK of a drug if drug disposition is rate-limited so that the whole body cannot be considered as a single, homogenous distributional space. This could be caused, e.g., by a pronounced distribution into slowly perfused tissues such as adipose (perfusion-rate limited distribution) or poor diffusion across membranes (permeability-rate limited distribution), active transporters, saturable protein binding, etc..

Physiology-based pharmacokinetic modelling

While the classical compartmental PK models are empirical, newer methods have been developed that are considered to be mechanistic or mechanism-based. The model structure and model parameters are defined in terms of the anatomical and/or physiological characteristics of the organism and some properties of the drug under consideration. The most promising and most popular mechanistic modeling technique is physiology-based PK (PBPK) modeling.

In pharmacokinetics, currently, the most frequently used mechanistic models are wholebody physiology-based pharmacokinetic (PBPK) models.. Physiology-based pharmacokinetic (PBPK) modeling makes use of the knowledge about physiological, physical and biochemical processes that are involved in drug disposition in order to predict the time course of drug concentration in various organs and tissues of the body. PBPK models are mechanistic in nature; the model structure and parameters are determined by anatomical and/or physiological characteristics of the species and physicochemical properties of the drug under consideration. Typically, a PBPK model consists of multiple compartments that represent the most relevant anatomical spaces of the body, e.g., single organs or tissues. The interconnections of the compartments represent transport fluids such as the blood flow or the lymph flow. The parameters of a PBPK model are classified to be either species- or drug-specific. Drug-specific data include physico- and biochemical properties of the compound that are ideally independent of the species, e.g., lipophilicity, ionization, protein binding, permeability, microsomal clearance. Species-specific data are related to the species only, e.g., organ volumes, blood flow rates, etc. Replacing the species-specific data, allows for extrapolation to different species or to human. To date, most PBPK models have been developed to be applied to small molecule drugs.

The other aspect of PBPK models is to use in vitro data to predict in vivo disposition. Thus, PBPK models aim at incorporating the most relevant ADME processes involved in drug disposition and can be used to predict the time course of drug concentration in plasma or blood as well as in various organs and tissues prior to any in vivo studies, solely based on in vitro data. If gradually refined and evaluated against preclinical and early clinical data, a PBPK model can be seen as reflecting a coherant collection of parts of the current knowledge about a drug candidate. Such models, however, are more complex than the empirical pharmacokinetic models in terms of number of equations and parameters.

Applications of Various Modeling Techniques

In drug discovery and development, empirical, low-dimensional compartment models and physiology-based pharmacokinetic (PBPK) models are successfully used to analyze and predict the pharmacokinetics of drugs. In the pharmaceutical industry, modeling and simulation is used to support decision-making processes, e.g., drug candidate selection, dose selection, clinical trial design, and benefit/risk assessment for new drugs. Yet, for a given drug, the ultimate goal is to determine the optimal dose and dosing regimen for a target population of patients to obtain the maximal desired effect while minimizing adverse events. The description and prediction of the time course of the drug effects in the patient play the most crucial role to achieve this attempt.

Due to the increased complexity, PBPK models are less suitable, e.g., for application in a population analysis of clinical trials in later developmental stages, and for this reason, the empirical models are prevalently employed in this field of application. So far, the classical, empirical and the physiology-based pharmacokinetic approaches are used independently or in parallel, with little to no overlap or cross-fertilization; and none of the approaches takes advantage of the other approach. In drug discovery and preclinical development, PBPK modeling is frequently used, e.g., to optimize the selection of drug candidates based on in silico and in vitro data that are likely to have the desired in vivo pharmacokinetic properties, and to determine the first dose in man based on preclinical data. After entry into clinical development, there is a shift from mechanistic to empirical modeling. In particular, mechanistic PBPK modeling is underrepresented in the analysis of clinical data and is rarely used to support or guide empirical model development.

Widely Used Models in Clinical Trials

One-Compartment Open Model

A simple example of a pharmacokinetic dissection and evaluation is the pharmacokinetic analysis of a molecule whose plasma concentration decreases exponentially with time after intravenous bolus administration as depicted in Figure 1. The rate of decline depends on the concentration of the drug in the respective compartment. Thus, one or more first-order processes describe's the kinetics of drug disposition. Most of the treatments in the earlier stages of drug discovery with new drug substances atleast in very unsophisticated laboratories or methodologies use this model. This is like a very preliminary, simple and good fit of the plasma data. This type of data fit is also helpful in the comparison of individual dosage forms for a single drug which most of the times is utilized in the generic product development processes. However, as the time progresses with new drug discovery processes, more sophisticated modelings such as convolutions, statistical fits, etc. could be routinely used. In addition, there are several other pharmacokinetic methodologies currently used and developed routinely to assess the pharmacokinetic behaviour of a new drug substance. The model mentioned in this section is described in the Figure 2a. This is a one-compartment open model in which C1 is the plasma concentration, V1 is the apparent volume of distribution, K_{10} is the overall elimination rate constant. It is called as an open model because it is assumed that the drug passes freely into and out of compartments in an open model. Apparent volume of distribution is defined as the total volume of the body in which the drug is distributed. In this situation, the decay is a first-order process and is therefore,

Derivations Related to One-Compartment Open Model with First-Order Elimination

$$-dC1/dt = K_{10}*C1$$

Upon integration,

$$C1 = C1*e^{-k10t}$$

$$= D*e^{-k10t/v1} \quad .....(12.1)$$

Upon further derivation,

$$T1/2 = 0.693/K_{10} \quad ......(12.2)$$

Where $T_{1/2}$ is the half-life and is defined as the time required for a given plasma concentration to be halved. The equation suggests that the plasma half-life of this molecule is inversely proportional to its elimination rate constant. At any given time, provided K_{10} is determined from plasma-time profile, the concentration of the drug in the plasma could be predicted. The logarithm of plasma-time curves is a linear graph as shown in Figure 1B. This is similar to a first order process. A first order process can describe many processes in pharmcokinetics accurately. This means that the rate of a drug biotransformation, the rate of transfer of a drug between compartments, and the rate of absorption and elimination of drugs from the body are directly proportioned to the size of the dose administered. It is also true that passive diffusion is responsible for the tranfer of a drug in the body and there is a directly proportional relationship between the administered dose and the resulting drug concentration in the body. This dose proportionality is often used as an indicator of linear pharmacokinetics. It is the parameters that most of the time are the indicators of a drug movement and termination in the body. This may be either of the parent drug or the metabolite. Thus, this type of derivations is always of immense help.

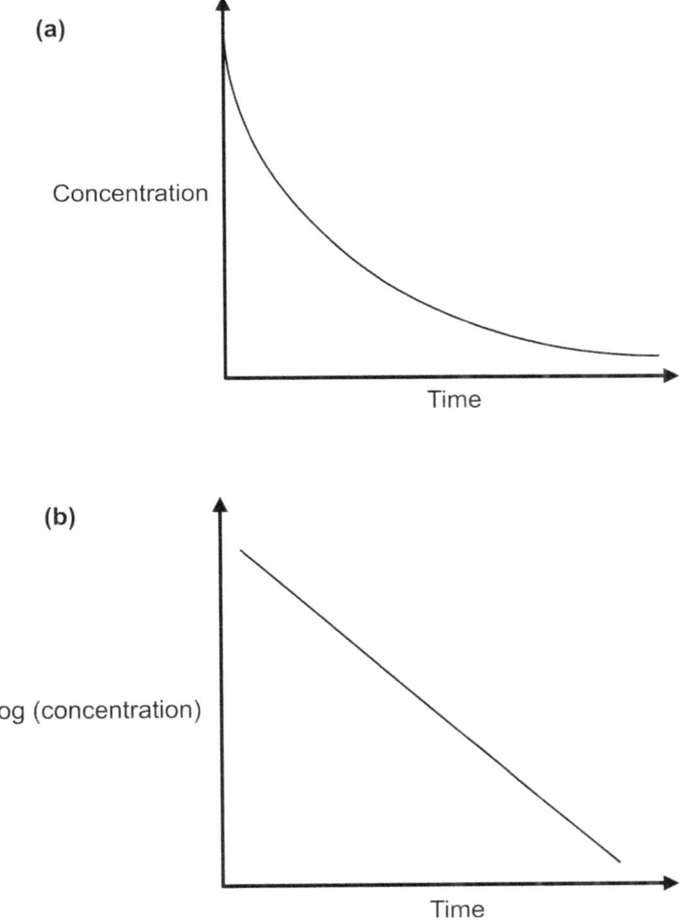

Figure 12.1A A typical plasma- time profile after intravenous bolus administration. B. A semilogarithmic plot of plasma concentration versus time for a one-compartment model.

Applications

Before entering the topic in detail, a brief mention of the application of oral pharmacokinetics would help to better appreciate this topic. Oral pharmacokinetic studies are applied in:

1. The evaluation of the movement of a new chemical entity in the body in preclinical and clinical studies.
2. Demonstrating the pharmacokinetic promise of a novel chemical entity for further investigations.
3. The selection of the best suitable formulation for preclinical and clinical studies and further in the identification of a market potential formulation.
4. Providing the information that is useful to predict the effect of alterations in the dose, dosage regimen, route of administration, and physiological state on the preclinical pharmacokinetics.
5. Clinical studies such as dose fixing, chrono-pharmacokinetics, dosage regimen identification and drug interactions.

Multicompartment Models

As mentioned before, in a compartmental model, the body is divided into several compartments. Plasma is generally the central compartment. The movement of a molecule from central compartment to the other compartments is described by rate constants. After a drug is administered by oral or i.v. route, the plasma and the tissues such as liver, lungs, brain, kidney, muscles, are separated at specific time intervals and the drug extracted and assayed. Theoretically, the profiles obtained from individual tissues are fit into tissue-time profiles. Elimination rate constants are obtained. Absorption patterns are determined. The tissues with similar absorption patterns and same elimination rate constants are considered as a single compartment. For instance, if plasma and liver show similar absorption profiles and same elimination rate constant and lungs, brain, kidneys and muscle show similar absorption profiles and same elimination rate constant, the pharmacokinetics of the molecule could be considered as a two-compartment model with plasma and liver as one compartment and the rest of the tissues the other compartment. Similarly if the disposition of a drug in different tissues is different then the system is termed as a multicompartment system. Generally, in a compartmental modeling one compartment is first fit to the data and statistics is used to validate the data. If this model, do not fit then either two or three compartmental modeling will be investigated. As previously mentioned, statistics is again used to validate the mode. Although very complicated models have been described in the literature, the general practice is to validate the data for one or two or three compartment models. Once the model is finalized, the pharmacokinetic parameters are determined. Based on the parameters, the dose and dose interval will be determined. Again, more complicated multicompartment models are not seen practically with drugs. A picture of a one-compartment and a multicompartment model is depicted below and is self-explanatory:

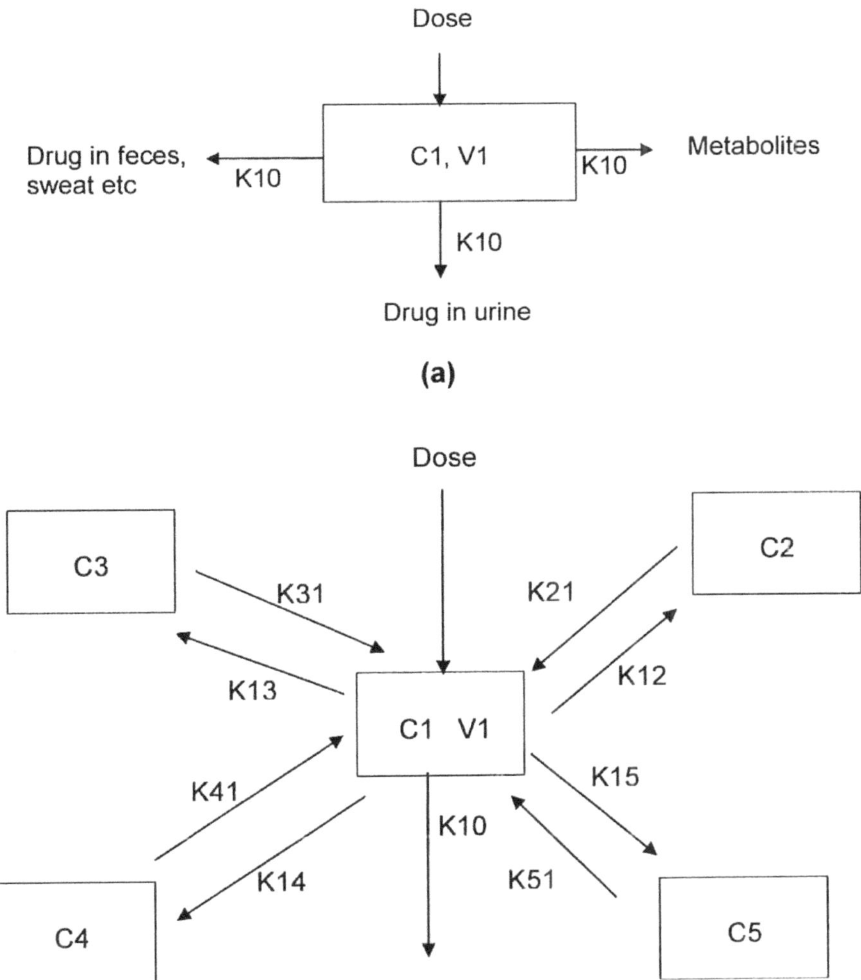

Figure 12.2 A One compartment open model (C1 is the plasma concentration, V1 is the volume of distribution, K10 is the elimination rate constant); B. Multicompartment model (C1 is the plasma concentration, V1 is the volume of distribution, K10 is the elimination rate constant; Various Ks are the disposition constants between the tissues).

Derivation of Rate Constants for Simple one Compartment Model, Simple Two Compartment Model, One compartment Model with Oral Absorption and Two Compartment Model with Oral Absorption

Drug distribution is generally a reversible process. The partition of the drug from plasma to individual tissues depends on the type of the tissue, existence of the transporters and the properties of the molecule. In a ***simple one-compartment model***, the movement of a drug into various tissues is rapid and the entire body acts as one single compartment. A single exponential adequately defines the plasma-time course. The derivation of rate constants and appropriate equations and calculations is shown in the fundamentals section of this chapter. On the other hand, the kinetics of drug disposition is often multi-exponential. Each additional exponential represent groups of tissues requiring progressively more time in which to achieve a steady state in drug distribution. In all the situations discussed, absorption is assumed to be a first order process. The following equations depict a biexponential decay and derivation is for a ***simple two-compartment model***:

$$C1 = Ae^{-\alpha t} + Be^{-\beta t}$$

The plasma profile shows an initial curvature that eventually becomes log-linear with a terminal slope $-\beta/2.303$ (Figure 3). The intercept B is obtained by extrapolation back to time zero. Taking the logarithm of the difference between

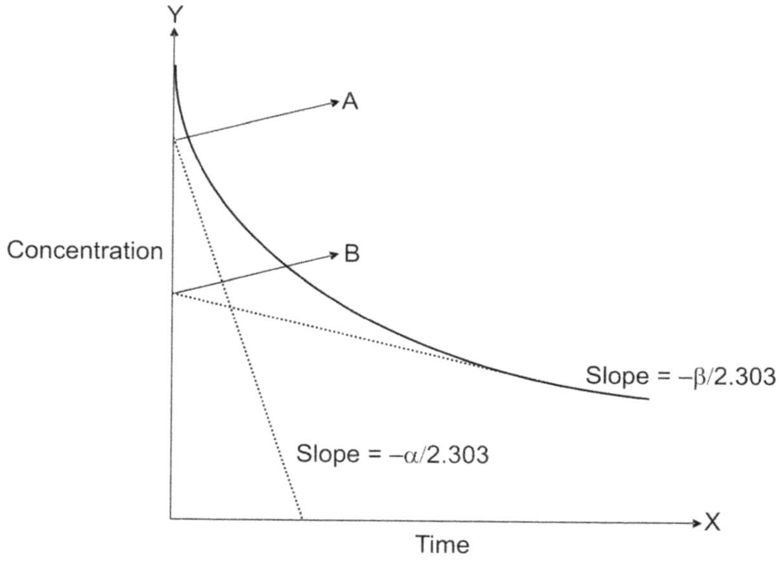

Figure 12.3 Semilogarithmic plot of plasma concentration vs. time for a two-compartment model.

plasma concentration C1 and the value of $Be^{-\beta t}$ yields another straight line from which A and alpha could be evaluated. This technique is called as curve stripping and could be repeated as often as necessary and is generally useful in obtaining eigenvalues (slopes) and eigenvectors (intercepts) of a polyexponential function. In addition, these values could also be obtained by appropriate mathematic derivations. An example of these kinds of derivations is presented for a two-compartment model where in the decay is shown in the figure 4. The system is perceived as two kinetically distinct compartments. A central comparment 1, which includes plasma and from which elimination occurs, is linked to a peripheral compartment 2 by first-order processes having rate constants K12 and K21.

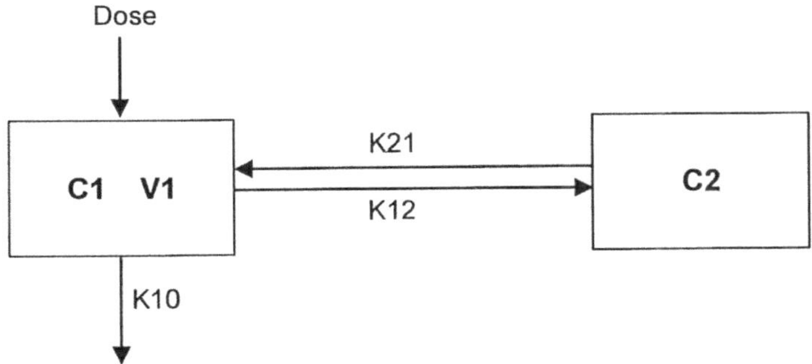

Figure 12.4 Two-compartment, open model.

Derivations Related to Two-Compartment Open Model with First-Order Elimination

$$dC1/dt = -K12C1 + K21C2 - K10C1$$

$$dC2/dt = K12C1 - K21C2$$

$$dU/dt = frK10V1C1$$

Upon appropriate derivations integration, the equations the following equations could be drawn,

$$V1 = D/(A + B)$$

$$K10 = A + B / (A/\alpha + B/\beta)$$

$$K21 = \alpha * \beta/K10 \qquad .....(12.3)$$

$$K12 = \alpha + \beta - K10 - K21 \qquad .....(12.4)$$

The simplest way of pharmacokinetic studies in preclinical or clinical studies is to administer the drug by oral route and then performing pharmacokinetic analysis. The oral formulation could be a solution, suspension, tablet or a capsule. Wagner-Nelson proposed methods to determine the pharmacokinetic parameters in this situation. The model is best described as a *one-compartment model with oral absorption*. These equations are still very commonly used in this kind of data analysis. According to this method, at any time after a drug is administered, the amount of the drug administered is the amount of the drug eliminated, the total drug that is eliminated and that metabolized.

Derivations Related to One-Compartment Open Model After Oral Absorbtion and First-Order Elimination

If $A_{(t)}$ is the amount of the drug absorbed at any time, $A_{b(t)}$ is the amount of the drug present in the body, X_E is the eliminated drug, then

$$A_{(t)} = Ab_{(t)} + X_E \quad \text{.....(12.4)}$$

When the drug disposition follows a one-compartment open model (equation 12.2),

$Ab_{(t)}$ = V1C1 (t), where V1 is the volume of distribution and C1(t) is the plasma concentration of the drug, respectively.

X_E, the total amount of the drug eliminated is calculated using,

$$X_E = K10^*V1^* \int_0^t C1.dt$$

And thus the above equation becomes,

$$A_{(t)} = V1C1_{(t)} + K10^*V1^* \int_0^t C1.dt \quad \text{.....(12.5)}$$

$\int_0^t C1.dt$ is the area under the plasma concentration versus time curve from time zero to t.

This equation is called as the Wagner-Nelson equation and is used to determine drug absorption parameters.

An equation for the amount of the drug absorbed from zero to infinity could be obtained using the equation,

$$XE\infty = K10^*V1^* \int_0^\infty C1.dt$$

Fraction absorbed to time t could be calculated using the equation,

$$Ft = A_{(t)/} XE\infty = (V1C1_{(t)} + K10^*V1^* \int_0^t C1.dt) / (K10^*V1^* \int_0^\infty C1.dt)$$

.....(12.6)

Upon simplification,

$$Ft = A_{(t)/} XE\infty = (C1(t) + K10^* \int_0^t C1.dt) \; / \; (K10^* \int_0^\infty C1.dt) \qquad .....(12.7)$$

The above equation relates the cumulative amount of drug absorbed at a certain time to the amount of drug ultimately absorbed rather than to the dose administered.

After a single oral dose the blood is collected analyzed for the drug, elimination rate constant is determined, and the fraction absorbed for various time after administration could be calculated. A plot of percent unabsorbed versus time on semi-logarithmic coordinates yields a straight line suggesting an apparent first-order absorption and the absorption rate constant is estimated from the slope of this linear curve, which is equal to –ka/2.303. The absorption is zero-order if the plot of percent unabsorbed versus time is a straight line.

The most serious limitation of the Wagner-Nelson method is that it applies to the drugs with one-compartment characteristics. For all other models, Wagner-Nelson method is only an approximation. This equation is generally used in the bioavailability studies. In the situation where Wagner-Nelson method is not applicable, where the concentration-time curve shows multicompartment characteristics after oral absorption, Loo-Riegelman method is used and this is discussed in several other textbooks. This model could be applied to a ***two-compartment model with oral absorption*** to calculate absorption rate constants.

Non-Compartmental Models

In a non-compartmental model, pharmacokinetic parameters Area under the concentration time curve (AUC), mean residence time (MRT), concentration maximum (C_{max}), time to reach maximum concentration (T_{max}), Fabs% (absolute bioavailability) are calculated and used in the evaluation of the pharmacokinetics of a molecule. The methods of determination of pharmacokinetic parameters in a non-compartmental analysis are usually based on the estimation of the area under a plot of drug concentration versus time. Provided that the pharmacokinetics is linear, non-compartmental models could be applied to any compartmental model. No assumptions are made based on the shape of the blood or plasma drug concentration verses time curve. The assumption is this kind of calculations is that the drug undergoes first-order (unsaturable) elimination. The clearance is always constant and the rate of drug elimination from blood or plasma is linearly proportional to its concentration.

The basis behind the non-compartmental models is the statistical moment theory. According to this theory, the time course of drug concentration in plasma is usually regarded as a statistical distribution curve. The first three moments (zero to second) of this distribution curve are defined by AUC, MRT, and VRT respectively.

Pharmacokinetic Parameters in a Non-Compartment Model

Accordingly,

$$AUC = \int_0^\infty C.dt$$

$$MRT = \left(\int_0^\infty tC.dt\right) \Big/ \int_0^\infty C.dt$$

$$= AUMC/AUC$$

$$VRT = \left(\int_0^\infty t^2C.dt\right) \Big/ \int_0^\infty C.dt$$

$$= \left(\int_0^\infty (t-MRT)^2 C.dt\right) \Big/ AUC$$

AUMC is called as area under first moment curve and is the area under the curve of a plot of the product of concentration and time versus time from zero time to infinity.

$$AUC = \int_0^\infty C.dt = C/\beta \qquad .....(12.8)$$

Where beta is the slope of the terminal exponential phase of a plot of log(concentration) versus time. The sum of the two partial areas is AUC.

AUMC is similarly calculated.

$$AUMC = \int_0^\infty tC.dt = C^*t/\beta + C/\beta^2 \qquad .....(12.9)$$

Volume of Distribution at Steady-State (Vss)

Volume of distribution, Vss, can be calculated from intravascular PK data using the following equation.

$$Vss = CL^*MRT \qquad .....(12.10)$$

Where MRT is the mean residence time. Therefore, a steady-state parameter can be calculated without steady-state data.

Mean Residence Time (MRT)

Mean residence time is the average of the duration of each molecule residing in the body. It is calculated using the following equation.

$$MRT = AUMC/AUC$$

MRT could be considered as the overall apparent t1/2 of a drug. For a drug that displays a single elimination phase,

$$t1/2 = 0.693*MRT \quad .....(12.11)$$

Bioavailability

Bioavailability is the fraction of extravascularly-administered dose that reaches the system circulation. Absolute bioavailability is determined using the equation

$$F = (AUC_{ext}/Dose_{ext})/AUC_{iv}/Dose_{iv} \quad .....(12.12)$$

Clearance

Clearance is a proportionality constant relating the rate of drug eliminatin to blood or plasma concentrations.

$$\text{Rate of elimination} = CL *C$$

Integrating,

$$\text{Total drug eliminated} = CL \int_0^{\infty} C.dt$$

Assuming that the entire drug entering the body is eventually eliminated, the total amount of drug eliminated equals the amount administered (for an i.v. dose). Therefore,

$$Dose_{iv} = CL *AUC_{iv}$$

$$CL = Dose_{iv}/AUC_{iv} \quad .....(12.13)$$

C_{max} and t_{max}

After intravenous (iv) or extravascular drug administration, the maximum observed concentration in the concentration-time profile (C_{max}) and the time to reach that concentration (t_{max}, equals 0 for i.v. bolus dosing) are the important descriptors of the extent and nature of drug exposure. C_{max} an indicator of maximum drug exposure some times relates better to pharmacological or toxicological effects than other measures of exposure.

In this chapter the very commonly used oral pharmacokinetic parameters are described and elucidated. However, several other parameters are not discussed here and are detailed in several textbooks and publications.

Allometric Scaling

In preclinical stage of drug development, pharmacokinetic parameters are generally obtained using one or more animal species. Allometric scaling helps in the extrapolation of these parameters to human clinical trials based on body weights. These conversions would help in answering several questions including,

1. Will the drug support once a day dosing in humans?
2. Will the drug be well absorbed?
3. What dose of the drug will be required to achieve efficacious concentrations?
4. What dose of the drug results in toxic concentrations?

Because of the huge investments in the drug discovery process it is always advisable to have efficient drug discovery program. Accurate pharmacokinetic scaling could reduce the chances of a drug to be killed due to poor pharmacokinetic properties while scaling from animal studies to human trials thereby taking this drug efficiently into the market place. Based on data using several compounds, the following equation has been proposed and is practiced in allometric scaling.

$$Y = a*W^b \quad .....(12.14)$$

Where Y is the physiological parameter that is being measured, W is the weight of the animal and a and b are constants. This is a very impressive way of avoiding a compound that is likely to be dropped later in human clinical trials thereby reducing the cost of the drug discovery process. Some companies choose not to develop compounds with low half-life and greater clearance. Allometric scaling helps in identifying these compounds from the small animal data and would help in avoiding these compounds for further investigations.

Software Programs to Determine Pharmacokinetic Programs

Several software programs programs have been developed lately to determine the pharmacokinetic parameters. As the mathematics of the pharmacokinetics is advanced and different compartments developed using different modeling concepts, like wise the software was also developed. Two software programs currently in use in various aspects of industry are WinNonlin and NonMem.

Currently, several other softwares are also marketed. However, for the convenience of the readers and the applicators, a brief introduction of the two software packages WinNonlin and Nonmem is described henceforth.

WinNonlin

WinNonlin is a soft ware program used commonly now a day for pharmacokinetic data analysis. Pharsight Corporation, California, currently markets this program. This program is useful in pharmacokinetic pharmacodynamic data and non-compartmental data analysis. According to the software developer, the most powerful functions of WinNonlin is its ability to solve non-linear regression problems, constrained parameter estimation problems, and systems of differential equations and as well as mixtures of differential equations and functions. The effects of different doses and dosage regimens could be clearly observed in this program. WinNonlins extensive storage of the models allows the pharmacokinetic data to be fit very appropriately with accurate predictions of various pharmacokinetic parameters.

NonMem

NonMem project at University of California, San Fransisco, produced the UCSF NonMem software. This software helps in data analysis techniques and exportable software for fitting non-linear mixed effects (statistical regression – type models). These techniques are particularly useful when the data are pharmacokinetic/pharmacodynamic data and when there are only a few PK/PD measurements from some individuals sampled from the population, or when the regression design varies considerably between individuals. This software was updated several times and the current version is UCSF Non-mem version V is licensed and distributed by Globomax. There should be plans for this software people to update this version of NonMem for better marketing abroad.

New Drug Reporting and Approval: Pharmacokinetic Perspective

Once a new chemical is identified to be a potential therapeutic agent, its formulation is developed and safety determined in animal models. To obtain the required evidence that will demonstrate the drugs safety and effectiveness for its proposed use, a carefully designed and progressive sequence of preclinical (e.g. cell culture, whole animal) and clinical (human) studies are investigated. Only when the preclinical studies demonstrate adequate safety and the new agent shows promise as a useful drug, will the drugs sponsor file an Investigational New Drug Application (IND) with the FDA for initial testing in humans. If the drug demonstrates adequate safety in these initial human studies, termed Phase I, progressive human trials through Phases 2 and 3 are investigated to assess both safety and efficacy. As the clinical trials progress, laboratory work continues toward defining the agents basic and clinical pharmacology and toxicology, product design and development, manufacturing scale-up and process controls, analytical methods development, proposed labeling and package design, and initial plans for marketing. At the completion of the carefully designed preclinical and clinical studies, the drugs sponsor may file a New Drug Application (NDA) seeking approval to market the final new product. The FDAs approval for an NDA indicates that the body of scientific evidence submitted sufficiently demonstrates that the drug/drug product is safe and effective for the proposed clinical indications; that there is adequate assurance of its proper manufacture and control; and that the final labeling accurately presents the necessary information for its proper use. The content of a products approved labeling; represented by the package insert, is a summary of the entire drug development process because it contains the essential chemistry, pharmacology, toxicology, indications and contraindications for use, adverse effects, formulation composition, dosage and storage requirements, as ascertained during the research and development process. As a part of this reporting of the new drug and its use, currently pharmacokinetics is playing a key role.

The new investigational drug is applied as a formulation to small number of human beings generally healthy patients as Phase I studies. This selection is based on very systematic study based on the previous results in animal models and cell culture studies. The end result is to move forward if the results are positive. Very safe trials are these. During this stage and during the earlier investigations the correlation of blood levels of the drugs with the end result is the key issue. In this aspect allopathy goes futher in the step of investigation of a new drug. If fortunately everything is correlating the next step is continued. However, if unfortunately this does not happen the new drug is generally dumped at this stage. The basics of pharmacokinetics are described in the entirety of this chapter. The same principles are applied to the current new drug research. The correlation of pharmacokinetics from animals to human beings is a good sign. On the other hand, if the correlation is not proper, definitely it is an unfortunate situation and needs to be rectified. Alternatives could be executed. This is the key issue as related to the role of pharmacokinetics in early drug discovery phases.

Clinical Trials

Application part for a clinical trial process for US FDA is all set for a new drug with rules and regulations properly laid. However, this is always a dynamic process. It is always being changed as per the requirements. Once a drug is tested in animal models and cell culture studies for safety and efficacy and produced positive results, it is then ready to be administered into human beings for phase I studies. Under the Food, Drug, and Cosmetic Act as amended, the sponsor of a new drug is required to file with the FDA and Investigational New Drug Application (IND) before the drug may be administered in human beings. After submission of the IND, the sponsor must delay use of the drug in human beings for not less than 30 days from the data the FDA acknowledges receipt of the application. An IND automatically goes into effect following this period unless the FDA notifies the sponsor, the period is waived (and the sponsor may initiate the study early). An IND automatically goes into effect following this period unless the FDA notifies the sponsor that, based on its review of the submission, the period is waived (and the sponsor may initiate the study early), or the investigation is being placed on a clinical hold. A clinical hold is an order issued by the FDA to delay the start of a clinical investigation or, in the case of an ongoing investigation, to suspend the study. During a clinical hold, the investigational drug may not be administered to human subjects (unless specifically permitted by the FDA for individual patients in an ongoing study). A clinical hold is issued when there is concern that human subjects will be exposed to unreasonable and significant risk of illness or injury; where there is aquestion over the qualifying credential of the clinical investigators; or in instances in which the IND is concerned incomplete, inaccurate, or misleading. If the concerns raised are addressed to the FDAs satisfaction, a clinical hold may be lifted and clinical investigations resumed; if not, an IND may be maintained in a clinical hold position, declared inactive, withdrawn by the sponsor, or terminated by the FDA. FDA is a very old organization involving several authorities professional in several area and is established to perform the clinical trials and thus after several years with lot of practice and experience has laid down a constitution for new drug approval processes. Currently, this is also monitoring clinical trials that are taking place in several countries along with very systematic clinical trials performed in the USA. Entire evaluation is definitely a tedius and time consuming process. Unfortunately or fortunately, this is a very big subject in itselves. The details of this section are excerpts from the agencies rules to conduct clinical trials. Further details could be conveniently obtained from www.fda.gov website. However, a brief description of a clinical protocol for the convenience of the readers of this textbook will be illustrated here. This definitely gives a complete idea of what is needed by the research organization and FDA as a part of new drug investigation research. A step by step following these rules definitely helps any investigator of pharmacokinetics from early phase I clinical trials to phase III clinical trials.

As a part of the IND application, a clinical protocol must be submitted to ensure the appropriate design and conduct the investigation. Clinical protocols include:

(a) Statement of purpose and objectives of the study

(b) Outline of the investigational plan and study design, including the control group and methods to minimize bias on the part of the subjects, investigators, and analysis;

(c) Estimate the number of patients to be involved;

(d) Basis for subject selection, including inclusion and exclusion criteria;

(e) Description of the dosing plan, including dose levels, route of administration, and duration of patient exposure;

(f) Description of the patient observations, measures and tests to be used;

(g) Clinical procedures, laboratory tests and monitoring to be used in minimizing patient risk;

(h) Names, addresses and credentials of the principal investigators and subinvestigators;

(i) Locations and descriptions of the clinical research facilities to be used; and

(j) Approval of the authorized Institutional Review Board.

Conclusions

Oral pharmacokinetics involves lot of mathematical and statistical concepts and involves dynamic and static movement of a molecule in the body after oral administration. Everyone involved in this field should have an idea of its precedence in filing of new drug application process. Previously it was reported that the clinical development of 40% of drug candidates was discontinued due to unacceptable pharmacokinetic properties. Thus, this chapter becomes crucial in new drug approval and acceptance process. This subject is a very vast area and USA and European authors publish several textbooks. The repetition of the entire role of this subject would be taxing to the readers and thus very small introduction has been furnished in this chapter. The significance of this chapter is very well illustrated in literature with various new drugs. As such the safety of new drugs is the criteria for any pharmaceutical company, thorough understanding is essential for the body involved in this kind of investigations.

Questions for Practice and Exercise

1. Explain compartmental models.
2. Derive equations for rate constants for simple-one compartment and two-compartment models.
3. What are noncompartment models? Explain.
4. Briefly mention about the various pharmacokinetic parameters routinely used in the new drug development processes.
5. What is allometric scaling?
6. Mention about various softwares available in the market to calculate the pharmacokinetic parameters.
7. Describe "New Drug Reporting and Approval: A Pharmacokinetic Perspective".
8. How is the investigation associated with the pharmacokinetic evaluation of new drug substances performed?
9. Mention a brief note on clinical trials from oral pharmacokinetic perspective.

Bibliography

1. The Theory and Practice of Industrial Pharmacy, Third Edition, Edited by Leon Lachman, Herbert A. Lieberman, and Joseph L. Kanig, Lea & Febiger Publications, 1986.
2. New Drug Development: Regulatory Paradigms for Clinical Pharmacology and Biopharmaceutics (Drugs and the Pharmaceutical Sciences: a Series of Textbooks and Monographs), First Edition, Edited by Chandrahas G. Sahajwalla, Marcel Dekker Inc., 2004.
3. The Practice of Medicinal Chemistry, Second Edition, Edited by Camille Georges Wermuth, Elsevier Publications, 2003.
4. Foye`s Principles of Medicinal Chemistry, Fifth Edition, David A. Williams and Thomas L. Lemke, Lippincott Williams & Wilkins, 2002.
5. Generic Drug Product Development: Solid Oral Dosage Forms (Drugs and the Pharmaceutical Sciences: a Series of Textbooks and Monographs), First Edition, Edited by Leon Shargel and Isadore Kanfer, Marcel Dekker, Inc. 2005.

6. Code of Federal Regulations, Title 21, Part 320-Bioavailability and Bioequivalence Requirements.
7. Gibaldi M. Biopharmaceutics and Clinical Pharmacokinetics. 4th Edition. Philadelphia: Lea and Febiger, 1991.
8. Rowland M, Tozer T, Clinical Pharmacokinetics: Concepts and Application. 3rd ed. Philadelphia: Lea and Febiger, 1994.
9. Wagner J. Do You Need a Pharmacokinetic Model, and, if So, Which One? J Pharmacokin Biopharm 1975; 3(6), 457-478.
10. Welling P. Pharmacokinetics: Processes and Mathematics. Monograph 185. Washington DC: American Chemical Society, 1986.

CHAPTER 13

CLINICAL TRIALS AND BIOAVAILABILITY STUDIES

- **Introduction**
- **Common Definitions in Biopharmaceutics**
- **Biopharmaceutics, an Overview**
- **Clinical Trials**
- ***In Vivo* Bioavailability Trials**
  - Basic Trial Designs and Analysis
  - Pilot Trials
  - Pivotal Trials
  - Bioequivalence
- **Inferences**
  - Acceptability Assessment
  - Bioequivalence Assessment
  - Challenges in Decision Making Process
- **Treatments**
  - Statistics
  - Scale Effects
  - Jackknife Evaluations
  - Interfering Factors
- **Conclusions**

Introduction

An extension of the receptor theory of drug action is an increased emphasis on the importance of physico chemical properties of the drug and the relationship of such properties to the pharmacologic responses. Because these properties play an important role in determining biological action of pharmaceuticals, it is appropriate to refer to these properties as biopharmaceutical properties of drug substances. Examples of such properties include solubility, partition coefficients, diffusivity, degree of ionization, polymerization, etc., which, in turn, are determined by the chemical structure and stereochemistry of drug substances. A consideration of these biopharmaceutical properties is fundamental to discussing several important aspects of the overall effects. For a given chemical entity (drug), there will often be a difference in physiological availability and, presumably, in clinical responses. This is primarily because drug molecules must cross various biological membranes and interact with intercellular and intracellular fluids before reaching the elusive region called the "site of action.". Under these conditions, the biopharmaceutical properties of the drug must contribute favorable to facilitate absorption and distribution processes to augment the drug concentration at various active sites. Furthermore, equally important is the fact that these biopharmaceutical properties of a drug must ensure a specific orientation on the receptor surface so that a sequence of events is initiated which leads to the observed pharmacological effects. Drug molecules deficient in the required biopharmaceutical properties, may generally display marginal pharmacological action or be totally ineffective. Almost any alteration in a drug delivery system is likely to alter the drug delivery rate and the amount of the drug delivered to the desired place in the body. All of these are related to biopharmaceutics.

The study of the physical and chemical properties of drugs and their proper dosage as related to the onset, duration, and intensity of action is called biopharmaceutics. This property may not be purely dependent on drugs only but also several times might depend on the physiology of the system in which the drug is moving and acting. Some times it depends on the psychology of the patient too. Not taking medicine continuously as needed might lead to altered onset, duration and intensity of action, although apparent. However, all these could be clubbed under biopharmaceutics. Thus, biopharmaceutics is a vast subject. Bioavailability, bioequivalence and other miscellaneous parameters, methods of estimation of parameters for bioavailability and bioequivalence, physicochemical factors affecting the bioavailability of drugs also constitue biopharmaceutics. Dissolution rate and methods of enhancing dissolution rates, Official and unofficial methods of estimation of dissolution/ invitro release of drugs from dosage forms; *in vitro in vivo* correlation and its significance, the clinical trials associated with bioequivalence, clinical trials associated with drugs action, the entire statistical gamut of bioequivalence are also currently considered under biopharmaceutics. On the other hand, its counterpart pharmacokinetics deals with the extent of the amount of the drug in a particular compartment in the system. Because action is related to the level, both these concepts are definitely interrelated. However, for the convenience and for better understanding of the students, the science of biopharmaceutics and pharmacokinetics is dissected and discussed in this textbook. Some of the issues related to biopharmaceutics are discussed in this chapter.

Common Definitions in Biopharmaceutics

Bioavailability and Bioequivalence

The term bioavailability describes the rate and extent to which an active drug ingredient or therapeutic moiety is absorbed from a drug product and becomes available at the site of drug action. The term bioequivalence refers to the comparison of bioavailabilities of different formulations, drug products, or batches of the same drug product.

Dissolution and Drug Absorption

For a drug to be absorbed, it must first be dissolved in the fluid at the absorption site. For instance, a drug administered orally in tablet or capsule form cannot be absorbed until the drug particles are dissolved by the fluids at some point within the gastrointestinal tract. This process is called dissolution. On the other hand, drug absorption is the entry of a drug particle into the systemic circulation from the gastrointestinal tract.

Drug Forms

Solid drug substances occurs as pure crystalline substances of definite identifiable shape or as amorphous particles without definite structure. The amorphous or crystalline character of a drug substance may be considerably important to its ease of formulation and handling, its chemical stability, and, as has been shown, even its biological activity. These different forms are termed drug forms. Salt forms of drugs are also different forms that may terminate the existence of already available drug if proven to be very effective compared to the drug in the market. The state of hydration of a drug molecule could affect both its solubility and pattern of absorption.

Route of Administration

The ultimate aim of a therapy is that the drug reaches the tissue of interest (also called target tissue). This could be achieved after administering it in any form into any cavity. The drug then slowly travels across the membrane to reach the systemic circulation. The injection of the drug into this specific site is termed as route of administration.

Parameters

In the evaluation of pharmacokinetics of drug substances, several estimations of the movements of drugs in the system are calculated and applied. These terms are called parameters. The parameters that are routinely used include peak height, time of peak, area under the seum concentration time curve and finally tissue uptake.

The Investigational New Drug (IND) Application

Under the Food, Drug, and Cosmetic Act as amended, the sponsor of a new drug is required to file with the FDA an Investigational New Drug Application (IND) before the drug is administered to human subjects in order to protect the rights and safety of the subjects and for very proper study conduction. The sponsor of an IND takes responsibility for and initiates a clinical investigation.

New Drug Applications (NDAs)

A section of each NDA is required to describe the human pharmacokinetic data and human bioavailability data, or information supporting a waiver of the bioavailability data requirement. When the first three phases of clinical testing yields positive results demonstrating safety and therapeutic efficacy, then a New Drug Application is filed.

Abbreviated New Drug Applications (ANDAs)

An application in which in vivo bioavailability data are required unless information is provided and accepted supporting a waiver of this requirement is termed an ANDA. These are required for duplicate products like generic products. Competing companies following the expiration of patent term protection of the innovator drug/drug product generally file these.

Bioequivalent Drug Products

Bioequivalent drug products are pharmaceutical equivalents or pharmaceutical alternatives whose rate and extent of absorption do not show a significant difference when administered at the same molar dose of the therapeutic moiety under similar experimental conditions, either single dose or multiple doses.

Power of a Statistical Test

The power of a statistical test is the ability of this test to detect a difference if such a difference really exists. The statistical test could be anything. It is not uncommon to set the sample size in a clinical trial to attain specified power at a value for the treatment effect deemed likely by the experimenters, even though a smaller treatment effect would still be clinically important. Recent publications on clinical trials have addressed the situation where such a study produces only a weak evidence of a positive treatment effect at an interim stage and the organizer wish to modify the design in order to increase the power to detect a smaller treatment effect than originally expected. Raising the power at a small treatment effect usually leads to considerably higher power than was first specified at the original alternative.

Biopharmaceutics, an Overview

Once a drug is administered and drug absorption begins, the drug does not remain in a single body location, but rather is distributed throughout the body until its ultimate elimination. For instance, following the oral administration of a drug and its entry into the gastrointestinal tract, a portion of the drug is absorbed into the circulatory system from which it is distributed to the various other body fluids, tissues, and organs. From these sites the drug may return to the circulatory system and be excreted through the kidney as such or the drug may be metabolized by the liver or other cellular sites and be excreted as metabolites. On the other hand, drugs administered by intravenous injection are placed directly into the circulatory system, thereby avoiding the absorption process, which is required from all other routes of administration for systemic effects. The various body locations to which a drug travels may be viewed as separate compartments, each containing some fraction of the administered dose of the drug. The transfer of drug from the blood to other body locations is generally a rapid process and is reversible; that is, the drug may diffuse back into the circulation. The drug in the blood therefore exists in equilibrium with the drug in the other compartments. However, in this equilibrium state, the concentration of the drug in the blood may be quite different (greater or lesser) than the concentration of the drug in the other compartments. This is due largely to the physiochemical properties of the drug and its resultant ability to leave the blood and traverse the biological membranes. Certain drugs may leave the circulatory system rapidly and completely, whereas other drugs may do so slowly and with difficulty. A number of drugs become bound to blood proteins, particularly the albumins, and only a small fraction of the drug administered may actually be found at locations outside of the circulatory system at a given time. The transfer of drug from one compartment to another is mathematically associated with a specific rate constant describing that particular transfer. Generally, the rate of transfer of a drug from one compartment to another is proportional to the concentration of the drug in the compartment from which it exits; the greater the concentration, the greater is the amount of drug transfer.

Metabolism is one of the major biopharmaceutic property by which foreign substances, including drugs are eliminated from the body. Most often the structure of the drug leads to appropriate metabolism. In the process of metabolism a drug substance may be biotransformed into pharmacologically active or inactive metabolites. Often, both the drug substances and its metabolites are active and exert pharmacological effects. For example, the antianxiety drug prazepam (Centrax) metabolizes, in part, to oxazepam (Serax), which also has antianxiety effects. In some instances a pharmacologically inactive drug (termed a prodrug) may be administered for the known effects of its active metabolites. Dipivefrin, for example, is a prodrug of epinephrine formed by the esterification of epinephrine and pivalic acid. This increases the lipophilic character of the drug, and as a consequence its penetration into the anterior chamber of the eye is 17 times that of epinephrine. Within the eye, dipivefrin HCl is converted by enzymatic hydrolysis to epinephrine. The metabolism of a drug to inactive products is usually an irreversible process that culminates in the excretion of the drug from the body, usually via the urine. The pharmacokineticist may calculate an elimination rate constant (termed Kel) for a drug to describe its rate of elimination from the body. The term elimination refers to both metabolism and excretion. For drugs that are administered intravenously, and therefore involve no absorption process, the task is much less complex than for drugs administered orally or by other routes. In the latter instances, drug absorption and drug elimination are occurring simultaneously but at different rates.

There are several factors that may affect the biopharmaceutics of chemical agents. Several new factors are always introduced into the literature. However, some of the factors that affect the biopharmaceutics of therapeutic agents as related to the clinical trials and bioequivalence studies, as of today, are henceforth discussed. These include:

1. Molecule Topography as Related to the Drug Absorption into Different Compartments

Topography is a very important feature of a molecule as related to absorption into various membranes. Definitely absorption into biological membranes is one of the key factors for drug absorption into any of the compartments in human system, thereby affecting its pharmacokinetics most of the times and pharmacodynamics sometimes, especially when the activity of the molecule is on the surface of the cell. A very specific example that relates molecular topography, as a determining factor of membrane affinity and transport will be illustrated with the help of hematoporphoryin analogs investigated by Bronshtein I, (2005). This study is purely a physico-chemical study. However, it could be very conveniently extrapolated to the affects of drugs with different topographies on the biological system. The effect of the acidity of the environment on the topography and photophysics of sensitizer molecules embedded in a lipid microenvironment, was studied. A crucial factor in choosing a porphyrin or analogous photosensitizer for photodynamic therapy (PDT) is its ability to incorporate into the cells. For hydrophobic compounds that partition passively into the cytoplasmic membrane, a partition coefficient between an organic solvent and water, *P*, is one factor that could be used to predict the molecule's ability to diffuse into biomembranes. Four hematoporphyrin (HP) analogs were investigated on these lines. These have chemical "spacers" of varying lengths between the chromophoric tetrapyrrole and the carboxylate moiety. These derivatives have essentially the same chemical attributes and reactivity as the parent compound, hematoporphyrin IX, which is used in clinical procedures of photodynamic therapy. The binding constants of these HP derivatives to membrane model systems increase with the length of carboxylate chain in the pH range 3-6.6. This effect of chain length is attributed to an increase in the hydrophobicity of the molecule upon elongation of the alkyl chains. A strong pH dependence of the quenching efficiency of the porphyrins' fluorescence by iodide ions was observed in aqueous solution, and is attributed to a unique electrostatic interaction between the fluorophore and the quencher. The quenching efficiency in liposomes, relative to the quenching in buffer, as a function of pH, shows that porphyrins in the neutral form penetrate deeper inside the lipid bilayer and are less exposed to external quenching than when negatively charged at the carboxylic moiety. This vertical displacement in the membrane is also evidenced in the effect of pH on the photosensitized oxidation efficiency of a membrane-bound chemical target. Increasing the pH causes a significant decrease in the sensitization efficiency in liposomes. This trend is attributed to the vertical localization, and protonation of the carboxylic groups upon lowering the pH leads to sinking of the sensitizer into the lipid bilayer and to a consequent generation of singlet oxygen at a deeper point. This increases the dwell time of singlet oxygen within the bilayer, which results in greater photodamage that is caused to a membrane-residing singlet oxygen target. The conclusion of the key of this study in terms of pharmacodynamics is that a therapeutic molecule could leave or enter a system definitely depending on its topological properties. As mentioned in this study pH is one of the key factors that determine the extent of ionization and membrane solubility. In addition, pH is definitely one property that influences the porosity of physiological membranes, the binding of a substrate to its target, it does not matter whether this target is a transporter or this target is a protein that affects a disease condition. Very similar properties affect the biopharmaceutics of molecules and thereby skew the clinical outcomes observed in clinical trials. Such an investigation that comes into the arena of the clinical trial is partially associated with pharmacogenomics. Similar to the topographic situation at a particular pH that might occur in one patient and which is not found in another patient could be found in other cases. This is mainly because of the variations in the genetics. This topic would be better cited with other examples. Pharmacogenetics deals with inherited differences in the response to drugs. The best-recognized examples are genetic polymorphisms of drug-metabolizing enzymes, which affect about 30% of all drugs. Loss of function of thiopurine S-methyltransferase (TPMT) results in severe and life-threatening hematopoietic toxicity if patients receive standard doses of mercaptopurine and azathioprine. Gene duplication of cytochrome P4502D6 (CYP2D6), which metabolizes many antidepressants, has been identified as a mechanism of poor response in the treatment of depression. There is also a growing list of genetic polymorphisms in drug targets that have been shown to influence drug response. A major limitation that has heretofore moderated the use of pharmacogenetic testing in the clinical setting is the lack of prospective clinical trials demonstrating that such testing can improve the benefit/risk ratio of drug therapy.

2. Molecular Topography as Related to the Drug Actions in Knock-out Animal Studies

Knockout (KO) mice lacking the orphan nuclear receptor steroidogenic factor 1 (SF-1) exhibit marked structural abnormalities of the ventromedial nucleus of the hypothalamus (VMH). In one study, Davis et al., (2004) sought to determine the molecular mechanisms underlying the VMH abnormalities. To trace SF-1-expressing neurons, this study used a SF-1/enhanced green fluorescent protein (eGFP) transgene. Although the total numbers of eGFP-positive cells in wild-type (WT) and SF-1 KO mice were indistinguishable, cells that normally localize precisely within the VMH were scattered more diffusely in adjacent regions in SF-1 KO mice. This abnormal distribution is likely due to the loss of SF-1 expression in VMH neurons rather than secondary effects of deficient steroidogenesis, as redistribution also was seen in mice with a CNS-specific KO of SF-1. Thus, the absence of SF-1 alters the distribution of cells that normally form the VMH within the mediobasal hypothalamus. Consistent with this model, the hypothalamic expression patterns of the transcription factors islet-1 and nkx2.1 also were displaced in SF-1 KO mice. Independent of gene expression, birthdate analyses further suggested that cells with earlier birthdates were affected more severely by the loss of SF-1 than were later born cells. The conclusion is that the absence of SF-1 causes major changes in cellular arrangement within and around the developing VMH that result from altered cell migration. This is a very simple example that illustrates how a change in the expression of a cellular protein may affect the entire network. On several occasions, a patient or a subject with such situations, that might have affected with the birth or due to the disease conditions or due to the drug abuse, may after a prolonged exposure leads to the differential physiological status, although he is very fine in terms of day to day activities. In these situations, this could be termed an abuse and the clinical trial oucome may be different compared to a normal subject. In these situations, a molecule of the same series may be effective on a healthy subject, whereas a molecule with different topography of the same series may be effective in a knockout patient situation. This is a specific example of the physiological alterations. Pharmacodynamics of a drug candidate is definitely affected. On the other hand, if a transporter is lost then it may totally alter the biopharmaceutics and pharmacokinetics of molecules. In clinical trial experiments this may lead to an outlier. Definitely, the results of the clinical studies may be skewed and such results should be very properly evaluated in terms of clinical trial designs and experiments.

Many of these type of study`s are in the very beginning stages as far as their application in clinical trial goes. However, keeping in perspective of the clinical investigation developments at the cellular levels in near future, this topic is very briefly mentioned here. Only a very few leading journals in clinical investigations area are currently focusing on this aspect. Similarly many topics of this chapter could be mentioned about. At its zenith, clinical trial investigation may encompass this topic in full detail. However, this factor is still in the beginning in clinical trial discussions at this time.

3. Age of the Subject

The elderly comprise 12 percent of the U.S. population but consume 33 percent of all prescription drugs. The incidence of adverse drug reactions is significantly higher in persons over age 65 than in younger population groups. The increased risk of adverse drug effects is related to decreased organ reserve capacity, to altered pharmacokinetics and pharmacodynamics, and to polypharmacy with associated drug-drug and drug-disease interactions. An organized therapeutic plan and critical evaluation of the list of drugs an elderly patient is taking will help in establishing a safe and effective drug regimen. In these patients, the clinical trial design is definitely different from normal subjects or young patients. In a study design, when patients of all ages are included the statistical outcomes with this drug needs to be carefully evaluated.

In the same way, the clinical trial design for children needs to be designed in a different way compared to adults. This is better illustrated with the following example. In most cases, childhood leukaemia has a fetal origin, but multiple molecular events are required after birth for pre-leukaemic cells to progress to leukaemia. Cure rates for acute lymphoblastic leukaemia (ALL) now approach 80%. A high level of minimal residual disease detected by polymerase chain reaction in patients with ALL in remission has profound prognostic importance and is the focus of a major Australian study attempting to prevent relapse in these children. Greater awareness of the late effects of chemotherapy has led to changes in the treatment protocols for ALL, with improvement in neurocognitive outcomes and reduced rates of secondary malignancies. Pharmacogenetics is a new field of research that aims to enhance treatment efficacy by assessing the individual's metabolism and response to chemotherapeutic agents. Targeted therapies currently being developed show some promise of being able to further improve cure rates. Adolescents with ALL have a better prognosis if treated with paediatric rather than adult protocols.

4. Disease Conditions

Chronic diseases are disruptive for patients and place considerable demands on health service costs and manpower. In addition, these play a major role in clinical trial outcomes and designs. In the estimation of the efficacy of drugs for these categories of patients, the best volunteers are the patients themselves. The controls are normal subjects. The physicians, the drugs and the society abuse these classes of subjects in a different manner. Thus, after prolonged subjugation, these candidates either become more tolerant in terms of interpretation, physiology or resistance. Thus, the design of clinical trials, the interpretation of the outcomes is very challenging. Dr. Kennedy et al., (2003; 2003), investigated a clinical trial design and interpretation for a group of diseased candidates. This group used inflammatory bowel disease (IBD) as a suitable example of a chronic disease to test this kind of approach. IBD (Crohn's disease and ulcerative colitis) affects approximately 175 000 people in the UK (symptoms include bloody diarrhoea, abdominal pain, and weight loss, and follow a relapsing course with periods of remission). The aetiology is unknown and medical treatment is ameliorative rather than curative; many patients need maintenance treatment with drugs whose dose varies according to disease severity. Although recently developed national management guidelines state that patients with IBD should be provided with information on treatment options, recent surveys reveal that patients still feel insufficiently informed and want greater involvement in their treatment.

The study design was a multicentre trial with randomisation by treatment centre (cluster randomisation). This method was chosen to avoid the risks of contamination within centres, as staff training, an essential part of the intervention, could only be delivered to entire clinical teams. All 24 district hospitals in the North West of England (population 6.7 million; **UK census data 2002**) with gastroenterology departments were approached and 19 agreed to participate (of the other five sites, including one teaching hospital, three failed to reply and two were already engaged in IBD research and declined to participate). The 19 hospitals (seven teaching hospitals and 12 non-teaching hospitals) were then randomly allocated either to continue to provide treatment as usual (10 sites) or to deliver the self-management programme to eligible patients attending the outpatient clinics (nine sites). At the time of recruitment, 15 centres had a policy of following up all patients with IBD on a long term basis (six randomised to intervention), two sites discharged patients when their symptoms had been quiescent for more than one year (both randomised to intervention), and at two sites there was no consistent follow up policy (one randomised to intervention).

Three outcome measures were constructed from medical records: number of appointments kept during the trial year; number of made appointments not attended; and percentage of patients who failed to attend at least once. The records also allowed comparative figures to be derived for the pre-trial year. When computing these outcome measures, the recruitment appointment was excluded, as it would be inappropriate to class this as either a pre-trial or in-trial appointment. The pre-trial period is therefore taken as the 364 days prior to the recruitment date and the in-trial period as the 364 days following recruitment. In conclusion, adoption of guided self-management was generally popular both with patients and clinicians, reduced use of hospital services without burden to primary care, and increased quality of care without an adverse effect on disease control at the same time as reducing cost. More widespread adoption of this programme for patients with IBD and other chronic medical disorders, particularly those with relapsing remitting patterns, now seems indicated. The very simple lesson from this study is that the disease state of the patient definitely affects the biopharmaceutics and pharmacokinetics outcomes of drug therapy both in terms of drug levels and the clinical measures.

5. Effect of Composition and Quality of Diet and Feeding Time on the Kinetics and Efficacy of Drugs

A recent example by Ali et al., (2004), illustrates this effect better. Ali et al., published the literature dealing with the effects of composition and quality of diet and feeding time on the pharmacokinetics and efficacy of some anthelmintic drugs in ruminants. Various studies suggested that greater availability, and therefore improved anthelmintic activity is possible through temporary feed restriction. It is also recommended that anthelmintic drugs should not be given to animals whilst they are maintained on large feed intakes, particularly of lush pasture that promotes rapid gastric transit, as this may reduce drug availability and anthelmintic efficacy. Generally, feeding animals low-quality fibrous diets reduces the passage rate of digesta and allows more time for absorption of several anthelmintic drugs and their metabolites from the gut. Some kinetic data of drugs given to animals on such diets may be slightly different, but this does not necessarily indicate alteration of the dosages of the anthelmintic drug. Nonetheless, due consideration should be given to anthelmintic dosages under various dietary regimes if optimum efficacy is to be achieved at all times.

Clinical Trials

A clinical trial is designed to test an intervention in a human system. The objective of the intervention could be prophylactic/preventive, diagnostic, or therapeutic. As a process these agents could be delivered as pharmacological agents with routine experiments as conducted in a physiology or pharmacology lab, using devices, as regimens or with the application of several miscallaneous procedures. Many of the basics as mentioned in the above section should be enough for further elucidation and understanding the basic reasons why clinical trials are conducted. Other reasons and explanations could be extrapolated. Several kinds of clinical trials are currently in use. These include Phase I (dose tolerance (MTD)), Phase II (biologic effect or activity of treatment; rate of adverse events) and Phase III/IV (clinical effectiveness (short term), long-term effect +safety (phase IV)). These intervention studies could be ***uncontrolled*** (pre/post test) or ***controlled***. Uncontrolled intervention studies are conducted as comparisons to controls in the very early stages of an investigation with a new chemical agent or an outcome. These studies are generally not yet relevant or clinical studies are not feasible. Most of the pilot works are of this type. For instance, a positive outcome with the consumption of a particular chemical, such as gutka and pan in India and chewing gum, etc. in other countries in a particular group of patients could be termed an uncontrolled intervention study. The clinical outcomes are either proxy or the presumed mechanism (s) of intervention is the outcome. On the other hand, control studies are very systematic investigations. Most of the clinical studies fall in this category. These studies could be further classified into non-randomized or randomized.

A Non-Randomized Clinical Trial

Generally, a non-randomized study does not have systematic control experiments conducted together with the intervention. A ***historical control*** or a ***concurrent control*** is generally used in these studies.

A historical control has the following salient features:

1. "Control" treatment data come from databases, existing literature, or medical records
2. Strengths
   (a) No one denied new treatments (more ethical)
   (b) Easier to recruit
   (c) More efficient (less costly)
3. Weaknesses
   (a) Poor control for bias (due to e.g. selection, changes in patient population and disease management)

A concurrent control has the following salient features:

1. Control group receives control treatment at about same time as intervention group
2. Strengths
   (a) Treatment is not left to chance, and may be more acceptable to participants (also favoring recruitment)
   (b) Cross-over of treatment is better managed
   (c) Better control of differences in patient populations or in disease management
3. Weaknesses
   (a) Still potential for serious bias due to differences between patients in intervention and control groups

A Randomized Clinical Trial

Generally, a randomized study has a very systematic control experiment conducted along with the intervention. The design is very appropriate. The inferences are very appropriate. The conclusions are definitely concrete at the end of the intervention. Different kinds of randomized clinical trials include parallel designs, factorial designs and crossover designs. A parallel design has either 2 or greater than 2 treatment arms. These kinds of designs are the simplest ones. One group is treated for the intervention and the other group is generally a control. A factorial design is generally a 2X2 design or it may be a combination greater than 2 different treatments. In a factorial design, a combination of groups is used for the interventions and for the controls. This is somewhat more sophisticated in terms of the designs and interpretations and inferences. In a crossover design the treatment is offered to the experimental group first followed by the control group. If the various aspects as ideal requirements for clinical trial designs are considered, the following comes to the picture: simplicity, statistical efficiency, scientific relevance, validity of assumptions, cost and ethical advantages. To target each of the idealnesses of the designs in a concordant way for a lay man, parallel designs are simple, statistically efficient, assumptions are more valid, and cost effective. On the other hand, factorial designs are very complicated, less statistically relevant, and costly. However, these kinds of designs are more scientifically relevant. In terms of validity of assumptions and the ethical advantages, these designs are neutral. Cross-over designs are the most commonly used clinical trial designs. These are simple, statistically efficient, scientifically relevant, cost effective and offer more ethical advantages. There is definitely a compromise in the validity of assumptions. However, these are the very often and more usually used methodologies in clinical trial designs. At this time, several modifications and modernizations in all round aspects of biopharmaceutics and clinical trial designs are in existence in the literature and practice. Some of the specifics are further discussed in the subsequent sections.

A General Protocol for a Clinical Trial Experiment

As indicated before, a clinical trial group or methodology occupies a significant place in a pharma industry. Although very brief introduction to the designs that are routinely used is mentioned, definitely there are several of these designs currently in existence and practice. However, most of the designs follow very similar steps that include:

1. Selecting or assigning subjects to experimental units
2. Selecting or assigning units for specific treatments or condition of the experiment (experimental manipulation)

3. Specifying the order or arrangement of the treatment or treatments
4. Specifying the sequence of observations or measurements to be used.

Thus, in any clinical protocol, the execution is to follow the above steps in a systematic manner, however complex or simple the design is. Blinding is very commonly used in the clinical trial investigations. These are of two types: double blind trials and single blind trials. In a double blind study, the participant and investigator are unaware of treatment assignment, mostly used for drug efficacy studies and "gold" standard is commonly used. In a single blind study, either the participant, investigator/interventionist, outcome assessor or the outcome event adjudicator are blinded. The follow-up of a clinical trial design includes duration, frequency and intensity. Expected onset or duration of treatment benefit, available funding and power, or the amount of change in or number of outcome events has to be taken care as a part of the duration. In addition, frequency of contact with participant and amount of follow-up assessment are also determined. Once the experiments are conducted as per the above protocol, the results are obtained. Most of the times the design as well as the conduction is statistically designed to obtain very appropriate data. The data is then subjected to analysis. Different types of analysis include intention-to-treat analysis, on-treatment analysis, secondary analysis (pre-specified and exploratory) and the analysis of presumed mechanisms.

Target Population

Most of the times, the target population selection is the important aspect as straightly related to clinical trials or invertly related to the outcome of the experiments. Thus, the selection of this population for a clinical trial is crucial. Before even the experiments are conducted in human subjects, lot of data has already been generated with the help of animal experiments. Toxicity profiles and pharmacological outcomes are already in place. This is how systematic clinical trials are conducted. Then, once the molecules are very effective and safe in these preliminary studies, a clinical trial in humans is designed. The sequence of the clinical trials is as mentioned in the section of the protocol for a clinical trial study. In this regard, a clinical trial could be conducted in patient population or in general population (healthy). Patient population could be further classified into disease specific vs generic or high-risk vs all. Healthy population is either one with elevated diseases risk or it is not defined by disease risk. Treatments or interventions are administered, results obtained and proper conclusions drawn. This is how an ethical study is designed, conducted and concluded.

In Vivo Bioavailability Trials

In vivo bioavailability trials are conducted to determine the extent of drug reaching the systemic circulation or sometimes the site of action of this drug. These studies are the part of clinical trial protocols. Earlier when the means of assay`s were not available or it was not convenient to obtain volunteers for drug pulling from the systemic circulation, only the disease effects were taken as the end points. However, a better correlation of drug levels with pharmacodynamics is always a criterion. Not all the times appropriate drug levels in the system means that the drug is effective. In this regard, the current trend is to determine the amount of the drug in the systemic circulation and at the same time correlate the action of this drug for a particular disease. Similarly when generics are compared and the judgement of a better formulation of a drug from a set of the formulations of the same drug is made, comparisons of the bioavailabilities of the drugs is the criterion. Bioavailability is the part of biopharmaceutics as discussed previously and is definitely a part of clinical trial protocols. The clinical trial designs are thus always spoken in terms of bioavailability and disease end points. However, keeping in view the nature of this chapter, from now on this chapter will be discussed totally in a clinical trial, statistical and bioavailability perspective.

Basic Trial Designs and Analysis

A well-planned arrangement of volunteers to determine very best the efficacy of a treatment or intervention is termed a trial design. A volunteer is the very appropriate term to be used in the context of clinical trials. To determine the efficacy of a drug, it is definitely not possible to conduct these tests in the entire population. Thus, only a bunch of the subjects are obtained and the treatment or the intervention is administered. Once the experiment is conducted results are obtained. Then the results obtained from these volunteers are extrapolated to the population. Thus, it becomes imperative that these methods are very close to the ideal possibility. The basic trials designs could be a parallel group, in series designs, factorial designs or sequential designs. A basic introduction to this concept is discussed in the section "Clinical Trials". The first very systematic clinical trial is that of field trial of salk polio vaccine conducted in 1954. In this situation, the comparison was made between a randomized controlled double blind clinical trial and a non-randomized open trial. In any case the ethical situation is the priority. In ethical considerations, treaty of Helsinki (1960 +amendments) is carefully weighed. Ethics are then considered between individual and collectives conducting the clinical trial. A badly planned or executed experiment could be termed unethical. For example, comparison of treatment A with treatment B when the group is genuinely unsure if the treatment

A and treatment B are effective. Currently, there are no such terms. However, an unethical situation could lead to a jail term, however influential or powerful the investigator or the group of clinical trial conduction. In any situation local ethics committees are responsible for the conduction of fair clinical trials. The clinical trials are first licensed (hospital/city/region). Informed consent is needed. It is very unethical to perform a trial that has little prospect of reaching any conclusion. This may be because of insufficient numbers or poor design. Contributors then must sign to declare: full responsibility for conduct of study, had access to data and should get controlled decision to publish. Phase I trials are performed to determine the pharmacology and toxicity (n=10-50); Phase II trials are performed for safety and efficacy studies (n=50-100); Phase III trials are performed for treatment comparisons (n=100-1000); Phase IV trials are for post-marketing surveillance (n=as many as possible); Blind trials (double or single are conducted preferably to reduce the bias); Placebo trials (to assess the controls).

A randomized controlled trial is conducted for comparative (new vs. standard); remove bias (conscious or unconscious) and control group (as similar as possible to treated group). In a **parallel group** design each volunteer group receives 1 treatment. Comparison is between the volunteers. Average difference between groups needs to be much larger than between the patient volunteers. For 2 groups t-test, Mann-Whitney test etc. are applied and when the group size is greater than 2 1-way ANOVA or Kruskal-Wallis test are applied. In **series designs** comparisons are within patient volunteers. Differences between patient volunteers do not affect differences between treatments. For 2 groups paired t-test (t-test on differences), Wilcoxon signed rank test are applied. For greater than 2 groups 2-way ANOVA and Friedmans test are applied. The advantages of these kinds of tests include patients can state preferences; may be applied to treatments simultaneously; comparisons within patients are made (reduces variability thereby precise comparison is made; suitable for rapidly evaluated outcomes and finally minimizes number of subjects when clear differences between treatments are noticed. The disadvantages of such a design include trend in results may complicate the analysis; treatments may persist; not suitable if treatment cures subject (only suitable for chronic conditions) and withdrawals complicate the analysis. **Crossover designs** are similar to in series designs but different groups have treatments in different orders. The advantages and disadvantages are similar to those for parallel group and in series designs. In **factorial designs** patient volunteers generally receive combination of treatments. These designs are more appropriate because interactions between the drug treatments are noticed. The other advantages are in terms of biopharmaceutical perspective. As mentioned before, several factors may confound the results in clinical trials. All these factors are considered or the interaction of the treatment with a particular biopharmaceutical aspect may be clarified. If there are more interactions very complicated factorial designs are performed to clarify and indicate the more responsible factor that is interacting with the outcome. Controlling these factors becomes very important in case of controllable factors. If that is not possible, generally it leads to the generation of dropouts. In these situations dropouts cause difficulties. Thus, a constant surveillance is necessary. However, the ballpark in these kinds of designs is that the patient volunteers or the normal volunteers are to be treated like animals if there are two treatments in one regimen. But, definitely these statistical designs have several advantages. In any of the design cases, time is the criteria. If the volunteer groups are complicated or if the comprehension of the protocols is not proper, it may lead to lot of waste of time of everyone involved in the project.

Pilot Trials

As mentioned earlier, statistics are used right from the beginning of clinical trial studies. Most statistical methods for clinical trials are based on the frequentist paradigm of hypothesis testing (and the dual concept of confidence intervals), in which long-run probabilities for false positive and false negative test decisions are controlled by fixing significance levels and sample sizes based on power calculations. In early stage formulation development, exploratory or pilot trials are performed on 8-12 healthy male (usually in a pilot study the number of volunteers is very limited) subjects to evaluate the acceptability of the test drug products as candidates for further bioequivalence evaluation. This is because the in vitro dissolution profile of the test product usually cannot provide a reliable prediction of the in vivo bioavailability. Pilot studies provide an estimate of the test-reference ratio for the primary bioavailability measures: AUC and C_{max}, and their intrasubject variability. Unfortunately at this level several statistical tests could be used for estimating pharmacokinetic parameters and for comparison purposes. However, planning of the study is the very essential feature. These pilot studies are not only used for the evaluation of the various parameters of a new chemical moiety but also for pharmacological, therapeutics, medical or surgical uses. A very simple example as illustrated would be an indicative of a careful and planned pilot study. Very recently as of January 2003 a prospective randomization pilot study to evaluate predictors of response in serial core biopsies to single agent neoadjuvant doxorubicin or placlitaxel for patients with locally advanced breast cancer was investigated.

Despite the widespread utility of anticancer therapy, the molecular signatures of the activity of individual agents on tumor cells during therapy are not well characterterized. So during the early stages of a clinical study for cancer patients, it becomes difficult to determine whether a treatment in positive or negative. Traditionally treatment efficacy for breast cancer such as time to progression, disease-free survival, and overall survival, which requires large database, is used. However, definitely this is a difficult process. In this situation, elucidating surrogate markers of efficacy of traditional agents may provide earlier insights into drug sensitivity and resistance. Stearns et al., (2003), after signing an informed consent approved by the Institutional Review Board at George town University Medical Center, selected volunteers in the study. The women (n=29) were randomized before the study. One group was treated with doxorubicin and other group with paclitaxel. To make sure equivalence between two arms, the randomization was stratified by menopausal status and lesion stage and the study conducted in blocks of 4 patients as suggested in RANLST module of the STPLAN software package. Breast biopsy, apoptosis assays, markers of proliferation assays, expression of ER, HER2/neu, bcl2, and p53 were used as the end points. Before even conducting the trial the baseline end point biomarkers were estimated before and after the exposure. The selected regimen was effective. The markers were effective in the evaluations. The conclusion of the study is that the clinical design could serve as a model for combining standard chemotherapy and novel agents. Further, studies are needed to be conducted.

Pivotal Studies

Bioequivalence studies are used in a variety of situations, most often when a sponsor proposes manufacturing a generic version of an approved off-patent product. A bioequivalence study may also be part of a new abbreviated drug application (NADA) or supplemental NADA for approval of an alternative dosage form, new route of administration, or a significant manufacturing change that may affect drug bioavailability. A pivotal trial is the required bioequivalence study that is performed to establish bioequivalence between test and reference drug products when submitting an abbreviated new drug application (ANDA). Immediate release (IR) drug products are generally tested in single-dose bioequivalence studies, whereas extended release (ER) drug products require both single-dose and multiple-dose studies. In general, bioequivalence studies are performed under fasting conditions. However, for ER drug products and certain IR drug products single-dose bioequivalence studies are performed under both fasting and fed conditions. The food effect studies are performed to assess the comparative effect of food on the bioavailability of the test and reference drug products. In a pivotal fasting study, equivalence is accepted if the 90% geometric confidence interval for the test-reference ratio is completely contained within the range of 0.80-1.25 for both the AUC and Cmax. The fixed range (0.80-1.25) used in the bioequivalence evaluation is normally referred to as the bioequivalence range that is set by regulatory authorities. In addition, the food effect study requires test-reference ratios of arithmetic means for AUC and Cmax to fall between 0.80 and 1.20. Bioequivalence between the test and reference products is concluded when equivalence has been established in all three types of bioequivalence trials.

Failure in establishing the bioequivalence for a successful product in a pivotal trial may be the result of an insufficient sample size. The width of the confidence interval is negatively correlated to sample sizes. The sample size in a pivotal trial is normally estimated, based on the power function of the parametric test procedure that is sensitive to the input values of the test-reference ratio and intrasubject variance, particularly the test-reference ratio. The test-reference ratio and the intrasubject variability are mainly derived in pilot trials that are subject to large sampling variation. Use of a lower intrasubject variance and a test-reference ratio that is closer to unity than that observed in pivotal trials will lead to sample size estimates for pivotal studies that are insufficient to reduce the confidence interval into the bioequivalence range.

Bioequivalence

Bioequivalence is the term very often used when comparing different formulations of the same drug (generally containing the same amount of a drug in the formulation). Generally for drugs that are routinely used in the pharmacies and routinely used by the patient's, small variations in the drug absorbed or the drug bioavailable to the target may not affect the efficacy of the dosage form. However, for some categories of drugs this becomes a very important factor. Slight variation in the extent of absorption or extent of the drug reaching the target may cause tremendous problems. A slight difference, for instance, instead of a standard 56% oral bioavailable formulation, if a formulation with 60% oral bioavailability is administered, the case may become toxic rather than pharmacologic. Pharmacists and physicians noticed these situations long time ago when switching from one brand to the other. Not only the examples of two formulations may be helpful in deciphering this situation, but definitely needs further elaboration and investigation. For instance if a very common treatment has 5-10 products of the same drug with the same dosage with the same formulation type in the market, and definitely there is a significant variability in terms of the extent of therapeutic benefit, then it definitely becomes imperative to investigate these situations and formulate rules and laws accordingly. Currently, science and mathematics in this area is very significant. However, keeping in view its historical and current situations, this section needs to be further elucidated with very specific examples along with the statistical and mathematical concepts.

Another example of the importance of bioequivalence studies is illustrated by a very severe case which clearly depicts the importance of long-distance, mathematical, statistical and probability oriented directive study for these investigations. Pharmacological treatment of CNS disorders often requires perfect dosage titration to achieve satisfactory symptom control whilst minimizing the risk of adverse effects. Relapses requiring hospitalization are an important potential source of additional cost for the health service and any inadequate symptom control increases the indirect costs of CNS relating support, for example the need for sheltered accommodation of intensive social services support. There are several previous cases as observed by physicians over several years. Currently, there are several products in the market to treat CNS disorders. For the same drug and for the same dosage form and for the same dose, different products may result in different extents of CNS absorptions, maximum plasma concentrations, different extents of bioavailabilities and different times to peaks. Unfortunately or fortunately, generic drugs may differ from branded drugs in their formulation and may not show precise bioequivalence with the branded product. A higher maximum plasma concentration (C_{max}) could lead to increased or emergent adverse effects, whereas a decreased absorption or minimum plasma concentration (C_{min}) may result in a reduced therapeutic effect. In the situations where the drug is incorporated in chewing gums, say for example nicotine chewing gums to treat nicotine addiction, the time of chewing also plays a major role. The other example is that of another CNS drug, clozapine. Plasma levels of clozapine are critical to therapeutic response. Opportunistic treatment doesnot hold well for the treatments involving clozapine, say for instance schizophrenia. Symptom aggravation occurred in approximately 10% of patients switched from branded to generic clozapine in a small, randomized, crossover study. Patients with schizophrenia may also show suspicion and hostility regarding their treatment. This may result in unwillingness to take an unfamiliar medication and decreased compliance, thus increasing the risk of a relapse. Unfortunately, the standard protocols are not the same for all the patients in this category and lessons from one study different from lessons for other study. Definitely the regimens are developed but the practice has not been there by physicians in this regard. Thus, psychiatrists should take great care when switching patients with schizophrenia from branded to generic antipsychotic drugs; this entails monitoring clinical outcome closely and adjusting the treatment in case of symptom aggravation or emergence of adverse effects. Prevention is better than cure is the ballpark statement for this situation. The basic causes for these effects are demonstrated and indicated in the section of the biopharmaceutics. Further, a very brief overview of bioequivalence terminology, FDA guidelines for bioequivalence, general considerations regarding bioequivalence as published by Daniel Baker (2003) in the “Reviews In Gastroenterological Disorders”, Vol 3. No. 4 as part of New Drug Review will be exerpted henceforth.

Several terms are exclusively used in **bioequivalence jargon**. *Bioavailability* refers to the rate and extent that a drug is absorbed from various dosage forms. *Reference product* is generally the first branded product. It could also be a new formulation in a different dosage form or using a different delivery system that is considered the testing standard for a particular drug. *Bioequivalence* is determined by a comparison of the bioavailability of different drug products (a reference product and a comparator product) using the same dosage form (eg, tablet vs tablet, sustained-release tablet vs sustained release tablet, capsule vs capsule). If two formulations are shown to have equivalent bioavailability, then the formulations are said to be bioequivalent. *Individual bioequivalence* is determined through comparison of the bioavailability of various products to determine intrasubject variability associated with the different drug products. Bioequivalence and individual bioequivalence should not be confused with *pharmaceutical equivalence*. Drug products are considered pharmaceutically equivalent when they contain the same active ingredient in the same concentration, dosage form, and route of administration. However, these products may differ in shape, scoring configuration, release mechanisms, packaging, excipients, and expiration date. These are currently the minimum requirements to describe bioequivalence. Several statistical and mathematical concepts are currently in use and research. **The Food and Drug Administration (FDA) guidelines for bioequivalence** require a number of parameters to be in place for two drugs to be considered bioequivalent. The differences in the means of the AUC and the Cp_{max} must be 0.8% to 1.25%. Data from the FDA indicate that most drugs fall within 3% to 7% compared to the reference agent. It is estimated that there is a 5% change that a generic could be approved whose actual mean values fell outside the 80% to 125% range. Most of the information on bioequivalence of medications is based on controlled clinical trials with defined patient populations. These studies provide the general demographics of the study population, but generally provide no information regarding genetic variations within the study population that might have influenced some or all of the study results. The **current standards for bioequivalence** were implemented before most of the information regarding pharmacogenomics and its potential impact on drug metabolism were established with some specific examples. It is very unfortunate that current standards are implemented mainly out of developed countries. Indian pharmaceutical situation in terms of bioequivalence is not upto the mark. **The current Indian scenario** would be to implement many of these FDA type of guidelines with regard to bioequivalence, drug safety and patient benefit. India has large patient populations for almost all major indications and hence the patient recruitment rates in India are 2-3 times higher than in the US or Western Europe. India has a large and growing pool of clinical investigators who are highly qualified (many trained in the West), fully conversant with GCP and who have extensive experience conducting bioequivalence studies. India has huge genetic diversity among its population. Thus results from studies conducted here are easily transferable to other ethnic and geographical milieus. Although genetics play a major role, very careful statistical designs, evaluations, and guidelines would definitely rule out the effects of genetic factors in the bioequivalence studies and their evaluations.

Inferences

Inference in the bioequivalence studies is important both in terms of marketing aspect as well as the clinical efficacy. This inference mostly depends on the statistical principles. Marketing aspect is the decision by a company whether to develop a generic equivalent for patent expired compound or simply set up the development of a new chemical moiety. Since the goal of any company is to earn profits. This is the first step in this direction. The next step then is to identify a therapeutic molecule that could give enough profits for this new company to compete enough in the market for further development.

Acceptibility Assessment

An observed test-reference ratio of close to unity may indicate test formulations of value for further evaluation in bioequivalence trials. The test formulation is accepted for further evaluation in pivotal trials when the test-reference ratio of geometric means obtained in pilot trials falls within an acceptable range, such as (0.9, 1.11), otherwise the test formulation may require modification. The acceptable range is determined by the bioequivalence range, the permissible sample size of pivotal trials; and the intrasubject variability, apart from several other statistically acceptable factors. New techniques are always published in the literature. Selection of the subjects for investigation is also an important criteria.

The subject population for bioequivalence studies should be selected with the aim to minimise variability and permit detection of differences between pharmaceutical products. Therefore, the studies should be performed with healthy volunteers. The inclusion/exclusion criteria should be clearly stated in the protocol. Subjects could belong to both sexes; however, the risk to women of childbearing potential should be considered on an individual basis. In general, subjects should be between 18 – 55 years old, capable of giving informed consent and of weight within the normal range according to accepted life tables (cf. Supplement I) or Body Mass Index (BMI) of 18 - 30. They should be screened for suitability by means of clinical laboratory tests (cf. Supplement II), an extensive review of medical history, and a comprehensive medical examination. Subjects should preferably be non-smokers and without a history of alcohol or drug abuse. If moderate smokers are included (less than 10 cigarettes per day) they should be identified as such and the consequences for the study results should be discussed. If the purpose of the bioequivalence study is to address specific questions such as investigation of differences in bioavailability in different subsets of the population or drug-drug interactions the selection criteria and the statistical analysis should be adjusted accordingly.

Bioequivalence Assessment

Three types of pivotal trials – single-dose fasting, single-dose food effect and multiple-dose fasting are normally performed on separate occasions to minimize the risk of selecting an unsuccessful test formulation in pilot trials. When equivalence is successfully established in the initial pivotal trial (s), the remaining trial (s) will follow. A single-dose fasting study is normally first to be performed. Each of the above studies have their own advantages. Generally it is thought that multiple-dose fasting are normally more powerful than other kinds of studies. T-test (both one-sided and two-sided) and ANOVA are used in the bioequivalence assessment. In one study it was shown that the standard two one-sided tests procedure for bioequivalence is a biased test. Several other tests were proposed and were found to be effective in bioequivalence assessments. In another study an unbiased alpha-level test and other tests that are uniformly more powerful than the two one-sided test procedures were constructed. The power of this test was noticeably larger than that of an alpha-level two one-sided test procedures. The experimental designs used in bioequivalency assessments are the same as those mentioned in the previous sections. A commonly used experimental setting in clinical trials is the two-period, two-sequence cross-over design. The other important aspect is the sample size calculation. Several methods are available in the literature as well as several experts in the area have their own methods of deciding upon sample sizes used in the bioavailability assessments.

Challenges in Decision Making Process

The very important criteria facing decision makers in generic drug product development is the identification of successful test products based on the results of individual trials. The pharmacokinetic data set may contain outlying observations that could lead to wrong rejection of bioequivalence. There is always a possibility of the outliers because of the several reasons mentioned previously. In addition, there could be a wrong decision making process because of the inappropriate models that could have been selected because of the ignorance of the connecting fields of pharmaceutics, clinical trials, statistics and physicians. In these situations, a very well trained person in the medical field, pharmacy, pharmaceutics, pharmaceutical technology, statistics and engineering would be a very appropriate person to make a proper decision or, a group of body consisting of individuals specialized in these areas could be a very right replacement in this perview of decision making process.

Treatments

Treatment of the data that results from bioequivalence studies is a very important aspect. Several times situations may arise where in a company`s product is superior than the competitor`s product; however, it could be discarded because the results and interpretations may indicate that the superior product is inferior. This situation arises when the treatments are not properly done. In pilot studies, the likelihood of correctly concluding the acceptability of a test formulation is usually low. As mentioned previously, several factors may come into the picture. In any case, some of the peculiarities are not avoidable. The best way in this situation is to treat the data very judiciously and appropriately. In small size crossover trials, estimation of the test-reference ratios is sensitive to the influence of extreme individual ratio observations. The acceptability assessment based on the test-reference ratio of geometric means from pilot trials may present a considerable risk of rejecting a successful test formulation or accepting an unsuccessful test formulation. Similarly several other treatments are used and are in vogue with the bioavailability data. Some of these peculiar treatments and relevant statistics are very briefly discussed henceforth.

Statistics

The test statistics that are generally used in the bioequivalence evaluations are the mean of the studied population and the variability among the individuals. The intrasubject variability is normally expressed as intrasubject variation of coefficient (CV). As per several investigations, requirements and the needs, the data is derived from various pharmacokinetic studies and it is then subjected to statistical evaluations. Mean and CV are routinely used. However, to appropriately conclude the data several other techniques are also in vogue. Before introducing some of the very basic statistical methods, the pharmacokinetic parameters that are routinely used for test statistics equivalence studies are the maximum drug concentration (C_{max}), time to reach C_{max} and the area under the concentration time curve (AUC). These are derived from the plasma drug concentration-time curve, and are used as the measure of the rate and extent of drug absorption for bioequivalence evaluations. The square root of the residual mean squares from the analysis of variance (ANOVA) on log-transformed data is normally used as an approximation of intrasubject CV. Since the residual of the standard ANOVA model for crossover trials reflects intrasubject variation, log transformed data is sometimes very pinpointing. Once this data is transformed, the sample estimates and their deviation from the originial estimate may be depicted by using histogram charts. Arithmetic mean is a generally used test statistic. However, geometric mean could be an alternative to provide appropriate end result as per the requirement.

Scale Effects

The problem of drug interchangeability among a brand-name drug and its generic copies is considerably significant. Under current Food and Drug Administration (FDA) regulations, a patient may switch from the brand-name drug to a generic drug if the generic drug is shown to be bioequivalent to the brand-name drug based on bioequivalence testing. After the patent of a brand-name drug is expired, usually there will be a number of generic copies available on the market. The FDA does not indicate that a patient may switch from a generic to another even though both of the generic drugs are bioequivalent to the brand-name drug. As a result, drug interchangeability among the brand-name and its generic copies is a safety concern. A meta-analysis for an overview of bioequivalence provides an assessment of bioequivalence among generic copies of a brand-name that could be used as a tool to monitor the performance of the approved generic copies of the brand-name drug. In addition, the meta-analysis provides more accurate estimates of inter- and intrasubject variabilities of the drug product. Although the trial is fine, the design is fine, and the subjects involved in a trial may share very similar pharmacokinetic characteristics, some times it is a possibility that the resulting response may result in a skewed average response in bioavailability that is relative to the population average response. Although crossover design may maintain a relative constant difference between the test and reference amoung studies, geometric means that are much lower than the population average may also result in unacceptable ratio estimates. This situation is termed the "scale effects". This topic is currently delved in length in the bioequivalence circles. In practice, it is not uncommon for a drug product to have a 15-30% variation in average bioavailability across studies with the same design settings. Thus, when assessing relative bioavailability, scale effects should be definitely considered. Few more details with a specific study example are discussed.

Wang et al. (1998), investigated the scale-effects in bioequivalence evaluations. The objective of their study was to evaluate the relationship between the magnitude of the sample means for a bioavailability measure and the ratio of the sample means in bioequivalence evaluations. It was assumed that bioavailability data were obtained from crossover trials on a test and a reference drug product. The true test-reference ratio was constructed as a function of dosage strength under specified dose-response relationship assumptions, and was used for deriving analytical results of assessing the scale effects due to dosage strength. In addition, the test-reference ratio of sample means was constructed as a function of the true test-reference ratio and the correlated sampling deviation in the sample means, was used in a deterministic simulation for quantifying the scale effect due to the correlated sampling deviation. The results indicated that the major systematic factors that influence the magnitude of the sample means include the dosage strength, dose-response relationship, and the positively correlated sampling deviation in the sample means. Results of this study showed that the true test-reference ratios could be improved with increasing dosage strength in most of the situations studied, but at a diminishing rate. The correlated sampling deviation can alter the test-reference ratio of the sample means through changing magnitude of the sample means, especially for drug products with low bioavailability. Thus, for extended release drug products with multiple dosage strengths, the development efforts should focus on the lowest strength if there is little or no formulation by dose interaction effect. Pilot studies should be conducted for both the highest and the lowest strength instead for possible formulation by dose interaction effect. The magnitude of observed means for bioavailability measures on the reference drug product can indicate the degree of systematic variation in the ratio of means. The expected mean values of the reference drug product could be derived from previous trial(s) and from other information sources. If the sample mean for the reference drug product in a failed bioequivalence trial is lower than expected, the investigator should consider repeating the trial.

JackKnife Evaluations

One way of avoiding misinterpretations generated out of bioequivalence studies is to use Jackknife evaluations. The bootstrap, Efron and Tibshirani, Tukey and the Jackknife are well known tools for estimating standard errors of statistics. They create artificial replicates by randomly resampling or sequentially deleting data values, to simulate the sampling variability of a statistic. Kunsch (1989) and Liu and Singh (1992) independendetly proposed the moving blocks boot-strap and the moving blocks jackknife for dependent data. Park and Willemain (1999) introduced the threshold bootstrap and threshold jackknife for stationary and weakly dependent time series. Park et al., (2001) also established the asymptotic unbiasedness and consistency of the threshold bootstrap and threshold Jackknife estimates. The context of this section is not to discuss these issues. However, a brief introduction to the use of jackknife evaluations in bioequivalence studies is discussed.

Shortly, Jackknife sampling techniques were used in the evaluation of outliers like data in the bioequivalence investigations (Ulrich and Miller, 2001; Bonate et al., 2004; Liu and Sambol, 1999; Loeys and Goetghebeur, 2003; Liu and Singh, 1992). These situations may not be adopted to the statistical tests in the beginning of the bioequivalence evaluations with the data obtained from bioequivalence evaluations, respectively. However, when the data is further intensified and conclusions properly made, Jackknife sampling techniques are used. Jackknife samples are generated by sequentially deleting one resampling unit from the initial data. The resampling unit may be one observation or a combination of several observations. The sample derived from sequentially deleting one observation at a time is called the 'delete-one jackknife sample', and this may be used in the assessment of the influence of individual observations on a target statistic value. The delete-two-or more subjects jackknife samples are used for the evaluation of their joint influence on the statistic value. There are several types of such jackknife evaluations. The delete-one jackknife sample is the simplest type compared with other types of jackknife samples. Once the statistic value has been computed for all the jack knife samples, jackknife influence profiles for the statistic value could be constructed as bar charts to display the statistics corresponding to jackknife samples and to the initial data. The initial estimate is included to measure the magnitude of the influence of individual observations. From these jackknife influential observations one can directly obtain the statistic value without the influence of the individual influential observations. Currently, several other techniques are in vogue with regard to very proper evaluations of the test statistics. Further discussion is out of perview of this textbook.

Interfering Factors

In the cases when two or more influential observations are encountered, the joint influences of these individual ratios should be accounted for at the same time, particularly when they are clustered. The idea of trimmed means could be used for the assessment of the joint influence of the two extreme individual observations in opposite directions. The trimmed mean is computed based on the subset of the initial data by deleting the largest and the lowest observations. The subset data for the trimmed mean could serve as an additional jackknife sample. The computed statistic value from such a delete-two jackknife sample may be more reliable than that from delete-one samples in situations in which the individual influence of the two observations is large. The joint influence could be approximated based on the sum of the individual influences obtained from delete-one jackknife samples. The number of deleted observations should be restricted, because deleting too many observations at a time may sacrifice the statistical power of the assessment.

Conclusions

In any number of experiments conducted in physics, chemistry or biology, the key factor is the randomization. Similarly randomization is a very common phenomenon even in the biological system. In a biological system there are several interfering factors. Randomization and interfering factors together result in variabilities in drug effects. This results in inter and intra-subject variabilities. These are the key factors in any clinical investigation and definitely this rule is extrapolated to biopharmaceutics and bioequivalence studies. This chapter very briefly introduces the concept of biopharmaceutics oriented towards the clinical trial investigations.

Questions for Practice and Exercise

1. Define
    1. Pharmacokinetics and
    2. Biopharmaceutics. Explain the differences between the two.
2. Define the following:
    1. Bioavailability and bioequivalence,
    2. Dissolution and drug absorption,
    3. Drug forms,
    4. Route of administration,
    5. Pharmacokinetic parameters,
    6. The investigational new drug application,
    7. New drug applications,
    8. Abbreviated new drug applications,
    9. Bioequivalent drug products,
    10. Power of a statistical test.
3. Why is there a difference in the hepatic and renal excretion ratio of the following groups of drugs? Pinpoint and mention in detail and with clarity. Pull out from literature if necessary. Class A: Low (<0.3) hepatic and renal extraction drugs, eg. tolbutamide, lithium, carbamazepine, warfarin, digitoxin, salicylic acid, theophylline, phenobarbital, gentamicin, tetracycline and digoxin; Class B: Intermediate (0.3-0.7), eg. cimetidine, aspirin, quinidine, and cephalothin; Class C: High (<0.7): propranolol, (some) penicillin, arabinosyl-cystosine, nitroglycerin, meperidine and pentazocine.
4. Explain based on their pharmacological effectiveness the differences in the biopharmaceutics of different barbiturates.

5. Briefly describe about the molecular topography of drug substances as related to the drug absorption into the different compartments.
6. Briefly describe about the molecular topography of drug substances as related to the drug actions in knockout animal studies.
7. Give the example of hematoporphyrin (HP) analogs as related to the changes in their topological structure with a change in the environment in which they are placed. How does this influence the biopharmaceutics of these molecules?
8. How does the age of the subject affect the biopharmaceutics of a new drug substance?
9. How do the disease conditions affects the biopharmaceutics of a new drug substance?
10. Elaborate about clinical trials keeping in view the biopharmaceutics perspective. Compare and contrast the several clinical trial designs currently in vogue among clinical trial investigators.
11. Define target population. Explain very briefly.
12. Compare and contrast the *in vivo* bioavailability trial designs currently in vogue among clinical trial investigators.
13. What is the sequential order of conducting a bioequivalence testing?
14. Describe
    1. basic trial designs and analysis,
    2. pilot trials,
    3. pivotal trials,
    4. bioequivalence.
15. Describe
    1. acceptability assessment,
    2. bioequivalence assessment,
    3. challenges in the decision making process.
16. Describe
    1. statistics,
    2. scale effects,
    3. jackknife evaluations,
    4. interfering factors.
17. How is the relationship between the dose and the effect related to biopharmaceutics?

References

1. Bronshtein I, Smith KM, Ehrenberg B. The effect of pH on the topography of porphyrins in lipid membranes. Photochem Photobiol. 2005 Mar-Apr;81(2):446-51.
2. Davis AM, Seney ML, Stallings NR, Zhao L, Parker KL, Tobet SA. Loss of steroidogenic factor 1 alters cellular topography in the mouse ventromedial nucleus of the hypothalamus. J Neurobiol. 2004 Sep 15;60(4):424-36.
3. Kennedy A, Robinson A, Hann M, Thompson D, Wilkin D; North-West Region Gastrointestinal Research Group. A cluster-randomised controlled trial of a patient-centred guidebook for patients with ulcerative colitis: effect on knowledge, anxiety and quality of life. Health Soc Care Community. 2003 Jan;11(1):64-72.
4. Kennedy A, Nelson E, Reeves D, Richardson G, Roberts C, Robinson A, Rogers A, Sculpher M, Thompson D. A randomised controlled trial to assess the impact of a package comprising a patient-orientated, evidence-based self-help guidebook and patient-centred consultations on disease management and satisfaction in inflammatory bowel disease. Health Technol Assess. 2003;7(28):iii, 1-113.
5. Ali BH. Effect of composition and quality of diet and feeding time on the kinetics and efficacy of some anthelmintic drugs: a mini-review. Acta Vet Hung. 2004;52(3):339-47. Review.
6. Stearns V, Singh B, Tsangaris T, Crawford JG, Novielli A, Ellis MJ, Isaacs C, Pennanen M, Tibery C, Farhad A, Slack R, Hayes DF. A prospective randomized pilot study to evaluate predictors of response in serial core biopsies to single agent neoadjuvant doxorubicin or paclitaxel for patients with locally advanced breast cancer. Clin Cancer Res. 2003 Jan;9(1):124-33.
7. Daniel Baker. New Drug Review: Reviews in Gastroenterological Disorders. Medical Reviews. 2003. Vol. 3. No. 4.
8. Wang Y, Eradiri O, Odidi I, Geng W, Odidi A, Muhuri G. Scale effect in bioequivalence evaluations. Int J Clin Pharmacol Ther. 1998 Oct;36(10):534-9.
9. Kunsch HR. 1989. The Jackknife and the bootstrap for general stationary observations. Annals of Statistics 17, 1217-1241.
10. Park, D., and Willemain, T., "The Threshold Bootstrap and Threshold Jackknife," *Computational Statistics and Data Analysis* 31 (1999), 187-202.

11. Park, D., Kim, Y., Shin, K., and Willemain, T., "Simulation Output Analysis Using the Threshold Bootstrap," *European Journal of Operational Research* 134 (2001), 17-28.
12. Ulrich R, Miller J. Using the jackknife-based scoring method for measuring LRP onset effects in factorial designs. Psychophysiology. 2001 Sep;38(5):816-27.
13. Bonate PL, Craig A, Gaynon P, Gandhi V, Jeha S, Kadota R, Lam GN, Plunkett W, Razzouk B, Rytting M, Steinherz P, Weitman S. Population pharmacokinetics of clofarabine, a second-generation nucleoside analog, in pediatric patients with acute leukemia. J Clin Pharmacol. 2004 Nov;44(11):1309-22.
14. Liu CY, Sambol NC. Pharmacodynamic analysis of analgesic clinical trials: nonlinear mixed-effects logistic models. J Biopharm Stat. 1999 May;9(2):253-70.
15. Loeys T, Goetghebeur E. A causal proportional hazards estimator for the effect of treatment actually received in a randomized trial with all-or-nothing compliance. Biometrics. 2003 Mar;59(1):100-5
16. Liu, R. and Singh, K. (1992). *Moving blocks jackknife and bootstrap capture weak dependence*, in Exploring the Limits of Bootstrap, R. LePage and L. Billard, eds. New York: John Wiley & Sons.

Bibliography

1. New Drug Development: Regulatory Paradigms for Clinical Pharmacology and Biopharmaceutics (Drugs and the Pharmaceutical Sciences: a Series of Textbooks and Monographs), First Edition, Edited by Chandrahas G. Sahajwalla, Marcel Dekker Inc., 2004.
2. The Practice of Medicinal Chemistry, Second Edition, Edited by Camille Georges Wermuth, Elsevier Publications, 2003.
3. Foye`s Principles of Medicinal Chemistry, Fifth Edition, David A. Williams and Thomas L. Lemke, Lippincott Williams & Wilkins, 2002.
4. Rowland M, Tozer T, Clinical Pharmacokinetics: Concepts and Application. 3rd ed. Philadelphia: Lea and Febiger, 1994.
5. Design and Analysis of Clinical Trials: Concepts and Methodologies (Wiley Series in Probability and Statistics), First Edition, Authored by Shein-Chung Chow, Jen-Pei Liu, Johny Wiley & Sons, 2004.

6. Fundamentals of Clinical Trials, Third Edition, Authored by Lawrence M. Friedman, Curt D. Furberg, David L. DeMets, Springer Mathematics Series, 1998.
7. A Manager's Guide to the Design and Conduct of Clinical Trials (Manager's Guide Series), First Edition, Authored by Phillip I. Good, John Wiley & Sons, 2002.
8. Complete Idiot's Guide to Statistics (The Complete Idiot's Guide), First Edition, Authored by Robert A. Donnelly Jr, Wiley Publishing Inc., 2003.
9. The Jackknife and Bootstrap (Springer Series in Statistics), First Edition, Authored by Jun Shao, Dongsheng Tu. Springer, 1996.
10. Bootstrap Methods and Their Application (Cambridge Series in Statistical and Probabilistic Mathematics, No 1), First Edition, Authored by Davison AC and Hinkley DV, Cambridge University Press, 1997.
11. An introduction to the Bootstrap, First Edition, Authored by Brad Efron and Rob Tibshirani, Chapman & Hall/CRC, 1998.

CHAPTER 14

PHARMACEUTICAL TECHNOLOGY

- **Tablet Manufacture**
  - Process and Instrumentation
  - Quality Control
- **Capsule Manufacture**
  - Process and Instrumentation
  - Quality Control
- **Tablet Coating**
  - Process and Instrumentation
  - Quality Control
- **Novel Drug Delivery Technology Platforms**
- **Conclusions**

Tablet Manufacture

Process and Instrumentation

Currently, tablet manufacture is very well advanced. The modern instrumentation is well suited for high production rates and continuous production applications. Modern rotary tablet machines look more sophisticated and have more instrumentation today, but the basic technology has not changed in several decades. Tablet technology still requires skill and art, primarily because of uncertainties in the physics of compression that correlates with simple correlation of raw material properties with finished tablet properties even with simplest direct compression processes.

The following are the steps involved in the tablet manufacture in the sequential order:

1. Granulation
2. Feeding the mixture into the die cavity
3. Compression
4. Ejection

Granulation

Evaluation of the efficacy of new drug entities is a very important aspect of a new drug discovery industry. The later investigations are for generic products where in patent expired drugs are manufactured and sold in the market. On the other hand controlled release tablet dosage forms are very actively involved. The development and the utility of the three technologies is definitely in tandem with each other. Although expensive the production of three platforms together in one company set up is definitely a money matter. Many multinational companies are currently very actively involved in this area. Because of the generation of several lead candidates from high-through put drug discovery process, it has become imperative that preformulation has become an important task of these companies. On the other hand, most of the active compounds are less compressible and poorly soluble. This makes things more complicated for preformulation scientists. Solutions, emulsions, suspensions whose manufacture is taught in B. Pharm and M. Pharm curriculum thoroughly are very often used in the manufacture of these products. However, with the current molecules, these formulations are not that docile. In this situation, solids are the best alternatives. Solid dosage forms include tablets and capsules. At this time, tablets are the most convenient dosage forms. In addition, enough evidence in terms of manufacture and selling is available with tablets. Thus, the most convenient dosage forms are tablets for new drug discovery process. In addition, tablets offer several advantages apart from manufacture as mentioned in several chapters of this textbook. Most of the generic products available in the market are either tablets or capsules. Opting these dosage forms for early drug investigations is still considered to be time saving and cost effective. Tablets are usually prepared by compression process. The compression process is either single punch or multi punch. The speed varies with the increase in the sophistication. As such tablet manufacture is currently quite convenient with several kinds of machinery available in the market for various purposes. However, in a preformulation setup very easy tablet compression machines such as single punch machines to several punch machines are used. Usually these punches are of medium speed. Whatever the speed is and however sophisticated the project is the essence of tablet manufacture is the same and the basic principles are the same. Unfortunately, this topic itself consumes several volumes of information. However, a brief overview of these technologies along with numerous machineries is described in this chapter.

Tablet compression is generally classified into three types

1. wet granulation,
2. dry granulation, and
3. direct compression.

For tableting purposes, drugs require excipients. These excipients include diluents, binders, disintegrants, and lubricants. The first requirement is that the blend of the drug and excipients should be able to flow free and fill the die to reduce the weight variations and other compaction, release and bioavailability variations from batch to batch. This situation remains the same either with wet granulation process, dry granulation process or direct compressible tablets. The dose of the drug in older cases was higher. However, with the recent introductions in new chemical entities, the amount of the new drug substance available to a preformulation scientist is becoming very low. This definitely makes the manufacture of a tablet challenging. In addition, because of the convenience, the size of the modern tablets is generally miniaturized. This is another challenge. The other peculiar situation is when the dose of the drug is very high and the excipients required are very low. This is a situation with high dose drugs like aspirin. In these cases, the modern requirement is to include all the size of the tablet into one single tablet for one dosing. Definitely, the requirement of the amount of the drug is always the same for a particular ailment. This cannot be reduced. The option is to reduce the amount of excipients used and punch one single tablet. Thus, compressed tablets may be prepared by wet granulation, dry granulation, and direct compression. In a ***wet granulation process***, the drug substance along with other excipients is mixed, the binding agent added as solution and the adhesion prepared. This adhesion thus obtained is screened to obtain smaller particles, passed through a sieve and the granules dried. These granules are mixed with lubricants and the tablet punched. In a ***dry granulation*** process, the drug is mixed with excipients slugged to obtain large tough slugs, which are then reduced to smaller size and sieved to obtain the granules of desired size. Modern equipment is designed to carry out both wet granulation and dry granulation in one step. In addition, currently several directly compressible excipients are available in the market. With these excipients, the drug and the excipients are thoroughly mixed and compressed to obtain tablets. This process is called ***direct compression***. Several granulators and mixers are available in the market for the use in the process of granulation. Unlike other formulation technologies, flexibility is definitely not a key in tablet manufacture. Thus, the technology is definitely very sophisticated. Each of these processes along with some illustrations will be described henceforth. The examples of very common equipment used in the tablet manufacture are exemplified with the following pictures.

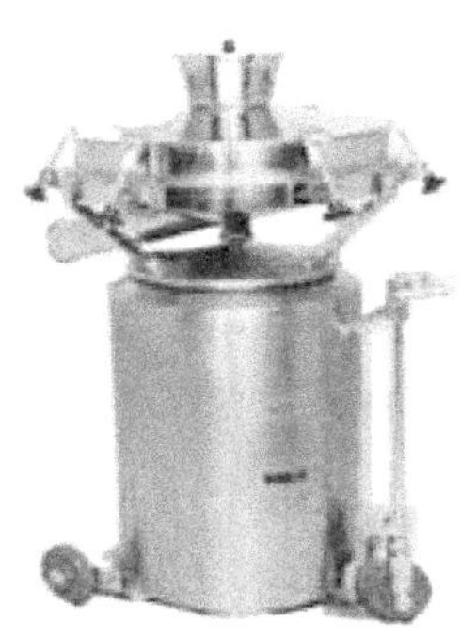

Seiving

Mfg: Karnavati Engineering Limited

Capacity: 25 L to 600 L

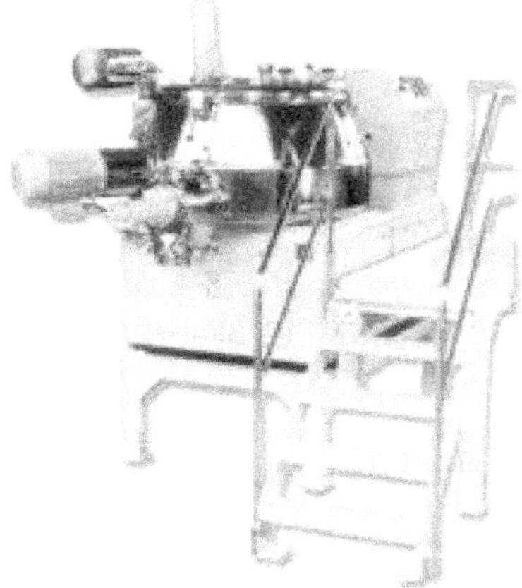

Rapid Mixer Granulator

Mfg: Karnavati Engineering Limited

Capacity: 25 L to 600 L

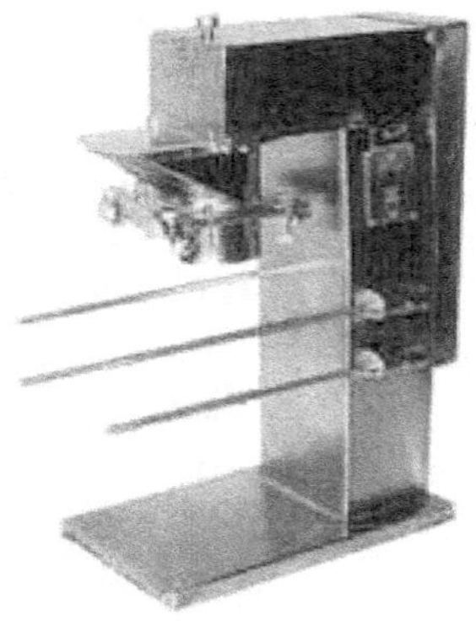

Oscillating Granulator

Mfg: Karnavati Engineering Limited

Max Output: 200 kg/hour to 400 kg/hour

Dry Granulator

A dry granulator is used to granulate tablet slugs and pellets. Two drive rollers with teeth force material to form slugs. Special design results in low proportion of powder. When using hard slugs, from 2 to 2.5 mm thick, the following granulation will be obtained, 45% - 16 mesh, 25% - 24 mesh, 10% - 70 mesh, 20% powder.

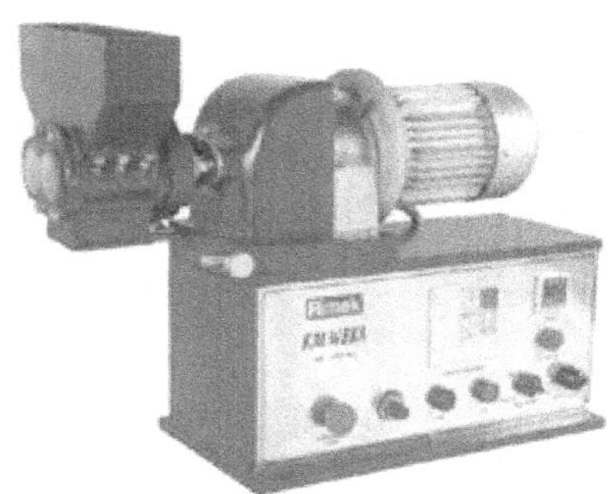

Dry Granulator

Mfg: Karnavati Engineering Limited

Capacity: 25 L to 600 L

Wet Granulator

This machine is equipped with an oscillating rotor suitable to manufacture wet granulates of various granule sizes. Sieves are easily interchangeable. Rotor, sieve and all parts coming into contact with the materials are constructed of stainless steel. Each apparatus is supplied with one sieve each of 1.0 and 1.6 mm mesh size. The following mesh sizes are available for the wet granulator type WGS: 0.315, 0.63, 0.8, 1.0, 1.25, 1.6, 2.0, 2.5, and 3.15 mm. The capacity of the machine depends on the material and the mesh sizes of the sieve and is maximum 20-25 Kg. per hour. The wet granulator is suitable for screwing on main Motor drive.

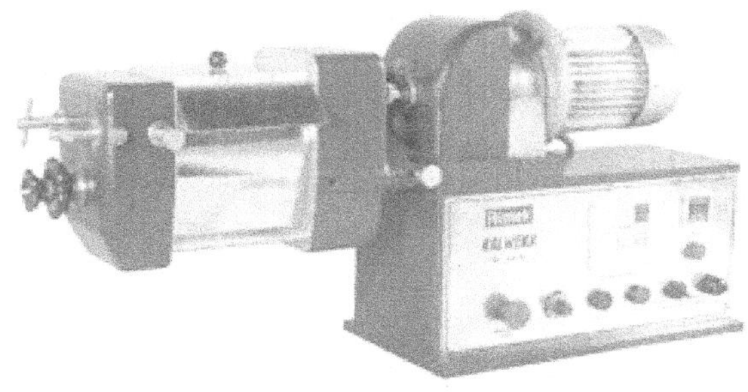

Wet Granulator Type

Mfg: Karnavati Engineering Limited

Capacity: 25 L to 600 L

Fluid-bed Granulator

A ***Fluid-bed* granulator** process is used in the process of wet granulation and a ***Roller Compactor*** is helpful in dry granulation process. The entire process of granulation is currently performed using one-single equipment called as a fluid-bed granulator. The fluid-bed granulator performs the following steps:

1. preblending the formulation powder, including active ingredients, fillers, disintegrants, in a bed by fluidized air,
2. granulating the mixture by spraying onto the fluidized powder bed, a suitable liquid binder, as an aqueous solution of acacia, hydroxypropyl cellulose, or povidone, and
3. drying the granulated product to the desired moisture content. An example of a fluid bed granulator and other granulators is shown below:

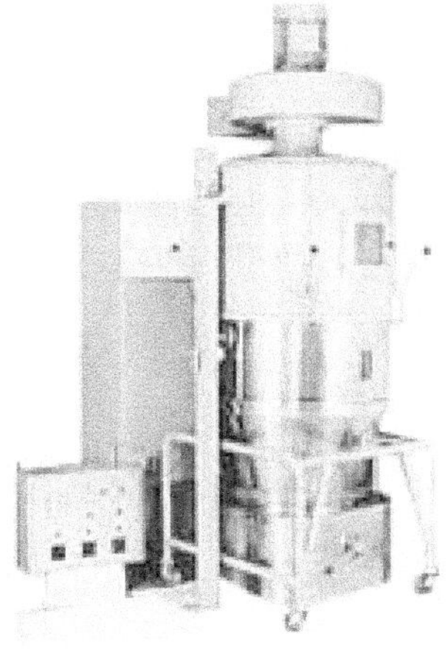

Fluid Bed Dryer

Mfg: Karnavati Engineering Limited

Capacity: 35 L to 430 L

Roller Compactor

The Roller Compactor is a versatile densification and dry granulation machine that produces uniform compacted sheets with consistent hardness and increased density by compacting powdered material between two uniquely designed rolls.

Free flowing granules for automatic packaging, compact granules for reduced packing sizes, and granules for high speed tableting or encapsulation are produced with consistent dust free purity and size. A tapered screw feeder inside the hopper precompacts and deaerates the powder for optimum product feeding. The screw feeder delivers deareated powder into the roll nip area and seal system. Roll seal system consists of top seal and side seals to confine powder to the roll nip area, and to minimize leakage of uncompacted powder. Three types of rolls provide maximum versatility for the particular material to be compacted. The DP and DPS series feature concave-convex roll surfaces with an outer rim, assuring even material feed and pressure distribution on the roll surface. The compacted sheets are milled to produce granules of the desired mesh size.

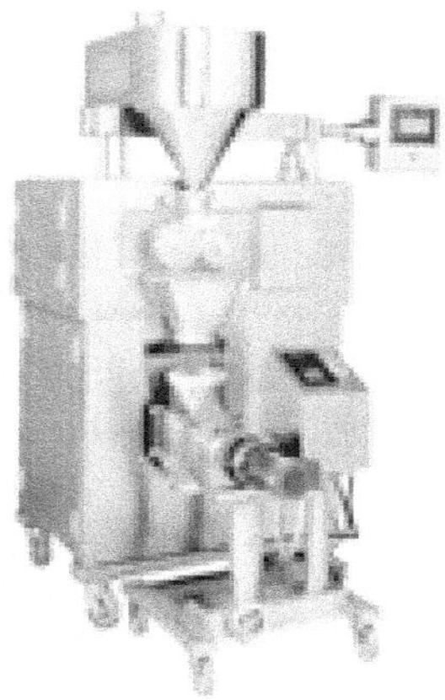

Roller Compactor

Mfg: Vector Corporation

Capacity: 15-45 kg/hour

Tablet Compression

The instruments used in the tablet manufacture are called tablet presses or tablet compression machines and the process is termed tablet compression. Along with several automations, the current instrumentation also has monitoring online devices. The components of the basic tablet instrumentation are:

1. Hopper for holding and feeding granulation to be compressed.
2. Dies that define the size and shape of the tablet.
3. Punches for compressing the granulation within the granules.
4. Cam tracks for guiding the movement of the punches.
5. A feeding mechanism for moving granulation from the hopper into the dies.

Tablet presses are either single-punch or multi-station rotary presses. A single punch machine is like a stamping press. The excipient mixture does not move from one place to other in the sequential line similar to in a steel plant or infact in any other manufacturing setup. Everything is automated on the entire line. In such sophistication online monitoring is also a crucial aspect. Thus, in this instrument's set up online quality control is also well placed and everything is documented and monitored with the help of computers. Similarly this happens in a multistation tablet manufacturing technology platform where in granule flow, tablet compression, tablet ejection, tablet packing, and finally tablet storing in the container occurs in the same line. Definitely this requires lot of engineering skills, in both the design and the mechanics. However, this instrument setup is used only for production purposes. The setup is not foreseen in a laboratory used for early clinical and preclinical investigations. Some time definitely a multi-station press is used for the convenience of a laboratory scientist. In a multi-station press, the upper punches, dies, and lower punches in place rotate. As the head rotates, the punches are guided up and down by fixed cam tracks, which control the sequence of filling, compression and ejections. That is the reason why a multi-station press is called a rotary machine. In this situation, this occurs at a very rapid speed. And several of the tablets are produced at one time period. This is very important because to manufacture a batch process, the process has to be very carefully controlled. Otherwise, the entire batch goes waste. However, the steps involved in the tablet manufacture are the same in both a single punch machine and a rotary machine. The first step is the manufacture of the granules or drug excipient mixture. This is placed in front of the die and the punch sequence in an enclosure. The blend could reach this enclosure by using a hopper. A chopper helps in filling this blend in the die. In a rotary press, there is a scale up in all the sizes. In addition, instead of one die and punch, there are several of these dyes and punches. Once the die is filled, the punch enters, compresses the blend into a tablet and retracts back to its original position. The compressed tablet then is ejected and the tablet collected. Several modifications according to the requirement could be made in both single station and rotary machines. Special adaptations of tablet machines allow for compression of "layered" tablets and coated tablets. If the process is not controlled there definitely could be problem of chipping and lamination of the tablet process. Some of the equipment pictures along with the volumes etc. currently used in the Indian production unit are as below. The degree of sophistication ranges from low to high.

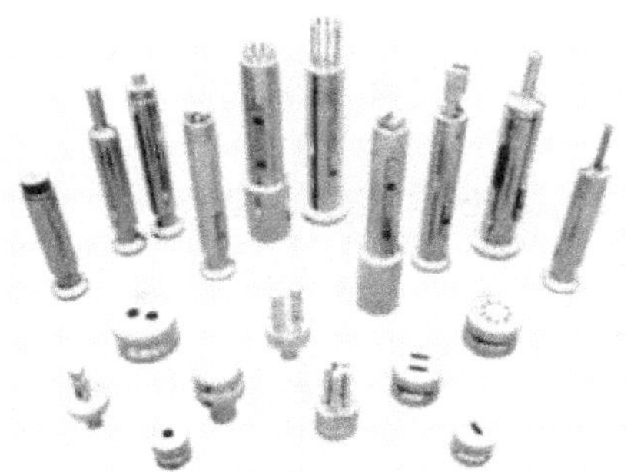

Dies and Punches

Mfg:	Karnavati Engineering Limited		
Models:	RSB4-1;	MP2K-16;	MP2K-20
No. Stations:	10	; 16	; 20
Max. Output:	18,000	; 28,800	; 36,000
Rotary:	Single		

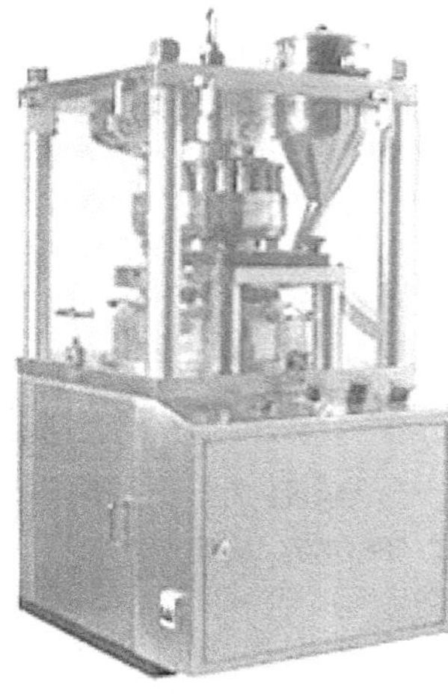

Table Top Mini-Rotary Press – Mini Press 1

Mfg:	Karnavati Engineering Limited		
Models:	RSB4-1; MP2K-16; MP2K-20		
No. Stations:	10	; 16	; 20
Max. Output:	18,000	; 28,800	; 36,000
Rotary:	Single		

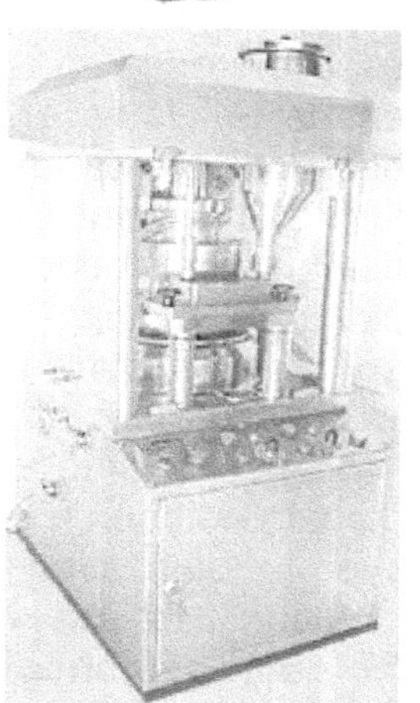

Table Top Mini-Rotary Press – Mini Press 1

Mfg:	Karnavati Engineering Limited		
Models:	RSB4-1; MP2K-16; MP2K-20		
No. Stations:	10	; 16	; 20
Max. Output:	18,000	; 28,800	; 36,000
Rotary:	Single		

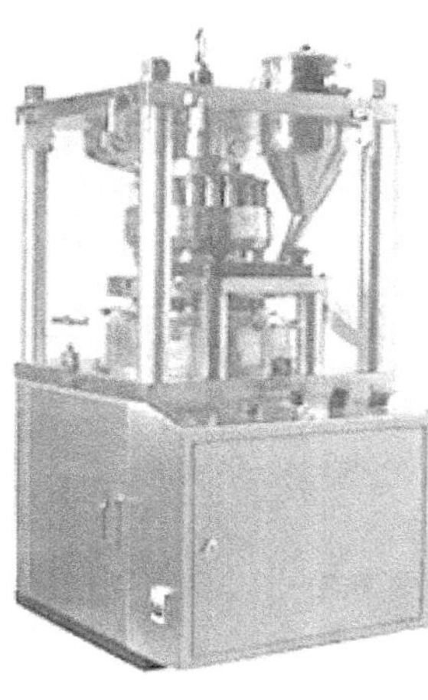

Table Top Mini-Rotary Press – Mini Press 1

Mfg:	Karnavati Engineering Limited		
Models:	RSB4-1; MP2K-16; MP2K-20		
No. Stations:	10	; 16	; 20
Max. Output:	18,000	; 28,800	; 36,000
Rotary:	Single		

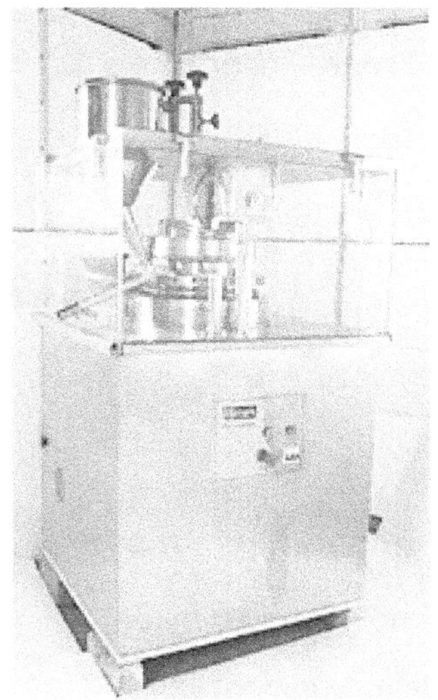

Table Top Mini-Rotary Press – Mini Press 1

Mfg:	Karnavati Engineering Limited		
Models:	RSB4-1;	MP2K-16;	MP2K-20
No. Stations:	10	; 16	; 20
Max. Output:	18,000	; 28,800	; 36,000
Rotary:	Single		

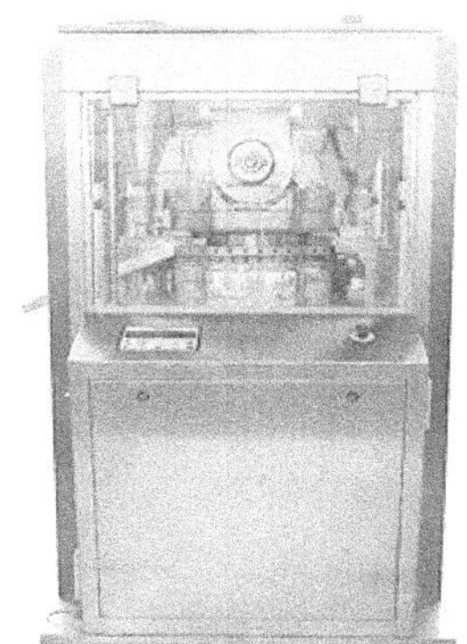

Table Top Mini-Rotary Press – Mini Press 1

Mfg:	Karnavati Engineering Limited		
Models:	RSB4-1;	MP2K-16;	MP2K-20
No. Stations:	10	; 16	; 20
Max. Output:	18,000	; 28,800	; 36,000
Rotary:	Single		

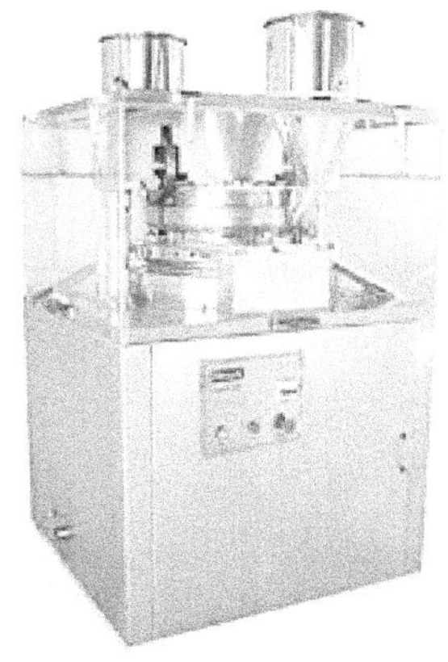

Table Top Mini-Rotary Press – Mini Press 1

Mfg:	Karnavati Engineering Limited		
Models:	RSB4-1;	MP2K-16;	MP2K-20
No. Stations:	10	; 16	; 20
Max. Output:	18,000	; 28,800	; 36,000
Rotary:	Single		

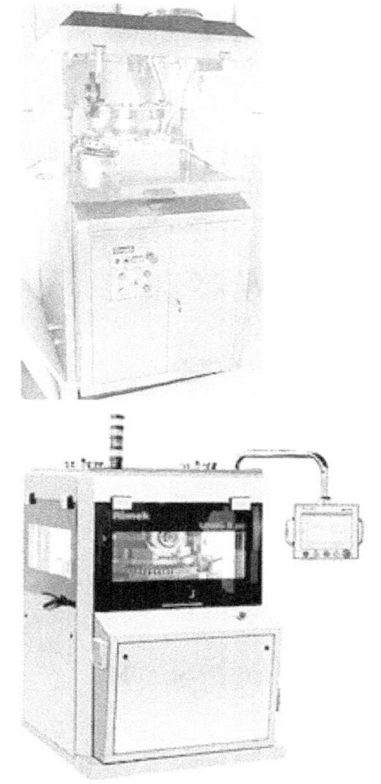

Table Top Mini-Rotary Press – Mini Press 1

Mfg:	Karnavati Engineering Limited		
Models:	RSB4-1;	MP2K-16;	MP2K-20
No. Stations:	10	; 16	; 20
Max. Output:	18,000	; 28,800	; 36,000
Rotary:	Single		

Table Top Mini-Rotary Press – Mini Press 1

Mfg:	Karnavati Engineering Limited		
Models:	RSB4-1;	MP2K-16;	MP2K-20
No. Stations:	10	; 16	; 20
Max. Output:	18,000	; 28,800	; 36,000
Rotary:	Single		

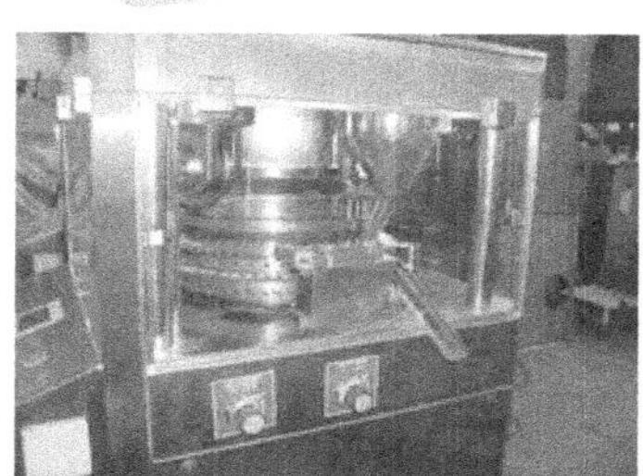

Table Top Mini-Rotary Press – Mini Press 1

Mfg:	Karnavati Engineering Limited		
Models:	RSB4-1;	MP2K-16;	MP2K-20
No. Stations:	10	; 16	; 20
Max. Output:	18,000	; 28,800	; 36,000
Rotary:	Single		

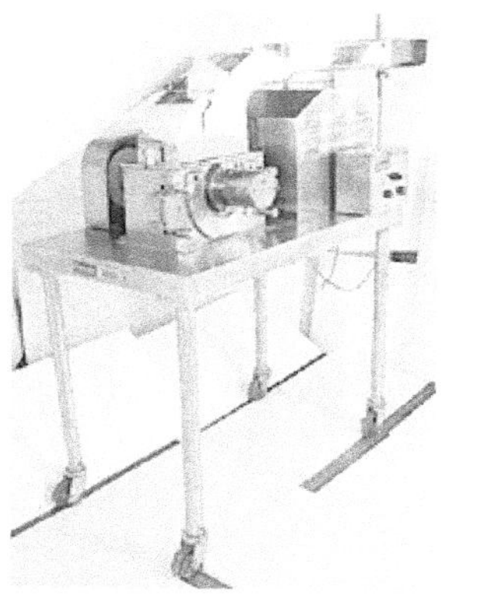

Table Top Mini-Rotary Press – Mini Press 1

Mfg:	Karnavati Engineering Limited		
Models:	RSB4-1;	MP2K-16;	MP2K-20
No. Stations:	10	; 16	; 20
Max. Output:	18,000	; 28,800	; 36,000
Rotary:	Single		

Quality Control

Once the tablets are manufactured or during the manufacture quality control is a very important aspect. Currently, online monitoring is the trend. However, keeping in view the goal of the current chapter to make it simpler, very briefly quality control of the tablets is discussed here. The different quality standards and compendial requirements include tablet weight and USP weight variation test, content uniformity, tablet thickness, tablet hardness and friability, tablet disintegration and tablet dissolution. Weight variation is a very important quality control parameter. Since several tablets are punched at one time using any of the current instruments, it is always likely that the weight of the individual tablets vary. This may affect the disintegration time, the dissolution time and potency. Thus, these quality control parameters are the key sets to ensure tablet manufacture tightness. Each of these tests are described very briefly in one or two lines. **Tablet Weight and USP Weight Variation:** The quantity of fill placed in the die of a tablet press determines the weight of the resulting tablet. In a USP weight variation test, 10 tablets from a batch are weighed individually and the average weight calculated. The tablets are assayed and the content of active ingradient in each of the 10 tablets is calculated assuming homogenous drug distribution. **Content Uniformity:** By the USP method, 10 dosage units are individually assayed for their content uniformity according to the assay method described in the individual monograph. Unless otherwise stated in the monograph, the requirements for content uniformity are met if the amout of active ingradient in each dosage unit lies with the range of 85% to 115% of the lable claim and the relative standard deviation is less than 6.0%. **Tablet Thickness:** The thickness of a tablet is determined by the diameter of the die, the amount of fill permitted to enter the die, the compactibility of the fill material, and the force or pressure applied during compression. Tablet thickness may be measured by hand gauge during production or by automated equipment. **Tablet Hardness and Friability:** It is not unusual for a tablet press to exert as little as 3,000 and as much as 40,000 pounds of force in the production of tablets. Generally, the greater the pressure applied, the harder the tablets, although the characteristic of the granulation also has a bearing on tablet hardness. **Tablet Disintegration:** For the medicinal agent in a tablet to become fully available for absorption, the tablet must first disintegrate and discharge the drug to the body fluids for dissolution. Tablet disintegration also is important for those tablets containing medicinal agents (such as antacids and antidiarrheals) that are not intended to be absorbed but rather to act locally within the gastrointestinal tract. In these instances, tablet disintegration provides drug particles with an increased surface area for localized activity within the gastrointestinal tract. **Tablet Dissolution:** *In vitro* dissolution testing of solid dosage forms is important for a number of reasons that are discussed in the dissolution-testing chapter.

Capsule Manufacture

Process and Instrumentation

At this moment, capsule manufacture is very well advanced. The current equipment is well suited for high production rates and continuous production applications. Modern capsule production machines look more sophisticated and have more instrumentation today, but the basic technology has not changed in several years. Capsule technology consists of two parts shell manufacture and drug filling, primarily because of requirements of a shell that correlates with drug release from finished capsules both with hard gelatin and soft gelatin capsule manufacture.

The following are the steps involved in capsule manufacture in sequential order:

(a) Shell manufacture
(b) Feed manufacture
(c) Filling of the capsules
(d) Sealing and packing

Hard Gelatin Capsule Manufacture

Determination of the efficacy of new drug entities is a key aspect of any new drug discovery process. Capsules are the important formulations used in such investigation for oral delivery of drugs. Products where in a patent of a drug is expired are manufactured and sold as generic compounds. In this regard hard gelatin capsules are the most convenient dosage forms. On the other hand soft gelatin capsules are also very actively involved. Several new chemical entities are investigated using capsule dosage forms. Because of the requirement of capsule manufacture from gelatin, it has become imperative that gelatin processing has become an important task for the manufacture of capsules. The reasons for their use in preclinical formulations are simply the same as that of the use of the tablet formulation. As a reiteration, most of the active compounds are less compressible and poorly soluble. This makes things more complicated for preformulation scientists. Liquid dosage forms basically taught in pharmacy undergraduate courses are very often used in the manufacture of these products. However, with the recent innovative molecules, these formulations are not that applicable. In this situation, solids dosage forms are the best choices. These dosage forms include powders, tablets and capsules. Apart from their routine use, capsules offer more convenience in terms of their uses compared to other dosage forms. The capsules could include solid powders, sustained released pellets, microparticles, nanoparticles etc. The other advantage is that these dosage forms could be locally released by sealing the capsule with an enteric coat. That way if a drug is degraded in particular location, it could be protected and thus capsules would further help in the local release of the drug. In addition, enough evidence in terms of manufacture and selling is available with capsules. Thus, the most convenient dosage forms are capsules along with tablets for new drug discovery process. On the other hand, compression is not used in the capsule manufacture and thus protects drugs like proteins and peptides, which are susceptible to hydrolysis upon compression.

Gelatin is obtained by the partial hydrolysis of collagen obtained from the skin, white connective tissue, and bones of animals. Commercially, it is available in the form of a fine powder, a coarse powder, shreds, flakes, or sheets. Gelatin is stable in air when dry but is subject to microbial decomposition when it becomes moist. However, if stored in an environment of high humidity, additional moisture is absorbed by the capsules, and they may become distorted and lose their rigid shape. In an environment of extreme dryness, some of the moisture normally present in the gelatin capsules is lost and the capsules may become brittle and crumble when handled. Because gelatin capsules can affect hygroscopic agents contained within may absorb moisture, many capsules are packaged along with a small packet of a desiccant material to protect against the absorption of atmospheric moisture. The desiccant materials most used are dried silica gel, clay, and activated carbon. Hard gelatin capsules are prepared using an industrial setup. However, the filling of the powder into hard gelatin capsules is done manually or by automatic filling equipment. A brief description of hard gelatin capsule shell manufacture is demonstrated here.

Once raw materials have been received and released by Quality Control, the gelatin and hot demineralized water are mixed under vacuum to obtain gelatin solution. After aging in stainless steel receiving tanks, the gelatin solution is transferred to stainless steel feed tanks. Dyes, opacification agents, and any needed water are added to the gelatin in the feed tanks to complete the gelatin preparation procedure. The feed tanks are then used to gravity-feed gelatin into the Capsule Machine. From the feed tank, the gelatin is gravity fed to specially engineered Dipper section. Here, the capsules are moulded onto stainless steel Pin Bars that are dipped into the gelatin solution. Once dipped, the pin bars rise to the upper deck allowing the cap and body to set on the pins. The pin bars pass through the upper and lower kilns of machine drying system. Here gently moving air that is precisely controlled for volume, temperature, and humidity, removes the exact amount of moisture from the capsule halves. Precision controls constantly monitor humidity, temperature, and gelatin viscosity throughout the production process. Once drying is complete, the pin bars enter the table section which positions the capsule halves for stripping from the Pins in the Automatic section. In the Automatic section, capsule halves are individually stripped from the Pins. The cap and body lengths are precisely trimmed to a ±0.15 mm tolerance. The capsule bodies and caps are joined automatically in the joiner blocks. Finished capsules are pushed onto a conveyer belt that carries them out to a container. Capsule quality is monitored throughout the production process including size, moisture content, single wall thickness, and colour. Capsules are sorted and visually inspected on specially designed stations. Perfect capsules are imprinted with the client logo on high-speed capsule printing machines. Capsules are now ready to be sterilized and packaged. The next step is to fill the capsules with appropriate fillers.

Manufacture of Capsule Fill

In the manufacture of capsule fill, the aim is to develop a capsule formulation with accurate dosage, good bioavailability, ease of filling and production, stability, and elegance. The active and the filling material must be blended thoroughly to obtain a uniform mix to be filled in the capsules. Care in blending is especially critical for low-dose drugs since lack of homogeneity could result in significant therapeutic consequences. Preformulation studies are performed to determine if all of the formulations bulk powders may be effectively blended together as such or if they require reduction of particle size or other processing to achieve homogeneity. A diluent or filler are added to the formulation to produce the proper capsule fill volume. Lactose, microcrystalline cellulose and starch are commonly used for this purpose. In addition to providing bulk, these materials often provide cohesion to the powders, which is beneficial in the transfer of powder blend into capsule shells. Very often lubricants or glidants like fumed silicon dioxide, magnesium stearate, calcium stearate, stearic acid, or talc are added to increase the flow properties.

Capsule Filling

The speed of the manufacture of capsules containing medication increases with an increase in the sophistication of capsule filling. As such capsule filling is currently quite convenient with several kinds of machinery available in the market for various purposes. However, in a preformulation setup very easy capsule filling process such as manual filling is used. The other method, which is also manual, is the use of hand-operated capsule filling machines. Usually this method is of medium speed. The various types of filling machines have capacities ranging from 24 to 300 capsules and when efficiently operated are capable of producing from about 200 to 2000 capsules per hour. Automated equipment is used in an industrial set up. These capsules are filled upto 165,000 capsules per hour.

Whatever the speed is and however sophisticated the capsule fill is the essence of hard gelatin capsule manufacture is the same and the basic principles are the same. Unfortunately, this topic itself takes several volumes of information. However, a brief overview of this technology is described in this section.

Soft Gelatin Capsule Manufacture

The two methods used in the soft gelatin capsule manufacture are called plate processes and productive rotary or reciprocating die process and the process is termed soft gelatin capsule manufacture. Along with several automations, the current instrumentation also has monitoring online devices. An overview of these instruments is simply described for the convenience of the reader. Companies that are manufacturing these dosage forms routinely especially in India has procured most of the instruments from the local markets. Usually liquids are incorporated into soft gelatin capsules. Liquids that migrate across the capsule shell cannot be incorporated into soft gelatin capsules. These materials include water above 5%, and low molecular weight water-soluble and volatile organic compounds like alcohols, ketones, acids, amines and esters. Currently different manufacturing equipment is available in Indian, US and European markets. Couple of pictures of soft gelatin capsule manufacturing equipment is demonstrated in this section. These are also sold in Indian markets at this time. As a simple illustration, the components of the basic soft gelatin capsule manufacture are self-explanatory and are:

1. Manufacture of liquid gelatin to form a sheet of gelatin.
2. Pouring of liquid drug feed onto the gelatin sheet.
3. Layering one more layer of gelatin sheet.
4. Pressing to obtain soft gelatin capsules.

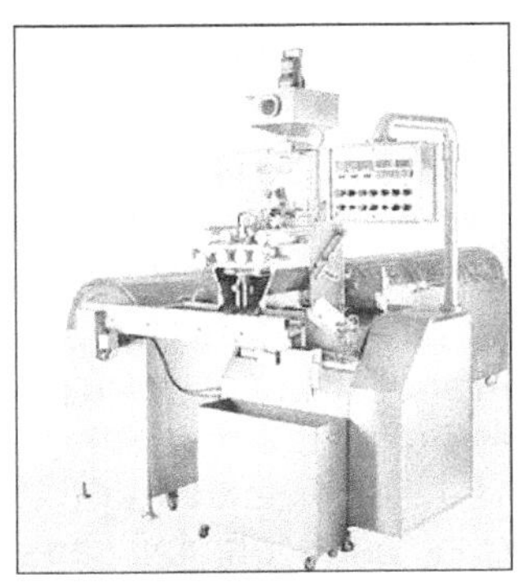

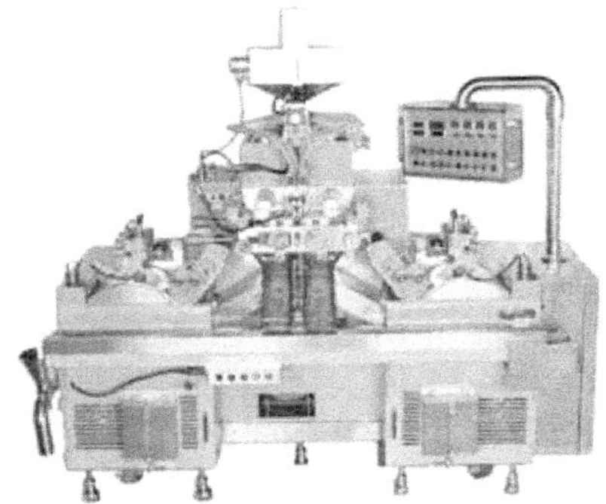

Soft Gelatin Capsule Manufacturing Equipment (CAPPLUS TECHNOLOGIES)

Soft gelatin capsules are prepared to contain a variety of liquid, pasty, and dry fills. Liquids that may be incorporated into soft gelatin capsules include:

1. Water-immiscible volatile and nonvolatile liquids like vegetable and aromatic oils, aromatic and aliphatic hydrocarbons, chlorinated hydrocarbons, ethers, esters, alcohols and organic acids.
2. Water-miscible, nonvolatile liquids, such as polyethylene glycols, and nonionic surface-active agents as polysorbate 80.
3. Water miscible and relatively nonvolatile compounds, as propylene glycol and isopropyl alcohol, depending on factors as concentration used and packaging conditions.

Quality Control

Once the capsules are manufactured or during the manufacture quality control is a very important aspect. Currently, online monitoring is the trend. However, keeping in view the goal of the current chapter to make it simpler, very briefly quality control of the capsules is discussed here. The different quality standards and compendial requirements include USP container specification, disintegration test, dissolution test, weight variation and content uniformity, content labeling requirement and moisture permeation and stability testing. **Weight variation** is a very important quality control parameter. Since several capsules are manufactured at one time using any of the current instruments, it is always likely that the weight of the individual capsules varies. This may affect the disintegration time, the dissolution time and potency. Thus, these quality control parameters are the key sets to ensure capsule manufacture tightness. Each of these tests for hard capsules and soft capsules are described very briefly in one or two lines. **Hard capsules and Soft capsule weight variation:** The quantity of fill placed in a capsule determines the weight of the resulting capsule. In a capsule weight variation test, 10 capsules from a batch are weighed individually and the average weight calculated. Extraction of the contents is thoroughly obtained especially for an active ingradient. The capsules are assayed and the content of active ingradient in each of the 10 capsules is calculated assuming homogenous drug distribution. **Content Uniformity:** By the USP method, 10 dosage units are individually assayed for their content uniformity according to the assay method described in the individual monograph. Unless otherwise stated in the monograph, the requirements for content uniformity are met if the amout of active ingradient in each dosage unit lies with the range of 85% to 115% of the lable claim and the relative standard deviation is less than 6.0%. **USP container specification:** There are specifications listed in the USP prescribing the type of container suitable for the repacking or dispensing of each official capsule and tablet. Depending on the item, the container might be required to be tight, well-closed and light container. **Tablet Hardness and Friability:** It is not unusual for a tablet press to exert as little as 3000 and as much as 40,000 pounds of force in the production of tablets. Generally, the greater the pressure applied, the harder the tablets, although the characteristic of the granulation also has a bearing on tablet hardness. **Capsule Disintegration:** For the medicinal agent in a tablet to become fully available for absorption, the capsule must first disintegrate and discharge the drug to the body fluids for dissolution. Capsule disintegration also is important for those tablets containing medicinal agents (such as antacids and antidiarrheals) that are not intended to be absorbed but rather to act locally within the gastrointestinal tract. In these instances, tablet disintegration provides drug particles with an increased surface area for localized activity within the gastrointestinal tract. The capsules are placed in the basket-rack assembly, which is repeatedly immersed 30 times per minute into a thermostatically controlled fluid at 37°C and observed over the time described in the individual monograph. **Capsule Dissolution:** The compendial dissolution test for capsules uses the same apparatus, dissolution medium and test as that for uncoated and plain coated tablets. However, in instances in which the capsule shells interfere with the analysis, the contents of a specified number of capsules can be removed and the empty capsule shells dissolved in the dissolution medium before proceeding with the sampling and chemical analysis. **Moisture permeation and stability testing:** USP requires determination of the moisture-permeation characteristics of single-unit and unit-dose containers to assure their suitability for packaging capsules. Thus, moisture permeation is a very important test for both hard and soft gelatin capsules. Stability testing is a very routing test performed on any dosage form. The same principles are applicable to capsule dosage forms.

Tablet Coating

Tablets are the very common dosage forms useful to treat the patients. In addition, these are also useful in preclinical investigations with new chemical moieties. Most often just tablets are sufficient for the above-mentioned application. However, very often the need for tablet coating may arise. The reasons may include:

1. Protection of a new chemical agent against destructive exposures. This is similar to a prodrug approach, where in the active drug is cleaved in the system to elicit a therapeutic role. However, this drug still is a prodrug during all the formulation steps. This is especially true with to protect an active drug intestinal destruction.
2. Masking the taste of a drug. Very often new chemical moieties are bitter in taste and often times are smelly. In the initial evaluations in Phase I clinical studies, the bitter taste may mask the therapeutic benefits over the organoleptic properties.

3. Providing a drug with appropriate release properties. New chemical moieties are often times more soluble in water. They often times have very low half-life. In this situation, one of the ideal ways of protecting these chemicals is to prepare a tablet of the drug and coat it with a sustained release coat,
4. Providing aesthetics or distinction to the product. This is very often with colored new chemical moieties, which are irresistible because of their persistant and promising pharmacological role. However, these lack aesthetics with color mottling to the tablets, etc. In these situations, to cover up these properties, a coat is laid on the tablet surface to shield the mottled color surface, and
5. Preventing inadvertent contact with nonpatients with the drug substance and the consequent effects of drug absorption. Often times this is very important. Some times may need repeated coating. Despite of several warnings with this kind of drug, its role remains the same, unfortunately. For example, Proscar tablets (finasteride, Merck) are coated for just this reason. Men to treat benign prostatic hyperplasia use the drug. The labeling instructions warn that women who are pregnant or who could be pregnant should not come into contact with the drug. Drug contact can occur through the handling of broken tablets. If a woman who is pregnant carrying a male baby absorbs finasteride, the drug has the potential capacity to adversely affect the developing male fetus. The very general categories of tablet coating will be discussed in this section. Tablet coating could be conveniently classified into
    1. Sugar coating,
    2. Film coating,
    3. Enteric coating,
    4. Air suspension coating and
    5. Compression coating.

Sugar Coating

The very first developed and practiced coating method was sugar coating. Because of the time consumption, cost-ineffectiveness, borderline advantage, tablet weight accumulation, this coating is not very often used at this time. However, because of its significance in terms of tablet coating methods definitely this has to be very amply discussed. Sugar coating method could be conveniently placed into the following sequential order

1. Water proofing or sealing,
2. Subcoating,
3. Smoothing and final rounding,

4. Finishing and coloring and
5. Polishing.

The entire coating process is performed in a series of round vessels, mechanically operated and surface coated with different resistant material. A series is required because of the time consumed in cleaning each and every container after the step is completed; this often times saves time and work productivity. The small pans are used for experimental purpose and the larger ones are used for manufacturing purposes. The pans operate at an angle to contain the tablets and help the operator visualize the process of coating. In the process of tablet coating, the pans are very often moved at a desired speed to aid in the uniform coating of the tablets. Unfortunately, it takes several validations to fix the size of the pan, the speed and the angle of the movement. In addition the size of the coat is also an important aspect. The validation is thus fixed because of these reasons. The coat is formed over a period of time. In this regard, each layer is laid over the tablet followed by blowing to obtain a uniform thickness. This process is continued till a desired coat is obtained. Each steps of the process are explained in brief.

Water Proofing and Sealing Coat

Most often this coat is used for enteric coating to protect acid labile drugs. Thus, the first coat this tablet needs is to protect it from moisture. One or more coats of a waterproofing substance as pharmaceutical shellac or a polymer, is applied to the compressed tablets before the subcoating application. The water proofing solution is prepared and is generally poured into the pan when the pan is rotating. Warm air is then applied to hasten the drying and thus a coat is formed. This could be continued as per the reservation requirements with two to four layers.

Subcoating

After the tablets are waterproofed (if needed), 3 to 5 subcoats of a sugar-based syrup are applied. This bonds the sugar coating to the tablet and provides rounding. The sucrose and water syrup also contains gelatin, acacia, or polyvinylpyrrolide (PVP) to increase the coating of the tablets. When the tablets are partially dry they are sprinkled with a dusting powder, usually a mixture of powdered sugar and starch but sometimes talc, acacia, or precipitated chalk as well. Warm air is applied to the rolling tablets, and when they are dry, are of the desired shape and size. The subcoated tablets are then scooped out of the coating pan and the excess powder is removed by gently shaking the tablets on a cloth screen.

Smoothing and Final Rounding

After the tablets have been subcoated, then they are ready for smoothing and rounding. About 5 to 10 additional coatings of thick syrup are administered to complete the rounding and smoothing the coatings. Basically this coat is to seal any abnormalities that are found on the tablets. This syrup is sucrose-based with or without additional components as starch and calcium carbonate. As the syrup is applied, the operator moves away from the pan and keeps in controlled environment to protect the previously laid coat. This process is done several times before smoothing and final rounding occurs. A dusting powder is often used between syrup applications. Warm air is applied to hasten the drying time of each coat. Very efficient technicians and personal who are very much familiar with the process are required at this time. Skill is one of the criteria for not using sugar coating very often in the pharmaceutical industry. Sugar coating definitely requires tremendous skill as is desired for any qualified profession like a cardiologist or an internal medicine practitioner. Very often very potent medicaments are introduced into the coat as the first layer. This is the same as used in the case of homeopathy pills. This coat helps in the release of very minute quantities of potent therapeutic agents followed by the release of the drug. Generally, the next coat is a very thin coat and is basically used for finishing and coloring.

Finishing, Coloring and Embossing

The final layer is to obtain proper finishing and coloring. This coat generally contains color in thin syrup. During all the stages the steps are achieved in different pans in a sequential order. Once the finishing, coloring and drying are achieved, then subsequently, embossing or imprinting is achieved. Different codes could also be achieved on the tablets based on the requirement. This very often is helpful for differentiating different tablets groups, thereby increasing the efficiency and makes easy to a pharmacist in the administration and prescription of drugs to patients.

Polishing

It is very unfortunate that the process of tablet coating with the help of sugar coating techniques often time results in not that polished tablet surface. Definitely this requires polishing as the final step. Most of the times it may not consume that much time. However, in every likely the final texture of the tablet at the end of polishing step results in a decent looking tablet.

Film Coating

The film coating process is often times used to obtain the final tablets after coating to have the same tablet size. Several types of film coatings could be used. The film generally is not seen as a thick bulge when the coated tablets are broken down. Enteric coating is possible with film coating. In addition, local delivery of new molecules could also be achieved with film coating. Because of the diversity of film coating, definitely it resulted in the prominence in the area of tablet coating. Tablets are film coated by the same technique as is used for sugar coating. However, in the case of film coating rather than skill, it is the sophistication of the machinery that helps. Film-coating solutions may be nonaqueous or aqueous. The excipients in a film coating solution generally are film former, alloying substance, plasticizer, surfactant, opaquants and colorants, sweeteners, flavors and aromas, glossant and volatile solvent. Because of the expensive nature of the film coating technique this is not very often preferred. In addition, environmental contamination is the major problem. Repeated coating that may result in the instability of the drug is not generally investigated. A very common aqueous film-coating formulation contains the following along with their percentages, respectively:

1. Film-forming polymer (7-18%). Examples: Cellulose ether polymers as hydroxypropylmethylcellulose, hydroxypropyl cellulose, and methylcellulose.
2. Plasticizer (0.5 –2.0%). Examples: glycerin, propylene glycol, polyethylene glycol, diethyl phthalate, and dibutyl subacetate.
3. Colorant and opacifier (2.5-8%). Examples: FD & C or D & C Lakes and iron oxide pigments.

Several problems as listed below are envisaged with film coating technique. However, proper understanding of the technique will be definitely of help in the film coating process. These problems are the same for all kinds of drugs and definitely a very common understanding would help this process. In addition, more than experience, instrumentation and machanization process understanding are very important for film coating technique. In addition, selection of appropriate film would also help in reducing the toxicity of drugs for local action in the gut. Very briefly, the problems associated with film coating are described. The appearance of small amounts (picking) or larger amounts (peeling) of film fragments flaking from the tablet surface; roughness of the tablet surface due to failure of spray droplets to coalesce (orange peel effect); an uneven distribution of color on the tablet surface (mottling); filling-in of the score-line or indented logo on the tablet by the film (bridging); and the disfiguration of the core tablet when subjected for too long a period of time to the coating solution (tablet erosion). Each of these problems is solved by necessary alterations in formulations, equipment, technique or the process of coating.

Enteric Coating

Crack in a coated tablet is very often the results of sugar coating and film-coating. However, these problems could be corrected upon proper treatment. On the other hand, some situations such as when the drug is supposed to pass the gastrointestinal tract and then disintegrate and release, sugar coating and film coating are not sufficient. The problem lies in the local delivery and release of the drug. Only the drug that is required to be release in the intestinal tract needs the requirement for an enteric coating. This is definitely a very peculiar situation. Despite several techniques were adopted after the development of sugar coating and film-coating, the lessons in the area of sustained release of the drugs was the same. In these situations, the next technique that was adopted was enteric coating. Coating theory definitely helps, however practice is an issue. It is altogether a different ballpark. However, the entire process of coating could be conveniently clubbed into coating process. The technique of utility of enteric coating process is the same as that of sugarcoating and film coating. But the enteric coating results in the coat around a tablet that protects the tablet from gastic pH. The design of an enteric coating is based upon the transit time required for the passage of the dosage form from the stomach to the intestines and is generally accomplished through coatings of sufficient thickness. The principles definitely remain the same until a very thorough coat is given. The process of enteric coating could be administered to tablets or to granules that are then used to manufacture tablets or capsules. Tablets or capsules containing granules is like a double trouble, but it may is useful for time release of the drug in the small intestines. Usually an enteric coating is based upon factors of pH, resisting dissolution in the highly acid conditions of the stomach but yielding to the less acid environment in the intestines. Some enteric coatings are designed to dissolve at pH 4.8 or greater. The coating systems are often times thin. The coating systems may be aqueous-based or organic-solvent based and are effective so long as the coating material resists breakdown in the gastric fluid. The most common materials used in enteric coatings are pharmaceutical shellac, hydroxypropylmethylcellulose phthalate, polyvinyl acetate phthalate, diethyl phthalate, and cellulose acetate phthalate. Several other materials could be used.

Fluid-Bed or Air Suspension Coating

In a fluid bed or air suspension coating, the tablets are suspended in a stream of air and then the coat is administered. It is totally a mechanized process and each and evey parameter could be controlled. Not only tablets but also powders, granules, beads, pellets also could be coated with the help of this technique. In addition, the equipment used in fluid-bed coating is also useful for various other purposes. Several kinds of fluids bed or air suspension coating methods are available. The most widely known technique is called Wurster Process. In all of the techniques, the different formulations could be coated from the top or from the bottom. In some of the fluidized process, the spray could also be achieved from an angle. These several fold options are helpful to coat several fold application purposes. The variables that are required to control in order to produce product of desired and consistent quality are: equipment used and the method of spraying (e.g., top, bottom, tangential), spray-nozzle distance from spraying bed, spray (droplet) size, spray rate, spray pressure, volume of fluidization air, batch size, method (s) and time for drying, air temperature and moisture content in processing compartment.

Compression Coating

In a manner similar to the preparation of multiple compressed tablets having an inner core and an outer shell of drug material, core tablets may be sugarcoated by compression. The coating material, in the form of a granulation or powder, is compressed onto a tablet core of drug with a special tablet press. Compression coating is an anhydrous operation and thus may be safely employed in the coating of tablets containing a drug that is labile to moisture. Compared to sugarcoating using pans, compression coating is more uniform and uses less coating materials, resulting in tablets that are lighter, smaller, easier to swallow, and less expensive to package and ship. Irrespective of the method used in coating, all tablets are virtually or electronically inspected for physical imperfections.

Quality Control

Once the tablets are coated or during the coating quality control is a very important aspect. Currently, online monitoring is the trend. However, keeping in view the goal of the current chapter to make it simpler, very briefly quality control of the tablet coating is discussed here. The different quality standards and compendial requirements include checks for color (both hue and continuity), size, appearance, and any physical defects in the coating that could affect the performance or stability of the product. The very standard disintegration and dissolution tests are routinely needed. In addition, the *in vitro – in vivo* correlation is also required. Additional testing may also include mechanical strength, resistance to chipping and cracking during handling. All the methods are the same as those used for tablets. Borderline is that the necessary tests have to be performed both in and out to make sure that proper coating on tablets is done. This ensures perfect batch release of coated tablets into the market. The culmination of these tests is especially true for sustained release coated tablets.

Novel Drug Delivery Technology Platforms (NDDTPs)

Although tablets and capsules are there in the market for several years, there is definitely a need for sophistication in this area. This is because of the requirement and the need of continuous progress. The origins of these novel drug technologies definitely lie in the histories of conventional dosage forms like tablets and capsules. Repeated dosage, one of the oldest theories of pharmacy practice, through continous administration was in practice for over several years. Historical evidence dates back atleast to the time of Higuchi. Higuchi constructed several plots of drug release from different kinds of sustained release dosage forms and applied these to various matrix systems and reservoir devices (Desai et al., 1966; Desai et al., 1966; Sierra et al., 1976). On the other hand, several other scientist theories of sustained release dosage forms were practiced and researched. It took several years from then on to allow sustained release dosage forms into the market and these people realized the importance of sustained release dosage forms as such and not exactly sustained administration of drugs, which had several drawbacks. Most of the technologies in sustained released systems were shared by Europe and the America at this time. Altogether these systems resulted in rapid strides in drug delivery. It took several innovations in the area of sustained release tablets and capsule platform technologies before finally the technology resulted in the very appropriate sustained release tablet and capsule that entered the market. During the same time sustained released systems such as liposomes, nanoparticles and microparticles and other kinds of novel systems advanced to leaps and bounds. However, the basics of sustained release as proposed by Higuchi and his group are still the same. Several Indian companies are now supplying all the advanced sustained release tablets and capsules that are available in west at this time. More than 70% of small molecule drugs are absorbed almost exclusively in the transit time duration limited to 3 to 4 hours. In order to extend the time of action, it is necessary to increase the duration of absorption by maintaining the drugs longer in the small intestinal tract. Some companies have developed gastro-retentive systems with sizable tablets. Problems inherent to these monolithic systems, large tablets are generally not useful for children and present swallowing problem for elderly people. Thus, a need arises for sustained and convenient release dosage systems for these drugs. However, these systems are of limited utility and the resulting innovation lead to the development of Novel Drug Delivery Technology Platforms. In this regard, the Indian pharmaceutical companies also have considerable progress. For instance, Ranbaxy India Ltd., an Indian multinational company has 4 Patented Platform Technologies. These are Aerogel, Gastric Retention, pH Independent Matrix, and Microencapsulation and particle coating. Currently, sustained release capsule and tablet platform technologies are very advanced and some of these progresses will be discussed in this section. Ranbaxy India

Limited is currently using these technologies for the development of Novel Drug Delivery Systems for anti-infectives, cardiovasculars, respiratory, NSAIDS and central nervous system drugs.

As mentioned about the progress of sustained release tablets and capsules, with time they entered the market. The theory behind these systems is mentioned in the chapter titled "Novel Drug Delivery Systems". However, it was realized that in the area of sustained release tablets and capsules, more has to be accomplished because of the rising needs. In this regard, the following parameters are considered prior to the design of a sustained release tablet and capsule platforms. These include immediate release, sustained release, enteric release, pulsed release, delayed release, low solubility, high solubility, low drug load, high drug load, high interpatient variability, gastrointestinal irritation, low oral bioavailability, gastrointestinal degradation, targeted delivery, side effects associated with high C_{max}, alternative to the parenteral administration, food effect and first pass metabolism. All these terms are self-explanatory in terms of sustained release tablets and capsules (SRTCs). However, with the routine SRTCs, the above properties cannot be tailored as per the requirements. For instance, SRTCs that contain drugs to prevent gastrointestinal degradation, cannot achieve other properties required. In addition, some systems need drugs to be low oral bioavailable, low gastrointestinal degradation, require targeted delivery and prevent first pass metabolism, very specially designed systems are required. These systems could be termed sustained release tablet and capsule platforms (SRTCPs). Altogether all these new systems could be abbreviated as NDDTPs.

Originally, these technologies were developed in either large Universities or small companies. This was because of the realization of the need for these kinds of systems that are advantageous compared to the sustained release tablets or capsules. Several small labs sprung up to develop these technologies. Once a platform technology with a model drug has been developed, then the technology is usually applied for a patent followed by marketing. These small companies license the controlled release products early in the development cycle to pharmaceutical companies that controlled clinical trials, regulatory process, manufacturing and sale of their products in a number of international markets. In the pharmaceutical industry the word "innovative" can have two meanings. In the general sense, it can mean inventive, creative and the first to try something new. In industry jargon, it refers to a unique patented brand name drug developed and owned by an innovator company. On a general level, when these labs or small companies pioneer and innovate the controlled release drug delivery, they come in license agreement with the company that is interested. These are then termed "proprietary technology platforms". The term that is used for these systems is "Novel Drug Delivery Technology Platforms (NDDTPs)". Basically, the small companies involved in such development have the following motive "The companies new drug application (NDA) pipeline is dedicated to the development of innovative branded products, to be marketed directly by this company and also to select marketing partners". Some advantages of these systems over the conventional sustained and controlled release systems are illustrated using the following examples:

1. One of the technical challenges in the development of multiple-particulate dosage forms with a variety of active ingredients is to achieve an acceptable uniformity and reproducibility of a product. NDDTPs like concentric Multiple-Particulate Delivery Systems (CMDS) of Global Pharmaceuticals, ensures that each of the active ingredient is released at predetermined time intervals and desired levels on a consistent basis. The system provides the ability to control the release rate of multiple ingredients in a multi-particulate dosage form.
2. Many of the controlled-release technologies available today are designed for the release of only one active ingredient with one rate of release (typically a zero-order or single mode release). Such a release pattern may not be adequate for drugs in certain therapeutic categories. Timed Multiple-Action Delivery System (TMDS) of Global Pharmaceuticals allows for more than one active component in a single tablet formulation to be released in multiple profiles over time. The system provides the ability to control the release rate of multiple ingredients within a single tablet in a programmed manner.
3. Many traditional controlled-release tablets lose their "controlled" mechanism of delivery once broken. The Dividable Multiple-Action Delivery System (DMDS) of Global Pharmaceuticals Programmed-Release Technology allows the patient to break the tablet in half and each respective portion of the tablet will achieve exactly the same release profile as the whole tablet. This allows the patient/physician to adjust the dosing regimen according to clinical needs and without compromising efficacy. The system accommodates greater dosing flexibility, especially during titration, helping to improve efficacy and reduce side effects.

Examples of some of these platform technologies available in the market are dual polymer platform, electrolyte platform, aminoacid platform, ProPhile, ProScreen, OptiScreen, Microtrol IR, Microtrol XR, Microtrol PR, Microtrol DR, Consurf, Flash Dose, Shearform, Solutrol, EnSoTrol, Micropump I, Micropump II, Aerogel, Gastric Retention, pH Independent Matrix, Microencapsulation and particle coating. Currently, ample progress is being made around the world in this area of pharmaceutical technology.

Conclusions

Pharmaceutical technology consists of several aspects of innovations. The older medicines that were in existence survived along with allopathy therapy, despite lack of efficacy and sideeffects. However, many of the basic concepts that are currently used in the sustained release delivery systems are derived from these older therapies. The coordinated effort survived along with the existing allopathy therapy. The basics of technological advances of tablets, capsules, tablet coating and novel delivery systems definitely are derived from the older therapies in practice. However, with coordinated effort of the age-old therapies and the industrial growth and modernization, pharmaceutical technology saw tremendous growth. In this aspect, currently India is making lot of progress in this area. This chapter covered the basic concepts of tablets, capsules and tablet coating as related to the modern allopathy medicine. Along with these, there was definitely a brief introduction to novel drug delivery technology platforms. Currently, ample progress is being made around the world in this area of pharmaceutical technology.

Questions for Practice and Exercise

1. Mention in detail about the steps involved in the tablet manufacture in a sequential order.
2. Write a note on:
    1. Dry granulation method,
    2. Wet granulation method,
    3. Fluid-bed granulator, and
    4. Roller compactor.

    At what stage of drug discovery these methods are generally used for tablet manufacture? How is the scale-up conducted from preformulation stages to the manufacturing stages? What are the main differences of these stages? When are each of these techniques used in the drug development methodologies? Enumerate and elaborate keeping in view the Indian background if you have industrial experience. Otherwise, ignore.
3. Write a detailed note on tablet compression.
4. How is the quality control for the tablets conducted? Define elegance keeping in view the perspective of tablet manufacture. Explain in general. Specify in detail. Give very specific supportive examples.

5. Mention in detail about the steps involved in the
   (a) hard gelatin capsule and
   (b) soft gelatin capsule manufacture in a sequential order. Mention in your own words very briefly.
6. Briefly introduce tablet coating.
7. Write a note on:
   1. Sugar coating,
   2. Film coating,
   3. Enteric coating, and
   4. Fluid-Bed or Air suspension coating and
   5. Compression coating.
8. How is the quality control for the capsules performed?
9. Write a note on novel drug delivery technology platforms (NDDTPS).

References

1. Desai SJ, Singh P, Simonelli AP, Higuchi WI. Investigation of factors influencing release of solid drug dispersed in inert matrices. 3. Quantitative studies involving the polyethylene plastic matrix. J Pharm Sci. 1966 Nov;55(11):1230-4.
2. Desai SJ, Singh P, Simonelli AP, Higuchi WI. Investigation of factors influencing release of solid drug dispersed in inert matrices. IV. Some studies involving the polyvinyl chloride matrix. J Pharm Sci. 1966 Nov;55(11):1235-9.
3. Sciarra JJ, Patel SP. In vitro release of therapeutically active ingredients from polymer matrixes. J Pharm Sci. 1976 Oct;65(10):1519-22.

Bibliography

1. The Theory and Practice of Industrial Pharmacy, Third Edition, Edited by Leon Lachman, Herbert A. Lieberman, and Joseph L. Kanig, Lea & Febiger Publications, 1986.
2. Essentials of Physical Pharmaceutics, First Edition, Authored by CVS Subramanyam, Vallabh Prakashan Publications.
3. Pharmaceutical Engineering, First Edition, Authored by CVS Substramanyam et al., Vallabh Prakashan Publications.
4. Pharmaceutical Industrial Management, First Edition, Authored by RM Mehta, Vallabh Prakashan Publications.

CHAPTER 15

PRODUCT PROCESSING AND EVALUATION

- **Introduction**
- **Production**
    - Equipment
    - Manufacture
    - Lab NoteBook Maintenance and Data Handling
    - Batch Record
    - Process Validation
    - Packaging and Storage
- **Quality**
    - What is Control and Assurance?
    - What is meant by high Quality?
    - How is Quality and Control achieved?
- **Personal**
    - Managerial Duties
    - Validation
- **Conclusions**

Introduction

A pharmaceutical industry incorporates manufacture, extraction, processing, purification and packaging of chemical substances to be used in human beings or animals for demonstrating a therapeutic benefit. These companies could be classified into bulk drug companies, new drug formulation development companies or generic companies. Apart from these there are several other contract research organizations which mainly does the activities associated with the above three companies. Bulk drug companies deal with the manufacture of an API (Active Pharmaceutical Ingradient). An API is an active chemical substance that has therapeutic role. Definitely it cannot be administered orally and needs the development of various formulations. The most common pharmaceutical formulations include liquids, tablets and capsules. A new formulation development company develops a formulation for new drugs coming out of bulk drug industry. On the other hand, a generic company copies the formulations of new drug substances already in the market. They do this after the patent for the formulation and the new drug substance expires. The other way is to have an agreement with the innovator of the new drug substance to copy and sell this product, so called the generic version of the new formulation of the new drug substance. A contract research organization takes up small projects from these three companies and delivers the goods to them as per the agreement. On the other hand, the other most common pharmaceutical companies deal with Research and Development. In these these companies, the product is developed right from the very beginning to the end, however, in small and research scale. These companies are not incorporated into the list of the pharmaceutical companies because they are better called R & D organizations rather than companies. However, the steps involved in product processing and evaluation in all these four pharmaceutical set-ups is the same. For instance, most of the times the manufacture of liquids or solids for oral purpose may need only clean room environment. However, some occasions may mandate the use of sterile environment for the manufacturing purpose, and especially for liquids that are used for both oral and intravenous purposes. In all the four cases it is true. In addition, the person responsible has to follow proper protocols with diligence and the protocol designer should not have any bias to the manufacture process. This becomes especially important for new chemical entity formulation development, in which case, the company may loose lot of money and time on a project that may not fetch any result at the end. The protocol execution could be right from the very begin step to the very ending step. This is where product processing and evaluation comes. However, the production controls are seeing rapid changes during recent years. As per the needs, the changes have to be followed. The current regulatory standards that include 21 CFR 11 and cGMP guidelines govern all aspects of pharmaceutical manufacture. In addition, the current pharmaceutical manufacture has to manage increasing demands for improved customer service, leaner and quicker product development, and lower cost of goods through operational excellence. Recently, the FDA effectively combined the above factors and recommended the use of their combination. "There is need for greater flexibility and efficiency". This is what FDA emphasized in its Strategic Action Plan (August, 2003). It continued and said, "New standards are being designed to encourage cost cutting and precision enhancing innovation in manufacturing and technology". For the same reason the product processing and evaluation have to be followed with due diligence. Some of the sequential steps on these lines are listed below:

Process Development

- Route Assessment
- Recipe Development
- Pilot & Industrial Scale-up
- Environment Impact Assessment
- Site Evaluation
- Regulatory Compliance
- Technology Transfer
- Process Optimization

Supply Chain Planning

- Advanced Planning and Scheduling
- Demand Planning
    - Statistical, Casual and Collaborative
    - Product/Customer Segmentation Analysis
    - Sales & Operations Planning
- Inventory Planning
    - Safety Stock Optimization
    - Cycle Stock Optimization

Manufacturing

- Resource Management
- Product Definition Management
- Production Dispatching and Execution

- Historical Data Management
- Process, Production and QA Data Analysis
- Production Tracking and Performance

The other key issues in the product processing and evaluation are personal training and evaluation. This is termed personal management. This includes training routine employs and training managers. The next factor to be considered is validation. Validation includes validation of process, validation of quality, and validation of the personal. All these processing and evaluation steps could be conveniently clubbed into production, quality and man-power management.

Production

The product and process design starts at research and development, and includes preformulation and physical, chemical, therapeutic and toxicologic evaluations. Then comes production. In the fields of production as well as R&D, a perfect understanding of the production environment represents the best guarantee for optimum quality and productivity. It is also the key to ensuring that all procedures are in full compliance with FDA and GMP. Primary objectives of the product include assuring compliance with regulations imposed by the US Food and Drug Administration, the European Community Pharmaceutical Industry Commission and other regulatory authorities. Currently, these are conducted very diligently along with using sophisticated computer software packages, atleast in big pharma of developed countries. These involve adherence to current Good Manufacturing Practices (cGMP), electronic signature/approval (21 CFR 11), electronic batch records, and document management. They also involve lot tracking, handling of variances between planned vs. actual production, lot reconciliation, full material tracking and genealogy, and recipe management. The FDA's 1997 Electronic Signatures Rule has dramatically increased the demand for electronic Batch Record Systems (eBRS). This rule sent a clear signal that it is now an accepted, and even preferred, practice for manufacturers to utilize some kind of computerized system in managing their production and compliance processes. Currently, several loan licensing and small companies are privately taking up this aspect of production. Several new softwares are being generated and marketed that takes care of all the production requirements using a computer. One such system is Aspen Production Management. All the above duties are performed by Aspen Production Management system. Aspen Production Management is a model based Manufacturing Execution System (MES) covering four main business process: Coordinate (production, planning & scheduling), Ready (recipes definition and simulation, procedures definition), Execute (work orders, recipes and Procedures execution), and Analysis (production information and accounting). Aspen Production Management solution covers both the plant (bulk chemical, formulation and packaging) and the clinical trials production management needs. Further, information could be obtained from the innovators of these production management systems. Several such systems are available all over the world currently.

The development of manufacturing formula is the first step in the production of a particular dosage form for a particular drug. This is developed after rigorous considerations of preformulation, formulation, toxicological and clinical aspects. After preformulation formulation, preclinical formulation, clinical formulation and market formulations are thoroughly evaluated, the manufacture formula is developed. Each and every step is properly evaluated. This may take several years for new chemical entities. Several back and forths in the manufacture of the formulation right from the preformulation to the final formulation is usually performed till everything is optimized. Depending on how ease the formulation development is, this period varies. For generic formulations, the average time is generally lower. Once the final market formulation is finalized, the product is taken to the manufacturing set up. Scale-up is a big issue in the manufacturing setup. Production of a 5 Kg batch size of tablets in the laboratory set up with the help of small pans and low punch number tableting presses may give thorough content uniformity and very proper release kinetics. However, when it is taken to a manufacturing set up where in the routine practice the average batch size is more than 100 kg, the total assumption may be entirely different. Hypothetical or intuitive calculations or assumptions do not work in these kinds of set up. Several permutations and combinations of the manufacturing variables till the final manufacturing parameters are set up may be required. This process is termed as scale-up. Some times this could be a very big issue. Critical laboratory-scale experiments are required to obtain information for the design, operation, and control of commercial scale equipment for profitable manufacturing of solids and liquids. A logical procedure must be followed in designing these experiments, or the pertinent information will not be obtained and resources will have been wasted. The iterative performance of these steps is sometimes required before thorough scale-up of a batch process. In very long time ago when the solid or liquid manufacture was semi-automatic, then scale-up was definitely a tedious job. With the advances in the automation, the batch could be prepared with all the parameters set up very properly. These parameters could be validated using a statistical design process called factorial design, where in the number of repetitions could be considerably reduced in drawing proper conclusions. This technique is one of the optimization techniques in the pharmaceutical manufacturing. Optimization techniques could also be performed using regression analysis and including several other statistical techniques.

Pharmaceutical manufacturing is recognized to be a major industry in the United States of America. This industry employed 160,000 employees at one time. It had 13 billion dollar investment and with second largest sales return. In terms of profits, most pharmaceutical companies rank within top 100. These companies currently invest more on research compared to any other industry in the United States of America. All manufacturing in the pharmaceutical industry is done in compliance with FDA Good Manufacturing Practices Regulations (GMP); hence, all production personnel should understand GMP, at least as it applies to their particular area of responsibility. Production deligence right from the initial stages of the manufacture is necessary for the development of proper oral formulations.

Equipment

Manufacturing equipment has to designated, located, and maintained to facilitate thorough cleaning. Ensurance for its intended use and minimized potential for contamination during manufacture has to be made. Quality assurance personnel are responsible for this. Manufacturing equipment and utensils should be thoroughly cleansed and maintained based on specific written directions. From time to time, equipment should be disassembled and thoroughly cleaned to avoid the carryover of drug residues and traces from previous operations. Monitoring adequate records of such procedures and tests should be accomplished by quality assurance personnel. Routinely swab tests on the equipment have to be performed to detect if there are any traces of drugs at end of the specific cleaning of an instrument. This is the part of Good Manufacturing Practice. Prior to the start of any production operation, the quality assurance personnel should ascertain that the proper equipment and tooling for each manufacturing stage are being used. All the equipment must be identified with labels bearing the name, dosage form, item number, and lot number of the product to be processed. Equipment used for special batch production should be completely separated in the production department. All dust-producing operations should be completely separated in the production department, and all dust-producing operations should be provided with adequate exhaust systems to prevent cross-contamination and recirculation of contaminated air. Weighing and measuring equipment used in production and quality assurance processes, such as thermometer and balances, should be calibrated and checked at suitable intervals by appropriate methods. Records of such tests should be maintained by quality assurance and production personnel. The equipment is now ready and the batch manufacture could be proceeded. Definitely all the steps that are mentioned here are after the validation of the equipment is completely achieved and standard operation procedures (SOPs) are in place.

Manufacture

Manufacture is accomplished after the equipment is ready. The series of steps in the manufacture is quality assurance at start-up, raw materials processing, labels control, packaging materials control, compounding, quality assurance during packaging operation and auditing. Label control, quality assurance at start-up, packaging materials control and raw materials processing could be accomplished prior to the manufacture or during the manufacture. However, all these should be ready before the manufacture batch record is finalized. Manufacture batch record finalization involves all the steps that are mentioned previously and the corresponding validations. The situation of the manufacture of a formulation, whether solid or a liquid, specifications should be in place, in a manufacture batch record. For instance, the quality and performance of solid oral dosage forms depends on solid phase, formulation design and also on the manufacturing process. A crucial aspect of the relationship of dosage form processing to product quality is the potential for process-induced solid phase changes of a drug candidate during the manufacturing. Therefore, rational formulation and process designs require an integrated knowledge of polymorphism, interconversion mechanisms and available processing options. In order to make sure consistent product quality, it is essential to anticipate, control or prevent phase transformation in process design and development. However, as per manufacture, these preliminary basic investigations are already in place before even the manufacture is started. However, keeping in view, these important formalities, a few statements are added in this context. Retrospectively speaking "Process design and specification used to be a somewhat unstructured process; now there's a language and a methodology that allows everyone involved in design and process control to communicate with each other." Now, everything is automated. Today, most of the leading automation vendors serving the pharmaceutical industry have control-design software or related IT tools to help clients specify and code their control systems. Despite the lack of sophisticated software, all the manufacturing procedures are quite routine. A skilled person could accomplish the manufacture quite conveniently. In this regard, three different kinds of methods as per the investment and sophistication of the manufacturer could be investigated and routinely used and are discussed here. Recommendations have been made in this regard.

Group I. Manufacture by Educational plus Software Training

This is the conventional treatment: a standard course, plus another course on the use of the practical manufacture to implement the techniques taught once the students have "understood" them. A pharmacist, may be with a M.Pharm or Ph.D. degree in pharmaceutical sciences with proper training in manufacturing set up includes group 1. The skill rate for this group is high. A M. Pharm and

Ph.D. degrees gives enough fundamentals and should be conveniently handle manufacturing even without training in a manufacture plant. Troubleshooting could be easy for this kind of background. The same could be extrapolated to the process with the manufacture plant. Highly qualified and most of the cases multi-national companies manufacture use these kinds of set up. Basic research also becomes a part of this kind of manufacture.

Group 2. Manufacture by Training with a Software

This group is taught exactly the same as the first group (i.e., they are exposed to the theory and to the use of the manufacturing set up), but the teaching is done by an intelligent and generally well-learned person, esp. qualified in manufacture with several years of experience with a Ph.D. degree preferably in pharmaceutical technology. B. Pharm and M. Pharm degrees or B. Tech in chemical engineering should be enough along with training in sophisticated computer manufacturing packages currently available. Execution and following each and every step of a protocol with due diligence is essential for this group of manufacture process. The same is true with the manufacturing set up. A medium size company with a proper collaboration with a medium scale set up is a good example for this kind of pharmaceutical manufacture.

Group 3. Manufacture with Little Training May Include Software

The third group does not attend a basic training in technology at all. Instead, they are provided with a package that assists them with statistical analysis as and when they need it. The manufacture would be very simple with very limited manpower with limited training, may incorporate software for the training and manufacture. Generally, a B. Pharm should be fine for such manufacture handling. The help of external support could accomplish troubleshooting. Mostly these companies are small sized companies. However, what ever the size of the company is the manufacture has to be accomplished in clean room and GMP set up. Everything at the end has to be approved by FDA or other regulatory agencies.

Lab Notebook Maintenance and Data Handling

Recording data is essential and is one of the biggest issues with any research, whether school or industrial research. Since the entire project and the protocols and the reports and the publications depend on the data recording, this becomes a crucial issue. A project moves forward with data generation, protocols are generated with previous experiments, reports are generated from the data obtained by conducting the experiments using these protocols, and finally the data is organized and the outcomes of the project are published and routinely viewed. This is a common practice for any research project (s). Recently, this issue has cropped up because of the introduction of intelligent electronic laboratory notebooks. However, in this regard, a brief overview on lab notebook management and data handling will be henceforth presented.

Recording data on paper (Laboratory Note Book) has always served as the central element of organic process R & D activities. Process R & D data must be recorded for archiving. Further, quality experimental information is especially critical during scale-up and technology transfer to manufacturing. Paper laboratory notebooks have been the primary methods. With the generation of patents and increased business competitiveness, this becomes more important. The initial pages of any laboratory notebooks will have instructions of maintenance. The author and the issuer makes sure that the instructions are properly taken care and thus forth signed before writing anything on the note book. For instance, some of the instructions from a well-established laboratory notebook (From Ranbaxy Research Laboratories, Gurgaon) are as follows:

(a) For Research and Development to secure adequate Patent-Rights are the primary purposes of this book. Only properly kept records will assure the company of such protection. Record your work as you progress for a project, giving sufficient details. Hand-write directly in the book. Do not make notes elsewhere to be copied later.

(b) All entries should be in permanent black/blue ink. Do not use pencil.

(c) Record batch number as ...., based on the standard operating procedure of that particular organization.

(d) In chronological order give a complete, accurate account of what you did and what resulted. Enter all results, both good and bad. In case of error, draw a single line through the incorrect words and sign.

(e) Complete calculation in detail should be written in this book.

(f) All experiments should be signed and dated by the author and the verifier.

(g) Note new ideas, procedures, sketches, etc immediately when they come into your mind.

(h) All the material of the notebook is exclusive property of the research lab.

(i) All projects should be recorded currently and up to date that any co-worker may comprehend the operation in your absence or on re-assignment.

However, presently the paper laboratory notebook is slowly being replaced by intelligent electronic laboratory notebook (ELN), especially in big pharma of developed countries. An intelligent ELN solution enables higher quality data storage, use, analysis, and management leading to the excellence of pharmaceutical companies in the current scenaria as indicated before the importance of data and its management in the form of a lab notebook. Introduction of intelligent electronic laboratory notebook is still not well adopted by regulatory agencies. It is definitely long way to go. However, the basics of a lab notebook still remain the same. The four main thrusts of direction for the intelligent ELN in the future are

1. increasing levels of intelligence,
2. increasing levels of integration,
3. continued strides in ease of data entry, and
4. improved management reporting and data mining.

Batch Record

Batch production records should be prepared, maintained, and controlled for each batch of product. In generally, they should be retained for a period of about five years after distribution has been completed. The idea is that if something happens after the product has reached the market, it always boils down to the batch record mistakes. Since the shelf-life is fixed and if for example, the shelf-life is for 3 years and this batch of product was not bought by any customer for what so ever the reason is and all of a sudden if one doctor prescribes this medicine and a patient consumes it and notices more toxic effects, the origins have to be determined, debated and discussed. This is generally an unfortunate situation. On the other hand, definitely there are cases where in there is a deliberate contamination. Even in these situations, it definitely helps to scroll back onto the batch records and further investigate the origins of this accident.

The batch production record shall contain an accurate reproduction of the manufacturing formula, procedure, and product specifications from the correct master formula procedure to be used in the production of a batch of product. Generally, the manufacture of a placebo is essential as a control. Thus, any manufacturing batch includes a placebo batch record and an active batch record. These batch records are then sent to each of the departments involved in the production, packaging, and control of the product. The records include dates, specific code or identification numbers of each ingradient employed, weights or measures of components and products in the course of processing, results of in-process and control testing, and the endorsements of the individual performing and supervising each step of the operation. In addition, a lot number is assigned that permits the identification of all procedures performed on the lot and their results. This lot number appears on the label of the product. This has been a practice that was done earlier. However, lately, the trend is electronic batch record and record keeping.

The US FDAs finalization of part 11 of Title 21 of the Code of Federal Regulations (CFR), which governs the use of electronic batch records and outlines the conditions that they are considerable acceptable replacements for papers. As this was introduced, several companies started adopting electronic batch records over paper batch records. Apart from FDA guidelines, electronic batch records are in place because of their several fold advantages. Electronic Batch Record systems are implemented to automate batch-oriented production processes and provide electronic records and signatures. These systems not only improve a manufacturer's performance but also improve their regulatory compliance. Currently, very complex algorithms are used in the generation of these batch records. Very sophistical computer software and hardware professionals along with experts in the field of pharmaceuticals are being accredited for the generation and introduction of electronic batch records on day-to-day basis in the pharmaceutical industry. It would take several volumes of information along with several parallel software informations to basically understand the concept of electronic batch record. Still in third world countries these are not yet in place. Together things will make better with the help of these software packages. Definitely their introduction helps the pharmaceutical companies in these countries. The advantages an electronic batch record offer include:

1. Reduced cycle times
2. Improved accuracy and consistency of batch record
3. Reduced costs of compliance
4. Increased productivity
5. Cost avoidance
6. Increased speed of product changes and product introductions

Process Validation

The validation department writes and executes validation protocols to demonstrate that equipment, activities, and processes consistently produce products or results that meet approved specifications. Validation is conducted on manufacturing processes, aseptic operations, equipment cleaning procedures, equipment, and computerized systems. The validation group also evaluates proposed changes to determine if additional studies need to be done. Validation is also conducted on analytical methods used in laboratories; sometimes a lab methods validation group is responsible for doing these.

Qualification is a term that was used for long time and is related to proper function of an instrument. Reproducibility is a main function of any machinery. The production and selling of inferior goods has been a major problem in any market. With industrial output, the main source of such defects was focused on the machinery in the beginning. Thus, the performance of instrument and the reproducibility were very well considered on these lines. The term that was used was qualification. Qualification is generally related to equipment and is used to determine whether the equipment operates as it was designed to in a reproducible manner. Quality is definitely a factor that is affected due to the entire manufacture process and not only due to the machinery. Subsequently, the term validation was introduced, elaborated and applied with several rules and regulations. Thus, validation is a term related to the entire manufacturing process. The FDA definition for validation goes like this, "A validated manufacturing process is one that has been proved to do what it purports or is represented to do. The proof of validation is obtained through collection and evaluation of data, prefereably, beginning from the process development phase and continuing through into the production phase. Validation necessarily includes process qualification (the qualification of materials, equipment, systems, building, personnel), but it also includes the control of the entire processes for repeated batches or runs".

Process validation includes the demonstration of a process that controls the critical steps of a process results in products of repeatable attributes (e.g., content uniformity) or causes a reproducible event (e.g. sterilization). Prior to the introduction of the methods of validation, quality control of the finished products was used as the quality of the production. However, it was subsequently realized that several factors influence the quality of the finished goods. These include raw material quality, process quality, manpower quality and instrument quality. Each of the methods of qualification is subsequently termed validations. These validations include raw material validation, process validation, manpower validation and instrument validation.

The FDA defines process validation as follows:

"Process validation is establishing documented evidence that provides a high degree of assurance that a specific process will consistently produce a product meeting its pre-determined specifications and quality characteristics".

Manufacturer prepares a written validation protocol that specifies the procedures (and tests) to be conducted and the data to be collected. The purpose for which the data are collected must be clear. The data must reflect facts. The data must be collected carefully and accurately. The protocol should specify a sufficient number of replicate process runs to demonstrate reproducibility and provide an accurate measure of variability among successive runs. The test conditions for these runs should include upper and lower processing limits and circumstances, including those within standard operating procedures, which pose the greatest chance of process or product failure compared to ideal conditions; such conditions have become widely known as "worst case" conditions. (They are sometimes called "most appropriate challenge" conditions.) Validation documentation should include evidence of the suitability of materials and the performance and reliability of equipment and systems. Key process variables should be monitored and documented. Analysis of the data collected from monitoring will establish the variability of process parameters for individual runs and will establish whether or not the equipment and process controls are adequate to assure that product specifications are met. Finished product and in-process test data can be of value in process validation, particularly in those situations where quality attributes and variabilities can be readily measured. Where finished (or in-process) testing cannot adequately measure certain attributes, process validation should be derived primarily from qualification of each system used in production and from consideration of the interaction of the various systems. In addition, the following validation terminology is routinely used. These include validation, prospective validation and retrospective validation. The definition and description of validation is mentioned before. Validation conducted prior to the distribution of either a new product, or product made under a revised manufacturing process, where the revisions may affect the product's characteristics is termed prospective validation. Validation of a process for a product already in distribution based upon accumulated production, testing and control data is called retrospective validation. A thorough investigation of data from all the three-validation steps results in thorough validation process of the entire batch and thus saves lot of time and money and prevents market damage and public damage. Definitely this helps in a long run. This concludes the validation involved for the entire batch process.

Packaging and Storage

Packaging and storage are key aspects in oral drug formulations. Basically, these steps are to protect the active moiety. The very common oral dosage forms are liquids, capsules and tablets. A variety of material in a variety of container types is used to pack these formulations. For any external stress to reach the active moiety, it has to penetrate the atmosphere, and then it has to penetrate the container material, reach the formulation, then penetrate the formulation contents and then reach the active moiety. In most of the cases, the current pharmaceutical manufacture techniques results in very thorough protection of the active moiety from the external stress. Despite all these efforts and proper care taken, in several instances, the active moiety may not be protected. The reasons for this process could be the package material is not appropriate for this preparation or the stress is more or the drug is actively prone to degradation. Checking on the packaging is important because toxicity profile of a degradation product may be very severe compared to the originial compound. In earlier days of drug discovery, only the safety and toxicity of the new drug substace was investigated. However, with advances, it was realized that in some instances, the degradation product in the packaged material might be more toxic compared to the original drug. What is the best solution in this situation? Selection of appropriate packaging material, selection of appropriate container, selection of appropriate storage conditions, are all important conditions for proper packaging control of drug substances. If very systematic study has been conducted from very early times with regard to packaging and storage, this would not be a major problem. However, if proper care has not been taken during this process, definitely, the drug stored in this container is not stable and may be very deleterious. On the other hand, if everything has been properly taken care, the only way this active moiety could be destroyed is by tampering, i.e., by applying outward forced degradation conditions. In that situation, the culprit could be caught and proper action could be meted.

At some time before the manufacture of a product is completed, a packaging record bearing an identification number is issued to the packaging section. This record specifies the packaging materials to be used, operations to be performed, and the quantity to be packaged. Simultaneous, requisitions are issued for the products to be packaged and for the packaging and the printed materials, such as labels, containers, inserts, brochures, cartons, and shipping cases. The packaging process unites the product, container, and label to form a single finished unite. Along with the individual package components, the assembly in which these formulations are packed must be correct. The packaging may be the packaging of the raw material or the packaging of the finished products. Packaging of the raw material is very important for both stability and safety purposes. The raw material includes the API and the material used in the preparation of the tablets. With regard to the API, the stability is the main issue. Most of these molecules in the generic companies are already established. However, in the manufacture of products with new chemical entities, the stability of NCEs in the storage conditions, and in the containers have to be properly studied and validated. These NCEs especially in big and new pharma if enormous, cross contamination would be a major issue. For the safety investigations, proper indexing and labeling of each and every new chemical entity has to be cross-checked. Unfortunately, if not properly indexed and caged, the spillage would lead to enormous damage both in long term and short term case sceniarios. Whatever the reason for such happening, definitely the key is the safety to the scientists conducting the experiments who are directly handling. In this regard, labeling and the authenticity of the scientists handling these chemical entities becomes the main issue. Some times this could lead to community hazard and thus definitely proper care has to be taken in handling these chemicals. Spillage could cause enormous damage to the surroundings. Once the damage has been done, any amount of money or safety will not help the surroundings and the community in general.

Once the manufacture of the dosage forms is completed, control inspector and packaging supervisor takes the opportunity of packing the dosage form into an appropriate container. Several innovations currently in place in tablet and capsule industry are resulting in automated packaging process. This could be said as automated caging. The process is in advanced stage that it could be either automated or semiautomated. The seal is automatically placed. Example of such packaging system is blister packaging system. Several millions of tablets or capsules could be packed into individual pouches in a very short time. The main concern with regard to the stability of any pharmaceutical drug substance is the exposure to the moisture. It is inevitable that moisture is definitely absorbed through the packing on most occasions. The best way early on is to conveniently investigate several kinds of packaging materials and containers for determining the stability of the drug substance in a final packaging system. Interestingly, on many occasions, more than two different containers are adequate as proper storage measures, currently. In this regard, very brief basics with little manufacture orientation will be illustrated along with some recent examples.

A novel mathematical model was recently developed for predicting moisture uptake by packaged solid pharmaceutical products during storage. High-density polyethylene (HDPE) bottles containing the tablet products of two new chemical entities and desiccants were investigated. Permeability of the bottles was determined at different temperatures using steady-state data. Moisture sorption isotherms of the two model drug products and desiccants at the same temperatures were determined and expressed in polynomial equations. This is done by regression analysis. The isotherms are used for modeling the time-humidity profile in the container, which enables the prediction of the moisture content of individual component during storage. Predicted moisture contents agree well with real time stability data. The current model could serve as a guide during packaging selection for moisture protection. That way the cost and cycle time of screening the study are reduced.

Alternatively, as mentioned before an active drug could be protected for external environment using dessicant in the package. This could save a lot of time on simple investigations with several containers. Desiccants protect the drug in the pouch. The sorption--desorption moisture transfer (SDMT) model is used to predict the effect of desiccant quantity, tablet quantity and tablet initial moisture content on the relative humidity inside high density polyethylene (HDPE) bottles. The drug stability could be determined once the tablets are inside the container. This gives the basic results, which demonstrates the affect of moisture content on the stability of the drug. In one recent study a very moisture sensitive drug roxifiban was used for these investigations. Roxifiban tablets were manufactured using the common procedures. The tablets were stored in HDPE bottles and the stability of the drug inside the container was investigated. Monitoring of moisture content with time was accomplished. The effect of these variables on the stability of roxifiban tablets in the HDPE bottles was investigated. Good correlation between the calculated relative humidity values inside the package and stability results was found. Tablet degradant concentration increased with the increase in the relative humidity calculated by the SDMT model. Desiccant quantity was the most important factor in controlling degradation rate. The degradation rate decreased as the quantity of desiccant in the bottle was increased. For a given desiccant quantity, degradation rate increased with an increase in the weight of tablets in the container. The inclusion of a desiccant in the package dramatically reduced the effect of initial tablet moisture content on stability. Nevertheless, the effect of initial moisture content was still observed. This study demonstrated the practical utility of a desiccant in comprehending the correlation between packaging variables and the stability of a moisture sensitive product. This is when the tablets are stored in bottles. However, in current situations, tablets and capsules are stored in blister packs that are made of different polymer contents. The results would be illustrated using a specific example. Packages that provided stability (less than a 10% loss in potency) of a moisture sensitive compound (PGE-7762928) in tablet form at accelerated conditions for 6 months were determined using equilibriation moisture content studies. The equilibrium moisture content of the tablets at 25 degrees C/60%RH, 30 degrees C/60%RH and 40 degrees C/75%RH as determined were 2.3,2.4, and 2.9%, respectively. The tablet equilibrium moisture content, degradation rate of unpackaged product, and the moisture barrier properties of the packages were used in the prediction of the stability of the packaged product. The physical and chemical stability (HPLC assay) of the products were measured after 2,4,6,8,12, and 24 weeks at ICH conditions. The containers permeation of polyvinyl chloride blisters, cyclic olefin blisters, aclar blisters, cold-form aluminum blisters was 0.259, 0.040, 0.008 and 0.001 mg per blister per day, respectively. At 6 months at 40 degrees C/75%RH, the percent active was 84% in polyvinyl chloride blisters, 91% in cyclic olefin blisters, 97% in aclar blisters, 100% in cold-form aluminum blisters and 99% in an high density polyethylene bottle with a foil induction seal. The stability results for the packaged product were fairly consistent with the predictions based on the moisture sensitivity of the product and the moisture barrier properties of the respective package. To gain a better prediction, the flux value determined by the Containers-Permeation procedure was adjusted for the internal moisture concentration of the blister.

Several other factors that could be considered in determining the stability include temperature, contact area with film, excipients and moisture contents in the preparation on the remaining amount of a drug in polyethylene packaging. Usually granules and tablets are packed in this kind of packaging material. The decrease of bromhexine HCl contents in granules and tablets was determined when the preparations were stored in these films. In this case, the effects of temperature, contact area with film, excipients and moisture contents in the preparation on the remaining amount of bromhexin HCl were studied in order to investigate the interaction mechanism between bromhexine HCl and polyethylene film. It was observed that the decrease of bromhexine HCl was due to the sorption to the polyethylene film. The results indicated that the moisture contents of the dosage forms determined the rate of sorption predominantly, and that removal of adsorbed water from dosage forms was effective to prevent bromhexine HCl content decrease. Selecting an appropriate manufacturing process or an appropriate packaging material or container, especially for drugs that are not that stable could protect the drug.

Not only is the stability affected because of the container used to store the final products but also several physical features of the final products may be affected. An example is the dissolution of the active drug from a dosage form is sometimes affected by various containers used. Thus packaging is an important factor in pharmaceutical processing of oral formulations. The bulk of the product and each of the packaging components should be checked, endorsed, and dated by qualified packaging personnel. This should be done with the cooperation of the control inspector. In practice, only the exact number of labels required for a batch, including small excess, should be delivered to the labeling area after careful and meticulous inspection of each label. Everything has to be properly checked. Proper on-line inspections and end product monitoring and evaluation would be very crucial to ensure proper product output. The common approach is for key personnel to prevent distribution of the batch in question, and other batches of products that were packaged during the same period of time, until the product output quality is very fine.

The other key issue is storage. Seeing is believing in any technological situation is not valid. Thus, storing of substances in refrigerators and in well-defined places does not mean that a drug is protected and is stable in this condition. Very systematically, the affect of storage conditions should be investigated. Commonly, this is a part of stability protocol. The stability of a drug substance is investigated very early on in the process of formulation development and thus by the time this product reaches the market, enough stability data has been generated to fix the storage atmosphere of the drug substance and the corresponding formulation. This not only helps in the determination of drug substance in a shelf, but also determines its stability during transit. Thus, packaging and storing are the very important factors of product processing and evaluation. Again as mentioned before, storage of NCEs is also a main issue. This is definitely a part of formulation development. In addition proper storage is also important for security purposes. This is important not only for the person who is handling the chemical or the formulation, but also prevents if any, the ulterior motives in mishandling the stored chemicals. Proper indexing, regular evaluation of shelves, security and the tight control are the key issues related to the storage of drugs and formulations. However, proper precautions have to be taken from the angle of safety.

Quality

What is Control and Assurance?

"To achieve the quality objective reliably there must be a comprehensively designed and correctly implemented system of Quality Assurance (QA) incorporating Good Manufacturing Practice (GMP) and thus quality control (QC)." Good Manufacturing Practice (GMP) is that part of Quality Assurance (QC) which ensures that products are consistently produced and controlled to the quality standards appropriate to their intended use and as required by the Marketing Authorisation or product specification. GMP is concerned with both production and quality control. The basic requirements of GMP are that:

1. all manufacturing processes are clearly defined, systematically reviewed in the light of experience and shown to be capable of consistently manufacturing medicinal products of the required quality and complying with their specifications;
2. critical steps of manufacturing processes and significant changes to the process are validated;
3. All necessary facilities for GMP are provided including:
   (a) Appropriately qualified and trained personnel;
   (b) Adequate premises and space;
   (c) Suitable equipment and services
   (d) Correct materials, containers and labels
   (e) Approved procedures and instructions
   (f) Suitable storage and transport
4. instructions and procedure are written in an instructional form in clear and unambiguous language, specifically applicable to the facilities provided;
5. operators are trained to carry out procedures correctly;
6. records are made, manually and/or by recording instruments, during manufacture which demonstrate that all the steps required by the defined procedures and instructions were in fact taken and that the quantity and quality of the product was as expected. Any significant deviations are fully recorded and investigated;

7. records of manufacture including distribution which enable the complete history of a batch to be traced, are retained in a comprehensible and accessible form;
8. the distribution (wholesaling) of the products minimises any risk to their quality;

What is meant by high Quality?

Quality in this context means a product which is pure and which is consistent. Medicines need to avoid any kind of contamination from other substances since this could have damaging effects upon the person taking the medicine. Also it is vital that each dose contains exactly the correct amount of ingredients. Maintaining high quality is particularly important in pharmaceutical manufacture. This is because the consumer will often be ill and weakened when they use the product. There are a number of overseeing bodies worldwide, such as the Medicines and Healthcare products Regulatory Agency (MHRA) in the UK and the Food and Drugs Administration (FDA) in the USA. Their representatives can come and inspect a factory at any time. Medicines are made in batches and the results of the checks are recorded. These results are inspected by a Qualified Person at the end of the process, and if satisfactory, the batch is released. The records are then kept in an archive so that the progress of all the medicines in every batch can be traced at a later date, if necessary. Note that records are begun when the raw materials are drawn from the store. These records then follow the batch through every stage of manufacture with additional information added at each stage. It is very important to get these procedures right. If the quality of a medicine is not up to standard or impurities find their way into the product during the manufacturing process, then the result could be disastrous. The medicine might be ineffective or in the worst case actually harmful.

How is Quality and Control achieved?

The personal involved at the manufacturing site has to very properly understand the complicated links between several of the output and the input feedbackers in a manufacturing unit. These interlinks could be conveniently called internal customers and external customers. Thus, control and assurance is not only achieved by the personal involved in the manufacturing but also several of the interlinking functionalities. Control results in the best quality of the final product. Assurance is the ensurance of the best quality of the final product. These two are interrelated terms and very often used together in the description of quality control in any industry. In addition, the other aspect that is worth mentioning at this stage is retailing which is closely linked to the concepts of external and internal customers. The other word that is closely related not only to the customer concept but also to the quality and assurance is retail management, and definitely not as a reiteration. The word 'retail' is derived from the French word 'retaillier', meaning to cut off or to break bulk. In simple terms, it implies a first-hand transaction with the customer. Retailing involves a direct interface with the customer and the co-ordination of business activities from end- to end- right from the concept or the design stage of a product or offering, to its delivery and post-delivery service to the customer. Generally, every industry strives to obtain perfect end product. However, on every attempt perfection may not be achieved. This process has been investigated eversince industrialization began. However, quality is not only with industrial goods. It could also be any good that is available in the market. Thus, together these terms are used very commonly in any industry and especially in pharmaceutical industry. Herewith, very comprehensively these two terms will be described one by one. The concept of total quality control refers to the process of striving to produce a perfect product by a series of measures requiring an organized effort by the entire company to prevent or eliminate errors at every stage in production. Quality control is mainly the responsibility of the quality assurance department. However, quality assurance involves many departments and disciplines within a company. It is definitely a team effort. Quality must be built into a drug product during product and process design, and it is influenced by the physical plant design, space, ventilation, cleanliness, and sanitation during routine production. The assurance of product quality depends on more than just proper sampling and adequate testing of various components and the finished dosage form. Every mistake as described in the entirety of this chapter has to be properly controlled. It is not always easy to determine the mistake if proper control is not maintained. Sources of quality variation are determined and these serve as checkpoints for determining the quality of the product. Thus, several checkpoints to monitor the quality of the product as it is processed and upon completion of the manufacture are documented in the quality control protocols. Subsequently, these are investigated to determine and ensure the quality of the pharmaceutical products. If these protocols are not laid down properly or the person who is the incharge of their maintenance or the deliverer are not following the instructions properly, it is always a tricky situation in terms of the quality of the final products.

Control includes raw materials control, in-process items control, validation of manufacturing equipment, validation of the entire process, quality assurance at start-up, packaging materials control, labels control, finished product control, bulk product testing, qulity assurance during packaging operations and auditing are the key steps in control and assurance. Currently, each of these steps is scientifically controlled and assured. Various statistical and mathematical principles are used. Statistical methods of investigation based on the theory of probability is used for estimating parameters, for performing tests of significance, for determining the relationship between factors, and for making meaningful decisions on the basis of experimental evidence. Quality control charts are used in the determination of variables responsible for the quality of a product. Quality control incorporates personnel, equipment and building, batch production record, control of production procedures, manufacturing control, packaging control and validation. As steps to ensure total quality product identification systems, adulteration, misbranding and counterfeiting, maintenance, storage, and retrieval of records, complaints, return of goods, recall procedures and adverse effects are all needed to be monitored.

Personal

Managerial Duties

Managerial duties are very important roles in a pharmaceutical manufacturing firm. This could include management on a production ground, on a research ground or on a market ground. Several volumes of information have been written in several textbooks. However, for the most precise understanding as per the perfect reference to context of the chapter of oral drug delivery, very brief overview will be presented here. It is a common knowledge that all management personnel require to posses a number of essential skills and characteristics in order to efficiently perform and fulfill managerial duties. Skills like leadership, communication, mentoring and planning are always seen, as imperative requirements for all types of management roles whether they are in the upper, the middle or the lower-management.

In this day and age of the high tech society, there has been a steady increase in the number of managerial positions that are filled, not with MBA or Business graduates, but with people from technical backgrounds such as pharmaceutical or medicine or engineering degrees. This is 100% true with the management of pharmaceutical production floor. There is definitely an advantage in terms of management of a pharmaceutical floor as related to a pharmaceutical background. The role of a manager is more lucrative than other roles and as such there is a significant competition among pharmaceutical personal to go onto the production floor in an industry. In order to climb the proverbial career ladder many people from technical backgrounds are compelled to take on managerial positions that involve little or no technical duties. Furthermore technical managers, who generally have limited knowledge and experience of management, are expected to perform administrative managerial tasks. Some additionally, even try to fulfill their personal interests by continuing to perform technical duties/responsibilities that are no longer required by them. This is like a Professor conducting every day research in the laboratory. As a result, this can lead to a number of problems and trends. Technological degrees like B. Pharm,

M. Pharm and Ph.D. in pharmaceutical sciences generally attract people who are technically sound and who want to pursue high-tech careers. It can therefore be seen that many of the problems faced by pharmaceutical graduates working on the production floor are in fact a lack of exposure to the management practices.

There are a number of common issues and problems faced by Technology Managers like staff management, project planning and ethical issues to name a few. In an industry where deadlines are the driving forces to the success, effective management of employees and their output is important. As a result, Technology Managers or workers must have strong leadership, mentoring and communication skills to guide employees through a stressful environment. Project planning is another very important aspect of Technology Management or staff – the planning of timelines and staffs requirements are mandatory tasks that need to be designed carefully and thoughtfully in order to attain the proposed goals. Another common problem that is faced by Technology Managers is the ethical issue. As they are responsible for the technology being used by employees, they must also ensure that the technology is being used appropriately. This raises some dilemmas on where to draw the line between invading staff privacy and ensuring that technology is being used responsibly. Although most companies do have Acceptable Use Policies defined, however the extent of monitoring is largely left to the Managers of Technology. During the mid 90s statistics showed that most technology security breaches were made by internal staff as opposed to outside hackers. Even though this trend is decreasing as nowadays most breaches are made from outsiders, managers are still faced with the ethical dilemma of monitoring.

A lot of responsibility lies upon the shoulders of pharmaceutical Managers. Not only are they expected to have a high level of technical knowledge and experience, but they also have to be business minded with strong leadership and communication skills. However, due to the nature of the technology industry and such roles in general, many technical personnel, who lack training, experience or knowledge of management principles, are required to take on managerial positions. Hopefully in the near future, as the industry further grows and matures, we will be seeing a new wave of technical managers who have good managerial skills. This definitely increases the pharmaceutical output. These are the some of the fundamental principles and duties of a manager working on product processing section of a pharmaceutical industry. In this section, only the functions and roles are mentioned. However, he has to be technically savvy, especially if he is working in the area of pharmaceutical sciences, he has to for sure be an expert in the area of theory and practice of product processing with relevant training. This ensures that production errors would not be foreseen. This is definitely useful in the long run to the company in general and to the patient force, in particular.

Validation

Since human nature is very fickle, and always prone to psychological stresses, it is always a nice idea for any company to validate the personal working in the organization routinely. This is especially true with pharmaceutical companies. The staff working in a pharmaceutical company has to deal with internal and external customers. Internal customers are the staff with whom this person is in constant touch. External customers are the ones who the staff is dealing with. This includes patients, vendors of raw material, machinery, engineers, technicians, assistants, sales personal, medical representatives, physicians and pharmacists. Thus, for an outcome to be positive personal validation becomes very important. As mentioned in the managerial roles, the same principles apply to any staff working in a company. Honesty and integrity along with intelligence and regular training ensures that things are moving smoothly leading to a cordial atmosphere. This includes personal validation. A company has to ensure that the people working in the company are routinely validated. This is a part of GMP in several developed countries. Several parameters and regular precisions and methods would be essential for proper personal validation.

Consultation, discussion, planning, delivery, conclusions and regular training, both within the organisation and with response partners are the steps involved in personal validation. Comprehensively, a validation strategy should contain the following elements:

1. Planning, consultation and discussion.
2. Exercises and Training.
3. Checking the continuity of the delivery of the validation.

Planning, consultation and discussion

The first step essential for the staff to work on a production or research unit is the planning. This may come through consultation and discussion. Thus, the staff has to be thorough with regard to the planning. Proper planning saves lot of time and often time results in effective end result. Personal validation process goes on throughout the plan preparation phase as the response objectives are developed, the internal and external customers identified and comments on the draft plan sought. For a pharmaceutical production, the initial stages are quite tedius and definitely requires lot of planning. As per the requirements, a plan is generated. Once a plan document is complete, consultation does not stop. Those responsible for maintaining and activating the plan should keep in regular touch with customers and try to be involved with their planning activities, eg as participants in, or observers at, training and exercises. Planners should be careful that in consulting others, the emphasis should be on the likely effectiveness of the plan rather than on conforming to a set pattern or simply ensuring that references are accurate. Several training methods or exercises may help in achieving this first goal of personal validation.

Exercise or Training

Exercise or training the staff is the next step. Validation exercises assume that staff have received the necessary training and are able to carry out their emergency roles, so that the lessons learnt relate to the effectiveness of the planned response and the responsible staff and not to the skills of the manager or the group or the organization. Exercises and exercise debriefs are key methods of validating plans. Normally there will be an exercise cycle set out for each plan, starting with simple exercises, perhaps of individual aspects of the plan (communication, production, planning, quality control, etc.) and developing over time into more complex, multi-functional exercises. The intention is normally to validate all aspects of the plan, both individually and as an integrated part of the whole, over a 3-5 year exercise cycle. The training could be the initial training, intermediate training or terminal training. Given that exercise budgets are normally very limited, it is often the case that exercises have to include elements of training and validation. Where this is the case, particular attention should be given to designing the exercise and setting objectives. That way clear lessons are learnt about the likely effectiveness of the plan. Thus, exercise and training are the very crucial elements of a personal validation.

Checking the continuity of the delivery of the validation

A pharmaceutical industry is always dynamic. New staff may come and old staff may leave. This movement makes things more complicated. Thus, validity of the plan in the light of changes to staff, new organisational structures, or the social and political environment in which the staff would operate becomes very important. In addition, attending various meetings, seminars and training sessions is also important to make sure the continuity of the delivery of the validation. The continuity would be ensured with the help of regular checking the continuity of the delivery of the validation. All exercises should be followed by debriefs – opportunities for all participants to comment on how well the response met the plan objectives and to share any lessons learnt from the exercise. How debriefs are organised will depend to some extent on the size and complexity of an exercise. Debriefs or these meetings could be divided into:

- 'Hot' debrief meetings held immediately after an exercise is complete, which give participants the opportunity to share learning points while the experience is still very fresh in their minds.
- 'Cold' debrief meetings, held days or weeks after an exercise, when participants have had an opportunity to take a considered view on the exercise and how effective the plan or plans were.

The evaluations, attendance and utility of these meetings become a very important part of staff training. Along with these issues, document management is also a very important aspect of personal validation. This is important because everything that is involved right from the step 1 to step last and day in and day out, it is all documentation in the production management of pharmaceuticals, and infact applies to other productions also. In this regard all the steps of validation of documentation are also important. Higher authority, responsible staff and managers are responsible that this aspect of validation is proceeding in an ideal way.

Conclusions

In the entirety of this chapter various aspects of pharmaceutical processing and evaluation are described. Most of the techniques described here are well placed in developed countries. However, these methods are adopted in few of the major pharmaceutical companies in India. With the introduction of several reforms in the area of industrialization, currently India is also picking up in this forefront and thus it is very essential not only for entrepreuners but also for all the staff working in the area of product processing and evaluation to know these concepts.

Questions for Practice and Exercise

1. Describe very briefly the sequential methodology in the development of drugs right from the first step to the last step.
2. List the steps involved if any of the manufacturing processes is stratified.
3. Define the following:
    1. 21 CFR 11 and
    2. cGMP.
4. Define the following:
    1. An internal customer and
    2. An external customer.
5. Briefly describe the relationships between the internal customers and the external customers.
6. Very briefly describe retailing.
7. Mention very briefly the pivotal role of retailing in the manufacturing methodologies right from the very beginning to the end of a production and a manufacturing process.

8. Write a note on the following:
    1. FDAs 1997 Electronic Signature Rule,
    2. Electronic Batch Record Systems (eBRS),
    3. Production Requirement Softwares,
    4. Standard Operating Procedures,
    5. Quality Assurance,
    6. Pharmaceutical Manufacture Sequence,
    7. Training to a Manufacturer,
    8. Lab Notebook Maintenance and Data Handling,
    9. Batch Record,
    10. Code of Federal Regulations,
    11. Process Validation,
    12. Process Qualification,
    13. Packaging and Storage,
    14. Stability of the Product and its Container Dependency,
    15. Managerial Duties,
    16. Validation,
    17. Planning, Consultation and Discussion,
    18. Exercise and Training,
    19. Checking the Continuity of the Delivery of the Validation,
    20. Control and Assurance.

Bibliography

1. The Theory and Practice of Industrial Pharmacy, Third Edition, Edited by Leon Lachman, Herbert A. Lieberman, and Joseph L. Kanig, Lea & Febiger Publications, 1986.
2. Retail Management, Functional Principles & Practices, Second Edition, Authored by Gibson G. Vedamani, Jaico Publishing House, 2004.
3. Pharmaceutical Jurisprudence & Ethics (Forensic Pharmacy), Third Edition, Authored by S.P. Agarwal and Rajesh Khanna, Birla Publications, 2004.
4. Pharmaceutical Dosage Forms and Drug Delivery Systems, Seventh Edition, Authored by H.C. Ansel, L.V. Allen, and N.G. Popovich, Lippincott Williams & Wilkins, 1999.

CHAPTER 16

PROCESS VALIDATION

- **Definitions**
- **Why to Do Process Validation?**
- **When to Do Process Validation?**
- **Classification**
- **Validation of Solid Dosage Forms**
- **Guidelines for Process Validation of Solid Dosage Forms**
- **Conclusions**
- **Questions for Practice and Exercise**
- **Bibliography**

Definitions

Different authors defined process validation differently. Some of these definitions are as below:

1. Validation is defined as "A documented program which provides a high degree of assurance that a specific process will consistently produce a product meeting its pre-determined specifications and quality attributes."
2. Validation is an essential procedure that demonstrates that a manufacturing process operating under defined standard conditions is capable of consistently producing a product that meets the established product specifications.
3. In its proposed guidelines, the U.S. Food and Drug Administration (FDA) has offered the following definition for process validation. Process validation is establishing documented evidence that provides a high degree of assurance that a specific process (such as the manufacture of pharmaceutical dosage forms) will consistently produce a product meeting its predetermined specifications and quality characteristics.

Why to do Process Validation?

There are several important reasons for validating a product and/or process. First, manufacturers are required by law to conform to CGMP regulations. In the early 1990s, the concept of preapproval inspection (PAI) was born and had as one of its basic tenets the assurance that approved validation protocols and schedules were being generated and that comprehensive development, scale-up, and biobatch and commercial batch validation data were required in order to achieve a successful regulatory PAI audit. Second, good business dictates that a manufacturer avoid the possibility of rejected or recalled batches. Third, validation helps to ensure product uniformity, reproducibility, and quality. The FDA has published a guideline for use by industry that outlines general principles considered acceptable parts of process validation. Pharmaceutical firms have been inspected against this standard and those found wanting have been cited or had approval to manufacture product denied. Indeed, statistics compiled by the FDA for fiscal year 1997 show inadequate process validation as one of the top 10 reasons for withholding approval.

When to do Process Validation?

Most discussions of product and process validation that have been published or that have been the subject of presentations at meetings have concentrated on validation associated with the full-scale manufacture of pharmaceutical processes and how equipment processing variables affect the overall quality of the finished product. Although this is certainly an important aspect of product validation, validation of numerous earlier aspects of development are critical to the subsequent phases of the process. Without proper characterization, specification, and control of these earlier development steps, the foundation will be weak and will not support the evolving product when it is challenged during the formal validation of pilot and production batches. Many individuals tend to think of validation as a stand-alone item or an afterthought at the end of the entire product/process development sequence. Some believe that the process can be considered validated if the first two or three batches of product satisfy specifications. However, process validation is of different types and it has to be performed at different stages as per the type of validation. Before discussing further on various types of process validations, it would be essential to describe one stereotype of the process in pharmaceutical industry. In this case the process is formulation developing of tablets. It is henceforth discussed below.

A Typical Pharmaceutical Process and the Essential Elements of Validation

Process validation is performed for all the processes with particular specifications and most of the times guidelines are followed. For designing an ideal process validation program, the pharmaceutical process should be thoroughly known. Here the example of formulation development of tablets is explained. The typical process will illustrate the various essentials of tablet processing. Here for the process is discussed further.

Formulation development should not be considered complete until all those factors that could significantly alter the formulation have been studied. Subsequent minor changes to the formulation, however, may be acceptable, provided they are thoroughly tested and are shown to have no adverse effect on product.

The process development program should meet the following objectives:

1. Develop a suitable process to produce a product that meets all
   (a) Product specifications
   (b) Economic constraints
   (c) Current good manufacturing practices (CGMPs)
2. Identify the key process parameters that affect the product attributes
3. Identify in-process specifications and test methods
4. Identify generic and/or specific equipment that may be required It is important to remember that cleaning procedures should at least be in the final stages of development, as equipment and facilities in the pilot or

proposed manufacturing plant are involved, and the development of the cleaning verification test methods must be complete.

Process development can be divided into several stages.

Design

Challenging of critical process parameters

Verification of the developed process.

Typical Variables for Table Preparation

Granulation:

Preblending (Blending time)

Load size

Order of addition

Amount of granulating agent

Solvent addition rate

Granulation time

Drying temperature

Moisture content

Air flow program

Drying time

Cooling time

Sieving:

Sizing Screen type

Granule size distribution

Screen size

Loose density

Feed rate

Packed density

Blending Load size

Blend uniformity

Flow characteristics:

Blending time

Particle size distribution

Tableting:
Compression rate
Granule feed rate
Friability
Precompression force
Hardness
Compression force
Thickness
Disintegration time
Dissolution
Dosage form uniformity

After the qualification trials have been completed, the protocol for the full-scale process validation runs can be written. Current industry standard for the validation batches is to attempt to manufacture them at target values for both process parameters and specifications. The validation protocol is usually the joint effort of the following groups:

Research and development

Pharmaceutical technology or technical services

Quality control (quality assurance)

Manufacturing

Engineering

One of these groups usually coordinates the activities.

A complete qualification protocol will contain specific sections; however, there can be considerable variation in individual protocol. Section content typical validation protocol may consist of the following:

Safety instructions
Environmental restrictions
Gas or liquid discharge limitations
Solid or scrap disposal instructions
Equipment
Description
Operation
Cleaning
Raw materials

Pertinent characteristics
Acceptance limits
Analytical methods
Packaging and storage
Handling precautions
Process flow chart
Critical parameters and related means of controls
Responsibilities of each of the groups participating
Cleaning validation/verification requirements
Master batch components (percentage by weight)
Production batch component (by weight)
Process batch record
Process sequence
Process instructions
Material usage
Product testing
In-process testing and acceptance criteria
Finished product testing and acceptance criteria
Test method references
Formulation
Validation sampling and testing
In-process
Finished product
Definition of validation criteria
Lower and upper acceptance limits
Acceptable variation
Cleaning sampling plan (locations, type, and number of samples)

It is expected that acceptable, salable products will be produced, since all qualification batches will be produced using a defined process under CGMP conditions with production personnel. A question that always arises is how many replicate batches or lots must be produced for a validation protocol to be valid or correct. There is no absolute answer. Obviously, a single batch will provide the minimum amount of data. As the number of replicated batches increases, the information increases. The FDA, however, has determined that the minimum number of validation batches should be three.

An extensive quantity of documents is generated at each stage of the development and validation of the final production process. Some of these documents will be directly related to the manufacture of the final products. Others may provide the basis for decisions that ultimately result in the final process. The documents that are required for manufacturing the product then become the master product document. This document must be capable of providing all of the information necessary to set up the process to produce a product consistently and one that meets specifications in any location. Items that will normally be included in the master product document are

Batch manufacturing record

Master formulation

Process flow diagram

Master manufacturing instructions

Master packaging instructions

Specifications

Sampling (location and frequency)

Test methods

Process validation data

Each of the above items must contain sufficient detailed information to permit the complete master product document to become an independent, single package that will provide all information necessary to set up and produce a product.

Classification

Process validation is of different types. These are as below:

1. Prospective Validation
2. Concurrent Validation
3. Retrospective Validation
4. Process Revalidation
5. Change Control

These are described one after the other:

Prospective Validation

In Prospective Validation, the validation protocol is executed before the process is put into commercial use. During the product development phase the production process should be broken down into individual steps. Each step should be evaluated on the basis of experience or theoretical considerations to determine the critical parameters that may affect the quality of the finished product. A series of experiments should be designed to determine the criticality of these factors. Each experiment should be planned and documented fully in an authorised protocol. All equipment, production environment and the analytical testing methods to be used should have been fully validated. Master batch documents can be prepared only after the critical parameters of the process have been identified and machine settings, component specifications and environmental conditions have been determined. It is generally considered acceptable that three consecutive batches/runs within the finally agreed parameters, giving product of the desired quality would constitute a proper validation of the process. It is a confirmation on the commercial three batches before marketing. Upon completion of the review, recommendations should be made on the extent of monitoring and the in-process controls necessary for routine production. These should be incorporated into the batch manufacturing and packaging record or into appropriate standard operating procedures. Limits, frequencies and actions to be taken in the event of the limits being exceeded should be specified. It may be possible and acceptable in particular circumstances for a manufacturer that uses the same process for several related products to develop a scientifically sound validation plan for that process rather than different plans for each product manufactured by that process. The matrix approach generally means a plan to conduct process validation on different strengths of the same product, whereas the “family” approach means a plan to conduct process validation on different products manufactured with the same processes using the same equipment.

Prospective validation is a requirement of US FDA, and therefore it makes validation an integral part of a carefully planned, logical product/process developmental program. An effective prospective validation program must be supported by documentation extending from product initiation to full-scale production. The complete documentation package can be referred to as the master documentation file. It will accumulate as a product concept progresses to the point of being placed in full-scale production, providing as complete a product history as possible. The final package will be the work of many individual groups within the organization. It will consist of reports, procedures, protocols, specifications, analytical methods, and any other critical documents pertaining to the formulation, process, and analytical method development. The package may contain the actual reports, or it may utilize cross-references to formal documentation, both internal and external to the organization. The ideal documentation package will contain a complete history of the final product that is being manufactured. In retrospect, it would be possible to trace the justification or rationale behind all aspects of the final product, process, and testing. The complete master documentation file not only provides appropriate rationale for the product, process, and testing, but also becomes the reference source for all questions relating to the manufacture of a product at any plant location. This master documentation file, however, should not be confused with the concept of the master product document, which is essential for routine manufacturing of the product. The validation process using these approaches must include batches of different strengths or products which should be selected to represent the worst case conditions or scenarios to demonstrate that the process is consistent for all strengths or products involved.

Concurrent Validation

Concurrent validation may be the practical approach under certain circumstances. Examples of these may be when:

- A previously validated process is being transferred to a third party contract manufacturer or to another manufacturing site
- The product is a different strength of a previously validated product with the same ratio of active/inactive ingredients
- The number of lots evaluated under the Retrospective Validation were not sufficient to obtain a high degree of assurance demonstrating that the process is fully under control
- The number of batches produced are limited (e.g. orphan drugs).
- Process with low production volume per batch (e.g. radiopharmaceuticals, anticancer)
- Process of manufacturing urgently needed drugs due to shortage (or absence) of supply.

It is important in these cases however, that the systems and equipment to be used have been fully validated previously. The justification for conducting concurrent validation must be documented and the protocol must be approved by the Validation Team. A report should be prepared and approved prior to the sale of each batch and a final report should be prepared and approved after the completion of all concurrent batches. It is generally considered acceptable that a minimum of three consecutive batches within the finally agreed parameters, giving the product the desired quality would constitute a proper validation of the process

Retrospective Validation

In many establishments, processes that are stable and in routine use have not undergone a formally documented validation process. Historical data may be utilized to provide necessary documentary evidence that the processes are validated. The steps involved in this type of validation still require the preparation of a protocol, the reporting of the results of the data review, leading to a conclusion and recommendation. Retrospective validation is only acceptable for well established detailed processes that include operational limits for each critical step of the process and will be inappropriate where there have been recent changes in the formulation of the product, operating procedures, equipment and facility. The source of data for retrospective validation should include amongst others, batch documents, process control charts, maintenance log books, process capability studies, finished product test results, including trend analyses, and stability results. Thus, one way for a firm to satisfy the requirement for validated processes is to identify those products that have been on the market for some time and use the wealth of production, testing, and control data to demonstrate that the process is reliable. This strategy is commonly referred to as retrospective validation. Historical data also may be used to augment an earlier validation in cases in which the product has changed. For a product to be considered for retrospective validation, it must have a stable process; that is, one in which the method of manufacture has remained essentially unchanged for a period of time. The first step in the product selection process is therefore to obtain a summary of changes in the method of manufacture. In most companies such information is part of the master batch record file. Then a time interval is selected that represents the last 20 to 30 batches. Products for which there is no record of a change in the method of manufacture or control during this period can be regarded as candidates for validation. The 20-to-30-batch rule originates from control chart principals, which consider 20 to 30 points that plot within the limits as evidence of a stable process. Once this criterion is met, the number selected is actually somewhat arbitrary, as there is no one number that is correct for every product. The ideal number of batches required to study a product is theoretically the number that permits all process variables to come into play. By process variables, we mean raw materials from different but approved vendors, introduction of similar but different pieces of equipment, personnel and seasonal changes, and the like. The second step in the product selection process addresses the situation in which a change in the method of manufacture or control was implemented during the last 20 or so production batches. The fact that a change has occurred does not automatically disqualify the product for retrospective validation. One must first know whether the particular modification has caused an expected result to be different to the extent that it is no longer comparable to previous batches. An example may be helpful. Suppose the method of granulating was changed midway through the series of 20 batches selected for the validation study. The number of batches representing the new process would be significantly reduced and could be insufficient to capture some of the interactions that can affect process reproducibility. A product found to be unsuitable for retrospective validation because of a revised manufacturing process is a likely candidate for prospective validation. Such a discovery, however, should be brought to the attention of the appropriate authority. In today's regulatory environment ignoring the matter would be imprudent.

Process Re-Validation

Re-validation is usually performed to the confirmation of initial validation for a periodic review. Re-validation provides the evidence that changes in a process and /or the process environment that are introduced do not adversely affect process characteristics and product quality. Documentation requirements will be the same as for the initial validation of the process. Re-validation becomes necessary in certain situations. The following are examples of some of the planned or unplanned changes that may require re-validation:

- Changes in raw materials (physical properties such as density, viscosity, particle size distribution, and moisture, etc., that may affect the process or product).
- Changes in the source of active raw material manufacturer.
- Changes in packaging material (primary container/closure system).
- Changes in the process (e.g., mixing time, drying temperatures and batch size)
- Changes in the equipment (e.g. addition of automatic detection system). Changes of equipment which involve the replacement of equipment on a "like for like" basis would not normally require a re-validation except that this new equipment must be qualified.
- Changes in the plant/facility.
- Variations revealed by trend analysis (e.g. process drifts).

A decision not to perform re-validation studies must be fully justified and documented.

Change Control

Clearly defined procedure is required in order to control any changes in the production processes. These procedures should control all the planned changes and ensure the presence of sufficient supporting data that show that modified process will result in a product of the desired quality. Significant changes to process (e.g. mixing time, drying temperature, etc.), using new equipments with different operating parameters, etc may require the pre-approval of the regulatory agencies. If a change is proposed in any of the procedures, product, processes, or equipment which may impact the quality, appropriate written procedures should be in place. All changes must be formally requested, documented and accepted by the Validation Team. The proposed changes were scientifically assessed and, depending on the changes, the need of re-validation will be determined. Commitment of the company to control all changes to premises, supporting utilities, systems, materials, equipment and processes used in the fabrication/packaging of pharmaceutical dosage forms is essential to ensure a continued validation status of the systems concerned. It is essential for a company to control all changes to ensure the validity of the continued assurance of validation. The change control system should ensure that all notified or requested changes are satisfactorily investigated, documented and authorised. Products made by processes subjected to changes should not be released for sale without full awareness and consideration of the change by the Validation Team.

Validation of Solid Dosage Forms

Validation of solid dosage forms has different steps. These are described one after the other as below.

Validation of Raw Materials

The validation process of a solid dosage form begins with a validation of the raw materials, both active pharmaceutical ingredients (APIs) and excipients. Variation in raw materials is one of the major causes of product variation or deviation from specification. The API may represent the most uncontrollable component in the complete product/process validation scheme, as key physical properties such as morphology and particle size/surface area may not be completely defined this early in the sequence. Often times the synthesis of the new API (drug substance) is not finalized, and changes occur during the development of the compound. The preformulation program initiated during the early exploratory phase of product development is rarely considered part of validation, but it represents one of the more critical steps in the development cycle. Chemical characteristics such as drug impurities and impurity levels can affect the stability of the product. Physical properties such as drug morphology, solubility, and particle size/surface area are important in assessing drug availability. The particle size, shape, and density of the drug can affect material flow and blend uniformity. The hygroscopic nature of the drug can be important in both the handling the material and the reproducibility of the manufacturing process. The certification/validation of excipients used in solid oral dosage forms is also extremely important. Excipients can represent less than 1% of a tablet formula or as much as 99%. It is no less important to validate the critical characteristics of the 1% material than of an excipient used in larger quantities. Factors to be aware of are

1. the grade and source of the excipients,
2. particle size and shape characteristics, and
3. lot-to-lot variability.

An example will illustrate this point.

Microcrystalline cellulose is widely used in solid dosage forms as a diluent. It is manufactured in different grades and by different companies. There can be significant differences in the chemical composition, crystallinity, and particle size/size distribution between different microcrystalline cellulose lots. Besides differences between manufacturers, differences can be seen with the same company using different manufacturing sites, raw materials, and/or manufacturing processes. Differences in the particle size/size distribution of microcrystalline cellulose can affect the wet granulation step and/or blend uniformity of a tablet formulation. With direct compression formulations, differences in particle size distribution between lots can result in

1. the initial mix not actually being uniform when using the validated processing parameters, or
2. materials segregating during compression. A smaller particle size will require additional binder solution to granulate the materials due to the greater surface area of the microcrystalline cellulose. This could result in granules having greater strength, which could decrease the tablet dissolution rate. The dissolution rate of prednisone was shown to vary due to the particle size and chemical composition of microcrystalline cellulose.

Analytical Method Validation

The following list of analytical criteria must be assessed prior to beginning any validation program:

1. *Accuracy of method*: The ability of a method to measure the true value of a sample.
2. *Precision of method*: The ability of a method to estimate reproducibility of any given value, but not necessarily the true value.
3. *Specificity*: The ability to accurately measure the analyte in the presence of other components.
4. *In-day/out-of-day variation*: Does the precision and accuracy of the method change when conducted numerous times on the same day and repeated on a subsequent day?
5. *Between-operator variation*: Repeat of the precision and accuracy studies within the same laboratory using the same instrument but different analysts to challenge the reproducibility of the method.
6. *Between-instrument variation*: How will different instruments within the same laboratory run by the same analyst affect the accuracy and precision of the method?

7. *Between-laboratory variation*: Will the precision and accuracy of the method be the same between the development and quality control laboratories?

Validation of Equipment

Process equipment used in the development phase is assessed relative to its suitability for large-scale manufacture. Alternate equipment is identified and evaluated and a final decision rendered. Existing or new equipment to be used to manufacture the new pharmaceutical product must then undergo a comprehensive evaluation called a validation protocol. This protocol can be divided into a number of components, but usually has design qualification, installation qualification, operation qualification, performance qualification, maintenance (calibration, cleaning, and repair) qualification, and closure qualification as integral components. Once the full-scale manufacturing equipment and process have been identified, it is important to either ensure that an existing physical facility is available in which the product can be manufactured or determine if a modified or new facility is required. Once these decisions have been made, a validation commissioning document (VCD) is prepared that identifies the shared responsibility and cooperation that must occur among the owner, construction manager, and vendors. A commissioning program that is well planned will facilitate the validation process, accelerate start-up, enhance documentation, and ensure that the pharmaceutical product is produced in a GMP-compliant facility. The VCD would usually be prepared by a validation specialist and approved by the facility's project manager. It would be very comprehensive and would include purchase orders, process flow diagrams, operation and maintenance manuals, installation requirements and factory acceptance testing results, heating, ventilation, and air conditioning (HVAC) requirements and test results, calibration procedures, software specifications, and staff training.

Validation of Tablet Compression Process

Once above steps are done, some other major steps in the development of a validation program are as follows:

1. Obtaining test data to determine the numerical range of each parameter e.g., assess the tablet hardness over a series of batches that achieves an acceptable friability, disintegration, and dissolution.
2. Establishing specification limits from the test data derived for a given parameter. Based on the data collected and using statistical techniques, determine the extremes of acceptable hardness (high and low) that would provide 95% assurance that the friability, disintegration, and dissolution specifications would be met (upper and lower control/release limits).

3. Determining how well the specification limit indicates that the process is under control. Challenge the process by producing product at the extremes of the specification limit to ensure all product specifications are met.
4. Certifying the equipment that is used in obtaining the data and controlling the process. Ensure that equipment operating conditions (e.g.,rpm, temperature, power utilization) are within specification limits under variations of product load.

Once this has been done, one can proceed to actual product testing utilizing these parameters and their specifications to validate that the process will produce acceptable product. The testing can be conducted on samples during the manufacture (in-process tests) or on the finished product (finished product tests). Each product may have its own idiosyncrasies requiring special tests, but generally the in-process and finished product tests that would be required for all solid dosage forms in process validation are as follows.

A. In-Process Tests

1. *Moisture content of "dried granulation"*: Loss on drying (LOD) can be used to determine whether or not the granulation solvent has been removed to a sufficient level during the drying operation (usually less than 2% moisture).
2. *Granulation particle size distribution*: An extremely important parameter that can affect tablet compressibility, hardness, thickness, disintegration, dissolution, weight variation, and content uniformity. This parameter, which can be done by sieve analysis, should be monitored throughout the tablet validation process.
3. *Blend uniformity*: Samples of the blend are taken and analyzed to ensure that the drug is uniformly dispersed throughout the tablet/capsule blend. The proper blend time must be established so that the blend is not under- or overmixed. The sampling technique is critical for this test to be valid.
4. *Individual tablet/capsule weight*: The weight of individual tablets or capsules is determined throughout compression/encapsulation to ensure that the material is flowing properly and the equipment is working consistently. The individual weight should be within 5% of the nominal weight. Weight fluctuations or frequent machine adjustments suggest that the formulation/process (e.g., poor granulation flow) is not optimized and/or that the equipment may need maintenance.
5. *Tablet hardness*: Tablet hardness is determined periodically throughout the batch to ensure that the tablets are robust enough for coating, packing, and shipping and not too hard to affect dissolution.

6. *Tablet thickness*: Tablet thickness is also determined periodically throughout the batch and is indirectly related to the hardness. It is another indication of whether or not the formulation has proper flow and compression properties.
7. *Disintegration*: Disintegration is determined during the manufacture as a predictor of tablet performance (e.g., dissolution).

B. Finished Product Tests

1. *Appearance*: The tablets should be examined for such problems as tablet mottling, picking of the monogram, tablet filming, and capping of the tablets. If the tablets are colored, the color quality needs to be examined.
2. *Assay*: This test will determine whether or not the product contains the labeled amount of drug.
3. *Content uniformity*: Samples are taken across the batch profile (beginning, middle, and end) and analyzed to ensure that the dosage forms comply with compendial standards (~15% of the labeled amount) or more stringent internal limits. It will indicate whether there is demixing during the manufacturing operation (i.e., segregation during flow of granulation from a storage bin).
4. *Tablet hardness*: A critical parameter for dosage form handling and performance.
5. *Tablet friability*: Friability is an important characteristic on the tablets' ability to withstand chipping, cracking, or "dusting" during thepackaging operations and shipping.
6. *Dissolution*: Dissolution is important to ensure proper drug release characteristics (in vitro availability) and batch-to-batch uniformity.

These key test parameters are the yardsticks by which the major processing variables in solid dosage forms are evaluated. Some processing variables are:

Mixing time and speed in blenders and granulators

Solvent addition rates in granulators

Time, temperature, and airflow conditions in dryers and coaters

Screen size, feed rate, and milling speed in mills

Machine speed and compression force in tablet presses

Machine speed and fill volume in encapsulators.

Process validation testing is generally done on the first three batches of product made in production-size equipment. Revalidation testing is only done when a "significant" change has occurred. A significant change is one that will alter the in-process or final product specification established during the validation program or a change in formula, process, or equipment.

Guidelines for Process Validation of Solid Dosage Forms

Numerous factors should be considered when developing and validating solid dosage forms. As a means of providing a broad overview of these validation criteria, the following checklist/guideline is provided for tablets for inclusion in an in-depth validation program. Some of these unit operations will not be applicable for every solid dosage form (e.g., direct compression tablets and uncoated tablets).

Tablets

A. Tablet Composition

Identify the key physicochemical properties of the drug substance that need to be considered in developing the formulation, such as the following:

Solubility of the drug substance throughout the physiological pH range: Depending on the solubility of the drug, a surfactant may be needed to enhance dissolution.

Particle size distribution and surface area: The particle size distribution of the drug may determine what grade of an excipient (e.g., microcrystalline cellulose) to use.

Morphology: If the drug is amorphous or has different polymorphs, certain excipients may be used to prevent conversion of the drug to other physical forms.

True and bulk density: An excipient (e.g., diluent) that has a similar bulk density as the drug may be selected to minimize segregation, especially with a direct compression formulation.

Material flow and compressibility: A free flowing, highly compressible material such as microcrystalline cellulose may be used for drugs with poor flow or compressibility properties.

Hygroscopicity: Special environmental working conditions may be required to ensure that moisture is not picked up during material storage or handling and during the manufacture of the tablet dosage form.

Melting point: If the drug has a low melting point, a direct compression formulation may need to be developed instead of a wet granulation formulation to avoid drying the material and potentially melting or degrading the drug.

Provide the reason for the presence of each ingredient in the formula.

Why was a particular ingredient (e.g., povidone) used from an excipient class (e.g., binder)? Performance? Supply? Cost? Indicate whether a particular grade or manufacturer is required for an ingredient and the reasons. Justify the level or range of each ingredient, especially the binder, disintegrant, and lubricant.

Explain the required unit operations in relationship to the tablet formulation.

For example Why was high shear wet granulation used instead of dry granulation?

Why is the tablet film coated?

B. Process Evaluation and Selection

Determine the unit operations needed to manufacture the tablets.

1. Mixing or Blending

   The mixing or blending unit operation may occur once or several times during the tablet manufacture. For example, a direct compression formulation may involve one blending step in which the drug and the excipients are blended together prior to compression. A wet granulation formulation may require two mixing/blending steps:

   1. prior to granulating to have a uniform drug/excipient mixture, and
   2. after milling the dried granulation to add other excipients, such as the lubricant. Some or all the items provided in this section may therefore be pertinent for validation, depending on the mixing or blending objective. The following physical properties of the drug and excipients are factors in creating a uniform mix or blend:

      Bulk density

      Particle shape

      Particle size distribution

      Surface area

   Materials that have similar physical properties will be easier to form a uniform mix or blend and will not segregate as readily as materials with large differences.

   Items to consider:

   Mixing or blending technique: Diffusion (tumble), convection (planetary or high intensity), or pneumatic (fluid bed) techniques can be used to mix or blend materials. Determine the technique that is required for the formulation or process objective. It may be different, depending on whether you are mixing the drug and excipients for a direct compression formulation or adding the lubricant (e.g., magnesium stearate) to the granulation.

Mixing or blending speed: Determine the intensity (low/high shear) and/or speed (rpm) of the mixing or blending. Mixing the drug and excipient will require more intense mixing than adding the lubricant to the final blend.

Mixing or blending time: How much mixing or blending is required to obtain a uniform mixture? The mixing or blending time will be dependent on the mixing or blending technique and speed. Experiments should be done to determine if the materials can be overmixed, resulting in demixing or segregation of the materials. Demixing can occur due to the physical property differences (e.g., particle size distribution and density). For example, demixing can occur in a direct compression formulation in which the drug substance is micronized (5 microns) and the excipients are granular (500–1000 microns).

Drug uniformity: Content uniformity is usually performed to determine the uniformity of drug throughout the mix or blend. Representative samples should be taken throughout the mix or blend. The sampling technique and handling of the materials are key in obtaining valid content uniformity results. Segregation of the sample can occur by overhandling, resulting in inaccurate results. For the final blend (blend prior to compression), the sample taken should be equivalent to the weight of a single tablet.

Excipient uniformity: Besides drug uniformity, excipients need to be uniform in the granulation or blend. Two key excipients are:

□□*Lubricant*: The lubricant needs to be distributed uniformly in the mixture/granulation for the high-speed compression operation. Uneven distribution of the lubricant can result in picking and sticky problems during compression. It can also lead to tablet performance problems (low dissolution due to excessive lubricant in some tablets).

□□*Color*: The colorant(s) need(s) to be evenly distributed in the mixture so that the tablets have a uniform appearance (e.g., color, hue, and intensity). The coloring agent may need to be prescreened or more uniformally dispersed in the blend prior to compression to avoid speckling or shading of the color.

□□*Equipment capacity/load*: The bulk density of materials or granules will affect the capacity of the equipment. If an excipient in the formulation affects the density of the final blend to a greater extent than any other ingredient, then a well-controlled density specification for that excipient may be warranted. Test different-sized loads in the mixer/ blender (e.g., 30, 50, and 70% of working volume) for optimal mixing or blending. Undercharging or overcharging a blender can result in poor drug or tablet lubricant distribution.

2. Wet Granulation

What type of wet granulation technique will be used? Will it be low shear (e.g., Hobart), high shear (e.g., Diosna, GEI-Collette) or fluid bed (e.g., Glatt, Fluid Air)? Each technique will produce granules with different physical properties and will require monitoring of different processing parameters. Wet granulation parameters to be considered during development and validation are:

Binder addition: Should the binder be added as a granulating solution or dry like the other excipients? Adding the binder dry avoids the need to determine the optimal binder concentration and a separate manufacture for the binder solution.

Binder concentration: The optimal binder concentration will need to be determined for the formulation. If the binder is to be sprayed, the binder solution needs to be dilute enough so that it can be pumped through the spray nozzle. It should also be sufficiently concentrated to form granules without overwetting the materials.

Amount of binder solution/granulating solvent: How much binder or solvent solution is required to granulate the material? Too much binder or solvent solution will overwet the materials and prolong the drying time. The amount of binder solution is related to the binder concentration.

Binder solution/granulating solvent addition rate: Define the rate or rate range at which the binder solution or granulating solvent can be added to the materials. Can the granulating solution be dumped into the mixer or does it have to be metered in at a specific rate?

Mixing time: How long should the material be mixed to ensure proper formation of granules? Should mixing stop after the addition of the binder or solvent solution or should additional mixing be required? Granulations that are not mixed long enough can form incomplete or weak granules. These granules may have poor flow and compression properties. On the other hand, overmixing the granulation can lead to harder granules and a lower dissolution rate.

Granulation end point: How is the granulation end point determined? Is it determined or controlled by granulation end point equipment (e.g., ammeter or wattmeter)? Is it controlled by specifying critical processing parameters? For example, a drug or excipient mixture may be granulated by adding a predetermined amount of water (granulating solution) at a certain rate. The granulation is completed after mixing for a set time after the water has been added.

3. Wet Milling

Does the wet granulation need to be milled to break up the lumps and enhance drying of the granulation? Wet granules that have a wide aggregate range can lead to inefficient drying (long drying times and partially dried large granules or lumps).

Factors to consider are:

1. *Equipment size and capacity*: The mill should be large enough to delump the entire batch within a reasonable time period to minimize manufacturing time and prevent the material from drying during this operation.
2. *Screen size*: The screen needs to be small enough to delump the material, but not too small to cause excessive heating of the mill, resulting in drying of the granulation.
3. *Mill speed*: The speed should be sufficient to efficiently delump the material without straining the equipment.
4. *Feed rate*: The feed rate of the wet granulation is interrelated to screen size and mill size and speed.
4. *Drying:* The type of drying technique (e.g., tray, fluid bed, microwave) required for the formulation needs to be determined and justified. The type of technique may be dependent on such factors as drug or formulation properties and equipment availability. Changing dryer techniques could affect such tablet properties as hardness, disintegration, dissolution, and stability. The optimal moisture content of the dried granulation needs to be determined. High moisture content can result in
   (i) tablet picking or sticking to tablet punch surfaces and
   (ii) poor chemical stability as a result of hydrolysis. An overdried granulation could result in poor hardness and friability. Moisture content analysis can he performed using the conventional loss-on-drying techniques or such state-of-the-art techniques as near infrared (NIR) spectroscopy.

Parameters to consider during drying are:

Inlet/outlet temperature: The inlet temperature is the temperature of the incoming air to the dryer, while the outlet temperature is the temperature leaving the unit. The inlet temperature is critical to the drying efficiency of the granulation and should be set high enough to maximize drying without affecting the chemical/physical stability of the granulation.The outlet temperature is an indicator of the granulation temperature and will increase toward the inlet temperature as the moisture content of the granulation decreases (evaporization rate).

Airflow: There should be sufficient airflow to ensure removal of moistureladen air from the wet granulation. Insufficient airflow could prolong drying and affect the chemical stability of the drug. Airflow and the inlet/outlet temperature are interrelated parameters and should be considered together.

Moisture uniformity: The moisture content could vary within the granulation. Heat uniformity of the dryer (e.g., tray), amount of granulation per tray, and incomplete fluidization of the bed are factors that could affectthe moisture uniformity of the granulation.

Equipment capability/capacity: The load that can be efficiently dried within the unit needs to be known. A larger load will require more moisture to be removed on drying and will affect the drying time. In the case of fluid bed drying, a maximum dryer load is that load above which the dryer will not fluidize the material.

5. Milling

The milling operation will reduce the particle size of the dried granulation. The resultant particle size distribution will affect such material properties as flow, compressibility, disintegration, and dissolution. An optimal particle size/size distribution for the formulation will need to be determined.

Factors to consider in milling are:

Mill type: What mill type (e.g., impact or screen) should be used? Each has several variants, depending on the means to reduce the particles.The type of mill can generate a different particle size/size distribution. Particle size testing will need to be conducted and the results examined when substituting mill types.

Screen size: The selected screen size will affect the particle size. A smaller screen size will produce a smaller particle size and a greater number of fines.

Mill speed: What is the optimal mill speed? A higher mill speed will result in a smaller particle size and possibly a wider particle size distribution. It can also generate more heat to the product, depending on the screen size and feed rate, which could affect the stability of the product.

Feed rate: The feed rate is dependent on the mill capacity, screen size, and mill speed.

6. Tablet Compression

Compression is a critical step in the production of a tablet dosage form. The materials being compressed will need to have adequate flow and compression properties. The material should readily flow from the hopper onto the feed frame and into the dies. Inadequate flow can result in "rat holing" in the hopper and/or segregation of the blend in the hopper/feed frame. This can cause tablet weight and content uniformity problems. As for the compressibility properties of the formulation, it should be examined on an instrumented tablet press.

Factors to consider during compression are as follows:

Tooling: The shape, size, and concavity of the tooling should be examined based on the formulation properties and commercial specifications. For intagliated (embossed) tablets, factors such as the position of the intagliation on the tablet and the intagliation depth and style should be examined to ensure that picking of the intagliation during compression or fill-in of the intagliation during coating does not occur.

Compression speed: The formulation should be compressed at a wide range of compression speeds to determine the operating range of the compressor. The adequacy of the material's flow into the dies will be determined by examining the tablet weights. Is a force feeder required to ensure that sufficient material is fed into the dies?

Compression/ejection force: The compression profile for the tablet formulation will need to be determined to establish the optimal compression force to obtain the desired tablet hardness. The particle size/size distribution or level of lubricant may need to be adjusted in order to have a robust process on a high-speed compressor.

The following in-process tests (as previously discussed) should be examined during the compression stage:

Appearance
Hardness
Tablet weight
Friability
Disintegration
Weight uniformity

Conclusions

Process validation is an essential part for pharmaceutical technologists to fulfill to get products approved in regulatory markets. It is a very systematic process. Some basics of the process validation along with some guidelines has been presented in this chapter.

Questions for Practice and Exercise

1. What is process validation? What is its importance in pharmaceutical product development?
2. Classify process validation and describe each components.
3. Elaborate the protocol for process validation of a tableting process.

Bibliography

Guidelines for *Process Validation* of. Pharmaceutical Dosage Forms. Version 2. Drug Sector. Saudi Food & Drug Authority. Kingdom of *Saudi Arabia.*

Current Good Manufacturing Practices. January 2011, USFDA. Guidance for Industry. Process Validation: General Principles and Practices.

Pharmaceutical Process Validation. Eds. Wachter and Nash. Informa Health Care. 2003.

CHAPTER 17

QUALITY CONTROL

- **Introduction**
- **Quality Assurance**
- **Quality Variation**
- **Control of Quality Variation**
  - A General Manufacturing Process
  - Raw Materials Control
  - In-process Items Control
  - Finished Products Control
- **Assurance of Quality**
  - Manufacturing Practices
  - Analytic Methodologies
  - Modern Sampling, Assay and Data Analysis Techniques
  - Regulatory Guidelines
- **Salient Features of Quality Control**
  - Stability Studies
  - Product Identification Systems
  - Adulteration, Misbranding, and Counterfeiting
  - Maintenance, Storage and Retrieval of Records
- **Marketed Software**
- **Conclusions**

Introduction

The quality control of goods of any type is the main part of a business organization. In ancient times, when complex mathematical theories and probability and statistical concepts were not introduced, quality was purely determined by sensory inspections or by simple mathematical determinants or measurements. Specially trained personnel were employed for these determinations. Some of the examples of such quality control inspections are performed even today in several fields. Examples include tasting of alcoholic beverages or tasting or visual inspection of rice or other food products, to determine and measure their quality. However, with the advancements in the mathematical and other statistical concepts, this area is now well advanced. In addition, the other aspect in this regard is the growth of industrialization. Most of the techniques that are currently used in these areas were introduced in tandem with the development of industries or so called industrialization. Simply and currently, total quality control could be defined as the process of striving for producing and reproducing a perfect output, may it be an intermediate product or an end product, by a series of measures requiring an organized effort by the entire company to prevent or eliminate errors at every stage in the production and the reproduction. Quality must be built into a drug product during product and process design, and it is influenced by the physical plant design, space, ventilation, cleanliness, and sanitation during routine production. In earlier days, during neutralization periods of modernization, there was lot of wastage of batches because of wrong output due to any of the reasons mentioned in the above lines, when perfect quality control and assurance was not available. Mental or sensory determinations and calculations did not help further progress in the industrialization in terms of quality control and assurance. To be effective, it must be supported by a team effort. The product and process design begins in research and development, and includes preformulation and physical, chemical, therapeutic, and toxicologic considerations. It considers materials, in-process and product control, including specifications and tests for the active ingredients, the excipients, and the product itself, specific stability procedures for the product, freedom from microbial contamination and proper storage of the product, and containers, packaging, and labeling to ensure that container closure systems provide functional protection of the product against such factors as moisture, oxygen, light, volatility, and drug/package interaction. Provision for a cross referencing system to allow any batch of a product to be traced from its raw materials to its final destination in the event of unexpected difficulties is required. Several measures are introduced during the progress of total quality assurance to be introduced in the field of manufacturing in general. The result is the continuous development of this field as of today as any field is considered. The ballpark is, nothing comes free either a product or a total quality control principle.

Thus, very judicious investigations along with strict application of the principles are the underlying outcomes. In this regard, some of the very basic principles of quality control and assurance as related to pharmaceutical industry are mentioned in this chapter.

Quality Assurance

In engineering and manufacturing, quality control or quality assurance is a set of measures taken to ensure that defective products or services are not produced, and that the design meets performance requirements. It includes the regulation of the quality of raw materials, assemblies, products and components; services related to production; and management, production, and inspection processes. Traditional statistical process controls in manufacturing operations usually proceed by randomly sampling and testing a fraction of the output. Variances of critical tolerances are continuously tracked, and manufacturing processes are corrected before bad parts can be produced. A valuable process to perform on a whole consumer product is failure testing, the operation of a product until it fails, often under stresses such as increasing vibration, temperature and humidity. This exposes many unanticipated weaknesses in a product, and the data is used to drive engineering and manufacturing process improvements. Often quite simple changes can dramatically improve product service, such as changing to mould-resistant paint, or adding lock-washed placement to the training for new assembly personnel. Many organizations use statistical process control to bring the organization to Six Sigma levels of quality, in other words, so that the likelihood of an unexpected failure is confined to six standard deviations on the normal distribution. This probability is less than four one-millionths. Items controlled often include clerical tasks such as order-entry, as well as conventional manufacturing tasks. Many different techniques and concepts have been tried to minimize defects in products, including Zero Defects, Six Sigma, and the House of Quality. Most of these techniques and concepts are controversial to one degree or another, since there are two opposing schools of thought with regard to quality. One school subcribes to a statistical approach to quality, measuring defects and then taking corrective action. The other school subscribes to a more organic approach, arguing that one should "design in quality" rather than trying to "test in quality". Historically speaking, there are atleast four phases in the current quality control concepts in terms of delivering their meaning and the interpretation. Simply, these are:

Conformance to Specifications

Phil Cosby has worked to significantly advance the cause of the quality movement through his many personal contributions over the past four decades.

His philosophies have been ingrained into the fiber of many corporations both large and small and his book *Quality is Free* was one of the initial signals of the decade of quality in the 1980's when quality emerged as a viable career and work movement. He has developed pragmatic concepts that are considered foundational elements of the body of quality knowledge, such as:

- Concept of Zero Defects as the goal of quality performance
- Customer requirements define the standard of quality performance
- Teamwork as the principle for work
- Leadership as the requirement to make progress
- Cost of poor quality as a measure of non-conformance
- Prevention as the means to eliminate quality problems

Fitness for Use

Army and Airforce Exchange Service (AAFES) defines quality in terms of "fitness for use", i.e., if an item is not fit for intended use, then it is not quality item. Anything that adversely affects appearance, serviceability, or salability of an item is considered a defect. Safety of an item is an integral part of quality because if an item is not safe to use, it is not fit for use.

A Two-dimensional Model of Quality

The quality has two dimensions: "must-be quality" and "attractive quality". The former is near to the "fitness for use" and the latter is what the customer would love, but has not yet thought about. Supporters characterise this model more succinctly as: "Products and services that meet or exceed customers' expectations". One writer believes (without citation) that this is today the most used interpretation for the term **quality**.

Value to Some Person

In his book *Quality Software Management: Systems Thinking*, Jerry **Weinberg** defines quality as "**value to some person**" [Weinberg92]. When quality is defined this way, it is far from immutable – in fact, it's quite subjective. So, who expects to get value and what value do they expect? In the broadest sense, the customers expect value in exchange for their money. The company's board of directors and stockholders expect profit. The value expected by the customer takes different forms in different products. Profit can be achieved through different business strategies, which also place value on different aspects of the product.

Quality Variation

Quality variation in any stage or in any practice may be the result of variegated reasons. For instance, in current pharmacy or medicine practice, the overwhelmingly bad situations may arise due to the misuse of these advanced medicines by very routine lay and common man, because of inappropriate pharmacy practices, and also by experts, with ample knowledge in this area to achieve their personal gains. In either case very strict control of pharmacies with a perfect legislation; and with very controlled practice of the law, these situations in this area could be improved. Similar situations may arise in the engineering sector, when the latest technologies such as microcameras, spy networking tools, tampering technologies etc. in the very viscinities of the target person, target knowledge, or the target innovation would result in dramatic alterations in the end product output, resulting in the quality variation of this output. It is better not to use the technology rather than use it for malpractices. The product output may not necessarily be an industrial output. It could be anything from a simple laboratory experiment to a very ethical social situation. These quality variations were identified for a long time and thus several theories and practices were proposed and are currently in place in this area. Same rules are currently used or in the process of introduction in the Indian pharmaceutical scenario.

In engineering and manufacturing sectors, quality variation is identified by the number of defective products or services or by the defective designs. The minimum requirement is that the design should meet performance requirements. Quality variation could be envisioned at raw materials, assemblies, products and components; services related to production; and management, production, and inspection processes. These variations are identified by several means. The general process is the random sampling at every stage and testing it. Quality variations are determined using a variety of approaches as per the type of the industry and the type of the output. These quality variations for critical tolerances are continuously tracked, and manufacturing processes are preceeded. Apart from this, several sampling, quality control and statistical techniques are in place. These include stressing the sample under increasing vibration, temperature and humidity. This exposes many unanticipated weaknesses in a manufacturing process, and the data is used to drive engineering and manufacturing process betterments. Many a times simple changes could dramatically improve product service. The same rules apply to the pharmaceutical industry. These are very routinely used methods and currently several innovations are in place. Because of the increasing complexity of modern pharmaceutical manufacture arising from a variety of unique drugs and dosage forms, complex ethical, legal, and economic responsibilities have been placed on those concerned with the manufacture of modern pharmaceuticals. An awareness of these factors is the responsibility of all those involved in the development, manufacture, control, and marketing of quality products.

Control of Quality Variation

A very systematic effective quality assurance program takes into consideration potential raw material, process, packaging material, labeling and finished product variables. To appreciate the processes involved in the control of quality variation, a very brief outlay of a general pharmaceutical manufacturing process would be essential. This section deals with some of the practices in place or could be adopted to improve the situations dealing with the control of the quality variation.

A General Manufacturing Process

A typical pharmaceutical manufacturing procedure right from the raw material picking to the finished product output includes pooling of raw materials, manufacturing design and process, validated processes, quality control of the raw materials, channeling raw materials to produce the output, in-process quality control, finished product collection, quality control of the finished products, labeling and final quality control. Many a times it is the manufacturing process that results in the variations in the quality of the output. Thus, before preceding this step further, it is better to give a brief idea of a typical manufacturing process and the likely sources of quality variation as a result of this manufacturing process.

In a typical process, say for example, several raw materials like A, B, C, D, E, F, G, H, I, J, K, and L may be included. Their manufacturers have determined their quality. The certificate of quality was given and it is said that these raw materials are ideal for this particular use. Say for example, A is the active principle, B, C, D, E, F, G, H, I and J are the excipients, and K and L are the packaging materials. A is produced in the medicinal chemistry labs or is produced by a bulk manufacturing unit. Its quality was determined and the certificate of analysis mentioned it to be perfect and contained impurities with compendial requirements. Online, A is weighed by scientists, it is again analysed in the labs of the quality control department of this particular pharmaceutical industry and a confirmation regarding the quality is given. Now it is the turn of B and C. B is used to neutralize the bad effects of C. C has good effects in terms of the manufacturing process. Thus, C could not be avoided in this process and thus C is definitely required. The first step is to mix B and C together. Mixing is accomplished using a mixer. The final mix is layered, but uniform. C comes near the mixer feed and then in current computer set up communicates with the sensor signalling that it has come. Then this sensor signals A to proceed onto the line. B automatically comes near the sensor and the mixing proceeds. Similarly, the sensor gives signals to the chambers associated with D, E, F, G, H, I and J. They are all ready to further act and enter the process of manufacture. D and F are similar to B and and C in terms of mixing. They are mixed in a separate chamber and G gives the feedback and H proceeds. G is a need and H is its neutralizer. Again the sensor plays a major role and gives further to the mix of A, B, C, D and F to proceed to the chamber where G and H are added to this mix. In this context everything is mixed. Here, in-process quality is determined. A well-accomplished group does this. Most of the times this needs intelligent feedback. Thus, experts are the responsible personnel. Now, the ball-park belongs to I and J. These are the kind of final output measures such as tableting machines etc. in case of tablet manufacture. The examples of similar excipients could be lubricants or glidants. Now, at this stage, A, B, C, D, E, F, G, H, I and J are processed and the final product is obtained, say in this instance a tablet. The current set up consists of a single sensor identifying all these steps giving very appropriate feed back to the respective manufacturing unit heads. Now comes packaging. K and L are the packaging material. The tablet slowly enters the packaging unit and the packing material is very appropriately packed. The tablet is produced as the final output in a very nice form. This simply suggests that several steps are involved in this manufacturing process and thus the chance of quality variation is very rampant. Any mistake at any stage either by deliberate tampering or sensor interference may lead to the wrong signal and thus many a times result in the bad output and thus results in the discarding of the batch. This example simply illustrates the complexity of a manufacturing process. Discarding or accepting a batch mainly results because of this simple equation associated with the several of the components and the manufacturing processess.

Raw Materials Control

Before finished pharmaceutical dosage forms are produced, the identity, purity, and quality of raw materials must be established with the use of suitable test methods. Pharmacopoeia and formulary monographs such as the US Pharmacopoeia – National Formulary (USP-NF), the European Pharmacopoeia, the Indian Pharmacopoeia, and the Japanese Pharmacopoeia provide standardized test methods for the most common and widely used materials. Manufacturers take various steps to raw materials testing compliance. Some qualify raw material suppliers by performing an initial detailed vendor audit followed by an annual qualification consisting of full pharmacopoeial monograph testing three lots of material. If the qualification lots test successfully, then subsequent materials shipments will require only monograph identification testing. However, companies that take a more conservative approach to raw materials release full monograph testing for each lot of supplied material. The most common tests performed in a raw materials laboratory include titrations, loss on drying, Karl Fisher moisture determination, heavy metals limit tests, and infrared spectrophotometry. Full monograph testing often requires as many as seven different analytical techniques. For example, to perform full USP monograph testing for methylparaben, eight different tests using six analytical techniques ranging from infrared absorption to gas chromatography are required. Therefore, the most efficient organization of a raw materials laboratory is by function, so that analysts can specialize in specific techniques. The most commonly specified instruments include pH meters, balances, gas chromatographs, high-performance liquid chromatographs (HPLCs), infrared spectrophotometers, UV-Vis spectrometers, Karl Fisher moisture titrators, general titration apparatus, vacuum ovens, melting point apparatus, thin-layer chromatography apparatus, polarimeters, refractometers, viscometers, muffle furnaces, flame atomic absorption spectrophotometers, differential scanning calorimeters and thermogravimetric analyzers. As far as the raw material qualifications, several leniencies are currently allowed by different regulatory organizations.

The publication of Annex-18 of the EU guide to good manufacturing practice formally brought active pharmaceutical ingredients within the scope of GMP. Historically there had been several attempts to establish appropriate international standards for APIs, culminating in ICH Q7a, the first internationally harmonized Good Manufacturing Practice guidance developed jointly by the industry and the regulators and published in November 2000. ICH Q7a establishes one global GMP standard for APIs. Annex-18 to the EU Guide to GMP based on this guidance was published in July 2001. The aims of ICH Q7a are to minimize variations in interpretation among industry and regulatory bodies worldwide. There are a number of topics in ICH Q7a that may be considered new, for example, starting material was formerly defined as the first step in which impurities are formed which are not removed at a later stage; starting material is now a material used in the production of an API which is incorporated as a significant structural fragment into the structure of the API. Starting material may be an article of commerce, a material purchased from contract suppliers, or may be produced in-house. Starting materials are normally of defined chemical properties and structure. The guidance contains definitions of reworking and reprocessing and the role of agents and brokers. Where agents or brokers are used, the origin of the material needs to be established. This leads to the requirement for certificates of analysis, a consideration that has important implications. In addition, this guideline gives a keynote as related to the manufacturing of the active ingredients. These include increasing GMPs directed towards the pure API, the production of a product quality review (a new EC requirement following the example of the United States Food and Drug

Administration), disallowance of blending "passed" and "failed" batches to form a larger "acceptable" batch, and specific directions on storage, distribution and any critical time limits on the manufacturing process.

In-process Items Control

As mentioned in the manufacturing process section, in-process items control is also a very important aspect. The wastage of a batch could be reduced by intermittently and intermediately stopping a batch production in the middle, if it is thought that this may result in a bad quality product at the end. However, this may be a waste of the resources. The key for this step would be either the instrument has stopped because of the drop in the power supply or loss of power or the assay of the intermittent products tells that this batch may lead to a bad finished product. Thus, in-process items control becomes crucial. As of now, compendial standards do not mention the quality control of the in-process items control as is mentioned for the raw material control. However, it mentions that proper care has to be taken right from the beginning of the batch production in terms of environmental control and by the use of very appropriate batch records etc. The issue of batch records was mentioned in detail in the chapter titled "Product Processing and Evaluation". Hence, it is not mentioned in detail in this chapter. Tacitly, understanding the issue of the necessity of good environmental practice is the key for in-process items control. However, as a whole, the assay and the quality testing of the in-process items control some times become important. Currently, artificial intelligence is used in a manufacturing process in developed countries and in the leading industries of some of the developing countries. Thus, the assay of the in-process goods in tandem with the manufacture would be of definite help as far as the reduction of wastage of a batch is concerned. Knowledge representation, expert, logic, fuzzy logic, neural network, and object approaches are some of the methods used in this process. An example of an in-process quality control test is the blend uniformity analysis in tablet production. The CGMP regulations, 21 CFR 211.110, do not require Blend Uniformity Analysis (BUA). It requires some type of test or examination on each batch, but that test or examination does not have to be BUA as described in the guidance document. Failure to perform BUA type testing on routine production batches should not be cited as a CGMP deficiency. BUA type testing is recommended for low dose powder blend products (e.g., less than 50% or 50 mg) but other approaches may also be used to satisfy this CGMP requirement. The draft guidance also permits the submission of a supplement to delete BUA testing. This is also an application filing issue and does not exempt a manufacturer from the CGMP requirement for some type of test or examination on each batch. If BUA type testing is discontinued, an alternate approach to comply with 21 CFR 211.110 should be implemented.

To assure batch uniformity and integrity of drug products, written procedures shall be established and followed that describe the in-process controls, and tests, or examinations to be conducted on appropriate samples of in-process materials of each batch. Such control procedures shall be established to monitor the output and to validate the performance of those manufacturing processes that may be responsible for causing variability in the characteristics of in-process material and the drug product. Such control procedures shall include, but are not limited to, the following, where appropriate:

1. Tablet or capsule weight variation;
2. Disintegration time;
3. Adequacy of mixing to assure uniformity and homogeneity;
4. Dissolution time and rate;
5. Clarity, completeness, or pH of solutions.

Valid in-process specifications for such characteristics shall be consistent with drug product final specifications and shall be derived from previous acceptable process average and process variability estimates where possible and determined by the application of suitable statistical procedures where appropriate. Examination and testing of samples shall assure that the drug product and in-process material conform to specifications. In-process materials shall be tested for identity, strength, quality, and purity as appropriate, and approved or rejected by the quality control unit, during the production process, e.g., at commencement or completion of significant phases or after storage for long periods. Rejected in-process materials shall be identified and controlled under a quarantine system designed to prevent their use in manufacturing or processing operations for which they are unsuitable.

Finished Products Control

The best product output is one without any flaws. However, during the initial trials before a batch record is established, experiments are conducted several times to get a final batch record released. During this period, a lot of efforts are needed to be invested by a technologist, in this case a pharmaceutical scientist. Once the batch record is established, a very strict quality control system may ensure perfect control over the batches released. Although a strict control of raw material, very strict GMP procedures of manufacture and handling of the manufacture process by experts, batch losses are not avoidable. The best thing in this case is to perform finished product assay before a product is released. Most of the times, a particular sample is picked from the final batch, then the drug is assayed along with making sure of several physical parameters to be perfect. Once the assay and the physical inspection are made sure, the batch is released accordingly.

As related to the assay and release of the finished products, currently several finished product testing criteria are supported by various pharmacopoeia. For active ingredient analysis identity tests, assays (active ingredients, excipients), infrared spectroscopy, liquid chromatography (HPLC), thin layer chromatography, gas chromatography (GC), atomic absorption spectroscopy (AA), wet chemistry procedures and biological assays are performed. Several other properties of finished products must be investigated. Monographs set limits on various contaminants and degradation products. Impurity testing is one of the important criteria supported by FDA. Biological assays check for contaminants of physiological significance. Limit tests, impurities tests, pyrogen/LAL bacterial endotoxins tests, general safety tests (biologics), content uniformity, preservative assays are performed. Moisture content estimation, particulate testing, tablet hardness testing, dissolution testing and disintegration testing are some of the physical tests performed on finished products. Preservative effectiveness tests, pathogenic screening tests, bioburden tests, and identification of bacterial and fungal organisms are some of the microbiological tests performed. Stability testing and sterility assurance testing are included as finished product testing methods along with several other routine tests conducted. Once the finished products are within the specifications, the batch is released.

Assurance of Quality

A very systematic effective assurance of quality takes into consideration the manufacturing practices, analytical methodologies, modern sampling and assay techniques and regulatory guidelines. Some of the details related to the assurance of the quality are henceforth discussed.

Manufacturing Practices

The control and assurance of the manuacturing practices is achieved by *quality assurance before start-up*, which includes environmental and microbiologic control and sanitation, manufacturing working formula procedures, raw material planning, manufacturing equipment preparedness, *quality assurance at start-up*, which includes raw materials processing, compounding, packaging materials control, labels control and finished product control, and finally *bulk product testing, quality assurance during packaging operations and auditing*.

Schedule M of The Drugs and Cosmetics Act, 1940 and Rules, 1945 mentions Good Manufacturing Practices (GMP). According to this, maintaining the quality of drugs is basically the responsibility of manufacturer and the Good Manufacturing Practices (GMP) guidelines are a means to assure this very quality. A draft of GMP regulations was prepared in 1975 which was finalised and implemented in 1988, in the form of amendment. Schedule M for the dosage forms have also been revised. The revised Schedule M also requires documentation at every stage of production, validation of processes and equipment; efficient Standard Operating Procedures (SOP) during different stages of manufacture and quality control operations; training of technical personal engaged in the manufacturing and testing. This is Indian Scenario. However, several of the FDA guidelines as related to the quality control and assurance are briefly mentioned in the "Regulatory Guidelines" section. Since the pharmaceutical industry is becoming global in terms of marketing and innovation it is always better to parallel both USFDA guidelines and Indian legislations as related to the manufacturing processess design and execution.

To assure that finished dosage forms meet high standards of quality and purity, an effective sanitation program is required at all facilities where such products are manufactured. This is often times, the first step in the quality assurance before start-up. A successful extermination program must be enforced within and outside the plant to control insects and rodents. People are the mainstay of any plant housekeeping and sanitation program. Consequently, personal cleanliness and proper haircovering and clothing should be required. Floors, walls, and ceilings should be resistant to external forces, capable of being easily cleaned, and in good condition. Adequate ventilation, proper temperature, and proper humidity are other important factors. Ventilation in manufacturing departments is usually designed so that dust can be contained and removed. In such departmental operations, dust collectors, air filters, and scrubbers to clean the air are checked on a routine schedule. Air quality monitoring at the work station could indicate the adequacy of these elements. Water supply may be potable, distilled, or deionized, and must be under adequate pressure to keep the water flowing. Deionization units should be monitored, and the resins changed or regenerated frequently, to deliver water of consistently high chemical and microbial quality as per written compendial or inhouse specifications. A working formula procedure should be prepared for each batch size that is produced. To attempt expansion or reduction of a batch size by manual calculations at the time of production cannot be considered good manufacturing practice. Quality assurance personnel must review and check the working formula procedures for each production batch before, during, and after production. If things are not taken care of at this time, this may lead to lot of erroneous results and very often result in batch dumping. The reason for dumping this batch could be either deliberate purposes or for personal gains. Thus, signature and date of issue given by a responsible production or quality assurance employee. Proper identification by name and dosage form, item number, lot number, effective date of document, reference to a superseded version, amount, lot, and code numbers of each raw material utilized. This has to be employed at every step of processing. In addition it ensures the skill of the personal involved in this process. Most of the times unit processes such as mixing are the main sources of errors, and so, these have to be weeded out at very early stages. Thus, skill of the personal involved at this level is the key. Raw material quality assurance and the containers used in such assurance have to be properly validated. Enough care has to be taken that this is not the source of the batch losses. The other issue regarding this is the cleanliness of the manufacturing equipment. Very often personnel employed are used in the cleaning and this process is validated at the beginning of the batch production. Thus, this step has to be very carefully undertaken. Most of the times after a batch is produced, the equipment is dis-assembled and is cleaned for convenience. Proper protocol should be in place with regard to the cleaning of the equipment. It is likely that regular wear and tear of the equipment are possible. These have to be regularly monitored to ensure an ideal batch output.

Only released, properly labeled raw materials are allowed in the in-processing area. Several issues are important during this step of *quality assurance at the start-up*. Depending on the nature of the product, quality assurance personnel should check and verify that the temperature and humidity in the area are within the specified limits required for the product. If temperature and humidity is beyond the specified limits, production must be informed and corrective actions taken. If it is in the control of the person incharge, it is better to be safe than to be sorry. Everything has to properly documented by this person at this stage. Proper labeling containing the product name, item number, lot number, and gross, tare and net weights of the contents have to be properly mentioned. The next step is compounding. Since the batch record is already established, raw materials already tested, the next best thing that has to be taken care of is the compounding. In-process quality control is the key in this area. Measures and characteristics such as physical appearance, color, odor, thickness, diameter, friability, hardness, weight variation, disintegration time, volume check, viscosity and pH are the minimum requirements. Current Good Manufacturing Practices require that in-process quality assurance be adequately documented throughout all stages of manufacturing. In addition, packaging materials control and labels control are very essential features. The final step is the *finished product control*. Specifications as related to the assay, bulk product testing have to be properly considered. Quality assurance during packaging is also an important aspect. Everystep has to be complied to the regulatory rules. Finally auditing is the essential feature. This comes from the very early stages of production to the release of the batch into the market. All the people who are involved are responsible for the batch output. If after a batch is released into the market and customers complain, then along with the company personnel everyone involved in the process is answerable. Thus, a very proper control has to be maintained at each and every step.

Analytical Methodologies

The importance of the analytical methods in quality control investigations is described with the help of a recently published example. High performance liquid chromatography (HPLC) is very routinely used in the pharmaceutical industries for finished product assay. The aim of one pharmaceutical company (Seatrace Pharmaceuticals, Gadsden, AL) was to develop a tablet formulation consisting of antihistamine and analgesic combinations. This combination is used to treat fevers and inflammation conditions. Our group has developed a stability indicating high performance liquid chromatography method for the simultaneous determination of acetaminophen, salicylamide and phenyltoloxamine, along with several degradation products and the impurities. These include the known potential degradation products of acetaminophen, p-aminophenol, p-nitrophenol, precursor impurities p-hydroxyacetophenone and ethylsalicylate and the potential degradation products salicylamide and salicylic acid. Two different gradients (Method I & Method II) were developed. Method I was developed for assay, content uniformity, and quantification of degradation products. Method II was developed for assay and content uniformity. Once the method was developed, robustness of the method, sensitivity factors, detection and quantitation limits were determined, and the applicability of the stability studies were evaluated. **Robustness** is defined as the capacity of a method to remain unaffected by deliberate variations in method parameters. **Precision** of the chromatographic system was determined using relative standard deviation of the response factors for the different peaks in the injections of the standard solutions. **Response Factor** was calculated as RF=DR/C where DR is the detector response (peak area) and C is the concentration of the analyte. **Sensitivity Factor** was calculated by dividing the response factor of the drug with the response factor of respective degradation product and impurity. **Detection Limit** for all the components was evaluated till response/noise ratio was 3. The **Limit of Quantification** for all the components was evaluated till response/noise ratio was 10. The conclusions of this investigation were that the methods are linear, robust, reproducible, sensitive and stability indicating. Thus, the quality of a method has to be characterized, monitored, measured and validated. The nature of the analytical methods may be physical, chemical, microbiological, biological, or a combination of these types. The quality of analysis is built during its design stage, validated in its development stage, and confirmed in its utilization stages. The other methods that are very routinely used in a pharmaceutical industry are electrometric methods, solvent extraction methods, spectrophotometric methods, chromatographic methods and other stability indicating methods.

Modern Sampling, Assay and Data Processing Techniques

The current trend that is followed in a production facility is to analyze the samples at each and every quality/quantity limiting step. This saves time, resources and results in a perfect output by reducing the number of quality/quantity limiting steps. When the speed of the manufacture has increased several fold compared to the previous manufacturing processes, it is a difficult task to sample, analyze and report during this stage, in tandem with the production/manufacture. In this regard the current trend is to analyze the samples on line with the speed equal to that of the manufacturing process. HPLC is a very routine technique used in the assay of the samples in a pharmaceutical production unit. The other simpler techniques such as UV-spectrophotometry, fluorescence spectrophotometry, zeta-meter, viscometer, particle size analyzer are also routinely used in the in-process assay evaluations. All of these could be used online with modern sampling, assay, and data processing techniques. Any of the techniques mentioned can be tailored as per the needs. Several other modifications such as LC-MS etc. are always in place and are used as per the sophistication of the needs of the production unit. Many a times, especially with sustained release systems or suspensions where polymers are used, sample recovery becomes very important. In this regard, specialized extraction equipment are also used on-line along with the several instruments that are used in a production unit. Automation also has to increase as the sophistication increases. Automation usually improves the quality, quantity, and efficiency of an operation. Its introduction into an analytical lab dramatically changes the traditional look, capability, precision, and acceptability of most of our conventional analytical disciplines. The use of automated instrumentation for pharmaceutical analysis, data handling, and data storage is certainly on rise. Currently, several companies are marketing these types of automated instrumentation. The design, manufacture and the working principle are based on robotic technologies.

Some of the robotic techniques are multifunctional. They are equipped to perform repetitive laboratory procedures in a wide range of application areas such as nucleic acid extraction and purification (solid phase extraction and magentic bead separation), mother-daughter plate replication, ELISA assays, immunophenotyping, LC injection, cell-based assays and separations and protein assays. These robots offer automation solution for the research laboratory, where consistent results are vital and bench space is limited. These techniques are designed to take on the challenges of reproducible pipetting and dispensing of volumes including sub-microliter, and also aid in handling a variety of sample containers including troughs, tubes, and 96 or 384-well microtiter plates. The decks hold upto 6 microtiter plates. Some of these could hold upto 12 plates. The equipment has tow pipetting arms, each of these could have different functionalites. In addition, most of these instruments offer powerful software. These work under various platform software programs such as Windows 2000 and XP. These computers meet the challenges of a production facility by involving in method development and optimization with easy-to-use dedicated methods and further helps a scientist master the art of liquid handling. Depending on the sophistication of the instruments high-throughput quantification of the samples is also possible. Thus, this type of automation facilitates the speed of the pharmaceutical manufacture process. However, it takes lot of money, resources and time before such a process could be installed on a manuacturing floor. Validation of the total line becomes very essential, which is the key to this automated process.

Regulatory Guidelines

Reading and understanding the regulatory guidelines is a very important aspect of pharmaceutical manufacturing. This has to be done prior to the initiation of a person into the manufacturing setup. Although a person is well trained in the basics of pharmaceutical technology, when it comes to the actual practice of the manufacture, the ballpark is that following regulatory guidelines would be essential for an ideal output of a product. Several regulatory guidelines are currently published by FDA and other regulatory organizations as related to the quality control and the assessment. It is better for all the pharmaceutical scientists to have a very brief knowledge. Some of the important guidelines are listed in Appendix 1 of this chapter.

Salient Features of Quality Control

As mentioned before, quality control of goods of any type is the main part of a business organization. Although lot of care has been taken and considered during the pre- and during-manufacturing process, it is always possible that the product may be inferior once in the shelves. These inferiorities are manifested as loss of stability of the active component in the pharmacy stores, the loss of physical shape of the container, or inappropriate mixing that might have led to its contamination before, in and after its pharmacies' journey, deliberate tampering to achieve local gains etc. Some of these things are traceable and somethings are unavoidable. However, the goal of any business organization is to see that the quality of goods it produces are of superior quality. As a consideration of oral drug industry the following are the salient features of quality control that are to be strictly followed or considered: stability studies, product identification systems, adulteration, misbranding, and counterfeiting, maintenance, storage and retrieval of records. Some of the details of these requirements are henceforth discussed in this section.

Stability Studies

There are legal, moral, economic, and competitive reasons, as well as reasons of safety and efficacy, to monitor, predict, and evaluate drug product stability. The aim of quality control stability testing is to ensure that batches of the released product are maintained within specification limits throughout their stated period of shelf storage. Stability testing of the product during development and scale-up stages is employed to define the recommended expiration date and storage conditions for inclusion on the label and to establish a product stability profile. Therefore, stability testing after product is released to the market is for the verification and confirmation of this profile.

The stresses and hazards to which products are exposed during their passage from the manufacturing plant to the distribution chain and to the consumer can be environmental, mechanical or contaminant in nature. Environmental stresses such as extreme temperatures, high moisture, intense light and radiation are common, and mechanical hazards such as vibration, sudden drop, inversion, shock, and deformation are not unusual. Elevated temperature, especially if coupled with high relative humidity, is known to cause and accelerate physical deterioration and chemical degradation. Mechanical stresses have shown to cause such problems as liquid spillage, tablet chipping, and package deformation and breakage. Therefore, quality control of the marketed product does not stop at the final release of the product from manufacturing site. A reserve sample of at least two times the quantity of product required to conduct all the quality control tests performed on the batch of the product should be retained for atleast one year after the expiration date.

Section 505-(b) of the CFR law as stated on the New Drug Application Form, USA, specifically describes the requirements for stability information as: "A complete description of, and data derived from the studies of the stability of, the drug, including information showing the suitability of the analytical methods used. Describe any additional stability studies under way or contempleted. Stability data should be submited for any new drug substance, for the finished dosage form of the drug in the container in which it is to be marketed, and if it is to be put in solution at the time of dispensing, for the solution to be prepared as directed. State the expiration date(s) that will be used on the label to preserve the identify, strength, quality, and purity of the drug until it is used. If no expiration date is proposed, the applicant must justify its absence".

Under the regulation for antibiotic drugs, an expiration date is required for the product label of any antibiotic drug. These regulations detailed in the Antibiotic Application, FD Form 1675 (1/71), as follows:

"A completed description of, and data derived from stability studies of the potency and physical characteristics of the drug, including information showing the suitability of the analytical methods used. Describe any additonal stability studies underway or contemplated. Stability data should be submitted for any new antibiotic, for the finished dosage form of the drug in which it is to be marketed, and if it is to be put into solution at the time of dispensing, for the solution prepared as directed. The expiration date needs to preserve the identify, strength, quality, and purity of the drug until it is used."

The most desirable stabilty data are from actual shelf-life studies using products in the container-closure systems stored under labeled conditions. For introducing new products to the market, however, or for making material changes in the process, formula, or container-closure system of existing products, one cannot wait until all the needed stability data at room temperature are generated. Therefore, appropriately designed and executed short-term (e.g. 3 month) accelerated stability studies have been accepted by the FDA as data bases for use in extrapolating longer room-temperature expiration dates. Use of accelerated data is obviously not a substitute for actual shelf-life study. It is a means of predicting shelf-life of a product based on scientific principles and guided by experience. This method of shelf-life prediction based on short-term accelerated stabitliy data is currently well-utilized by pharmaceutical scientists.

The manufacturer is asked to confirm the shelf-life stability of the product on production batches by taking the first several batches of the product or by taking batches at certain intervals of time during the first year of manufacture, and in subsequent years at least one additional production batch, and subjecting them to extended shelf-life testing at ambient storage conditions. At each sampling, which is generally performed on a yearly or semiannual basis, the samples are tested for physical, chemical, and biological properties according to the standards set forth in the monographs of the official compendia or to the specifications established by the manufacturer.

The stability of the product should be evaluated in the container in which it is marketed. The expiration date and storage conditions should appear on the label of the product. Experience in the pharmaceutical industry has shown that there can be a considerable delay between the manufacture of a product and its eventual utilization by the consumer. To avoid deterioration of drugs and finished products during storage, the adequacy of warehouse and other storage facilities requires proper attention. To assist during transportation and storage, indication of the proper storage condition should appear on the label. Since 1979, expiration dates have been required on the prescription and over-the-counter drug products with limited exceptions. The FDA considers a product misbranded when it is labeled with an expiration date not supported by suitable stability data. The expiration date of a drug product must appear on the immediate container and also on the outer package. When single dose containers are packaged in individual cartons, however, the expiration date may propely appear on the individual carton instead of on the immediate product container. Furthermore, the current GMP regulations provide specific information as to the stability characteristics of pharmaceutical products and their expiration dating. These GMP regulations indicate that "The interests of the consumers must be served by the establishedment of valid expiration dates for all the products, and Sections 211.166 of the GMP regulations set forth basic guidelines for stability studies for all drugs, which studies will be used to establish expiration dates. "

Product Identification Systems

Product identification system is a very important aspect of pharmaceutical manufacturing. These identification systems could help at any stage of production. These stages include from the early package of the raw materials, the package of intermittent material to the final package that enters a pharmacy. To avoid cross-contamination, product identification systems were always in place, eversince the business field has started. This business could include pharmaceuticals also. Especially when tablets and capsules occupied a major chunk of pharmaceutical output, their production was in millions, special packages were also developed and finally to identify, very new product identification systems were also in place. The simplest coding system is the use of alphabets and numericals. A drug product code composed of nine characters to be used by pharmaceutical manufacturers for inclusion in the National Drug Code Directory has been developed and has been used by the FDA to establish a uniform code system for dosage forms. The nine-character code would identify the labeler, the dosage form, the strength of the product, and the number of product units in the package. The other mode of coding is bar-coding including several other coding technologies. These techniques are important because permanent direct marking of products assures ease of tracking and record keeping.

Bar coding was formally introduced to the healthcare industry in the USA in March 1984. At that time, the union of Health Industry Bar Code Council (HIBCC) was formed by the American Hopital Association (AHA), the Health Industry Distributors Association (HIDA), the Health Industry Manufacturers Association (HIMA), the National Wholesale Druggists' Association (NWDA), and the Pharmaceutical Manufacturers Association (PMA) resulted in the introduction of bar coding system in the hospital arena. The bar-coding technique in the arena of pharmaceuticals is to avoid cross contamination in the pharmacies and hospitals, thereby reducing medication errors. The other techniques used in this area are computerized physician order entry (CPOE), automated dispensing machines (ADMs), bar coding, and computerized medication administration records

(CMARs). Very similar techniques are also used in pharmaceutical manufacturing. Of these bar-coding system can be very conveniently used. This is an automatic identification system and thus facilitates easy flow of the raw material, manufacturing components and the finished products. There are several types of bar-coding systems that include: the two-dimensional bar code and matrix code. Encryption (the formulation of codes), is carried out prior to bar and matrix coding using acid-etch and laser techniques respectively. Laser technique is used in the instrument identification system. 'Reading' of the two types of code was more difficult with bar-codes because of the high reflectivity of background polished stainless steel, and only large instruments have sufficient area for bar-coding. Consistent, accurate, automatic identification of the instruments was possible with the matrix code for which a surface of only 4 sq mm is necessary. In one study, after 50 cycles of decontamination and packaging, neither code showed obvious deterioration and it was possible to read the matrix code as easily as prior to this process. Automatic instrument identification is possible using recently developed methods and could facilitate economies in the processing of instruments in health facilities, pharmaceutical manufacturing systems and the automatic recording of instrument usage in the production facility.

Currently several new innovations are in place in the labeling systems. One such system is “Compressed Symbologies”, developed by Symbology Research Center, Huntsville, Alabama. SRC offers compressed symbologies as a way to automate inventory and cut warehousing costs and avoid part shortages. Other benefits of direct parts marking are updating the part's history in real-time, increasing read rates to virtually 100 percent, guaranteeing part/component integrity, and eliminating paper labels and tracking paperwork. No longer does a company have to face missing paper labels--labels that can fall off a high-value part or product due to heat, cold, rain, wind, and other inhospitable conditions. The permanent digital data matrix codes work on practically any surface, be it steel or metal, even plastics, glass, paper, fabric, ceramics, or other material. Compressed symbologies can withstand extreme fluctuations of temperatures, up to 2,200 degrees Fahrenheit and an airflow exceeding 18,000 miles per hour. Thus, this type of technology could also be used in other hard-ball industries and also in space technologies.

Adulteration, Misbranding, and Counterfeiting

An adulterated, misbranded or a counterfeited drug is a fraud to the public. Such products could be very seriously dangerous to the patients and may some times cost the physician’s role and profession, if not proper precautions considered. A situation of this nature may mislead the physician because his patient’s response may differ from the response expected. Several countries have several definitions regarding these. However, some of the definitions as related to the Indian scenario are presented. Although sounds tandem, these definitions are different and should be very carefully understood by a physician, a pharmacist, a nurse, a clinical trial volunteer and in fact a patient.

According to Drugs and Cosmetics Act, 1940,

A drug is termed as **misbranded**:

1. If it is so coloured, coated, powdered or polished that damage is concealed or if it is made to appear of better or greater therapeutic value than it really is.
2. If it is not labeled in the prescribed manner.
3. If its label or container or anything accompanying the drug bears any statement, design, or device that makes any false claim for the drug or which is false or misleading in any particular.

A drug is termed **adulterated**:

1. If it consists, in whole or in part, of any filthy, putrid or decomposed substance.
2. If it has been prepared, packed or stored under unsanitary conditions whereby it may have been contaminated with filth or whereby it may have been rendered injurious to health.
3. If its container is composed in whole or in part, of any poisonous or deleterious substance which may render the contents injurious to health.
4. If it bears or contains, for purposes of coloring only, a color other than one which is prescribed.
5. If it contains any harmful or toxic substance which may render it injurious to health.
6. If any substance has been mixed therewith so as to reduce its quality or strength.

A drug is termed as **spurious or counterfeiting**:

1. If it is imported under a name which belongs to another drug.
2. If it is an imitation of, or is a substitute for, another drug or resembles another drug in a manner likely to deceive or bears upon its label or container, the name of another drug unless it is plainly and conspicuously marked so as to reveal its true character and its lack of identify with such other drug.

3. If the label or container bears the name of an individual or company purporting to be the manufacturer of the drug, which individual or company is fictitious or does not exist.
4. If it has been substituted wholly or in part by another drug or substance.
5. If it purports to be the product of a manufacturer of whom it is not truly a product.

Maintenance, Storage and Retrieval of Records

Recording keeping is a very important part of pharmaceutical manufacturing. All the records of master formula, batch production, and packaging records in the manufacturing should be carefully managed and databased. Complete records of the distribution of each batch of product must be maintained in a manner that would facilitate its recall if necessary. The current trend is very organized maintenance, storage and retrieval of records, the reason being the introduction of the computer in all the aspects of pharmaceutical manufacturing. In general, records of data converted to digitalized form are stored on computer tapes, cards, or discs, or in case storage. Case memory is the fastest, most expensive and most accessible type of memory. Disc storage is available for large volumes of data, and its almost random access features are particularly useful. Currently, in most of the big pharma, data is stored in a centralized computer system. The validation of each of these routes becomes important. The current trend and various regulatory bodies specially emphasize on the validation of the software that further facilitates the use of computers in pharma industry.

Marketed Software

Currently several software companies are marketing their packages as related to Good Manufacturing Procedures and Quality Assurance Processes. One such company is Novatek International. The software it markets as related to quality is advanced quality Nova-LIMS. This is a 21 CFR Part 11 Compliant long-term solution that makes sure that a company which bought this software has a centralized control and maintenance of all the data handling software solutions. The different software applications as suitable to the current pharmaceutical setup include stability program, environment monitoring program, document, audit and training software application, the finished product analyzer, the raw material analyzer, the preventive maintenance and calibration software, the automated packaging component analyzer and the consumable inventory management system. The use of these softwares facilitates easy manufacure control. It is recommended and is advisable to have this software in any leading manufacturing unit, provided cost is not a constraint. Further, as a lesson, any technician with enough expertise can easily handle the unit or support the unit without much technical background. Some of the features of this software are very briefly mentioned henceforth.

Stability module is a software application that manages the day-to-day activities of the stability department within the quality control and R&D divisions. Its design takes into consideration the latest guidelines from the FDA, TPP, ICH and EU, among others, pertaining to pharmaceutical, chemical, biological and biotechnological fields. This software is designed for all types of products, from pre-clinical to post market, innovator or generic. The Stability module is 21-CFR part-11 compliant and has an extensive, independent audit trail. The **Environmental Monitoring Program** is an application capable of capturing all environmental data in a 21 CFR Part-11 Compliant, fully validated system. It is envisioned for sterile and non sterile health care industries (Pharmaceuticals, Biotech, Chemical, microbiological) food and any other sterile environment based on the latest guidelines from, FDA, EU, ISO 14644-1 and PDA Technical report 13. Data from viable and non-viable monitoring, water analysis, clean steam and compressed gases are securely captured and easily trended to ensure site "state of control". The investigation window allows the user to investigate Out of Specification "OOS" with capability to add any files such as picture, audio video, scanned documents etc to the report. The **DATA** is a 21 CFR Part-11 compliant application used to manage and exchange information in all industries. It is made of three distinct modules: a document management system, an audit module and a training module. DATA incorporates several customer-driven enhancements and innovations.

The **Finished Product Analyzer** module is a software application that is used for capturing the test data from finished product testing. This application consists of Product Registration, where the user can input pertinent information regarding the product and the type of packaging; Monograph, where the user can define the required tests; Certificate of Analysis: used for entering, verifying and approving the data; The Approved manufacturers and Suppliers list, where the user verifies that the product is from an approved source; Investigation, where the user can initiate an Out of Specification Investigation. The trending of lots is possible to ensure that the process is under control. The Finished Product module is also 21 CFR Part-11 compliant and has an extensive, independent audit trail. The **Preventive Maintenance and Calibration (PMC) module** is a software application that is used to track the status of equipments used in a regulated environment. The software allows registration of the equipment, the definition of the required tests to ensure that the equipments are within the specifications and a test report where the user can enter the obtained results.

The software will automatically show the equipments due for calibration. The inventory control window allows the purchase and update of the required spare parts for each calibration. The PMC module is also 21 CFR Part-11 compliant and has an extensive, independent audit trail. The **Automated Packaging Component Analyzer** (APCA) module is an application used to automatically verify the incoming printed components against a pre-approved master. This software is language independent and capable of detecting the smallest error within the test and the master scans. It is capable of analyzing a predefined number of samples against the master and providing the error in each and every test sample. The user will have the choice to accept or reject the printed components based on the type of errors obtained. The APCA is envisioned to replace the tedious task of manually verifying a printed component against the master. The APCA module is, once again, 21 CFR Part-11 compliant and has an extensive, independent audit trail. Novatek's **Consumable Management Software** (CMS) is a 21 CFR Part-11 compliant, comprehensive inventory management system. It allows management of purchase orders, receivables, inventory locations, transfers, and serialized item tracking. Each material item in the price book has corresponding inventory details that can show all purchases, sales, quantities on hand, quantities reserved, quantities at each physical location, and the latest costs and values. The strength of the product lies in its non-modular design that enables one to enhance business productivity significantly without ever having to add separate software.

Conclusions

It is always two or three blockbusters that matter for the progress of a pharmaceutical company. Although a pharmaceutical company in new drug discovery spends a lot of investment, it is always a risky business. In these situations, when the luck favors the company, the group of body that is involved in this business helps further growth of this company in any dimension. Thus, every aspect of the pharmaceutical business is a learning experience. In these situations, the focus should be to get the blockbuster out without any problems. The best thing that this group could do is to follow regulatory guidelines very properly, understand the people involved, the competitors, the associates and everyone who could potentially interfere with the business. Sometimes it may cost with the availability of the blockbusters. Thus, reiterating quality control investigations are the key to the pharmaceutical manufacturing industry. As of now, several statistical and other tools are in place and are being investigated and into the manufacturing sector. Some of these techniques include Six Sigma levels of Quality, Zero defects and the House of Quality.

Appendix 1

1. Biotechnology Inspection Guide (November 1991)
2. Container Closure Systems for Packaging Human Drugs and Biologics -- Questions and Answers (May 2002)
3. Draft Guidance for Industry: Comparability Protocols--Protein Drug Products and Biological Products--Chemistry, Manufacturing, and Controls Information
4. Guide to Inspections of Infectious Disease Marker Testing Facilities (October 1996)
5. Cosmetic Good Manufacturing Practice Guidelines
6. FDA's Cosmetic Labeling Manual (October 1991)
7. Guide to Inspections of Cosmetic Product Manufacturers
8. Inspections of Cosmetics (February 2003)
9. Compliance Program Guidance Manual For FDA Staff: Drug Manufacturing Inspections (February 2002)
10. Container Closure Systems for Packaging Human Drugs and Biologics -- Questions and Answers (May 2002)
11. Draft Guidance: Drug Substance: Chemistry, Manufacturing, and Controls Information (January 2004)
12. Draft Guidance for Industry: Comparability Protocols--Protein Drug Products and Biological Products--Chemistry, Manufacturing, and Controls Information (September 2003)
13. Guidance for Industry: Sterile Drug Products Produced by Aseptic Processing — Current Good Manufacturing Practice (September 2004)
14. Draft Guidance for Industry on Formal Dispute Resolution: Scientific and Technical Issues Related to Pharmaceutical Current Good Manufacturing Practice (September 2003)
15. Draft Guidance for Industry on Sterile Drug Products Produced by Aseptic Processing (September 2003)
16. Draft Guidance for Industry: Process Analytical Technology--A Framework for Innovative Pharmaceutical Manufacturing and Quality Assurance (September 2004)

17. Draft Guidance Current Good Manufacturing Practice Regulations (September 2004)
18. Guidance for Industry: and FDA — Current Good Manufacturing Practice for Combination Products (September 2004)
19. Guidance for Industry: PAT — A Framework for Innovative Pharmaceutical Development, Manufacturing, and Quality Assurance (September 2004)
20. Guidance for Industry: Sterile Drug Products Produced by Aseptic Processing — Current Good Manufacturing Practice (September 2004)
21. Guide to Inspections of Dosage Form Drug Manufacturers - CGMP's (October 1993)
22. Guide to Inspections of Oral Solutions and Suspensions (August 1994)
23. Guide to Inspections of Pharmaceutical Quality Control Laboratories (July 1993)
24. Guide to Inspections of Sterile Drug Substance Manufacturers (July 1994)
25. Guide to Inspections of Topical Drug Products (July 1994)
26. Guide to Inspections of Validation of Cleaning Processes (July 1993)
27. ICH Q7A - Good Manufacturing Practice Guidance for Active Pharmaceutical Ingredients Final Guidance (August 2001)
28. Presentation on ICH Q7A Good Manufacturing Practice Guidance for APIs and Its Use During Inspections (August 2002)
29. PET Drug Products - Current Good Manufacturing Practice (CGMP) (March 2002)
30. SUPAC -Immediate Release Solid Oral Dosage Forms - Scaleup and Post Approval Changes: Chemistry, Manufacturing, and Controls, *In Vitro* Dissoultion Testing, and *In Vivo* Bioequivalence Documentation (November 1995)
31. SUPAC - Modified Release Scaleup and Post Approval Changes: Chemistry, Manufacturing, and Controls, *In Vitro* Dissolution Testing, and *In Vivo* Bioequivalence Documentation (September 1997)
32. SUPAC - Questions and Answers on Current Good Manufacturing Practices (cGMP) for Drugs

33. General Principles of Software Validation (January 2002)for Industry: Quality Systems Approach to Pharmaceutical Current Good Manufacturing Practice Regulations (September 2004)
34. Guidance for Industry: and FDA — Current Good Manufacturing Practice for Combination Products (September 2004)
35. Guidance for Industry: PAT — A Framework for Innovative Pharmaceutical Development, Manufacturing, and Quality Assurance (September 2004)
36. Guidance for Industry: Sterile Drug Products Produced by Aseptic Processing — Current Good Manufacturing Practice (September 2004)
37. Guide to Inspections of Dosage Form Drug Manufacturers - CGMP's (October 1993)
38. Guide to Inspections of Oral Solutions and Suspensions (August 1994)
39. Guide to Inspections of Pharmaceutical Quality Control Laboratories (July 1993)
40. Guide to Inspections of Sterile Drug Substance Manufacturers (July 1994)
41. Guide to Inspections of Topical Drug Products (July 1994)
42. Guide to Inspections of Validation of Cleaning Processes (July 1993)
43. ICH Q7A - Good Manufacturing Practice Guidance for Active Pharmaceutical Ingredients Final Guidance (August 2001)
44. Presentation on ICH Q7A Good Manufacturing Practice Guidance for APIs and Its Use During Inspections (August 2002)
45. PET Drug Products - Current Good Manufacturing Practice (CGMP) (March 2002)
46. SUPAC -Immediate Release Solid Oral Dosage Forms - Scaleup and Post Approval Changes: Chemistry, Manufacturing, and Controls, *In Vitro* Dissoultion Testing, and *In Vivo* Bioequivalence Documentation (November 1995)
47. SUPAC - Modified Release Scaleup and Post Approval Changes: Chemistry, Manufacturing, and Controls, *In Vitro* Dissolution Testing, and *In Vivo* Bioequivalence Documentation (September 1997)
48. SUPAC - Questions and Answers on Current Good Manufacturing Practices (cGMP) for Drugs
49. General Principles of Software Validation (January 2002)

Questions for Practice and Exercise

1. Explain Quality.
2. Explain Quality Assurance.
3. What is
    1. Confirmation to specifications,
    2. Fitness for use,
    3. A Two-dimensional model of quality, and
    4. Value to some person?
4. Explain quality variation.
5. How is the quality variation controlled?
6. Give a brief idea about a typical manufacturing process.
7. How are raw materials controlled?
8. What is in-process items control?
9. What is the difference between quality assurance and assurance of quality?
10. Explain assurance of quality.
11. What are the salient features of quality control?
12. Explain briefly how stability studies are conducted.
13. Explain
    1. production identification systems,
    2. adulteration, misbranding and counterfeiting.
14. How are records maintained, stored and retrieved in a typical pharmaceutical company?
15. Write a note on
    1. finished product analyzer software,
    2. preventive maintenance and calibration module,
    3. automated packaging component analyzer (APCA),
    4. consumable management software,
    5. six sigma levels of quality,
    6. zero defects and
    7. the house of quality.

Bibliography

1. The Theory and Practice of Industrial Pharmacy, Third Edition, Edited by Leon Lachman, Herbert A. Lieberman, and Joseph L. Kanig, Lea & Febiger Publications, 1986.
2. Retail Management, Functional Principles & Practices, Second Edition, Authored by Gibson G. Vedamani, Jaico Publishing House, 2004.
3. Pharmaceutical Jurisprudence & Ethics (Forensic Pharmacy), Third Edition, Authored by S.P. Agarwal and Rajesh Khanna, Birla Publications, 2004.
4. Pharmaceutical Dosage Forms and Drug Delivery Systems, Seventh Edition, Authored by H.C. Ansel, L.V. Allen, and N.G. Popovich, Lippincott Williams & Wilkins, 1999.
5. Quality Control, Seventh Edition, Authored by DH Besterfield, Prentice Hall, 2003.
6. Computer-Integrated Manufacturing, Third Edition, Authored by JA Rehg and HW Kraebber, Prentice Hall Career and Technology, 1994.
7. Production Management, International Student Edition, Authored by RA Mayer, McGraw Hill Book Company, 1962.
8. What is Six Sigma? First Edition, Authored by Pande P and L Holpp, McGraw Hill Book Company, 2001.

CHAPTER 18

DISSOLUTION TESTING

- **Introduction**
- **History**
- **Mathematics**
  - Dissolution theories
    - Noyes-Whitney`s equation
    - Hixon-Crowell cube root law
    - Surface renewal and limited solvation theories
  - Dissolution profile analysis
    - Wagner`s theory
    - Kitazawa`s theory
    - El-Yazigi's and Cartensen's theory
- **Factors affecting dissolution testing**
  - Dissolution media
  - Hydrodynamic factors
- **Dissolution testing**
  - Purpose
  - Testing methods
  - Calibrator tablets
  - USP modifications
  - FDA modifications

- **Compendial methods**
- **Noncompendial methods**
- **In Vitro In Vivo Correlations**
- **Conclusions**

Introduction

The consistency of dissolution and release of the drug into the dissolution media with any kind of dosage form would be very important. As such, dissolution tests were introduced into various pharmacopeia as methods to ensure the consistency of drug release and optimization of formulation from a variety of dosage forms. These dosage forms include solid dosage forms such as tablets and capsules, sustained release dosage forms such as transdermal devices, nanoparticles, microparticles and implants. Amenably, the dissolution testing has been developed according to the development of various dosage forms. Thus, apart from compendial and highly acceptable dissolution tests, several other dissolution testing methods suitable to the needs of the delivery systems is in vogue. For the last 30 years, FDA has emphasized the importance of drug dissolution testing in assuring lot-to-lot performance and bioequivalence of drugs. These tests have been modified and new research has been performed to ensure ideal testing. In this context, intuitive estimations of the real drug release from dosage forms are not valid. Because very slight variations in the dimensions, the densities of the dosage forms, the temperature of the dissolution medium and the route of administration of the delivery system all affect the dissolution and eventually blood levels of the drugs, all these factors are valid in the design of a dissolution experiment. The most common methods used for drug dissolution testing are the United States Pharmacopeia (USP) Basket method (Apparatus I) and the USP Paddle Method (Apparatus II) (US Pharmacopeia XXIV, 2000). This chapter discusses brief the history, the theory and the methods of dissolution testing and factors that affect the dissolution testing.

History

The first mathematical theory published with regard to dissolution is by Noyes and Whitney in 1897 titled "The rate of solution of solid substances in their own solution". According to this paper, a layer of saturated solution around the drug particle controls the dissolution rate of a drug from a solid drug substance. A few years later in 1900, Brunner and Tolloczko proved that dissolution rate depended on the chemical, physical structures of the pharmaceutical solid, the surface area exposed to the medium, agitation speed, medium temperature and the overall design of the dissolution apparatus. In 1904, Nernst and Brunner modified the Noyes-Whitney equation by applying Fick's law of diffusion. A relationship between the dissolution rate and the diffusion coefficient was established. In 1930, experiments began with *in vivo-in vitro* correlations. In 1931, Hixon and Crowell develop the cube-root law of diffusion. In 1934, Switzerland's Pharmacopeia Helvetica introduced disintegration testing for tablets. In 1950, the correlation of the dissolution of drugs with the bioavailability of the dosage forms was made according to the physicochemical properties of the drug substance. The experiments with the release study of aspirin suggested that the rate of dissolution in the gastro-intestinal tract affects the extent of therapeutic action of a drug. Disintegration testing became an official USP method (USP 14) in 1950. In 1958, the rotating bottle method was introduced to study the release of the drug from an extended release formulation. In 1960s it was recognized that although disintegration affects the bioavailability, the basic key factor is the dissolution. Thus, a variety of testing methods were investigated during this time. In 1970s, USP 18 incorporated the first official dissolution test for solid dosage forms. Twelve monographs published in USP-NF with the official dissolution test-a rotating basket. Standardization, calibration and validation of dissolution testing methods were suggested during 1970 - 1975. Three calibrator tablets were proposed and used by USP in 1975. Prednisone (disintegrating), salicylic Acid (non-disintegrating) and nitrofurantoin (disintegrating) were introduced as calibration testers. The rest is all bigger than history and mathematics and discussed further in this chapter.

Mathematics

Dissolution of a solute is a multistep process involving heterogenous swinging reactions/interactions between the phases of the solute-solute, solute-solvent, solvent-solvent and solute-solvent interface. This is one of the most common mass transfer rate processes in chemical engineering processes. Since very early times these interactions have been observed and subsequently theories were investigated and various rules were laid down. Here in a few of the very fundamental theories of dissolution and the dissolution profile analysis will be discussed. Fundamental theories of dissolution would help to better appreciate their application process and dissolution profile analysis, and are discussed here keeping in view its importance in pharmaceutical dissolution testing.

Fundamental Dissolution Theories

Diffusion layer theories Noyes and Whitney theory, Hixson and Crowell Cube Root theory are the two very common theories of dissolution and will be discussed henceforth. The other theories that could support dissolution testing and that are briefly mentioned here include surface renewal theory and limited solvation theory.

Noyes - Whitney`s equation

Generally, Ficks First Law of diffusion and the Second Law of diffusion describes the steady state and non-steady state diffusions (when drug concentration decreases with time), respectively. Fick`s laws of diffusion are more basic for the dissolution testing and could be hence referred in standard textbooks. On the other hand, the basic Noyes and Whitneys equation describes drug dissolution based on constant surface area. Brunner and Tolloczko modified Noye`s-Whitneys equation by incorporating surface are term S and further proposed the formation of a stagnant layer around the dissolving particle, a layer through which solute diffuses through the bulk. The currently used equation is Noyes-Whitneys equation that incorporates this later modification.

When a tablet or a capsule is introduced into a beaker of water or into the gastrointestinal tract, the drug begins to pass into the solution from the intact solid. Unless the tablet is a contiguous polymeric device, the solid matrix also disintegrates into granules, and these granules deaggregate in turn into fine particles. Disintegration, deaggregation, and dissolution may occur simultaneously with the release of a drug resulting in the formation of a solution of the drug in the medium of dissolution. If the excipients used in the manufacture of the dosage form are water soluble, at the end of dissolution study, a clear solution may result. If the excipients are not water soluble, these would be floating and then there is a chance of interruption in the dissolution study. If the drug is poorly soluble then the amount of dissolution medium may not be sufficient. In addition, to maintain the sink condition the dissolution medium may need to have specific modification tailored according to the needs of the drug. In all the three cases, the solution is filtered and submitted for the assay. However, when Noyes and Whitney proposed their theory and in the subsequent modifications, the data was obtained from a solid drug and thus the second situation is ruled out and only the first and third observations are possible.

Noyes and Whitney proposed the rate at which a solid dissolves in a solvent in quantitative terms in 1897 and several other workers elaborated this equation subsequently. The currently used equation could be written as

$$\frac{dM}{dt} = \frac{DS\,(Cs - C)}{h}$$

or

$$\frac{dC}{dt} = \frac{DS\,(Cs - C)}{Vh}$$

where M is the mass of solute dissolved in time t, dM/dt is the mass rate of dissolution, D is the diffusion coefficient of the solute in solution, S is the surface area of the exposed solid, h is the thickness of the diffusion layer, Cs is the solubility of the solid, i.e., concentration of a saturated solution of the compound at the temperature of the experiment, and C is the concentration of solute at time t. The quantity dC/dt is the dissolution rate and V is the volume of the solution.

This equation and the derivation holds true for every drug in a suitable dissolution study design.

During its derivation, it was assumed that a solid substance is surrounded by an aqueous diffusion layer or stagnant liquid film of thickness h exists at the surface of a solid undergoing dissolution. This thickness h represents a stationary layer of solvent in which the solute molecules exist in concentrations from Cs to C. Beyond the static diffusion layer, at x greater than h, mixing occurs in the solution, and the drug is found at a uniform concentration, C, through out the bulk phase. At the solid surface-diffusion layer interface, x=0, the drug in the solid is in equilibrium with drug in the diffusion layer. The gradient, or change in concentration with distance across the diffusion layer, is constant. This gradient is represented in the equations and by the term (Cs-C)/h. In the calculations of diffusion coefficient and the dissolution rate constant, the above equations are used. In particular, the Noyes-Whitney equation illustrates that one of the main factors determining the rate of dissolution is drug solubility. According to this equation, it is understood that *in vivo* the dissolution process may become the rate-limiting step if the rate of solution is much slower than the rate of absorption. This would be the case when the drug in question has a very low solubility at both gastric and intestinal pH. This situation has been observed and noted over several years. For the interested reader, the very basic derivations and the problems associated with the calculations would be demonstrated in very standard textbooks like Martin`s Physical Pharmacy or other relevant publications from the literature. With the release of these fundamental theories, dissolution testing has progressed. However, any modifications made in this area by any pharmacopoeia in any edition, these fundamental laws hold true.

Powder dissolution: The Hixson-Crowell Cube Root Law

Dissolution phenomenons have been studied in a quantitative manner for more than a century. This has been published and reported as very fundamental laws and modified several times. As mentioned before one of the fundamental laws of dissolution testing is Noyes-Whitneys equation. However, this is not derived for all occasions of dissolution testing. The equation is applicable when the surface area of dissolution is constant. This is not always the case and is more profoundly not true in the case of disintegrating tablets as mentioned before. The dissolution of solid particles as is the case very common with disintegrating tablets. This dissolution is more complicated than that of constant surface area tablets because of surface area and/or shape changes during dissolution. Although particle dissolution models have been developed, discrepancies between the theory and the experimental data are present. However, one of the very ideal and commonly used theories is Hixson-Crowell cube root law.

Two steps are involved in solid particle dissolution: the first step is the detachment of molecules from the solid surface to form hydrated molecules at the solid-liquid interface; the second step is the mass transport from this interface to the bulk solution. Most dissolution processes are controlled by the second step, which is diffusion-convection-controlled. As mentioned before Noyes-Whitneys equations and its modification consider a stagnant diffusion layer around a drug particle and the diffusion across this layer is the rate-limiting step for dissolution. Although, this is not practically the case, this allows complex dissolution process to be analyzed in a tractable fashion. However, in practical picture, this layer need not be stagnant and could be a hydrodynamic boundary, which has a velocity as well as concentration gradient. The more turbulence at the boundary layer, the more is the use of this equation for dissolution rather than Noyes-Whitneys equation.

For a drug powder consisting of uniformly sized particles, an equation that is derived to express the rate of dissolution is based on the cube root of the weight of the particles. In this situation, the radius of the particles is not assumed to be constant. The dissolution profile is mathematically derived using The Hixson-Crowell Cube Root Law. Its derivation and several similar laws could be looked in various references and not detailed here. However, according to this equation,

$$M_0^{1/3} - M^{1/3} = Kt$$

Where

$$K = [N\rho(\pi/6]^{1/3}\ [2kCs]/(\rho)$$

$$= [[M_o]^{1/3}/d]*2kCs/\rho$$

Mo is the original mass of the drug particles and k is the cube root dissolution rate constant.

Surface renewal and limited solvation theories

The **surface renewal theory** assumes equilibrium at the solute-solution interface is attained and that the rate limiting step in the dissolution process is mass transport. The model is thought as of being continually exposed to fresh dissolution medium. The agitating medium consists of numerous eddies or packets into which the solute diffuses and is carried to the bulk medium, thereby getting separated from the drug and the dosage form. Due to turbulence at the surface of the solute, there is no boundary layer and therefore no stagnant film layer. In other words the surface is continually being replaced with fresh medium.

The equation that depicts dissolution in surface renewal theory is

$$V\ dc/dt = dW/dt = S(\gamma D)^{1/2}\ (Cs - Ct)$$

Where V is the volume of the dissolution medium; S is the surface area; D is the diffusion coefficient; Cs is the equilibrium drug constant and Ct is the drug concentration at time t.

The **limited solvation theory** predicts that a crystal undergoes dissolution through an interfacial process in the dissolving medium. The true surface area of the crystal must be considered since each face of the crystal may have different interfacial barrier. Hence each surface may provide a different contribution to the dissolution process. Thus, the drug release from each of these crystal forms of the drug is different from the different drug-formulation pairs and is contributed as the formulation in the continuous process drugs level.

$$G = K_I (Cs\text{-}Ct)$$

Where G is the dissolution rate per unit area; K_I is the effective interfacial transport constant; Cs is the equilibrium drug concentration; and Ct is the drug concentration at time t.

Theories of Dissolution Profile Analysis

Some of the prominent dissolution profile analysis include Wagner's, Kitazawa`s, El-Yazigi's and Carstensen's theory. Owing to the complexity of El-Yazigi`s and Cartensen`s theory, they are not discussed in detail here. The other two theories are further elaborated.

Wagners theory

According to the Wagner`s theory, the percent dissolved value at a certain time may be equivalent to the percentage surface area generated. Based on this principle the percent dissolved-time plots of tablets and capsules are plotted. These plots basically follow apparent first-order kinetics under sink conditions. Dissolution does not come into picture. In case of exponential decrease in surface area with time, the first-order kinetics could be related to dissolution data.

$$\text{Log}\,(W^{\infty} - W) = \text{Log}\,m - Ks/2.303\,(t - t^{\infty})$$

Where $M = (K)/(KsCsS^{\circ})$

Where,

W^{∞} = amount of drug in solution at infinity time

$W^{\infty} - W$ = amount of undissolved drug

K = first-order dissolution constant

Cs = aqueous solubility of the drug

Ks = dissolution rate constant

S° = surface area at time t°

Kitazawa theory

Kitazawa in 1977, using uncoated caffeine tablets of four different hardnesses, tested the dissolution rate of the drug by the Sartorius (S.S. method) and by the rotating basket method of the U.S.P. XVIII. They found that in both the methods the dissolution rate decreased with increasing hardness, and the rate obtained with the S.S. method was always less than that by the U.S.P. method. When they tried to correlate the data with the differences in the volume they were not able to comprehend. In addition, it was difficult to ensure that the characteristic changes in the process of dissolution paralleled the curves obtained from a plot of % caffeine dissolved vs time. However, they showed that biphasic straight lines were obtained when ln Cs/(Cs-C) vs. t was plotted. The first segment was due to the tablet disintegration or the disruption of the capsule shell, while the second segment was obtained from this point onward to the end of the dissolution. In 1987, Igwilo and Pilpel used Kitazawa equation in the analysis of the dissolution process of tablets produced from lactose powder coated with paraffin. Using this analysis, they suggested either an initial breaking of the tablets into particles that subsequently break down into smaller particles or a progressive breaking of the tablet into smaller particles. The former produces a change in rate constant from k_1 to k_2. Kitazawa\` concentration equation upon multiplication by volume the concentration terms were changed to weight as depicted in the equation below and is used in dissolution analysis. However, this theory was criticized and thus the conclusions should be carefully drawn, since it assumed a sudden increase in surface area rather than a continuous change. In either case, the data has to be carefully interpreted with coordinative conclusions using Wagners derivations to be on the safer side.

$$\ln W^{\infty}/(W^{\infty}-W) = k`t$$

k\` is the dissociation constant

W^{∞} is the amount of the drug in the infinite time

W^{∞}-W is the amount of the undissolved drug

El-Yazigi\`s and Cartensen\`s theory

The major difference between the approach of El-Yazigi and Kitazawa is that the former treats disintegration and dissolution as two kinetically distinct processes. The application of the equations in Cartensens approach generated curves that had skewed S shapes and followed Weibull or log-normal distributions when the percent dissolved was plotted against time. This may be attributed to the initial lag phase in the dissolution process (also expected from the proposed theory in terms of the time-dependent phases of disintegration, escape of particles through the basket, and dissolution of initial particles).

Theory

Before a drug is approved to use in humans for treatment of a specific disorder, it must undergo entensive studies to establish its efficacy and safety. Subsequently, a suitable formulation is prepared and is tested for preclinical, clinical and market potentialities. One main part of testing the efficacy of a formulation is the investigation of the appropriate dissolution of the drug from the dosage forms. Since very number of drugs are currently placed into the body by different routes of administration, the release of the drug from these dosage forms has to be thoroughly investigated as closely simulate as possible the *in vivo* situation. The need is the therapeutic efficacy and not utopian formulation development. Once a delivery system is placed in the body, the drug is slowly released as per the formulation. In the system the main factor that influences the therapeutic efficacy is the amount of the active drug. This is mainly controlled by metabolism of the drug in the system. Dissolution tests definitely indicate the amount of the drug released into the system. Thus, although the active drug is the key definitely it is the release from the formulation that indirectly controls the efficacy. In this regard, dissolution is the first investigation. Several theories, models, methods are currently available. Many of these basics are discussed in this chapter. However, keeping in view the transitional state of drug development at this time, it is better to slightly introduce to may be most likely direction this field may proceed in near future. The current transition is from oral route in the form of very conventional dosage forms to the several other routes of administration along with the introduction of several novel dosage forms. Thus, one factor or one direction that could be introduced at this stage would be metabolism control that may be mostly the main reason for the lack of *in vitro- in vivo* correlation however best the *in vitro* dissolution model would be. One way of doing this would be to add metabolic enzymes to the dissolution medium and investigate the dissolution in tandem with metabolism. The other way would be the use of microbial metabolism to simulate the body conditions with regard to the amount of active drug in the system. This area is still new on these lines. However keeping in view this field's likely direction, a brief introduction at this juncture would be essential.

Metabolism (biotransformation) can be defined as enzymatic conversion of natural and chemically synthesized product, into substance having specifically modified structure. Drug metabolism is generally considered as a detoxification process leading to the formation of more polar substances, which are easily excreted from the organism. Interestingly, in some cases, the metabolism of a drug can lead to the formation of pharmacological or toxicological active compound. Hence, the understanding of drug metabolism plays an important role in the development of new drug entities. In addition, this would also be of definite help with other studies such as dissolution as well as formulation development. Controlling this factor in dissolution investigation *in vitro*, *in situ* and *in vivo* would be very essential. Generally, metabolic studies are carried out on codified animal models, perfused organs and cell cultures. Microbial models may constitute an alternative or at least a complement to the use of animal systems, provided they can mimic the mammalian metabolism and afford any relevant information about the metabolic fate of the drug. Such methodology would have the advantage of reducing the demand for animals, particularly in the early phases of drug development. Initially microbial transformation of drugs, particularly steroids and antibiotics were performed in an effort to obtain more active or less toxic substances. These studies paved a way to the initiation of so called "Microbial models of mammalian metabolism" in the mid 1970s and "Use of microorganisms for the study of drug metabolism in the mid 1980s. Since then there have been several reviews and updates on this topic. Presently this concept is in use with the same intention to obtain more active or less toxic substances and some selective conversions of compounds to useful derivatives. In addition the same models could be used to study drug dissolution in the system by various dosage forms by various routes of administration. This small addition would definitely help scientists proceeding in the direction of new concepts of dissolution testing and thus were introduced at this place.

Purpose

Dissolution tests are one of the tests most used in the characterization of drugs and in the quality control of dosage forms. During the late 1960s it became recognized that dissolution data should be determined by studying the rate at which dosage forms allow their formulated drug to dissolve. Subsequently, dissolution tests for six products were introduced into the USP 18 (1969). This increased to about 600 tests in the USP 24, which also includes drug-release requirements for modified release products and transdermal dosage forms.

Although dissolution tests are mainly used as quality control methods to ensure end-product or batch-to-batch consistency and to identify good and bad formulations, dissolution data may also be correlated with *in vivo* activity. Dissolution tests become especially important if dissolution is the rate-limiting step in drug absorption. Dissolution tests are, therefore, used to confirm compliance with compendial specifications and are needed as part of a product licence application. Additionally they are used during product development and stability testing as part of the specification for the product. No universal dissolution test has been designed that gives the same rank order for *in vitro* dissolution and *in vivo* bioavailability from different formulations and batches.

In vitro dissolution testing is important for a number of reasons including,

1. Product optimization.
2. Performance of manufacturing process.
3. Bioequivalence of drugs.
4. Regulatory market entrance of products.
5. *In vitro-In vivo* correlations

Failed dissolution tests resulted in 14 product recalls (18% of non-manufacturing recalls for oral solid dosages) in 1999, and 20 product recalls in 2000 (24% of non-manufacturing recalls for oral solid dosages) were attributed to dissolution failure. Clearly, failure of a dissolution test can have significant financial ramifications for a pharmaceutical company and thus it is highly desirable to avoid such failures, especially if a failure is because of flaws in dissolution methods and unrelated to actual product performance. On the other hand, with the introduction of new very low soluble and potent molecules, the FDA requirements on dissolution tests would definitely become more stringent. In addition, the differences in physical dimensions of drug products, different release mechanisms, the environment of the release of the drug, would affect the release profile of the drug. Subsequently, rigorous dissolution testing becomes very essential. The physics of dissolution apparatus and the physico-chemical properties of the drug substance and the dosage form would govern the dissolution. Thus, a thorough understanding of these concepts would be essential for optimum dissolution testing.

Testing Methods

Most of the world's pharmacopeias currently require dissolution testing as a standard testing for pharmaceutical products as tablets or capsules. Dissolution testing is currently a requirement by US Food and Drug Administration (FDA). The standards for testing are put forth by the United States Pharmacopoeia (USP). The testing procedures are described in USP General chapters under dissolution <711> and Drug Release <724>. According to the requirement, these tests offer a variety of dissolution testing equipment and testing conditions. Generally, a typical buffer solution or a hydrochloric acid (HCl) solution is used as dissolution medium. The solutions are used with either basket apparatus also called as USP Apparatus 1, or a paddle apparatus also called as USP Apparatus 2. The basket speed is 100 rpm and the paddle speed is 50 rpm. For estimating dissolution, the samples are usually collected at 15, 30, 45, and 60 minutes when testing immediate-release products. The compendial time points are usually a single point of either 30 or 45 minutes.

As the complexity of the dosage forms increases-through changes in the solubility, changes in the release characteristics, or both – the traditional dissolution conditions are becoming more invalid. Currently, several thorough investigations are performed to evaluate dissolution suitable to a particular drug and a dosage form. Examples of such measures include using a surfactant in the dissolution media, changing the paddle or basket speed, and making the test apparatus more specialized. Several other methods of dissolution studies are investigated currently as per the USP, with the two older methods very commonly used. Blundered results may be obtained and may lead to product drop out in the case of unsuitable testing methods. Developing dissolution test procedures for new products is a continuous challenge, especially when the drug is poorly soluble in aqueous media. Keeping pace with new product developments requires the guidance and education provided by standards groups, regulatory agencies, associations and working groups, publications and websites. In the USA, the main regulatory bodies are USP and FDA. Since most of the other pharmacoepias are the copies of the USP and FDA formats and follow most of these body's modifications, the recent agendas in this area are discussed further.

Calibrator Tablets

Calibrator tablets are very often used in the calibration of dissolution equipment. There are many factors that will cause a dissolution analysis to give incorrect or errant results. Most dissolution apparatus will not pass calibration unless all conditions are optimal in the apparatus, the standards, the media, and the calibrator tablets. Therefore, it is possible to narrow down all possible causes of failure to only few conditions. The apparatus calibration and the standards verification that could also be called validation of the dissolution testing equipment are described later. However, very routinely calibration tablets are used to calibrate the equipment in a lab and to confirm that everything is proper before a dissolution experiment is conducted. As mentioned before, three calibrator tablets were proposed and used by USP. These are prednisone (disintegrating), salicylic Acid (non-disintegrating) and nitrofurantoin (disintergrating).

USP Modifications

Dissolution testing of the USP standards, the alterations and modifications that took over the past 20 years are required to be specifically addressed when dissolution testing is discussed. These changes were adopted as per the concerns of pharmaceutical manufacturers and the FDA. The USP is continuously revising the standards of dissolution testing and there are many recent changes. In one of the recent USP conventions held in 2000, the following were the resolutions that addressed dissolution testing:

1. To encourage USP to expand on-going harmonization in consultation with US FDA, Japanese Pharmacopoeia, European Pharmacopoeia and the pharmacopoeias of the Americas.
2. Concurrent coordination of biopharmaceutic principles with dissolution tests to ensure equivalent performances of immediate and modified release pharmaceutical products, taking into account their regulatory control.
3. Establish training programs to support appropriate use of the USP/National Formulary (NF) standards and compendial methods.

FDA Modifications

Further, the last 10 years of FDA decisions and requirements regarding the changes and alterations in dissolution testing needs to be mentioned too. These major guidelines are related to

1. Dissolution testing of immediate release solid oral dosage forms
2. Extended release dosage forms: development, evaluation, and application of *in vitro/in vivo* correlations
3. Waiver of *in vivo* bioavailability and bioequivalence studies for immediate release solid oral dosage forms based on biopharmaceutics classification system
4. SUPAC-IR: Immediate release solid oral dosage forms: scale-up and post approval changes: chemistry, manufacturing, and controls, *in vitro* dissolution testing, and *in vivo* bioequivalence documentation
5. SUPAC-MR: Modified release solid oral dosage forms: scale up and postapproval changes: chemistry, manufacturing, and controls, *in vitro* dissolution testing and *in vivo* bioequivalence documentation

A few of the contributions, meetings, publications will be mentioned hence forth that are of worth for the reader to keep pace of this continuous quest to obtain ideal dissolution testing methods. The associations include American Association of Pharmaceutical Scientists (AAPS), Pharmaceutical Research and Manufacturers of America (PhRMA) Dissolution Committee, publications include Dissolution Technologies, New Dissolution Technology and the Internet sites include Dissolution Discussion Group (DDG) and Dissolution Solutions.

Factors Influencing the Dissolution Testing

The factors influencing the dissolution testing include:

- Dissolution media
    - Dissolved gas
    - Dearating media
    - PH
    - Volume
    - Temperature
    - Sink conditions
    - Dissolution media composition
- Hydrodynamic factors

Dissolution Media

The truth is that dissolution media is more important than other factors that affect the dissolution study and hence has been researched for over several years with the introduction of several new kinds of dissolution media apart from distilled water or 0.1 N hydrochloric acid that were routinely used while in the initial stages. However, at this time, different media tailored according to the needs of the new drug candidate and the formulation are placed securely in the pharmacopoeia. The plans of media changes are very routinely under scrutiny by FDA, USP and other regulatory agencies and are routinely published. Some of the media considerations are henceforth discussed here.

Dissolved Gas

Liquids are in equilibrium with surrounding gas at the gas-liquid interface. At a given temperature and pressure, a portion of the gas is dissolved in the liquid. The amount of dissolved gas in equilibrium decreases substantially as the temperature increases. The equilibrium value of oxygen in water (measured in mg/L), for example, drops from 8.74 at room temperature (22°C) to 7.31 at 32°C and 6.73 at 37°C; i.e., 100% saturation at room temperature increases to 120% at 32°C and 130% at 37°C, the specified dissolution temperatures. The excess from this super-saturation accumulates as minute bubbles in the media. This release of dissolved gas is one of the more annoying variables responsible for distorted dissolution data in all specified or proposed dissolution apparatus. Scientists at National Center for Drug Analysis (NCDA) state that a silvery appearance occasionally arising on the flask, rotating shaft, or basket or paddle is a warning of the release of dissolved gases that may disturb the test. The silvery appearance is a result of microscopic air or gas bubbles released as the medium adjusts to equilibrium with the gas. Such a phenomenon provides a warning to check deaeration methods and the influence of the released gas on the dissolution rate of the test under observation.

One may speculate about the many ways in which released gas can affect dissolution, but most probably the small bubbles interfere with fluid dynamics and the area of the liquid-solid interface. The bubbles may attach to the rotating basket or the screen in the reciprocating cylinder thereby altering the effective porosity. They may accumulate on or in filters or the glass beads of the flow-through apparatus, affecting the flow rate. They may accumulate in flow cells, where they could interfere with absorbance measurements. They may attach to aggregates from disintegrating dosage forms, changing their effective liquid-solid interface and flow patterns in Apparatus 1 and 2. They may accumulate on the membranes in transdermal or percutaneous absorption tests.

Deaerating media

Release of dissolved gases could be prevented if the concentration of gases is kept below the saturation value of the media during the test. To avoid problems, a value at least 5% below saturation at the operating temperature should be provided. A crude method in use at some laboratories involves filling the flasks with media at a temperature of 40°C and operating the stirring device until the temperature reaches the prescribed 37°C. This provides a 5% margin below saturation.

pH

Media composition is specified in individual monographs. If not, the general requirement is distilled water. Unbuffered media may vary in pH. Checks on pH in the authors laboratory suggest usual levels of pH 6.0 for distilled water, pH 6.6 for deionized water (deareated or not), and pH 7.2 for distilled water deaerated by boiling. Variations in dissolution rate at different pH levels is to be expected if the drug has a steep pH/solubility curve, but the pH/solubility curve of various excipients should not be overlooked. Shortening or lengthening the disintegration and deaggregation lag periods can exert significant effect on the dissolution rate, even for drugs with relatively flat pH/solubility characteristics. Absorbance sometimes may vary with pH. If the pH is changed during the test, e.g., in studying delayed release, the standard should be checked at each pH used. If pH varies significantly, analysts should use multiple standards.

Volume

It is elementary, of course, that the volume of medium must be maintained constant. Volume lost from sampling may be corrected in calculations, provided the correction factor is less than 25%. In dissolution tested of extended-release preparations, the volume of samples may exceed this constriction. Sample volumes must therefore be replaced (at the same temperature); automated equipment is available to accomplish this. The amount of liquid lost by evaporation can be considerable and should be checked. In low-humidity environments, up to 15-mL losses from standard dissolution flasks have been measured. Environment should not be over looked. There would be huge alterations in the amount of dissolution fluid retained at the end of dissolution study accomplishment if the evaporation is not properly controlled. The current automatic dissolution testing has suitable curtain-type covers with reciprocating cyclinder and disk equipment with automated sampling that prevents the evaporation of the dissolution medium.

Temperature

Solubility is generally linear with temperature, and sometimes the curve is steep. The effects of temperature variations will, of course, depend upon the temperature/solubility curves of the active ingredient, as well as those of the binders and excipients. Dosage forms may differ widely, ranging as high as 5% change in the dissolution rate per degree Celsius. Because the compendia allow ± 0.5°C tolerances, a considerable variation within this range might be anticipated for some dosage forms. The proposals of the USP Revision Conference (1990) include a requirement to monitor temperature at suitable interval. This can easily be done by automated systems (Zymark, Erweka), and recording devices are available (VanKel, Hanson) that way this would be a routing procedure. When covers are used, there is little substantial differential between the temperature of the contents of glass flasks and the bath temperature. The critical apparatus parameter is therefore consistent temperature at all parts of the bath. This can be held within ± 0.3°C in a properly designed and installed bath and should be a part of every manufacturers warranty.

Sink Conditions

When a low-solubility drug is specified at a dosage level that causes saturation in the dissolution medium, accurate dissolution profiles become difficult or impossible to obtain. In dissolution testing, the rule of thumb has been that sink conditions are approximated if the saturation volume is 5-10 times the test volume. The flow-through cell apparatus provides an infinite or variable sink and is the method of preference in Europe for low-solubility drugs. An alternative apparatus for low-solubility drug testing specifies an increase in the medium volume in Apparatus 1 or 2. A 4-L flask has been used successfully in Europe and North America. Special modifications of Apparatus 1 and 2 for 2- and 4-L flasks are commercially available (Erweka, Hanson, Vankel). Finally, several suggestions have been put forth for media modification in order to increase the solubility of specific dosage forms. The most common uses a surfactant, sodium lauryl sulfate, in small amounts. Some have suggested that this is acceptable procedure because ionic bile salts are a part of the assimilation mechanism of the human. This proposal, therefore, is in harmony with the movement toward better *in vitro - in vivo* correlation in dissolution. The alternate situation, low concentrations of active ingredient but no approach to sink conditions, is a problem with some dosage forms, particularly transdermal and extended-release dosage forms. The test may require a greatly reduced media volume in order to obtain detectable concentrations. Adaptations of a miniaturized basket have been successful. Modifications of Apparatus 1 and 2 have been made for 100- to 200-mL beakers. A more elegant solution, however, is the use of the proposed reciprocating disk or cylinder apparatus using small test tubes for media and a dosage form container in miniature. Volumes as low as 20 ml can be practically achieved by appropriate design of the dissolution apparatus.

Dissolution Media Composition

Dissolution behavior of drugs in some particular cases is affected by the choice of dissolution media. This is especially true when dissolution study is used for predicting the *in vivo* performance of the formulations. Instead of detailing, couple of examples will be illustrated here to better appreciate the use of different media other than the standard medium. Further research in this area could one-day result in having a special media tailored to the needs of individual formulation if required. Galia et al., (1998) investigated the dissolution behavior of two class I drugs acetaminophen and metoprolol, and three class II drugs danazol, mefenamic acid and ketoconazole, using USP Apparatus 2. The following dissolution media were used:

1. Water
2. SGF
3. Milk
4. Simulated Intestinal Fluid without pancreatin (SIFsp)
5. Simulated small intestinal contents in fed state (FeSSIF)
6. Simulated small intestinal contents in fasted state (FaSSIF).

Class I drugs dissolved rapidly in all media tested. Acetaminophen dissolution in milk was slow from one tablet formulation. In all other cases dissolution was more than 85% complete in 15 minutes. The dissolution rate of metoprolol was shown to be dependent on formulation and manufacturing method. One of the three tablet formulations did not meet compendial specifications (80%/30 minutes). Dissolution behavior of class II drugs was greatly affected by choice of medium. Dissolution from a capsule formulation of danazol proved to be dependent on the concentration of solubilizing agents, with a 30-fold increase in percentage dissolved within 90 minutes upon changing from aqueous media without surfactants to FaSSIF. Use of FeSSIF or milk as the dissolution medium resulted in an even greater increase in percentage dissolved, 100 and 180-fold, respectively. Dissolution of the weak acid mefenamic acid from a capsule formulation is dependent on both pH and bile salt concentration. The weak base ketoconazole showed complete dissolution from a tablet formulation in Simulated Gastric Fluid without pepsin (SGFsp) within 30 minutes, 70% dissolution in 2 hours under fed state simulated upper jejunal conditions but only 6% dissolution in 2 hours under fasted state conditions. These results indicated that dissolution of class II drugs proved to be in general much more dependent on the medium than class I drugs. In a different study conducted by Quereshi and Mcgilveray (1999) the dissolution behaviour of two commercially available glibenclamide formulations in biorelevant media and standard media was determined. The purpose was to determine which of the media was ideal for predicting the *in vivo* performance of the two formulations. The dissolution tests were performed using USP 23 apparatus 2, Conventional buffers, USP media and two BDM`s containing different amounts of lecithin and sodium taurocholate were used in the dissolution testing. The dissolution of two drug powders was highly dependent on wetting, particle size, pH, and the composition of the medium used and the dissolution behaviour of the two glibenclamide formulations showed differences in all media tested. A bioequivalence study conducted by the central quality control laboratory of the German pharmacists (ZL) it was found that BDMs are better able to discriminate between glibenclamide formulations than standard dissolution media, suggesting that the choice of the dissolution media is sometimes very important in predicting *in vivo* performance of the formulations from a dissolution test.

Hydrodynamic Factors

One of the first factors that were found to affect the dissolution was hydrodynamics of the dissolution fluid. Most often, this results in an uncontrolled variability, typical of the dissolution testing process, and is likely the result of a small-agitated vessel operated at Reynolds numbers in the transitional regime. Under these conditions flow behavior in stirrer chambers is both time-dependent and strongly heterogeneous. Particularly in the lower parts of the dissolution chamber not much waves are visible and thus these areas are apparently not exposed to the hydrodynamic variability. In these conditions, sampling from these areas result in data variability. Some products that might have been recalled previously would have been the result of these obvious notices observed. Consequently, the hydrodynamics in the vicinity of a tablet in the dissolution device would be both affected by the size and the position of the sample and also is time-dependent. The frequency of these waves affect the shearing of the tablet surface, de-agglomeration of particles, mass transfer from the solid to the liquid, suspension and mixing of the tablet fragments. Occasionally these fluctuations in the results may be because of the immature release during the early sample points that could have been because of uncontrolled scheduled of sampling time points which also is very important in a dissolution study. In addition position of sampling is also very important. As long as these two basic factors are heeded most of the problems associated with dissolution study would be taken care. These are very empirical ideologies about the dissolution study. However, the recent trend is to very carefully dissect the flow patterns, the dimensions of the dissolution apparatus, operating conditions and mathematically correlate these to the release profile. A thorough review on drug release testing was recently published (Kukura et al., 2003). One recent study performed visualization studies with dye released from a non-disintegrating tablet in a rotating basket apparatus to show that shear patterns can be unstable across the surface of a tablet. They also explored the impact of tablet position to further characterize the hydrodynamics within the device.

A computational model was used to aid in the understanding of the hydrodynamics controlling dissolution in the USP Apparatus II. The spatial distribution of the shear forces within the device are calculated from the simulated velocity field to show the direct impact of the hydrodynamics on the boundary layer for dissolution. In addition, targeted experiments are conducted to demonstrate the impact of non-uniform shear forces on dissolution measurements. Dissolution pattern study is definitely not very easy. Currently, very sophisticated instruments are used in the study with these patterns. Previously dye experiments were done over several days by repeated sampling of the dye released. However, this is very tedious and the mathematical analysis is not very often easy. In this particular study, computational fluid dynamics in the dissolution apparatus II were investigated using several software programs. The visualization of the dye movement in the dissolution apparatus was accomplished by planar laser induced fluorescence. Three-dimensional geometry specification and mesh generation are accomplished using ICEM-CFD (ICEM CFD Engineering, Berkeley, CA). The commercially available AcuSolve program (ACUSIM software, Mountain View, CA) is used to solve the algebraic form of the

Reynolds-Averaged Navier Stokes equations at each of the nodes defined by the mesh. This solver uses a Galerkin least-squares finite element formulation that provides second order accuracy. Particle tracking was accomplished using commercially available software provided by Acusim. Subsequent mixing analysis was performed using custom software developed at the Pharmaceutical Engineering Program at Rutgers University.

A planar laser induced fluorescence (pLIF) technique was used in the visualization of the movement of the dye. This technique is a non-intrusive, visual technique that reveals the time evolution of a mixing process. The experimental set up is shown in Figure 1. Fluorescent dye (Rhodamine) is injected in a mixing system and illuminated with a planar laser so that mixing patterns created by the flow can be captured. The density of the dye must be properly matched to the density of the fluid to reveal the flow structures. As mentioned before the movement of the dye was not calculated by doing several day experiments, but were picturized using a camera in a continuous pattern. Images of the illuminated plane are captured using a CCD camera to unveil the emerging mixing patterns. The results of the study indicated well-mixed and poorly-mixed regions in the mixer region. Convection carries dye rapidly to regions where mixing is good while segregated regions of the mixer remain dark for a long time since diffusion is the primary mechanism to bring dye into them. The Flowmap software package with Flow Manager 4.0 (Dantec Dynamics, Mahwah, NJ) was used in the data acquisition and laser/camera synchronization. The results from this study indicated that the shear strain environment in an aqueous media within the USP Apparatus II is highly heterogenous. Changing the agitator speed from 50 to 100 rpm only increases the intensity of the shear force exerted by the fluid but it does not improve the homogeneity of the spatial distribution of shear. Experiments confirm that dissolution rates can vary substantially when tablets experience different shear environments due to their physical location within the device. These results aid in understanding the underlying hydrodynamics within the USP Apparatus II and demonstrate the impact the heterogeneity can have on dissolution measurements. These data help explain many of the problems typically encountered with dissolution testing in the USP Apparatus II.

Naproxen sodium tablets were used for the investigation of the release profile of the drug into the dissolution media in the USP apparatus II. The tablet was placed at two different positions in the dissolution apparatus as indicated in the picture. The medium was agitated at either 50 rpm or 100 rpm. Repeated samples were prepared over a period of 45 minutes with 5 minute regular sampling.

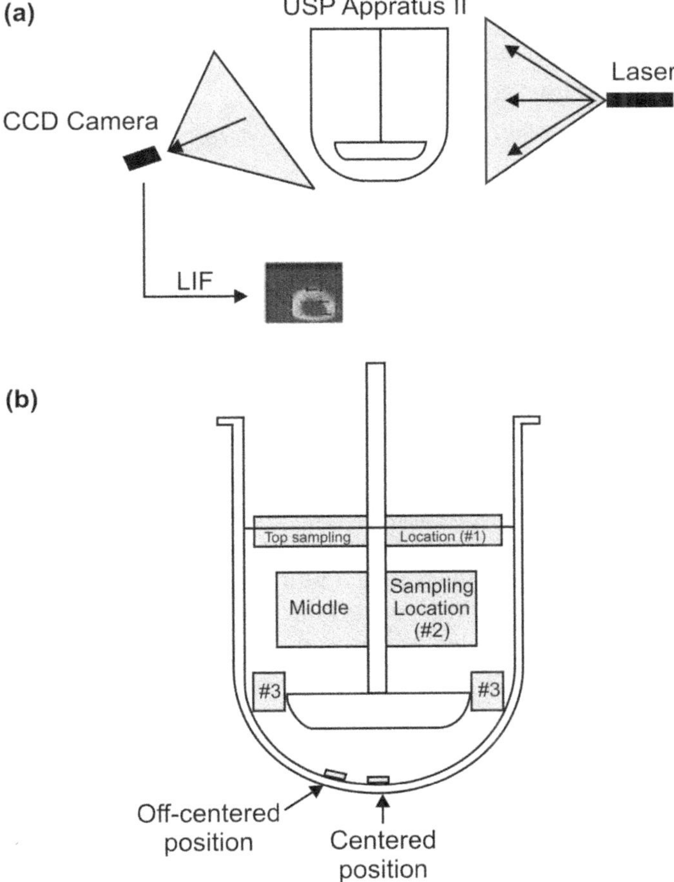

Figure 18.1

The mathematical data was fit and dissolution rates were determined. The results indicated that the dissolution rates are substantially lower for the tablets placed in the centered position than those observed for the case of off-centered tablets. The results in this study indicated that the shear forces exerted at the two tablet locations exhibit a three-fold difference. The impact of such a shear rate difference on dissolution was clearly evident in the experiments. There was also difference in the dissolution pattern with the sampling position. This study thus indicates the importance of hydrodynamics in the dissolution testing process.

Validation of Dissolution Testing Methods

Validation of an *in vitro* dissolution method is essential in

1. providing quality and process control,
2. determining stability of the relevant release characteristics of the product, and
3. facilitating regulatory determinations and judgements concerning formulation and process changes.

With the introduction of several new drugs with very complicated properties and very innovative and control delivery systems, it becomes very essential to device perfect dissolution testing in the very early stages of formulation development. In this respect, validation of the dissolution testing equipment becomes very essential. On the other hand, because of collaborative efforts that are lately very common in formulation development, it becomes imperative for lab-to-lab data reproducibility. In these two respects, the validation of dissolution testing equipment is very essential. As an illustration, couple of examples will be presented henceforth. A collaborative study participated by seven laboratories was carried out to develop a dissolution standard for evaluating vibration levels of dissolution apparatuses using enteric-coated granules of cefalexin (EG). Vibration levels in a dissolution apparatus are very key for reproducibility of the data and to confirm inter lab data. In this respect, dissolution apparatuses could be divided into two groups according to their vibration levels and the dissolution test results of EG by the rotating basket method at 50 rpm. The critical value of acceleration was about 0.05 m/s^2. The upper limit of normal dissolution rates of EG was calculated from the results of the rotating basket method at 50 rpm obtained from low vibration apparatuses. All high vibration apparatuses used in this study were distinguished by the limit from low vibration apparatuses, although current USP calibrators did not distinguish most of them. On some occasions, if it becomes invariable, the dosage forms could be entirely discarded if there are variations in the results due to not validation of the dissolution apparatus. The results from the experiments suggest that EG would be useful as a calibrator for detection of apparatuses on high vibration levels.

In a different experiment, to evaluate variability in drug dissolution testing 28 laboratories analyzed USP calibrators, US FDA prednisone tablets and a marketed glibenclamide tablet product were used. The experiments were conducted using paddle and basket methods at 50 (calibrators) and 75 (glibenclamide) rpm. The media employed were deaerated by equilibrating at 37°C for 24 h and by the USP recommended method. The 95% CI values for percent drug release for the USP calibrator tablets were similar to the reported tolerances for the USP Acceptance Ranges; however, individual results from 15 of 28 laboratories suggest that the apparatus would not comply with the USP

Apparatus Suitability Criteria. For FDA prednisone calibrator tablets, percent drug release using equilibrated medium was different (P=0.003) than by the USP recommended method. For the glibenclamide tablet results, a CV of 14-37% was observed, depending upon the sampling time and the type of apparatus employed. The results indicate that failure to meet the USP Dissolution Apparatus Suitability Test may not truly mean that the apparatus is 'out of compliance'. Due to the high variability in dissolution testing, in many cases the impact of formulation or manufacturing changes on drug release characteristics may not be observed, in particular with multi-point profiles. The calibrator tablets now used in the USP suitability test do not reveal common sources of systematic error associated with Apparatus 2. When the apparatus was operated under conditions near or beyond USP tolerances, changes in the results of the USP calibrators were slight, whereas those of several samples of commercial prednisone tablets were significant. Thus, the USP calibrators and requirements do not guarantee suitability of the equipment for general dissolution testing of drug products. The U.S.P./N.F. dissolution test (method I or rotating basket method) and the rotating flask technique (RESO-TEST dissolution method) were applied to four commercial prolonged release theophylline dosage forms. The dissolution data obtained were converted into dissolution efficiencies and submitted to a correlation analysis, the result of which demonstrates the equivalency of both methods with respect to the characterization of the dissolution behaviour of the dosage forms tested. It is suggested to consider replacement of the official dissolution technique, the shortcomings of which are well-known from the literature, by the rotating flask technique.

Compendial Dissolution Testing Methods

The USP includes seven apparatus designs for drug release and dissolution testing of immediate release and dissolution testing of immediate release oral dosage forms, extended release products, enteric-coated products, and trans-dermal drug delivery devices. In addition, other non-compendial methods are published in literature tailored according to the needs of the scientific endeavor. The compendial methods listed below are briefly discussed henceforth:

1. Rotating Basket Method
2. Paddle Method
3. Flow-Through Methods
4. Reciprocating Cylinder Apparatus
5. Paddle over Disk method
6. Rotating Cylinder method
7. Reciprocating Disk method

Rotating Basket Method (USP Dissolution Apparatus I)

Originally proposed by Pernarowski (1968) and modified to become the first official method adopted in USP XVIII and NF XIII in 1970, the rotating basket method has enjoyed more than 20 years of extensive testing for all types of dosage forms. Essentially, it consists of an approximately 1-in. diameter X 1 3/8-in. high stainless steel, 40-mesh wire basket rotated at a constant speed between 25 and 150 rpm. This method is now (1990) called Apparatus 1 and is illustrated in Figures 3-1 and 3-2. The more significant differences between USP and BP involve the dissolution flask: BP allows a flat-bottomed flask. The rotating basket apparatus is suggested for the European Pharmacopoeia and is included in all proposed or existing pharmacopoeias. The very detailed explanation of this kind of dissolution apparatus is found in the USP. Several modifications are available in rotating basket method and these include the use of gold plating of the baskets, which prevents the corrosion in the presence of 0.1 N HCl as the dissolution medium, basket mesh of sizes 10-, 20-, 30-, and 40-mesh screens in assays of aspirin tablets containing magnesium-aluminium hydroxide in one study to prevent the mesh clogging instead of the regular 40-mesh screen prescribed by the pharmacopoeia. The basket apparatus has been planed and used conveniently for several nonofficial tests that include tests for the release of the drug from suppositories and microencapsulated particles. Very simple modifications were used in these studies. However, these methods are not validated yet and thus are not official. On the other hand they are conveniently used for several dosage forms. The meshes and screens in this study could be used accordingly. These method alterations could be applicable to several other convenient modifications for other kinds of dosage forms also.

The Paddle (USP/NF Apparatus 2) Method

Apparatus 2 commonly known as paddle method, was originally developed by Poole (1969) and was refined by scientists at US FDA. The specifications for Apparatus 2 are identical with those for Apparatus 1 except that the paddle in substituted for the rotating basket. Compendial paddle specifications could be obtained from the latest USP. These specifications have been very widely used till recent times without any changes with the exception of a minor change (1985) in the arc radius that agrees precisely with the geometry of the other paddle dimensions. Some of the dimensions and tolerances for the paddle are critical if consistent results are to be obtained from flask to flask. USP/NF specifies that the paddle must rotate smoothly without significant wobble. The area of the paddle blade creates considerable flow, and wobble has the effect of increasing the angular velocity at the paddle tips in a manner that couples with the fluid much more significantly than would a comparable wobble in the basket. The contours of the paddle blade must not include any sharp edges – at the tips, for instance-that could produce turbulent instead of laminar flow.

Apparatus 3 (Reciprocating Cylinder)

The reciprocating cylinder apparatus is proposed as an alternative method for extended-release dosage forms. The instrumentation is not as complicated and is nicer looking than other dissolution apparatus. The apparatus uses a transparent cylinder capped on each end with a screen. The dosage form is enclosed, and the assembly is gently reciprocating up and down in media contained in a glass tube held in a water bath. The liquid flows through the cylinder, providing a solid-liquid interface shear where dissolution occurs. This apparatus is a modification of the USP/NF disintegration test. It was extensively used in Europe, and published data indicate remarkable correlation with the rotating bottle apparatus. The rotating bottle apparatus does not lend itself to automation and therefore is unsatisfactory for the extended-release dosage forms for which it otherwise is suitable. Apparatus 3 is currently commercially available with 6 columns of 6 rows and software to move from row 1 to row 6 successively with a drain period between each row. The active reciprocating time in each row may be programmed. After removal of the cylinder, samples were taken at a point halfway between the bottom of the tube and surface of the media.

Apparatus 4 (Flow-Through Cell)

Flow through methods involves constraining the dosage form in a cell and pumping dissolution fluid through that cell. This dissolution fluid is collected and assayed for the drug content. Flow dynamics affect the dissolution rate. Consistent and repeatable results will not be obtained with different pumping characteristics during different tests. This technique was developed at Ciba-Geigy in Switzerland under the direction of Dr. F. Langenbucher. It has been extensively evaluated in Europe before introducing as a USP method. The flow rate must be held constant, and, as might be expected, this is a difficult procedure that requires a careful watch involving pump setting, filter pore size, and dosage composition. If the filter clogs, the flow rate is reduced and pump pressure may increase to the point that it damages equipment. Fortunately this variable may be controlled by increasing the filter pore size and thereby reduces the flow rate. The open flow-through method provides a constant contact of fresh media with the dosage form and thus offers an infinite sink. For this reason it is particularly adaptable to testing low-solubility drugs. An easily automated switch of media source provides a change of pH environment without the hot spots that may appear while buffers are added to the media in Apparatus 1 or 2. The advantage of the flow-through method may be decisive when degradation occurs during dissolution, because the dwell time could be held to one minute.

Advantages

The following advantages are offered by the flow through system

1. Infinite sink for low-solubility drugs
2. great ease in precisely changing pH during test, avoiding hot spots that may appear with the basic basket and paddle apparatus
3. minimum dwell time, avoiding problems of degradation products during dissolution procedure
4. open system adaptable to controlled degrees of closed systems
5. easy sampling and automation of data reduction
6. adaptability to current USP calibrators

Disadvantages

The flow-through system entails certain disadvantages

1. large volumes of media are required
2. validation of flow rate during testing is difficult
3. difficulties can arise as a result of clogged filters

Apparatus 5 (Paddle Over Disk)

Apparatus 5 uses the same dissolution equipment as Apparatus 2 (paddle method) with the water bath kept at 32 C. The transdermal patch with the release side up is glued to a screen of inert material that is held at the bottom of the flask by a disk assembly so that the patch is parallel to and 25 ± 5 mm from the bottom of the paddle blade. The details of the disk assembly are not rigidly defined, but a Millipore disk is described as satisfactory. This assembly is limited to patches that can mount inside a diameter of 16 mm. The FDA researchers have suggested a less expensive and more universal disk assembly. It consists of watch glass and a screen held by plastic clips and is commercially available. This apparatus has the advantage of using standard equipment available to most pharmaceutical manufacturers. This method is likely to be further refined as collaborative studies are published.

Rotating Cylinder Apparatus (Apparatus 6)

Listed as Apparatus 4 in USP (1990) and changed to apparatus 6 in USP revision review (1990), this method also uses USP dissolution equipment. A special cylinder is attached to the rotating shaft and can accommodate various sizes of patches. The temperature is held at 32 C. The advantage of apparatus involving paddle over disk and rotating cylinder is that these techniques employ existing USP dissolution equipment. This not only reduces investment but also uses technology for which there is an extended database concerning variables. Most pharmaceutical companies already have dissolution equipment that can be easily adapted. A disadvantage of these methods, however, is the necessary large media volume, resulting in a dilute concentration of released active ingredient, which in turn complicates analysis. The long dwell time in the dissolution medium further increases the probability of degradation products. The reciprocating disk apparatus eliminates each of these problems.

Reciprocating Disk (Apparatus 7)

The reciprocating disk was listed as Apparatus 5 in USP (1990) and was changed to Apparatus 7 in USP revision. The proposed USP revision suggests this apparatus is also suitable for solid oral dosage forms. This technique was originated in Alza Corporation (Palo Alto, California, USA). In the reciprocating disk method, patches are attached to vertical holders that reciprocate up and down through a suggested stroke of 1.9 cm at a rate of 30 cycles/min, which is similar to the USP disintegration apparatus. Each patch reciprocates in a separate vessel for a prescribed period of time and then is transferred to a fresh vessel periodically during the test. A succession of tubes is analyzed for the released ingradient. An obvious advantage of this method is a convenient selection of solvent volume in order to maximize concentrations that could be analyzed accurately at the same time that optimum sink conditions are maintained. Further it allows test protocols that minimize dwell time in the media and hence reduce the probability of degradation products. Finally, by the nature of the instrumentation design, it is especially adaptable to massive sample treatment and automated control and sampling. The disadvantage of the reciprocating disk method is that it requires an investment in dissolution equipment that is totally different from the standard devices already in the possession of most pharmaceutical laboratories.

Non-Compendial Dissolution Testing Methods

Tracking of dissolution from different dosage forms is some times not possible with the already available compendial methods. In these situations, several companies and authors have designed non-compendial dissolution testing methods. These several non-compendial dissolution testing methods along with the already official compendial methods are routinely published in the literature. Very few of these are discussed briefly henceforth. These non-compendial methods some time become difficult to predict even after proper tracking and the availability of ample literature. Thus, definitely there is a limitation of the number of non-compendial methods. These methods could not be random and thus optimization of these methods also becomes important. These non-compendial methods include methods to determine percutaneous absorption of transdermal patches, dissolution of drugs from ointments, implants, and microparticles and dissolution of drugs from sustained release dosage forms. The techniques also are modified according to the needs of several other dosage forms depending on the convenience and suitability. Several methods are published in the literature. However, only a few important techniques are discussed here.

Percutaneous Absorption Techniques

Percutaneous absorption is related to the absorption across the skin. Percutaneous absorption methods are currently used to study transfer kinetics through membranes. These are useful for testing membrane characteristics and studying absorption through the skin. These techniques are popular in testing patch dosage forms. The patch is generally mounted in the same position as the simulated skin membrane and serves as the donor side of the system. Some of the techniques that are used in percutaneous absorption measurements include the side-by-side cell, the franz cell and the flow-through cell design. Currently, automating percutaneous absorption study systems are available in the market.

Rotating Bottle Method for Sustained Release Dosage Forms

This is probably the oldest dissolution apparatus used for solid dosage forms. However, it was used only lately for the dissolution investigations of sustained release dosage forms. The system consists of 12 small bottles attached to a horizontal shaft that rotates at a slow speed of 6-50 rpm. The whole assembly is placed in a constant water bath. Each bottle contains 60 mL of dissolution fluid that is decanted through a 40-mesh screen after each sampling period and is replaced by fresh fluid.

Dialysis Systems

In the case of very poorly soluble drugs, where perfect sink conditions would necessitate a huge volume of solvents with conventional methods, a different approach, utilizing dialysis membranes, was tried as a selective barrier between the fresh solvent compartment and the cell compartment containing the dosage form. The method however introduces its own arbitrary parameters that affect the dissolution process, and, therefore, has never gained enough acceptances to qualify as a principal alternate method for solid dosage forms. However, it has been used with some success in case of other dosage forms such as suspensions, creams and ointments.

In vitro Release of Drugs from Suppositories

Fortunately or unfortunately, no single ideal method has been used in the study of dissolution of drugs from suppositories. Many of the official compendial methods have been used for investigating the release of drugs from suppositories. Both dialysis and direct contact procedures have been used, with several modifications. Plaxco, et al., used dialyzing bags made from cellophane dialysis tubing tied with cotton thread and soaked overnight in distilled water before use. After rinsing each bag thoroughly, a certain volume of distilled water was introduced into the bag that was then placed in a wide-mouthed bottle containing a known volume of distilled water. The bottle was kept in a water bath at 39°C. The water in the bottle was mixed slowly using a magnetic stirrer. This prevents the water from evaporation or dripping outside. The bag size affects the dissolution. The smaller the bag, the greater is it unfit for dissolution testing and eventually not included in the compendial dissolution testing, respectfully. One suppository was suspended in each bag so as to have the level of the water inside even with the level of water outside the bag. The water in the bottle was mixed slowly using a magnetic stirrer. A sample was withdrawn from the bottle at fixed intervals and assayed for the drug. The sample could be filtered prior to the assay to get perfect data.

In Vitro In Vivo Correlation

In vitro dissolution is one of the vital tools for characterisation of biopharmaceutical quality of a dosage form at different stages of drug development. *In vitro* dissolution data helps in the evaluation and interpretation of possible risks especially in the modified release dosage form and the food effects on bioavailability that influence the gastrointestinal conditions. It also plays a great role while assessing changes in the manufacturing process. However none of these purposes will be fulfilled by *in vitro* dissolution testing without sufficient knowledge of its *in vivo* relevance. IVIVC have been defined in many ways and have been a subject to much controversy. A meaningful correlation must be quantitative so as to allow interpolation between data thus making the *in vitro* model predictive. IVIVC also ensures batch to batch consistency in the physiologic performance of a drug product.

USP defined five levels of correlation each of which denotes the ability to predict *in vivo* response of a dosage form from its *in vitro* property. Higher the level better is the correlation. The level of correlation is categorised as:

Level A Correlation

Among all the level of correlation defined, level A is of prime importance. It is defined as a hypothetical model describing the relationship between a fraction of drug absorbed and fraction of drug dissolved. In order to develop a correlation between two parameters one variable should be common between them. The data available is *in vitro* dissolution profile and *in vivo* plasma drug concentration profile whose direct comparison is not possible. To have a comparison between these two data, data transformation is required. The *in vivo* properties like percent drug dissolved or fraction of drug dissolved can be used while *in vivo* properties like percent drug absorbed or fraction of drug absorbed can be used respectively. It is considered as a predictive model for relationship between the entire *in vitro* release time courses. Most commonly a linear correlation exists but sometimes non-linear *In vitro- in vivo* correlation may prove appropriate. However, no formal guidance for non-linear IVIVC has been established.

When *in vitro* curve and *in vivo* curve are super imposable, it is said to be 1:1 relationship, while if scaling factor is required to make the curve super imposable, then the relationship is called point-to-point relationship. Level A correlation is the highest level of correlation and most preferred to achieve; since it allows bio waiver for changes in manufacturing site, raw material suppliers, and minor changes in formulation.

Level B Correlation

Here the mean *in vitro* dissolution time (MDT) is compared with either the mean *in vivo* residence time (MRT) or mean *in vivo* dissolution time derived by using principle of statistical moment analysis. Though it utilizes all *in vitro* and *in vivo* data, it is not considered as point-to-point correlation since number of *in vivo* curves can produce similar residence time value. Hence, it becomes least useful for regulatory purposes.

Level C Correlation

It is referred as single point correlation which is established in between one dissolution parameter (t50%) and one of the pharmacokinetic parameter (tmax, Cmax or AUC). However, it does not reflect the complete shape of plasma drug concentration time curve, which is the critical factor that defines the performance of a drug product. Level C correlation is helpful in early stages of development when pilot formulations are being selected.

Multiple Level C Correlation

It refers to the relationship between one or several pharmacokinetic parameters of interest and amount of drug dissolved at several time point of dissolution profile. It should be based on at least three dissolution time points that includes early, middle and late stage of dissolution profile.

Level D Correlation

It is a semi quantitative and rank order correlation and is not considered useful for regulatory purpose.

Predictability of Correlation

It can be calculated by Prediction error that is the error in prediction of *in vivo* property from *in vitro* property of drug product. Based on therapeutic index of the drug and application of IVIVC, evaluation of prediction error internally or externally may be appropriate. Internal error provides a basis for acceptability of model while external validation is superior and affords greater confidence in model. The % prediction error can be calculated by the following equation:

% Prediction error (P.E) = (C_{max} observed – C_{max} predicted) × 100/C_{max} observed

Reasons for Poor *In Vitro-In Vivo* Correlation

When *in vivo* dissolution is not the rate limiting pharmacokinetic stage, and when no *in vitro* test can simulate the drug dissolution along the gastrointestinal tract.

Study design: With inappropriate *in vitro* test conditions.

Dosage form: When the drug release is not controlled by the dosage form or is strongly affected by the stirring of synthetic liquid.

Drug substance: With a non- linear pharmacokinetics, for e.g, first-pass hepatic effect, an absorption window, a chemical degradation and a large inter or intra subject variability.

All these factors are of vital concern and should be kept in mind, especially the inter variability of patients' response to a drug.

Conclusions

Dissolution testing is a key aspect in pharmaceutical formulation development. It is an important step in all the stages of formulation development of new chemical entities and the development of generic formulations. Several compendial methods are used in the dissolution investigations of dosage forms. However, tailored to the needs, new dissolution methods are routinely investigated and introduced. The very important steps in the development of a dissolution test are measurement of the intrinsic dissolution rate, selection of a dissolution apparatus and dissolution data handling. In these experiments, different methods both compendial and noncompendial are routinely used. However, dissolution is a vast area and the current section of this textbook deals with very fundamentals of dissolution testing.

Questions for Practice and Exercise

1. Briefly introduce dissolution testing.
2. Define USP, BP, JP and FDA. Give a brief description of each of these?
3. What is a compendial method? What is a non-compendial method?
4. Write a brief history of dissolution testing?
5. Explain various theories of dissolution.
6. How is dissolution profile analysis performed?
7. What are the different factors that affect the dissolution testing?
8. What is a sink condition? Explain its significance.
9. Write a brief note on each of the following:
    (a) purpose of dissolution testing,
    (b) different dissolution testing methodologies,
    (c) calibrator tablets,
    (d) USP methods of dissolution,
    (e) FDA modification of dissolution testing,
    (f) compendial methods of dissolution, and
    (g) noncompendial methods of dissolution.
10. Write notes on in vitro in vivo correlations.

References

1. Galia E, Nicolaides E, Horter D, Lobenberg R, Reppas C, Dressman JB. Evaluation of various dissolution media for predicting in vivo performance of class I and II drugs. Pharm Res. 1998 May; 15(5):698-705.
2. Qureshi SA, McGilveray IJ. Typical variability in drug dissolution testing: study with USP and FDA calibrator tablets and a marketed drug (glibenclamide) product. Eur J Pharm Sci. 1999 Feb;7(3):249-58.

3. Kukura J, Arratia PE, Szalai ES, Muzzio FJ. Engineering tools for understanding the hydrodynamics of dissolution tests. Drug Dev Ind Pharm. 2003 Feb; 29(2): 231-9. Review.

4. Plaxco JM Jr, Free CB Jr, Rowland CR. Effect of some nonionic surfactants on the rate of release of drugs from suppositories. J Pharm Sci. 1967 Jul; 56(7): 809-14.

Bibliography

1. The Theory and Practice of Industrial Pharmacy, Third Edition, Edited by Leon Lachman, Herbert A. Lieberman, and Joseph L. Kanig, Lea & Febiger Publications, 1986.
2. Physical Characterization of Pharmaceutical Solids (Drugs and the Pharmaceutical Sciences: a Series of Textbooks and Monographs), First Edition, Edited by Harry G. Brittain, Marcel Dekker Inc., 1995.
3. New Drug Development: Regulatory Paradigms for Clinical Pharmacology and Biopharmaceutics (Drugs and the Pharmaceutical Sciences: a Series of Textbooks and Monographs), First Edition, Edited by Chandrahas G. Sahajwalla, Marcel Dekker Inc., 2004.
4. The Practice of Medicinal Chemistry, Second Edition, Edited by Camille Georges Wermuth, Elsevier Publications, 2003.
5. Foye`s Principles of Medicinal Chemistry, Fifth Edition, David A. Williams and Thomas L. Lemke, Lippincott Williams & Wilkins, 2002.
6. Physical Pharmacy: Physical Chemical Principles in the Pharmaceutical Sciences, Third Edition, Alfred Martin, James Swarbrick and Arthur Cammarata, Lea & Febiger Publications, 1983.
7. Pharmaceutical Dosage Forms and Drug Delivery Systems, Seventh Edition, Howard C. Ansel, Loyd V. Allen, Jr., and Nicholas G. Popovich, Lippincott Williams & Wilkins, 1999.
8. Pharmaceutical Salts: Properties, Selection, and Use, First Edition, Edited by P. Heinrich Stahl and Camille G. Wermuth, Wiley VCH, 2002.
9. Handbook of Dissolution Testing, Second Edition, by William A. Hanson, Aster Publication Corporation, 1991.
10. Pharmaceutical Dissolution Testing (Drugs and the Pharmaceutical Sciences: a Series of Textbooks and Monographs), First Edition, by Umesh V. Banakar, Marcel Dekker Publications, 1991.

CHAPTER 19

STATISTICAL QUALITY CONTROL

- **Introduction**
- **Statistical Process Control**
- **Monitoring Industrial Process**
- **Control Charts**
    - Sampling Plans
    - Variables Control Charts
    - Attributes Control Charts
    - Multivariate Control Charts
- **Time Series Analysis**
    - Basic Theory
    - Production Characteristics
    - Analytical Techniques
    - Model Applications
- **Salient Features of Statistical Quality Control**
    - Six Sigma Levels of Quality
    - Zero Defects Quality System
    - House of Quality
    - Scatter Diagrams
- **Marketed Software for Production Statistical Quality Control**
- **Conclusions**

Introduction

The statistical production quality control of the finished products of any type is the main part of a manufacturing facility. In earlier times (1920-1935), when the current techniques and modern concepts were not introduced, production quality was purely determined using the techniques proposed by HF Dodge and HG Romig. Plans for acceptance sampling were developed by these two. Four sets of tables were published in 1940: single sampling lot tolerance tables, double sampling lot tolerance tables, single sampling average outgoing quality limit tables and double sampling average outgoing quality limit tables. The sampling schemes they developed allowed inspectors to do more work with less effort, thus increasing their productivity. Specially trained personnel were employed for these determinations. Some of the examples of such production quality control inspections are performed even today in several fields. Examples include the inspections at Bell Labs or filling machines or automatic packaging, to determine and measure their every day performance. Acceptance sampling is the inspection of a sample from a lot to decide whether to accept that lot. There are two types: attributes sampling and variables sampling. In attributes sampling, the presence or absence of a characteristic is noted in each of the units inspected. In variables sampling, the numerical magnitude of a characteristic is measured and recorded for each inspected unit; this involves reference to a continuous scale of some kind. A specific plan that indicates the sampling sizes and associated acceptance or nonacceptance criteria to be used is called acceptance sampling plan. In attributes sampling, for example, there are single, double, multiple, sequential, chain and skip-lot sampling plans. In variables sampling, there are single, double and sequential sampling plans. Subsequently, in statistical quality control, it was the era of Shewhart, Walter A. and his control charts, called Shewhart Control Charts. He is referred to as the father of statistical quality control because he brought together the disciplines of statistics, engineering and economics. He described the basic principles of this new discipline in his book *Economic Control of Quality of Manufactured Product*. Shewhart worked for Western Electric and AT&T Bell Telephone Laboratories, in addition to lecturing and consulting on quality control. Now, it is the era of six-sigma, house of quality etc. We will learn some of these statistical quality control principles in this chapter. However, before proceeding lets mention the difference between quality control and statistical quality control. That would make a reader of this chapter appreciate statistical quality control. It is important to distinguish between the unsystematic inspection and supervision which often goes under the name of "quality control" and statistical quality control. The former does not say when or how samples should be taken or how large they should be. Also it does not have the advantages that go with graphic presentation and a clear objective standard is not enforced for "take action" or "skip it". The statistical quality control chart makes use of well-thought-out, tested rulesand avoids the indecision, inconsistency and arbitrariness of haphazard quality control. Statistical control is based on the fact that repeated random samples from a fixed population will vary, but in a predictable manner. Thus, statistical total quality production process could be defined as the statistical process of striving for producing and reproducing a controlled repetitive output, may be intermediate product or an end product, by a series of measures requiring an organized effort by the statistical production group to prevent or eliminate errors at every stage of production and reproduction. Drug Production quality must be built into a product during product and process design, and it is influenced by the physical plant design, instrument, metal used, cleanliness, and horsepower during routine production.

Statistical Quality Control

In production and manufacturing, statistical quality control or the monitoring of the process control is a set of measures taken to ensure that what is happening today will also happen tomorrow. It includes the regulation of quality of the equipment used, assemblies, products and components; services related to production; and management, production, and inspection processes. Traditional statistical process control as mentioned before involves routine inspection of the goods produced and the application of theories as proposed by Dodge and Romig. We take a snapshot of how the process typically performs or build a model of how we think the process will perform and calculate control limits for the expected measurements of the output of the process. Then we collect data from the process and compare the data to the control limits. The majority of measurements should fall within the control limits. Often quite simple changes can dramatically improve production quality, such as the use of high quality steel or good power supply. However, currently many organizations use control charts and time series analysis to bring organization to Six Sigma levels of quality, in other words, thus that the likelihood of an unexpected failure is confined to six standard deviations on the normal distribution. This probability is less than four one-millionths. Steps controlled often include establishment of initial snapshots of production or models, as well as sophisticated manufacturing tasks. In addition, many different techniques and concepts have been tried to minimize defects in products, including Zero Defects, Six Sigma, and the House of Quality. Most of the currently used techniques and concepts are controversial to one degree or another, and thus there are two opposing schools of thought with regard to quality. One school describes to a purely statistical approach to quality, measuring defects, developing control charts and then determining the quality of the production batch. The other school believes in time-series. Time series analysis accounts for the fact that data points taken over time may have an internal structure (such as autocorrelation, trend or seasonal variation) that should be accounted for. These two schools currently encompass quality control and are discussed like-wise in this chapter.

Monitoring Industrial Processess

Monitoring industrial processes in any stage or in any practice is required for a variety of reasons. For instance, in current pharmaceutical production, the overwhelmingly bad situations may arise due to the out of control situation, because of bad instrumentation or by the use of the sophisticated equipment by very routine lay and common man, because of inappropriate production practices, and also by experts, with ample knowledge in this area to achieve their personal gains. In either case very strict control of the production floors with a perfect legislation; and with very controlled practice of the law, these situations in this area could be improved. Similar situation may arise with medical and pharmacy sectors when the latest technologies such as diagnostic chemicals, inadequate cervical smears for monitoring purposes, inadequate diagnostic tools such as those for detecting AIDS etc. in the very viscinities of the target person, target knowledge, or the target innovation would result in dramatic alterations in the end product or end result output, resulting in the quality variation of this output. It is better not to use the technology rather than use it for malpractices. The product output may not necessarily be an industrial output. It could be anything from a simple laboratory experiment to a very ethical social situation. These quality variations were identified for a long time and thus several theories and practices were proposed and are currently in place in this area. Same rules are currently used or in the process of introduction in the legal ethics of industrial or any other productions. Thus monitoring industrial production becomes very important.

Process Control is the active changing of the process based on the results of process monitoring. Once the process monitoring tools have detected an out-of-control situation, the person responsible for the process makes a change to bring the process back into control. **Out-of-control Action Plans** (OCAPS) detail the action to be taken once an out-of-control situation is detected. A specific flowchart, that leads the process engineer through the corrective procedure, may be provided for each unique process. **Advanced Process Control Loops** are automated changes to the process that are programmed to correct for the size of the out-of-control measurement. If the process is out-of-control, the process engineer looks for an assignable cause by following the out-of-control action plan (OCAP) associated with the control chart. Out-of-control refers to rejecting the assumption that the current data are from the same population as the data used to create the initial control chart limits. Several techniques are used to determine out of control. For classical Shewhart charts, a set of rules called the Western Electric Rules (WECO Rules) and a set of trend rules often are used to determine out-of-control. "In Control" only means that the process is predictable in a statistical sense. What do you do if the process is "in control" but the average level is too high or too low or the variability is unacceptable? Process improvement techniques such as experiments, calibration, re-analysis of historical database can be initiated to put the process on target or reduce the variability. Note that the process must be stable before it can be centered at a target value or its overall variation could be reduced. It is definitely not a joke. An awareness of these factors is the responsibility of all those involved in control chart building and time series analysis in the development, manufacture, control, and marketing of quality products. Thus, monitoring industrial process is the crux of quality control.

Control Charts

A very systematic effective control chart program takes into consideration sampling plans, variables control charts, attributes control charts, and multivariate control charts. To appreciate the processes involved in the control chart design, a very brief overview of sampling plans would be essential. This section deals with some of the practices in place or could be adopted to improve the situations dealing with the utility of control charts in the statistical production quality control methodologies.

Sampling Plans

A typical sampling plan right from the inspection of incoming materials and parts, process inspection at various points in the manufacturing operations, final inspection by a manufacturer of his own product, and ultimately inspection of the finished product by one or more purchasers includes five types of acceptance sampling plans that could be classified into single sampling plan, double sampling plan, multiple sampling plan, sequential sampling plan and skip lot sampling plan. Many a times it is the improper selection in the sampling plan that results in the variation in the statistical quality control output.

The following five types of acceptance sampling plans are commonly used.

1. ***Single Sampling Plan:*** When the decision whether to accept a lot or reject a lot is made on the basis of only one sample, the acceptance plan is described as a single sampling plan. This is the simplest type of sampling plan. In any systematic plan for single sampling three things are specified,
   (a) Number of items N in the lot from which the sample is to be drawn,
   (b) Number of articles n in the random sample drawn from the lot,
   (c) Number of defective articles in the sample. More than this number will cause the rejection of the lot. Thus a sampling plan may be specified in this way; N = 200, n = 20 and c = 1. These three numbers may be interpreted as saying "Take a random sample of 20 from a lot of 200. If the sample contains more than 1 defective, reject the lot; otherwise accept the lot".
2. ***Double Sampling Plan:*** In the single sampling plan discussed above, decision with regard to acceptance or rejection of a lot is based on the evidence of only one sample from the lot. However, double sampling involves the possibility of putting off the decision on the lot until a second sample has been taken. A lot may be accepted at once if the first sample is good enough or rejected at once if the first sample is bad enough. If the first sample is neither good enough nor bad enough, the decision is based on the evidence of the first and second samples combined. In a double sampling plan 5 things are specified: n1, c1, n2, (n1 + n2) and c2, where n1 = number of pieces in the first sample; c1 = acceptance number of the first sample (the maximum number of defectives that will permit the acceptance of the lot on the basis of the first sample); n2 = number of pieces in the second sample; n1 + n2 = number of pieces in the two samples combined; c2 = acceptance number for the two samples combined (the maximum number of defectives that will permit the acceptance of the lot on the basis of the two samples). Thus, a double sampling plan may be N = 500; n1 = 20; c1 = 1; n2 = 60 and c2 = 4. This will be interpreted as follows:
   1. inspect a first sample of 20 from a lot of 500,
   2. accept the lot on the basis of the first sample if it contains 1 defective,
   3. reject the lot on the basis of the first sample if the sample contains more than 1 defective,
   4. inspect a second sample of 60 if the first sample contains 2, 3, 4 defectives,

5. accept the lot on the basis of combined sample of 80 if the combined sample contains 4 or less defectives and
6. reject the lot on the basis of combined sample if the combined sample contains more than 4 defectives. A double sampling plan has two possible advantages over a single sampling plan:
   1. It may reduce the total amount of inspection. The first sample taken is less than that called for under a comparable single sampling plan and consequently, in all cases in which a lot is accepted or rejected on the basis of first sample, there may be considerable saving in total inspection. It is also possible to reject a lot without completely inspecting the entire second sample,
   2. A double sampling plan has the physchological advantage of giving a lot a second chance. To some people, especially the producer, it may seem unfair to reject a lot on the basis of a single sample. Double sampling permits the taking of two samples on which to make a decision.

3. ***Multiple sampling plan:*** Just as double sampling plan may defer the decision on acceptance or rejection until a second sample has been taken, other plans may permit any number of samples before a decision is reached. Plans permitting from three or more number of samples are described as multiple or sequential. However, such plans are quite complicated and rarely used in practice.

4. ***Sequential sampling plans:*** This is the ultimate extension of multiple sampling where items are selected from a lot one at a time and after inspection of each item a decision is made to accept or reject the lot or select another unit.

5. ***Skip lot sampling plans:*** Skip lot sampling means that only a fraction of the submitted lots are inspected.

Selection of a sampling plan

All practical sampling plans have an operating characteristic curve, briefly called OC curve. The following points need emphasis regarding the OC curve:

(a) There is some chance that good lots will be rejected.

(b) There is some chance that bad lots will be accepted.

(c) These risks could be calculated by the theory of probability and depend on the number of samples inspected, the acceptance number, and the percent defective in the lots submitted for sample inspection. Given the amount of risks which can be tolerated, a sample plan can be devised to meet these requirements.

(d) The larger the sample used in sample inspection, the nearer the OC curve approaches the ideal. However, beyond a certain point, the added cost of inspecting a larger number of parts far exceeds the benefits derived.

Thus, the two parameters of an OC curve are the sample size and the acceptance number. The desired quality levels (p) and the probability of acceptance (Pa) must be selected so that the proper sampling plan could be designed. There are four factors that should be considered in a sampling plan:

1. P1, also known as AQL (the Acceptance Quality Level). This defines a good lot.
2. P2, also known as RQL (the Rejectable Quality Level) or LTPD (Lot Tolerance Per Cent Defective).
3. α, also known as Producers Risk. This is the probability of selecting a good lot.
4. β, also known as the Consumers Risk. This is the probability of accepting a poor lot.

There are several softwares currently in the market involved in identifying suitable sampling plans and thereby giving appropriate feed back to the respective concerned personalities. Now comes the development of control charts. Three different control charts are available. These are variables control chart, attributes control chart and multivariate control chart. This simply suggests that there are several steps involved in this statistical quality control process and thus the judicious sampling selection is the key to control chart utilization. Any mistake at any stage either deliberate tampering or package interference may lead to a wrong signal and thus many a times result in bad output and thus results in discarding of the batch.

Variables Control Charts

Before control charts are developed, the identity of the data must be established using suitable methods or classifications. Broadly speaking, control charts could be divided under two heads depending on the type of the data: control chart of variables and control chart of attributes. Control chart developers take various steps at this stage. Variables are those quality characteristics of a product that are measurable and can be expressed in specific units of measurement such as diameter of radio knobs that can be measured and expressed in centimeters, tensile strength of cement that can be expressed in specific measures per square inch of space etc. If the data is put into variables, the data could be summarized into statistical measures like the average, the standard deviation and the range. However, in establishing basic procedures for the operation of quality control programme, the manufacturer take the following preliminary steps: select the quality characteristics that are to be controlled (including the limits of variations), analyse the production process to determine the kind and location of probable causes of irregularities, determine how the inspection data are to be collected and recorded, and how they are to be sub-divided and chose the statistical measures that are to be used in the control chart. Full control chart development often requires as many as five different techniques. These include control charts for X and σ, X and R, control chart for X alone, control chart for σ or R alone, control chart for c and control chart for p or pn. Therefore, the most efficient organization of the data is by function so that analysts can further proceed in appropriate control charts. The most commonly used variable charts are the first three control charts. As far as the development of control charts is concerned, several leniencies are currently allowed because of the availability of several marketed softwares.

In this era of ever-growing competition it has become absolutely necessary for a businessman to keep a continous watch over the quality of the goods produced. Historically speaking the methods developed and used by W.A. Shewhart working for the Bell Telephone co. (During 1920s and 1930s) in America culminated into the very appropriate use of his control charts (Shewart Charts) in the production quality control assessments. X chart is used to show the quality averages of the samples drawn from a given process. The R chart is used to show the variability or dispersion of the quality produced by a given process. The aim of the development of X chart is to determine the means of each sample, obtain the mean of sample means and then establish the control limits set at UCL = X// + 3 sigma X and LCL = X – 3 sigma X. There are a number of correction factors that are considered in the development of X charts. The R chart is used to show the variability or dispersion of the quality produced by a given process. R chart is the companion chart to X chart and both are usually required for adequate analysis of the production process under study. The R chart is generally presented along with the X chart. The general procedure for constructing the R chart is similar to that for the X chart. The required values for constructing the R chart are:

1. The range of each sample, R;
2. The mean of the sample ranges, R and
3. UCL and LCL, where UCL = R + 3 std error and LCL = R – 3 Std error.

The value of std error may be estimated by finding the standard deviation of the ranges of the samples included in a chart, in practice, however, it is rather convenient to compute the upper and lower control limits by using the values D4 and D3 as provided from any of the statistical tables. It should be noted that the use of R chart is recommended only for relatively small sample sizes (rarely more than 12 to 15 units). For the large sample sizes ($n>12$) the standard error chart is generally used.

Attributes Control Charts

As mentioned in the introductory section, attributes control chart is also a very important aspect. The wastage of a batch could be reduced by intermittently and intermediately stopping a batch production in the middle, if it is thought that it may result in a bad quality product at the end. However, in this situation the data is not numerical. The key for this step is that the characteristic data cannot be represented by a particular numerical data or it is impractical to do likewise. Thus, attributes control charts become very important in these situations. An example of a common quality characteristic classification would be designating units as "conforming units" or "nonconforming units". Another quality characteristic criteria would be sorting units into "non defective" and "defective" categories. Quality characteristics of that type are called *attributes.* Note that there is a difference between "nonconforming to an engineering specification" and "defective" -- a nonconforming unit may function just fine and be, in fact, not defective at all, while a part can be "in spec" and not function as desired (i.e., be defective). Examples of quality characteristics that are attributes are the number of failures in a production run, the proportion of malfunctioning wafers in a lot, the number of people eating in the cafeteria on a given day, etc. Control charts dealing with the number of *defects* or *nonconformities* are called *c* charts (for count). Control charts dealing with the *proportion* or *fraction* of defective product are called *p* charts (for proportion). There is another chart that handles *defects per unit*, called the *u* chart (for unit). This applies when we wish to work with the average number of nonconformities per unit of product.

To assure the control on the number of defects per unit C-chart (Number of defects per unit) is commonly used, where in the opportunity for defects is large whole the actual occurance tends to be small which often occurs in the data distributed by poisson distribution. Such control procedures shall be established to monitor the output and to validate the performance of those manufacturing processes that may be responsible for causing variability in the characteristics of in-process material and the drug product. Such control procedures shall include, but are not limited to, the following, where appropriate:

1. The use of the C-chart is appropriate if the opportunities for a defect in each production unit are infinite but the probability of a defect at any point is very small and constant;
2. The formula is based on a normal curve approximation to the Poisson distribution;
3. Uniform sample size is highly desirable while using the C-Chart;
4. Where sample size varies particularly if the variation is large, the C-chart becomes difficult to read, and the p-chart provides a better choice;
5. Amongst control chart for attributes, the C-chart is most widely used in practice.

The p-chart is designed to control the percentage or proportion of defectives per sample, where in the number of defectives could be converted into a percentage expressed as a decimal fraction merely by dividing c by the sample size, the p-chart may be used instead of c-chart, thereby offering several advantages. Expressing the defectives as a percentage or fraction of production is more meaningful and more generally understood than would be the statement of the number of defectives. The latter concept must be related in some way to the total number produced. Where the size of the sample varies from sample to sample, the p-chart permits a more straightforward and less cluttered presentation. The p-chart requires, however, that the division c/n be made. This additional computation may be regarded as a slight disadvantage, the same data could be used for both c as well as p chart and when the sample size remains constant from sample to sample, the primary difference lies in the computation of the control limits.

Multivariate Control Charts

The best output is one without any flaws. However, during the initial stages of establishing relationship between variables, many a times the data could be multivariate thus making data analysis difficult. Univariate data consists of only one variable while multivariate data consists of more than one variables. For multivariate data, the data are represented by a vector X = (x1,..........xp) where p is the number of variables) or the dimension of the data. Hence it could be said that multivariate data are vectors while univariate data are numbers. Multivariate data is hard to see, utilizes the order and needs vector or matrix algebra. To effectively acquire the tools and techniques multivariate data needs to be interpreted. Interpreting the pattern of relationships among many variables rather than establishing causal linkages, and rely heavily on numerical examples, visualization, and on verbal, rather than mathematical exposition.

Currently, these are the most important types of data that could be visualized in any context and definitely are applicable to current industrial production and manufacturing processess. As of today there are several softwares available in the market that are helpful in the data analysis of multivariate data. Once such software is Aebel software. The following two pictures on a computer screen illustrates multivariate data and its analysis using Aebel software.

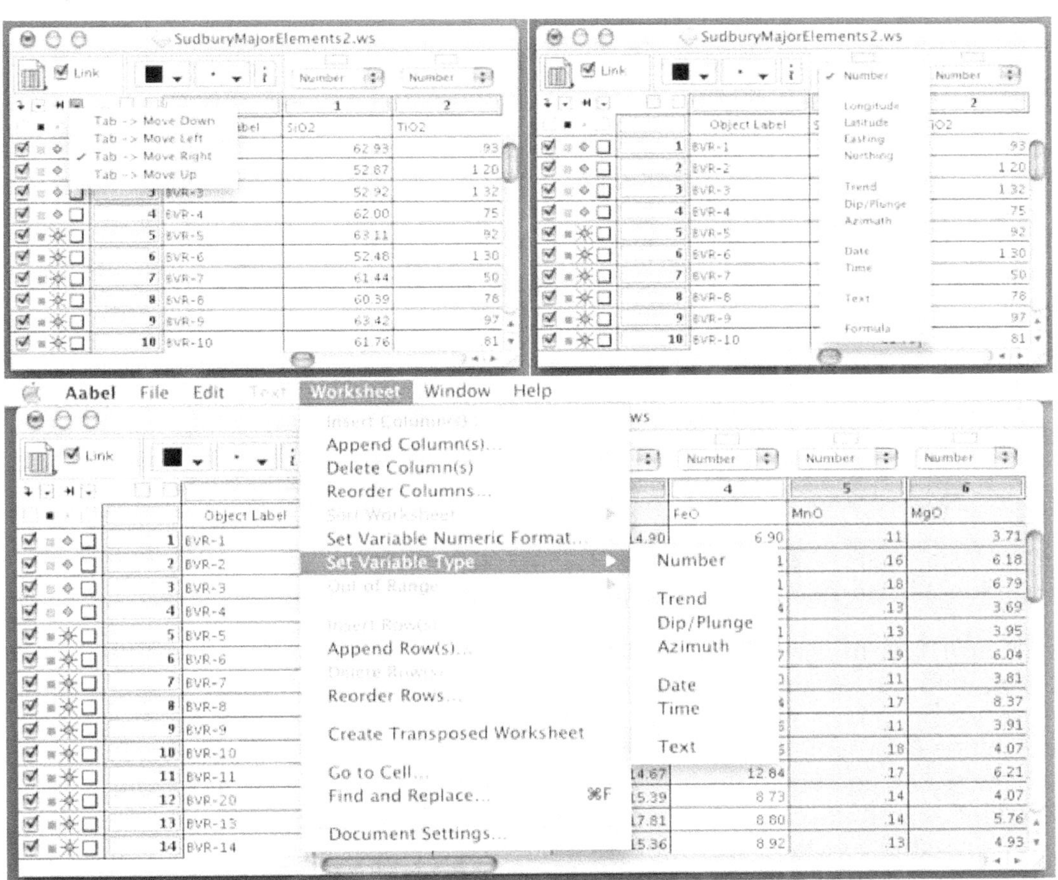

Figure 19.1 A spread sheet associated with data classification using Aabel software.

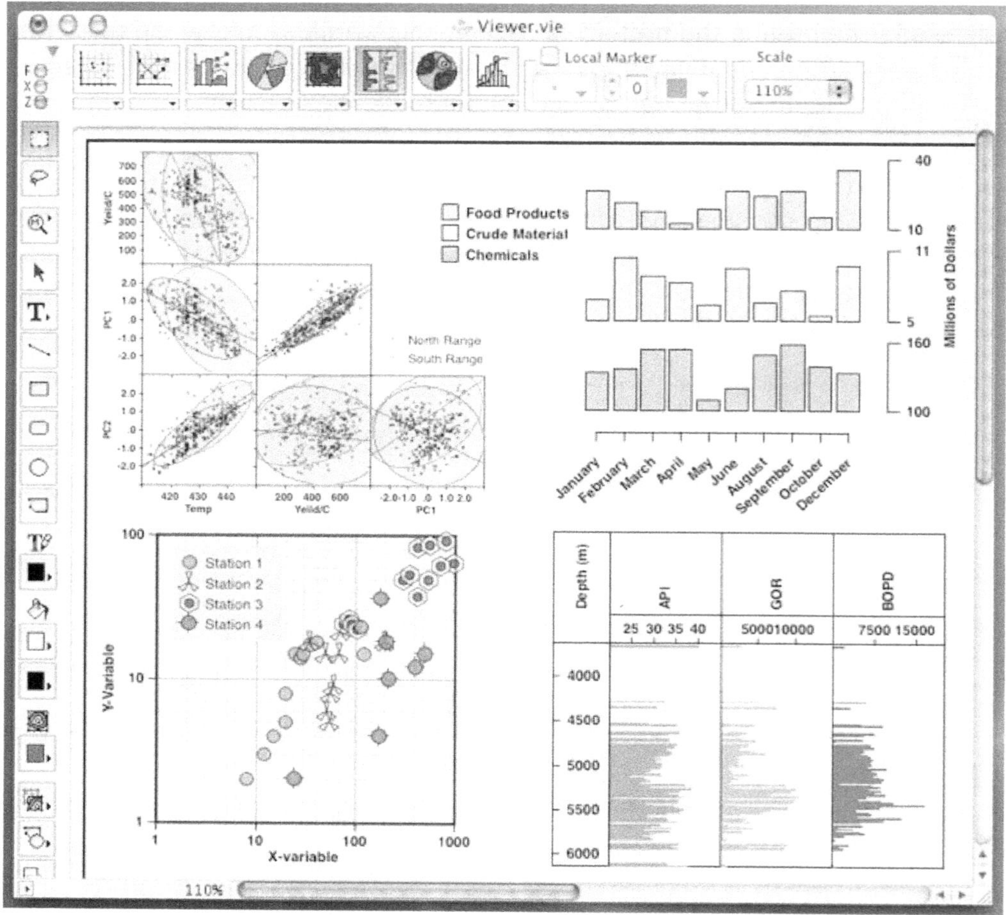

Figure 19.2 Multivariate Data Representation using Aabel Software.

It is a fact of life that most data are naturally multivariate. Hotelling in 1947 introduced a statistic that uniquely lends itself to plotting multivariate observations. This statistic, appropriately named Hotelling's T^2, is a scalar that combines information from the dispersion and mean of several variables. Due to the fact that computations are laborious and fairly complex and require some knowledge of matrix algebra, acceptance of multivariate control charts by industry was slow and hesitant. Nowadays, modern computers in general and the PC in particular have made complex calculations accessible and during the last decade, multivariate control charts were given more attention. In fact, the multivariate charts which display the Hotelling T^2 statistic became so popular that they sometimes are called Shewhart charts as well, although Shewhart had nothing to do with them. As in the univariate case, when data are grouped, the T^2 chart can be paired with a chart that displays a measure of variability within the subgroups for all the analyzed characteristics. The combined T^2 and T_d^2 (dispersion) charts are thus a multivariate counterpart of the univariate $\overline{X}$ and S (or $\overline{X}$ and R) charts.

Time Series Analysis

A very systematic effective time series analysis of production quality study should take into consideration, basic theory, production characteristics, analytical techniques, and models for investigation.

Basic Theory

The production quality control and time series analysis practices is achieved by *evaluation of production characteristics*, which includes determining the variations, their causes and the reasons, and data collection *analytical techniques*, which includes fitting the production data to models such as box-jenkins arima models, box-jenkins multivariate model, holt-winters exponential smoothing to conveniently have the production data behavior in the database and proceed to forcasting and monitoring, and finally *model using methodologies* for further proceeding to the determination of production quality control with the use of the identification, estimation, validation, prediction, forcasting and sample output generation. According to several statisticians and computer experts involved on the production floor, the five major characteristics of production value variations that could hold true for time series analysis of a pharmaceutical production floor include: average: production value tends to cluster around a specific level; trend: production value consistently increases or decreases with time; seasonality: production value shows peaks and valleys at consistent intervals. These intervals could be hours, days, weeks, months, years or seasons; cyclic: production value gradually increases or decreases over an extended period of time, such as years. Recession and expansion in the production and product (equipment, raw materials) life cycle influences the production value; and random error: production value fluctuations that cannot be explained. These are generally the causes of variations and should be definitely well understood before applying statistical principles of time series analysis in the quality control of industrial processes in an oral drug industry. Time series analysis also has several other applications. This statistical methodology could be used in economic forecasting, sales forecasting, budgetary analysis, stock market analysis, yield projections, process and quality control, inventory studies, workload projections, utility studies and census analysis.

To assure the production process meet high standards of quality and efficacy, an effective time series program is required at the facilities where the products are manufactured. This is often times the first priopity in the quality assurance in the production process before the manufacture in a plant preceeds. A successful quality control program must be enforced within and outside the plant to control the errors associated with the initial manufacturing batches. Consequently, expertise and innovation and program installation should be required. First, rate-limiting, and last steps should be properly monitored using appropriate steps in the early production batches. Adequate machinery, proper computer networks, and good manufacturing practices are the other important factors. As related to a pharmaceutical production unit, ventilation in manufacturing departments is usually designed so that dust can be contained and removed. In such departmental operations, dust collectors, air filters, and scrubbers to clean the air are checked on a routine schedule. Air quality monitoring at the work station could indicate the adequacy of these elements. The water supply may be potable, distilled, or deionized, and must be under adequate pressure to keep the water flowing. Deionization units should be monitored, and the resins changed or regenerated frequently, to deliver water of consistently high chemical and microbial quality as per written compendial or inhouse specifications. A working formula procedure should be prepared for each batch size that is produced. To attempt expansion or reduction of a batch size by manual calculations at the time of production cannot be considered good manufacturing practice. Quality assurance personnel must review and check the working formula procedures for each production batch before, during, and after production. If things are not taken care at this time, this definitely may lead to lot of erroneous results and very often result in batch dumping. The reason for dumping this batch could be either deliberate purposes or for personal gains it does not matter. Thus, signature and date of issue given by a responsible production or quality assurance employee has to be checked. Proper identification by name and dosage form, item number, lot number, effective date of document, reference to a superseded version, amount, lot and code numbers of each raw material utilized. This has to be employed at every step of processing. In addition, it ensures the skill of the personal involved in this process. Most of the times unit processes such as mixing are the main sources of errors. Definitely these errors have to be weeded out at very early stages. Thus, skill of the personal involved is the key. Raw material quality assurance and the containers used in such assurance have to be properly validated. Enough care has to be taken that this is definitely not the source of the batch losses. The other issue regarding this is the cleanliness of the manufacturing equipment. Very often personal employed are used in the cleaning and this process is validated at the beginning of the batch production. Thus, this step has to be very carefully undertaken. Most of the times after a batch is produced, the equipment is dissembled and is cleaned for convenience. Proper protocol should be in place with regarding to the cleaning of the equipment. It is likely that regular wear and tear of the equipments are possible. These have to be regularly monitored to ensure an ideal batch output.

Once the first several batches are manufactured, production characteristics are noted and the data is properly collected and pooled as per the needs of time series analysis using several statistical software packages. Several issues are important during this step of evaluation of the production characteristics. There are two main goals of time series analysis:

(a) identifying the nature of the phenomenon represented by the sequence of observations, and

(b) forecasting (predicting future values of the time series variable).

Both of these goals require that the pattern of observed time series data is identified and more or less formally described. Once the pattern is established, we can interpret and integrate it with other data (i.e., use it in our theory of the investigated phenomenon, e.g., sesonal commodity prices). Regardless of the depth of the understanding and the validity of our interpretation (theory) of the phenomenon, the data could be extrapolated and the pattern identified to predict future events. Analytical techniques are key in this area. Measures and characteristics such as identification of pattern, whether systemic or random, trend analysis and analysis of seasonality are important. These are the minimum requirements. Currently, in good production practices, the data is then fit into models using various statistical packages and some times the data is smoothed as per the requirements. In addition, forecasting becomes essential at this stage. There are no proven "automatic" techniques to identify trend components in the time series data; however, as long as the trend is monotonous (consistently increasing or decreasing) that part of data analysis is typically not very difficult. If the time series data contain considerable error, then the first step in the process of trend identification is smoothing. Smoothing always involves some form of local averaging of data such that the nonsystematic components of individual observations cancel each other out. The most common technique is *moving average* smoothing which replaces each element of the series by either the simple or weighted average of *n* surrounding elements, where *n* is the width of the smoothing "window". Medians can be used instead of means. The main advantage of median as compared to moving average smoothing is that its results are less biased by outliers (within the smoothing window). Thus, if there are outliers in the data (e.g., due to measurement errors), median smoothing typically produces smoother or at least more "reliable" curves than moving average based on the same window width. The main disadvantage of median smoothing is that in the absence of clear outliers it may produce more "jagged" curves than moving average and it does not allow for weighing. In the relatively less common cases (in time series data), when the measurement error is very large, the distance weighted least squares smoothing or negative exponentially weighted smoothing techniques can be used. All those methods will filter out the noise and convert the data into a smooth curve that is relatively unbiased by outliers (see the respective sections on each of those methods for more details). Series with relatively few and systematically distributed points can be smoothed with bicubic splines. Many monotonous time series data can be adequately approximated by a linear function; if there is a clear monotonous nonlinear component, the data first need to be transformed to remove the nonlinearity. Usually a logarithmic, exponential, or (less often) polynomial function can be used. Models such as box-jenkins arims, box-jenkins multivariate, holt winter exponential are also generated depending on the requirement. The final step is model-using methodologies. At this step (*Estimation or model-using methodologies*), the parameters are estimated (using function minimization procedures, so that the sum of squared residuals is minimized. The estimates of the parameters are used in the last stage (*Forecasting*) to calculate new values of the series (beyond those included in the input data set) and confidence intervals for those predicted values. The estimation process is performed on transformed (differenced) data; before the forecasts are generated, the series needs to be *integrated* (integration is the inverse of differencing) so that the forecasts are expressed in values compatible with the input data. This automatic integration feature is represented by the letter I in the name of the methodology (ARIMA = Auto-Regressive Integrated Moving Average). Finally auditing is the very essential feature. This comes from the very early stages of production to the release of the batch into the market. All the people who are involved are responsible for batch output. If after a batch is released into the market and customers complain, then along with the company personal everyone involved in the process are answerable. Thus, definitely a very proper production quality control has to be maintained at each and every step.

Production Characteristics

The importance of determining the causes of pharmaceutical production variations will be illustrated with a recent citation. One of the variabilities that may lead to variabilities in production characteristics in tablet production is blend analysis. Thus, the data from blend analysis is collected and then put into time-series analysis and the variabilities evaluated and the production characteristics are subsequently determined. In August 1999 the FDA issued a Draft Abbreviated New Drug Application (ANDA) Guidance for Industry titled "ANDA's: Blend Uniformity Analysis" that detailed blend uniformity sampling and acceptance criteria for the determination of final blend uniformity for generic drug products. Although this guidance was written specifically to address ANDA's, the guidance was also adopted as standard practice in the development of NDA's (New Drug Applications). The proposed release criteria established for blend uniformity were to be used in addition to, and independent from, the USP finished product uniformity release requirements. Based on the Blend Uniformity Guidance, batches that failed to meet the blend uniformity acceptance criteria should be rejected regardless of the products ability to demonstrate final product uniformity. In March 2002, the Product Quality Research Institute (PQRI) issued a proposal to the FDA with respect to both ANDA's and NDA's recommending the use of stratified sampling for final blend and in-process dosage units. The proposal recommended the use of final blend uniformity and dosage unit uniformity to demonstrate overall batch uniformity, with the possibility of using dosage unit uniformity in lieu of blend uniformity during routine commercial production. Consequently, in October 2003, the FDA issued a Draft Guidance for Industry titled "Powder Blends and Finished Dosage Units-Stratified In-Process Dosage Unit Sampling Assessment" that detailed the criteria for the use of stratified sampling and acceptance criteria to demonstrate batch uniformity. In response to the PQRI proposal, Endo Pharmaceuticals conducted an impact evaluation of the proposed PQRI sampling procedures and acceptance criteria on a product-by-product basis as compared to the 1999 Draft Guidance and current USP requirements. The evaluation of Product A demonstrates the benefit of implementing the 2003 Guidance for products that demonstrate questionable blend uniformity but acceptable finished product uniformity. Production characteristics of any other output could be as mentioned in the above case study.

Analytical Techniques

The current trend that is followed in a production facility is to fit the data to a perfect time series model at each and every quality/quantity limiting step before further moving. This definitely saves time, resources, and results in a perfect production quality control output by decreasing the number of tedius manipulations in the later stages of time series method of production quality control. When the speed of the output has increased many times compared to the previous production processing, it is definitely a daunting work to sample, analyze and report during this stage, in tandem with reporting/marketing. There are many methods of model fitting including box-jenkins arima models, box-jenkins multivariate models, and holt winters exponential smoothing (single, double and trible). This modeling of the data depends either on univariate time series models, that are based on the precinct that time series consists of singular observations recorded sequentially over equal time intervals e.g. monthly carbondioxide concentration, southern oscillations to predict elnino effects or a multivariate time series models (also called Autoregressing Moving Average Vector (ARMAV

Model)), that are based on the precinct that the time series consists of three different variables, e.g. {As an example, one gas furnace data will be illustrated. In one gas furnace, air and methane were combined in order to obtain a mixture of gases that contained CO_2 (carbon dioxide). The methane gas feedrate constituted the input series and followed the process. Methane Gas Input Feed = .60 - .04 $X(t)$, the CO_2 concentration was the output, $Y(t)$. In this experiment 296 successive pairs of observations (X_t, Y_t) were read off from the continuous records at 9-second intervals. A bivariate model of the data was fit using 60 pairs of data obtained from the above experiment and the results were investigated. Several software packages are currently available in the market to fit such a data}. The univariate data could be either stationary, in which the mean, the variance and the autocorrelation structure do not change with time (most of the time the data is without trend, constant variance over time, a constant autocorrelation over time and no periodic fluctuations) or seasonal, in which the data has periodic fluctuations (this type of data is quite common with economic time series). On the other hand, multivariate data is a matrix kind of data and the estimation of matrix parameter or the convariance matrix is complicated and is very difficult without computer software. Several scatter plots techniques demonstrate the relationship between the parameters (no correlation, positive correlation, negative correlation, quadratic correlation, exponential relationship, sinusoidal relationship, homoscedastic relationship, scatter plot matrix, conditional plot, spectral plot, heteroscedastic relationship, outlier detection, random data, star plot, sinusoidal model, weibull plot, Youden plot, 4-plot, 6-plot, lag plot, probability plot etc.) and are used as per the sophistication of the needs of the production unit. In many a times, a run sequence plot including several other techniques are used to demonstrate whether a particular time-series is stationary or seasonal, to interpret important data and detect the outliers. In this regard, specialized softwares are also used on-line along with the several other techniques that are used in the data analysis. Definitely the automation has to increase as the sophistication increases. Automation usually improves the quality, quantity, and efficiency of an operation. Its introdution into the time series data analysis techniques dramatically changes the traditional look, capability, precision, and acceptability of most of our conventional time-series techniques. The use of automated statistically softwares for time-series analysis, data handling, and production quality control is certainly on rise. Currently, several companies are marketing these types of softwares. The design and the production and the working principles are based on robotic technologies.

Some of the software techniques are multifunctional. They are equipped to perform several types of data analysis in a wide range of applications including to determine the seasonality, model identification, model validation, and finally model diagnosis. The softwares offer automated solutions for the production floor, where consistent results are vital and the software data is limited. Once stationarity and seasonality has been addressed, the next step is to identify the order, (i.e., the p and q) of the autoregressive and moving average terms. The primary tools for doing this are the autocorrelation plot and the partial autocorrelation plot including several other techniques. The sample autocorrelation plot and the sample partial autocorrelation plot are compared to the theoretical behaviour of these plots when the order is known. The using of the sample autocorrelation function helps identify the model. In practice, the sample autocorrelation and partial autocorrelation functions are random variables and will not give the same picture as the theoretical functions. This makes the model identification more difficult. In particular, mixed models could be particularly difficult to identify. Although experience is helpful, developing good models using these sample plots could involve much trial and error. For this reason, in recent years information-based criterial such as FPE (Final Prediction Error) and AIC (Aikake Information Criterion) and others have been preferred and used. These techniques can help automate the model identification process. Several software programs are currently available to provide ARIMA modeling capabilities, thereby helping in forcasting and monitoring. Depending on the sophistication of the production needs the model identification, validation and conclusion drawing is important. However, it definitely takes lot of money, resources and time before such a process could be installed on a manufacturing floor. Definitely validation of the total model becomes very essential, which is definitely the key to this automatic analytical technique in process engineering.

Model Applications

Interpreting and concluding the models generated is a very important aspect of pharmaceutical production quality control. This has to be done prior to the initiation of improper personal (who are not qualified to perform time series analysis of production batches) into the manufacturing setup. Although a person is well trained in the basics of pharmaceutical technology, still when it comes to the actual practice of the pharmaceutical manufacture, the ballpark is that following strict quality control measures such as control charts and time series analysis would be essential for an ideal output of a product. Several softwares are currently available in the market as related to the statistical methodologies in the quality control of the industrial processes that could be conveniently applied to the model generation and interpretation of pharmaceutical production data. It is better for all the pharmaceutical to have a brief awareness of these software packages. Some of the important software packages are:

(a) SPC software solutions

(b) STATISTICA

(c) JMP software
(d) Plant Master Statistical Quality Control
(e) Mitutoyo's new MeasurLink Statistical Process Control Software
(f) Marposs Quick Statistical Quality Control Software

Salient Features of Statistical Quality Control

As mentioned before statistical quality control of goods of any type is the main part of a business organization. Although lot of statistics, probability and mathematical concepts such as control charts and time series analysis are considered during the manufacturing stages, it is always a possibility that the quality control process may be entirely inadequate. These inadequacies are manifested as insufficiencies in team tools such as responsibility grid, threat versus opportunity matrix, action workouts ect., process improvement tools/techniques such as brainstorming, Pareto analysis, process mapping, cause and effect analysis, design of experiments, process mapping, cause and effect analysis, design of experiments, process FMEA, etc. and other adjuvant statistical tools such as hypothesis testing (t-test, F-test, Chi squared test), ANOVA, MANOVA, capability analysis, regression analysis etc. Some of these are currently used in many of the larger organizations in developed countries. As a current consideration as related to statistical production quality control the salient features that are to be strictly followed or considered are: six sigma levels of quality, zero defects quality system, house of quality and scatter diagrams. Some of the details of these methodologies are henceforth discussed in this section.

Six Sigma Levels of Quality

There are legal, moral, economic, and competitive reasons, as well as reasons of safety and efficacy, to monitor, predict, and evaluate production quality control. The aim of six sigma levels of quality is to identify and eliminate causes of errors or defects or failures in business processes by focusing on outputs that are critical to customers. Six sigma levels of quality of the production was originally developed by Motorola in the 1980s and has since been implemented by a number of world class organizations such as GE, Honeywell, ABB, Sony, Texas Instruments, Ford, Johnson Control Sysems, etc. with the purpose of reducing variability in processes, reducing quality costs, improving process capability and enhancing process throughput yield.

The stresses and hazards to which products are exposed during their passage from the manufacturing plant to the distribution chain and to the consumer can be environmental, mechanical or contaminant in natures. Thus, a healthy portion of Six Sigma training involves learning of the theory and the principles behind the methodology, i.e., DMAIC cycle. The elements of the DMAIC cycle inclues define phase, measure phase, analyse phase, improve phase, and control phase. Define phase involves understanding the customers, their needs and expectations, develop a project team charter (individual duties, project goals, key deliverables, project benefits, cost issues etc.), Measure phase involves the measurement of the performance of a process, determine what to measure and how to measure, measure current performance of the process and evaluate the contribution of variability contributed by the measurement system to the total variation. Therefore, statistical quality control does not stop at the control chart development and time series analysis. The next phase in this series is the Analyse phase that incorporates the identification of the root causes of defects or failures, understand the data, fit into statistical tools and select the vital few from trivial many for improvement phase.

As related to the Improve Phase and Control Phase, the main determinants are how can the causes of defects or failures removed, identification of the key variables which causes the problems, document solution statements, test solutions and measure results and during the control phase the key issues are how can the improvements be maintained or sustained, document new methods and select and establish standard measures to monitor performance. The employees must be capable of choosing the most appropriate tools and techniques for their situations. There are three major sets of tools/techniques that are required within the Six Sigma problem solving framework. These are outlined as follows.

"Six Sigma should begin and end with the customers. Projects should begin with the determination of customer requirements. The process of linking Six Sigma to the customers could be:

(a) identifying the core processes, defining the key outputs, and defining the key customers that they serve and

(b) defining the customer requirement. The first step that is then followed is based on Porters concept of value chains, which aim at representing the organization as a collection of activities. The next stage is to define the key outputs from the core processes and the key customers that these outputs serve."

Poorly selected and defined projects lead to delayed results and also a great deal of frustration. For the introduction of new projects business benefits criteria, feasibility criteria and organizational impact criteria are to be considered. Business benefits criteria thus include impact on meeting external customer requirement, impact on core competencies, financial impact and urgency. Feasibility criteria include resources required, complexity issues, expertise available and required and finall the likelihood of success within a reasonable timeframe. Use of organizational impact criteria involves learning benefits (new knowledge gained about the business, customers, processes etc.) and cross-functional benefits. For a lot of organizations, financial returns to the bottom-line is the main criterion and therefore the projects should be selected in such a way that they are closely tied to the business objectives of the organization.

Human resources-based actions need to be put into effect to promote desired behaviour and results. Some studies show that above 60% of the top performing companies practicing Six Sigma link their rewards to their business strategies. At GE, for instance, for any manager to be considered for promotion, they have to be Six Sigma trained. Likewise, upto 40% of top management bonuses are tied to their specific Six Sigma success.

Six Sigma is about change and change requires action from top management. Purposeful and useful action cannot occur without a system to monitor and control it. Effective Six Sigma implementation requires an IT system to receive, organize and help translate this information into effective decisions for the organization. To avoid lacking in activity and functionality, it requires an underlying IT infrastructure. To achieve effective IT system the team should support the collection of data from the process. IT infrastructure should provide a means for effective communication and sharing of data/information across the organization. It should provide an easily accessible database holding information regarding all ongoing and completed Six Sigma projects, provide an interactive training tool for employees to learn the Six Sigma methodology and the tools within the methodology for problem solving activities and finally should be able to provide on-line coaching for Six Sigma tools and techniques. In addition, many organizations that implement Six Sigma find it beneficial to extend the application of Six Sigma principles to management of their supply chain.

Zero Defects Quality System

Philip M. Cosby, a leading quality control champion, is one of the pioneers in the field of Zero Defects Quality System and his statements now part and parcel of quality speak – "zero defects" "do it right the first time". He is quite oriented and and felt we should "assume that people are vitally interested in the quality improvement process" and "assume the best and that is what usually happens". His four absolutes of quality are:

1. Quality is conformance to requirements,
2. The system of quality is prevention,
3. The performance standard is zero defect and
4. The measurement of quality is the price of non-conformance.

Zero defects advocates endorse continuous improvement. This is the never-ending effort to totally eliminate all forms of waste (the Japanese call it “muda”), including reworks, yield losses, unproductive time, over-design, inventory, idle facilities, safety accidents, and the less tangible factors of unrealized individual and societal potential. There are several lessons to be learnt in understanding Zero Defects Quality. These include:

1. Mathematics of the minimum total quality costs should be clearly understood,
2. Optimum quality costs depend on incremental, not total, elementary costs. At the optimum, nothing in general can be said about the relative levels of prevention and failure costs,
3. There is no mathematical requirement that the optimum occurs at $q<100\%$. There may be no optimum in the range of $q = 0$ to 100%. There might be a minimum rather than an optimum, and it could very well be at $q = 100\%$.
4. The optimum (or more correctly, the minimum) quality cost could lie at zero defects ($q=100\%$) if the incremental cost of approaching Zero defects is less than the incremental return from the resulting improvement, and
5. Does it really take infinite investment to reach zero defects”.

Currently several new innovations in the manufacturing sector are in place for an active achievement of zero defects quality system. Mennie Machine company (Mark, IL) adopting new, innovative gauging techniques and technology has helped grow an Illinois shop to a venture machining automotive and off-highway castings and forgings with “zero defects.” The quality level of products has improved tremendously over the last decade. The measurement standard for defective products has now dropped to Defective Part Per Million (DPPM). Is it possible to further improve quality and cut down on defects to reach a standard as low as Defective Part Per Billion (DPPB), or even better, Zero Defect Level? Dr. Shigeo Shingo, pioneer of the Mistake Proofing (Poka-Yoke) System in Japan, saw this as an achievable possibility. Human error is inevitable. However, these mistakes can in turn result in defects in the process of manufacturing. The Mistake Proofing System focuses on correcting the conditions for processing, thereby preventing human error from resulting in defects. The devices used by the Mistake Proofing System are easy to operate and cheap to install. Human error can therefore be eliminated, eventually leading to Zero Defect Level.

House of Quality

Suffering from customer complaint, struggle to turn business proposals into contracts, overrunning of project budgets, breaking delivery deadlines, throwing away good raw materials because of manufacturing errors, passing of tenders for the lack of ISO standards certification is a pain to any production or business organization. Such problems could be very deleterious to the growth of an organization, if not proper precautions considered. A situation of this nature may mislead the statistical production quality control manager because the reading from these mathematical and statistical concepts may differ from the output expected. Several methods are in place as regarding to avoiding these problems. House of quality is one of the new concepts that is covering these aspects. Although sounds tandem with other production control methodologies discussed in this chapter, the concept of house of quality is different and should be carefully understood by a production manager, pharmaceutical technologist, or definitely infact a customer.

As such this concept is new, some of the latest discussions as per several house of quality organizations and mostly as related to the pharmaceutical arena are:

Uptodate Comprehensive List

Major companies and all government-related organizations require that their suppliers with relevant industry standards and some of the major issues in this area are:

1. ISO 9001:2000 – Quality Management Standard
2. ISO 13485 – Medical Devices Standard (additions to ISO 9001 standard)
3. ISO 14000 – Environmental Management Standard
4. AS 9100 – Aeronautical Industries Standard
5. TL 9000 – Telecommunication Providers Standard
6. QS 9000 – Automotive Industry Standard
7. CMM – Software Standard
8. GMP – Food and Drugs Administration (FDA) Rules (USA)
9. OHSAS 18001 – Occupational Health And Safety Management Systems Standards

GMP - Food and Drugs Administration (FDA) Rules (USA)

1. The current Good Manufacturing Processes for the Food and Drugs Administration of the United States of America are a set of guidelines without which no drugs or food products can be commercialised in the USA.
2. The GMP standard is acknowledged the world over as generally the most stringent set of such rules.

3. Whether you are an international pharmaceutical firm or a small catering company, adopting the GMP rules will help you provide the highest quality products to your clients.

OHSAS 18001 - Occupational Health and Safety Management Systems Standard

1. Originally an English standard, OHSAS 18001 has been adopted worldwide as a complementary standard to the ISO 9001 (manufacturing or service processes) and ISO 14001 (environment) standards.
2. OHSAS 18001 is geared towards the continuous improvement of health and safety at work.
3. Based on local legislation, it requires extra, voluntary steps towards reducing occupational illness and accidents at work.
4. Together, the management and employees design an improved health and safety policy, plan an improvement process, train staff and implement the plan.
5. There are periodic audits to confirm the plan's success.
6. Experts can help a company design and implement OHSAS 18001.

Scatter Diagrams

Scatter diagrams are very important parts of statistical production quality control. A scatter diagram demonstrates a relationship between two variables. Any non-random structure reveals such a relationship in a statistical graph. The current trend is to fit the data into a computer software and then plotting a scatter diagram. The reason being the introduction of computer in all aspects of statistical production quality control. In general, records of data converted to statistical numbers are stored as different kinds of scatter diagrammatic relationships including no relationship, strong linear relationship (positive and negative correlation), exact linear relationship (positive correlation), quadratic relationship, exponential relationship, sinusoidal relationship, etc. Of these the simplest relationship is a strong linear relationship and most often found with production statistical quality control data. For large volumes of data several kinds of relationships such as quadratic, exponential and sinusoidal could be fit to get perfect modeling for further utilization. Currently, in most of the big pharma, production data is stored in a centralized computer system. The validation of each of these routes becomes important. The current trend is validation and various regulatory bodies specially emphasize on the validation of the software that further facilitates the use of computers in pharma industry.

Marketed Software for Production Statistical Quality Control

Currently several software companies are marketing their packages as related to the production statistical quality control methodologies. One such company is NWA quality analyst program. Numerous PC-based SQC software packages are readily available. Most, however, were created for discrete manufacturing such as auto parts machining, and consequently are limited in their application for other manufacturers. Chemical processors evaluating SQC software need to be aware of these shortcomings when making their selection:

- ***Limited usability:*** Can the software handle both process and laboratory data? Will you be able to select one package to meet the needs of all users?
- ***Data limitations:*** Can descriptive, measurement, and defect data be viewed in and analyzed from the same data file?
- ***Operator requirements*:** Can routine charting tasks be automated to reduce training time? Is unattended operation possible?
- ***Rigidity:*** Can charts be configured to precisely meet internal QC needs and still meet customer and regulatory reporting requirements?
- ***Data isolation:*** Can the software easily collect process data? Can it accept instrument data? Can it share or exchange data with corporate or plantwide information systems?
- ***Vendor awareness:*** Are the software developers knowledgeable about the issues and special requirements of the chemical processing industry?

With the introduction of NWA Quality Analyst in 1985, Northwest Analytical, Inc. (NWA) made the needs of the chemical processing industry a special focus. Because much of NWA's development staff began their careers in laboratory and chemical processing environments, they understand the needs and challenges faced in implementing SQC in the industry. As a result, NWA Quality Analyst is now a world leader in SQC software for chemical processors ranging from small independents to major multinationals. Their applications include internal QC and process improvement, vendor certification, and regulatory compliance. Similarly, any other software developed in such a manner could be the most ideal software for statistical quality control investigations.

Conclusions

It is always two or three companies (blockbuster) that matter for the progress of a country. Although a country in growth phase spends a lot of investment. It is always a tricky situation. In these situations, when the luck favors the country, the group of body that is involved in the development of any country helps further growth of this company in any dimension. Thus, every aspect of any company is a learning experience. In these situations, the focus should be to get the blockbuster out without any problems. In this regard, the best thing that this group could do is to follow perfect production statistical control methodologies very properly, understand the people involved, the competitors, the associates and everyone who could potentially interfere the business. Thus, reiterating quality control investigations are the key to the pharmaceutical production statistical quality control. As of now several production methodologies and other tools are in place are being investigated and introduction into the manufacturing sector of leading companies throughout the world.

Questions for Practice and Exercise

1. How the current methods in the statistical quality control culminated to?
2. Explain the significance of the term "Drug Production Quality".
3. State the meaning of the term 'statistical quality control' and its significance.
4. Define control chart.
5. What is contrl chart? Show a typical control chart. How are control charts for mean and range constructed when standards are given? Are not given?
6. What is time-series analysis?
7. What is advanced control?
8. What is
   (a) control engineering,
   (b) signal processing,
   (c) statistics,
   (d) decision theory,
   (e) artificial intelligence to hardware and software engineering?
9. How are industrial processes monitored?
10. (a) What are out-of-control action plans?
    (b) What are advanced process control loops?
11. What are Shewart Charts?
12. What do you do if the process is "in control" but the average level is too low or the variability is unacceptable?
13. What is control chart? How is it constructed and used for purposes of control of quality?

14. What is 'process control' and how is it achieved through control charts? Discuss the theoretical basis of p-charts. Given that the process fraction defective is 0.2 and n=25. Find the control limits for p-chart.
15. What are sampling plans? Explain
    (a) single sampling plans,
    (b) double sampling plans,
    (c) multiple sampling plans,
    (d) sequential sampling plans, and
    (e) skip lot sampling plans.
16. How is a sampling plan selected?
17. What are variable control charts?
18. What are attributes control charts?
19. What are multivariate control charts?
20. Write a note on Aebel software. How is it useful in regular checking of production quality variations? Explain.
21. Explain the use of time series analysis in quality control methodologies. Write a note on fundamental theory behind this concept.
22. What is Hotelling statistic?
23. How does recession and expansion in production and product life cycle influences the production value?
24. What are the cares that a production quality control manager takes to ensure quality control of a production process?
25. Explain in detail about all the methods involved in production forecasting.
26. What are the two main goals of application of time series in industrial quality control? Explain.
27. What is smoothing? How is production data smoothed? What is its application in quality control using time-series approach? Explain the expenses incurred by an industry in applying computers in statistical quality control using time-series analysis.
28. Write a note on production characteristics.
29. Explain systematically all the steps involved in the use of time-series analysis in control control.

30. Write a note on
    (a) six sigma levels of quality,
    (b) zero defects quality system,
    (c) House of quality,
    (d) quality control standards,
    (e) GMP,
    (f) OHSAS 18001,
    (g) scatter diagrams.
31. Write a note on the marketed software for production statistical quality control.

Bibliography

(a) Statistical Methods, Thirty Third Edition, Authored by Dr. SP Gupta, Sultan Chand and Sons, 2004.

(b) Statistics, Tenth Edition, Authored by James T. McClave and Terry Sincich, Prentice Hall, 2005.

(c) Management of Quality Control and Standardisation, First Edition, Authored by Atul Jaiswal, Kanishka Publishers, 1998.

(d) Business Mathematics and Statistics, Reprint, Authored by AP Verma, Asian Books Pvt. Limited, 2005.

INDEX

A

B

C

D

L

M

N

O

P

Q

R

S

T

V

W

X

Z

www.ingramcontent.com/pod-product-compliance
Lightning Source LLC
Chambersburg PA
CBHW080156170726
48282CB00005B/52

* 9 7 8 9 3 8 5 4 3 3 2 4 5 *